MCQs in
INFECTIOUS DISEASES
for DM Students

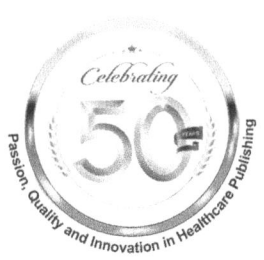

MCQs in
INFECTIOUS DISEASES
for DM Students

Editors

Om Shrivastav
MBBS MD (Med) Fellowship in Infect Dis and
Immunology (Australia)
Director
Department of Infectious Diseases
Jaslok Hospital and Research Centre
Visiting Professor
Department of Infectious Diseases
DY Patil University
Navi Mumbai, Maharashtra, India

Yatin Mehta
MD MNAMS FRCA FAMS FIACTA FICCM FTEE
Chairman
Medanta Institute of Critical Care and Anesthesiology
Medanta—The Medicity
Gurugram, Haryana, India
Adjunct Professor, National Board of Examinations (NBE)
Past President, Indian Society of Critical Care Medicine (ISCCM)

Forewords

TP Lahane
Sanjay Mukherjee

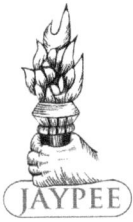

JAYPEE BROTHERS MEDICAL PUBLISHERS
The Health Sciences Publisher
New Delhi | London

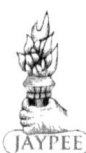 **Jaypee Brothers Medical Publishers (P) Ltd.**

Headquarters
Jaypee Brothers Medical Publishers (P) Ltd
EMCA House, 23/23-B, Ansari Road, Daryaganj
New Delhi 110 002, India
Landline: +91-11-23272143, +91-11-23272703
+91-11-23282021, +91-11-23245672
Email: jaypee@jaypeebrothers.com

Corporate Office
Jaypee Brothers Medical Publishers (P) Ltd
4838/24, Ansari Road, Daryaganj
New Delhi 110 002, India
Phone: +91-11-43574357
Fax: +91-11-43574314
Email: jaypee@jaypeebrothers.com

Overseas Office
J.P. Medical Ltd
83 Victoria Street, London
SW1H 0HW (UK)
Phone: +44 20 3170 8910
Fax: +44 (0)20 3008 6180
Email: info@jpmedpub.com

Website: www.jaypeebrothers.com
Website: www.jaypeedigital.com

© 2021, Jaypee Brothers Medical Publishers

The views and opinions expressed in this book are solely those of the original contributor(s)/author(s) and do not necessarily represent those of editor(s) of the book.

All rights reserved. No part of this publication may be reproduced, stored or transmitted in any form or by any means, electronic, mechanical, photocopying, recording or otherwise, without the prior permission in writing of the publishers.

All brand names and product names used in this book are trade names, service marks, trademarks or registered trademarks of their respective owners. The publisher is not associated with any product or vendor mentioned in this book.

Medical knowledge and practice change constantly. This book is designed to provide accurate, authoritative information about the subject matter in question. However, readers are advised to check the most current information available on procedures included and check information from the manufacturer of each product to be administered, to verify the recommended dose, formula, method and duration of administration, adverse effects and contraindications. It is the responsibility of the practitioner to take all appropriate safety precautions. Neither the publisher nor the author(s)/editor(s) assume any liability for any injury and/or damage to persons or property arising from or related to use of material in this book.

This book is sold on the understanding that the publisher is not engaged in providing professional medical services. If such advice or services are required, the services of a competent medical professional should be sought.

Every effort has been made where necessary to contact holders of copyright to obtain permission to reproduce copyright material. If any have been inadvertently overlooked, the publisher will be pleased to make the necessary arrangements at the first opportunity. The **CD/DVD-ROM** (if any) provided in the sealed envelope with this book is complimentary and free of cost. **Not meant for sale.**

Inquiries for bulk sales may be solicited at: jaypee@jaypeebrothers.com

MCQs in Infectious Diseases for DM Students

First Edition: **2021**

ISBN: 978-93-89776-71-3

Printed at

Contributors

Ajay Jhaveri
DNB (General Med) DNB (Gastroenterology)
Consultant
Department of Gastroenterology
Jaslok Hospital and Research Centre
Mumbai, Maharashtra, India

Altaf Patel
MD FRCP (Lon) FRCP (Edin) FCPS FCMT
Internist and Director
Department of Medicine
Jaslok Hospital and Research Centre
Mumbai, Maharashtra, India

Amita Athavale
MD (Tuberculosis and Chest Diseases)
Professor and Head
Department of Chest Medicine
GS Medical College and KEM Hospital
Mumbai, Maharashtra, India

Ashay Shingare MD DNB
Consultant
Department of Nephrology and
Transplantation
Jaslok Hospital and Research Centre
Mumbai, Maharashtra, India

Ayesha J Sunavala
DNB (Med) FNB (Infect Dis)
Consultant
Department of Infectious Diseases
PD Hinduja National Hospital and
Medical Research Centre
Mumbai, Maharashtra, India

Azad Irani MD DNB
Consultant Neurologist
Jaslok Hospital and Research Centre
Mumbai, Maharashtra, India

Chandresh Karnavat
Department of Radiology
Jaslok Hospital and Research Centre
Mumbai, Maharashtra, India

Darshana Rathod MD (Internal Med)
Chief Intensivist
Department of Critical Care Medicine
Sir HN Reliance Foundation Hospital and
Research Centre
Mumbai, Maharashtra, India

Dipsha Kriplani DNB Hematology
Breach Candy Hospital
Mumbai, Maharashtra, India.

Duru Shah
MD FRCOG FICOG FICS FCPS
FICMCH DGO DFP
Director
Gynaecworld—The Center for Women's
Health and Fertility
Mumbai, Maharashtra, India

Gaurav Kochar DA IDCCM IFCCM
Consultant Critical Care
Medanta—The Medicity
Gurugram, Haryana, India

Gautam Zaveri MS DNB DOrtho
Director of Spine Surgery
Jaslok Hospital and Research Centre
Head, Department of Orthopedics
Rajawadi Hospital
Mumbai, Maharashtra, India

Harshad Argekar MS (Ortho)
Associate Professor
Department of Orthopedics
University of Mumbai
Mumbai, Maharashtra, India

Hasnain Patel MD Medicine
Saifee Hospital
Mumbai, Maharashtra, India

Indraneel Raut
MBBS DNB (Med) IDCCM IFCCM EDIC
Additional Director
Department of Internal Medicine and
Critical Care
Jaslok Hospital and Research Centre
Mumbai, Maharashtra, India

Joy Desai MD DNB
Director
Department of Neurology
Jaslok Hospital and Research Centre
Mumbai, Maharashtra, India

Juhi Dhar MD
Senior Consultant
Department of Internal Medicine
Batra Hospital and Medical Research Centre
New Delhi, India

Ketan Kargirwar
MD (Anesthesia) FNB (Critical Care) IDCCM
EDIC Clinical Fellow Neurotrauma (Canada)
Consultant
Department of Critical Care Medicine
Sir HN Reliance Foundation Hospital and
Research Centre
Mumbai, Maharashtra, India

Krutarth Kanjiya
DNB (Internal Med) Fellowship in Infect Dis
PD Hinduja National Hospital and
Medical Research Centre
Mumbai, Maharashtra, India

Laxman Jessani
DNB (Internal Med) MNAMS FNB (Infect Dis)
FRSPH (UK)
Consultant
Department of Infectious Diseases
Apollo Hospital
Mumbai, Maharashtra, India

Mala V Kaneria
Professor and Unit Head
Department of Medicine
BYL Nair Charitable Hospital and
Kasturba Hospital for Infectious Diseases
Consultant
Department of Infectious Diseases
Jaslok Hospital and Research Centre
Mumbai, Maharashtra, India

Mayur Patel MD FCCP
Director
Department of Critical Care Medicine
Sir HN Reliance Foundation Hospital and
Research Centre
Mumbai, Maharashtra, India

Meghna Kabra MD
Senior Consultant
Department of Internal Medicine
Batra Hospital and Medical Research Centre
New Delhi, India

Contributors

Mehul Shah
DNB (Anesthesia) FNB (Critical Care)
IFCCM IDCCM MNAMS
Consultant
Department of Critical Care Medicine
Sir HN Reliance Foundation Hospital and Research Centre
Mumbai, Maharashtra, India

MM Bahadur MD DNB
Director and Head
Department of Nephrology and Transplantation
Jaslok Hospital and Research Centre
Mumbai, Maharashtra, India

Om Shrivastav
MBBS MD (Med) Fellowship in Infect Dis and Immunology (Australia)
Director
Department of Infectious Diseases
Jaslok Hospital and Research Centre
Visiting Professor
Department of Infectious Diseases
DY Patil University
Navi Mumbai, Maharashtra, India

Parikshit S Prayag
MD ABIM ABMS American Board Certified in Internal Med and Infect Dis AST Fellowship in Transplant Infect Dis
Consultant
Department of Transplant Infectious Diseases
Deenanath Mangeshkar Hospital and Research Center
Pune, Maharashtra, India

Pooja D Chaturvedy MS (Ophth)
Consultant Ophthalmic Surgeon
Department of Ophthalmology
Sir HN Reliance Foundation Hospital and Research Centre
Mumbai, Maharashtra, India

Pradip Kumar Bhattacharya
MD ACME FICCM FCCCM FCCM
Professor and Head
Department of Critical Care
Incharge (Trauma and Emergency Care Services)
Rajendra Institute of Medical Sciences
Ranchi, Jharkhand, India

Prasanna Shah MD DNB
Consultant Gastroenterologist
Jaslok Hospital and Research Centre
Mumbai, Maharashtra, India

Pritam Kataria MD (General Med)
Deputy Consultant
Department of Medical Oncology
Sir HN Reliance Foundation Hospital and Research Centre
Mumbai, Maharashtra, India

Rahul Bahot DNB (Respiratory Dis)
Consultant Chest Physician
Department of Chest Medicine
Jaslok Hospital and Research Centre
Mumbai, Maharashtra, India

Raj Kumar Mani
MD MRCP (UK) FCCP FICCM
CEO (Medical Services)
Chairman (Pulmonology, Critical Care and Sleep Medicine)
Nayati Healthcare and Research Pvt Ltd
Gurugram, Haryana, India
Visiting Honorary Consultant
Saket City Hospital
New Delhi, India

Rajesh Chandra Mishra
MBBS MD (Internal Med) FNB EDIC FCCM FCCP FICP
Consultant Intensivist and Internist
General Secretary
ISCCM (2019–20)
Ahmedabad, Gujarat, India

Reena Sharma MD (General Med)
Consultant Rheumatologist
Swastik Rheumatology Clinic
Ahmedabad, Gujarat, India

Rishit K Harbada MD DNB
Senior Resident
Department of Nephrology and Renal Transplant
Jaslok Hospital and Research Centre
Mumbai, Maharashtra, India

Ritu K Kashikar
Department of Radiology
Jaslok Hospital and Research Centre
Mumbai, Maharashtra, India

Rushi Deshpande
MD DM DNB (Nephrology)
Director Academics
Department of Nephrology
Jaslok Hospital and Research Centre
Mumbai, Maharashtra, India

Sabahat Rasool
MD MRCOG DNB MNAMS
FMAS (Obs & Gyne)
Consultant Gynecologist and Reproductive Medicine Specialist
Government Medical College
Srinagar, Jammu and Kashmir, India

Samir Shah MD MRCP MRCPath
Consultant Hematologist and Stem Cell Transplant Physician
Jaslok Hospital and Research Centre
Mumbai, Maharashtra, India

Shraddha Sinhasan
MBBS DNB (Radiology)
Consultant Radiologist
Department of Radiology
Jaslok Hospital and Research Centre
Mumbai, Maharashtra, India

Shrinivas B Desai MD (Radiology)
Director, Professor, and Head
Department of Radiology
Jaslok Hospital and Research Centre
Mumbai, Maharashtra, India

Sneha Gohil MD (Skin and VD)
Head
Department of Dermatology
Care Institute of Medical Sciences (CIMS) Hospital
Ahmedabad, Gujarat, India

Sujata Rege
MBBS, DNB, FID (Fellowship in Infectious Diseases)
Consultant
Department of Infectious Diseases
Bharati Vidyapeeth University and Medical College
Pune, Maharashtra, India

Sukanya Verma
MD (Microbiology) DNB (Microbiology)
Dip RCPath
Consultant
Department of Microbiology, Serology, and EIA
SRL Diagnostics Limited
Mumbai, Maharashtra, India

Surabhi Madan
MD (Med) Fellowship in Infect Dis
Head and Consultant
Department of Infectious Diseases
Care Institute of Medical Sciences (CIMS) Hospital
Ahmedabad, Gujarat, India

TP Lahane MS (Ophthalmology)
Professor and Director
(Medical Education and Research)
St George's Dental Hospital, Mumbai
Professor
Department of Ophthalmology
Sir JJ Group of Hospitals
Mumbai, Maharashtra, India

Vasant C Nagvekar
MD (Med) Fellowship in Infect Dis
Certificate ASTMH
Consultant
Department of Infectious Diseases
Lilavati Hospital and Research Centre
Global Hospital
Mumbai, Maharashtra, India

Vivek Kumar
MD (Med) DNB (Med) IFCCM EDIC
FICCM FICP FACP MNAMS (Critical Care)
Chief Intensivist
Department of Critical Care Medicine
Sir HN Reliance Foundation Hospital
and Research Centre
Mumbai, Maharashtra, India

VP Antia MD Dip in Hematology
Head
Department of Hematology
Breach Candy Hospital
Mumbai, Maharashtra, India

Yatin Mehta
MD MNAMS FRCA FAMS FIACTA
FICCM FTEE
Chairman
Medanta Institute of Critical Care
and Anesthesiology
Medanta—The Medicity
Gurugram, Haryana, India
Adjunct Professor
National Board of Examinations (NBE)
Past President, Indian Society of Critical
Care Medicine (ISCCM)

Foreword

It gives me great pleasure to write the foreword on the first book of *MCQs in Infectious Diseases for DM Students*.

It is also my privilege to be an author on Infections in the Eye which has an exhaustive array of all relevant clinical scenarios to both trainees and professionals. The book looks at elucidating all clinically relevant situations to the practitioners. This book should adequately provide a platform to those seeking the basics and advanced answers for everyday issues. I wish the book every success.

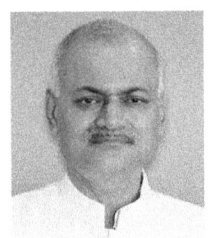

TP Lahane MS (Ophthalmology)
Professor and Director (Medical Education and Research)
St George's Dental Hospital, Mumbai
Professor
Department of Ophthalmology
Sir JJ Group of Hospitals
Mumbai, Maharashtra, India

Foreword

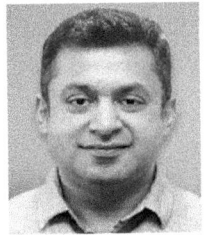

Infectious diseases have been present all along the history of mankind. In recent times, even with the advent of lifestyle diseases, infectious disease remains the cause of one-fourth mortality in India along with maternal, perinatal, and nutritional causes. Even after eradication of Smallpox and on-going efforts for polio eradication, bacterial diseases such as tuberculosis, viral diseases such as HIV/AIDS and Hepatitis B, water-borne and food-borne diseases leading to frequent outbreaks and epidemics remain a matter of concern. Emerging and re-emerging infectious diseases including the recent Coronavirus outbreak by 2019-nCoV cannot less emphasize the need of an in-depth knowledge regarding this deadly giant of infectious diseases.

MCQs in Infectious Diseases for DM Students presents a comprehensive collection of topics related to infectious diseases divided in 32 broad headings. The book introduces novel topics such as infection-related malignancies and fever in non-infectious settings. It provides a fresh perspective on well-known topics such as tuberculosis and sexually transmitted diseases. In addition, the book explores the dimension of infections in hematological disorders, renal transplants and other special conditions, which are more often than not ignored. A dedicated section on imaging in infectious diseases will catch the interest of most of the readers.

The book is designed keeping in mind the requirements of postgraduate and superspecialty aspirants of the medical field. The newer advances in the medical curriculum demands an approach of multiple-choice questions to be discussed. At the same time, faculties of clinical medicine and also of Public Health Department will find this book to update themselves with most of the important advances in infectious diseases. Undergraduate students interested in various projects by ICMR and inter-collegiate competitions will also find this book helpful.

This book, written in a lucid language to be easily understood by one and all, is the result of the collective effort of the subject experts. I am sure that it will provide the best of recent knowledge to the readers.

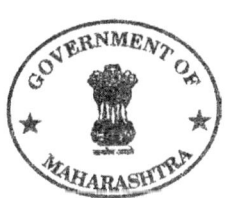

Sanjay Mukherjee
IAS
Secretary
Medical Education and Drugs Department
Government of Maharashtra

Preface

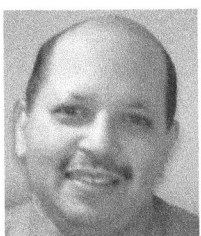 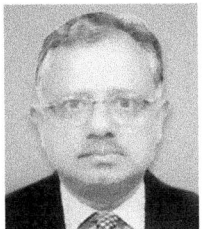

Om Shrivastav   **Yatin Mehta**

We are delighted to write the preface for the first edition of *MCQs in Infectious Diseases for DM Students*.

In this book, we have updated diagnostic and therapeutic modalities in a multidisciplinary approach which will be a clinical guidance book for practicing doctors. The content has been shaped with International Standards and Clinical Guidelines amongst all relevant disciplines. In addition, the discussions for the topics in-depth will serve as an educational resource, which is designed to serve as a reference book of infectious diseases for International Licentiate and National Entrance examinations as well. There are MCQs in each section with detailed and referenced explanations.

This book will provide an effective learning experience and referenced resource for all health professionals in the field of infectious diseases and also improve patient care.

We thank our families in whose time this book was written. We would also like to thank Dr Abhijit Moharkar; Dr Adarsh Shetty; Ms Poonam Anand, our secretarial staff; and Mr Sabarish Menon and M/s Jaypee Brothers Medical Publishers (P) Ltd, New Delhi, India, for their efforts.

Om Shrivastav
Yatin Mehta

Contents

1. Sepsis in 2020: Is it only Antibiotics? 1
   Gaurav Kochar, Yatin Mehta

2. Gram-negative Crisis 12
   Pradip Kumar Bhattacharya

3. Emerging Fungal Infections in Non-neutropenic Patients 25
   Ketan Kargirwar, Mayur Patel, Darshana Rathod, Mehul Shah, Vivek Kumar

4. Fungal Infections in Neutropenia 38
   Vasant C Nagvekar

5. Infection-related Malignancies 46
   Pritam Kataria

6. Fever in Non-infection Settings 52
   Reena Sharma

7. Immune Dysfunction and Infections 63
   Om Shrivastav

8. Approach to Cutaneous and Soft-tissue Infections 71
   Om Shrivastav

9. Sexually Transmitted Infections 82
   Surabhi Madan, Sneha Gohil

10. Tuberculosis and Its Variants 93
    Amita Athavale, Rahul Bahot

11. Central Nervous System Infections 100
    Joy Desai, Azad Irani

12. Respiratory Infections 123
    Rahul Bahot

13. Genitourinary Tract Infections 144
    MM Bahadur, Ashay Shingare

14. Bone and Joint Infections 155
    Gautam Zaveri, Harshad Argekar

15. Human Immunodeficiency Virus 167
    Om Shrivastav

16. Infections of Liver 175
    Prasanna Shah

17. Infections and Metabolic Sequelae 182
    Rajesh Chandra Mishra, Reena Sharma

18. Zoonosis 192
    Om Shrivastav

19. **Parasitic Infections** 202
    Ajay Jhaveri, Om Shrivastav

20. **Fever in the Returning Traveler** 212
    Juhi Dhar, Meghna Kabra, Raj Kumar Mani

21. **Pyrexia of Unknown Origin** 233
    Altaf Patel, Hasnain Patel

22. **Outbreaks** 240
    Laxman Jessani

23. **Nosocomial Infections** 247
    Ayesha J Sunavala, Indraneel Raut, Krutarth Kanjiya

24. **Hematological Disorders and Infections** 272
    VP Antia, Dipsha Kriplani

25. **Infections in Renal Transplants** 278
    Rushi Deshpande, Rishit K Harbada, Sukanya Verma

26. **Infections in Liver Transplants** 302
    Parikshit S Prayag, Sujata Rege

27. **Infections in Bone Marrow Transplants** 314
    Samir Shah

28. **Infections in the Eye** 323
    TP Lahane, Pooja D Chaturvedy

29. **Vector-borne Diseases** 338
    Mala V Kaneria

30. **Pregnancy and Gynecological Infections** 353
    Duru Shah, Sabahat Rasool

31. **Imaging in Infectious Diseases** 368
    Shrinivas B Desai, Ritu K Kashikar, Shraddha Sinhasan, Chandresh Karnavat

32. **COVID-19** 405
    Rahul Bahot, Om Shrivastav

Index 423

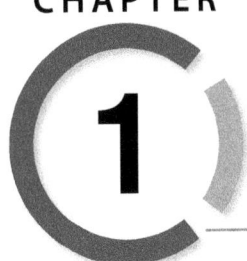

CHAPTER 1

Sepsis in 2020: Is it only Antibiotics?

Gaurav Kochar, Yatin Mehta

1. A 37-year-old male with immunodeficiency due to retroviral disease presents with chest infection diagnosed as *Pneumocystis jirovecii*. He is responsive to treatment but on 10th day in hospital he has massive hemoptysis and is intubated. His counts are 7,800/mm³ with 630 CD4 cells. X-ray shows multiple cystic lesions. The likeliest diagnosis is:
   A. *Pneumocystis jirovecii* disseminated disease
   B. Vasculitis and angiopathy of HIV
   C. Disseminated tuberculosis (TB)
   D. Angioinvasive aspergillosis

2. A 23-year-old man with history of childhood asthma presents with a 3-day history of shortness of breath and wheezing. His parameters are otherwise normal other than eosinophil count of 31%. His chest X-ray (CXR) shows bilateral infiltrative shadows. An *Aspergillus* precipitin test is negative and a galactomannan assay is unremarkable. Your next investigations to prove your diagnosis would be:
   A. Pulmonary function tests to show reversible airways disease
   B. CT chest in sitting and supine position to exclude aspergilloma
   C. Total serum immunoglobulin E (IgE) to establish allergic bronchopulmonary aspergillosis (ABPA)
   D. Bronchoscopy to exclude mechanical obstruction

3. In invasive aspergillosis:
   A. Surgical excision of fibrotic lung is gold standard
   B. Voriconazole dose needs close monitoring with immunosuppression
   C. Posaconazole and amphotericin are mainstay in initial treatment
   D. Immunosuppression in transplant patients should be withdrawn immediately

4. *Candida albicans* is a commensal at various sites, the most common being:
   A. Female genitourinary tract
   B. Central nervous system
   C. Pluripotent stem cells
   D. Macrophages and glial cells

5. In endophthalmitis, the most likely cause of endogenous candidemia is:
   A. Immunosuppression
   B. Total parenteral nutrition
   C. Gastrointestinal (GI) surgery
   D. Diabetes mellitus

6. A 44-year-old jute farm worker presents with a painless papular lesion on his forearm that is friable with a history of unproductive cough for 10 days associated with nonmigratory joint pains. A chest X-ray reveals moderate-sized right pleural effusion. Patient's CD4 count is 170 cells/mm³. Biopsy of the skin lesion areas of necrosis in epithelial cells with minimal inflammation. The likeliest diagnosis is:
   A. Cutaneous nocardiosis
   B. Disseminated cryptococcosis
   C. Systemic histoplasmosis
   D. Atypical mycobacterial infection

7. The biggest indicator of adverse clinical event in retroviral infection is:
   A. CD4 counts
   B. CD4 percentage of total leukocyte count
   C. CD4:CD 8 ratio
   D. Viral load of HIV.

8. A 21-year-old girl with a 3-month history of diarrhea presents with painful peripheral neuritis and headaches with blurred vision of recent onset. In the initial workup her western blot for HIV was positive and her CD4 count was 27 cells/mm³. Her likeliest diagnosis is:
   A. Cytomegalovirus (CMV) colitis and retinitis
   B. HIV neuropathy
   C. *Isospora belli* disseminated infection
   D. Salmonellosis bacteremia

9. A family of three test positive for H1N1 infection and are commenced on treatment. A fourth member with a renal transplant on immunosuppression is asymptomatic in contact with this family. The recommended treatment is:
   A. Isolation, oseltamivir after throat swab
   B. Prophylactic oseltamivir at half dose

C. Hospitalization for oseltamivir and Virenza dual therapy
D. Close observation for 7 days

10. An elderly farmer presents with a fracture of right forearm and index finger nonresolving abscess. Investigations reveal pathological fracture of radius-ulna, right carpal tunnel syndrome. Drainage of abscess and microscopy reveals gray brown smooth conidia. *Note*: He has failed treatment with caspofungin and amphotericin B. He has:
    A. *Mycobacterium abscessus* infection
    B. *Streptococcus milleri* infection
    C. *Scedosporium* infection
    D. Lujo hemorrhagic virus

11. A middle-aged man with flu-like symptoms has undergone a workup. His platelet count is ranging from 20,000 to 30,000 cells/mm^3. In further workup, his enzyme-linked immunosorbent assay (ELISA) for HIV is positive and his western blot is indeterminate. He needs:
    A. Single donor platelet (SDP) transfusion
    B. No therapy is indicated
    C. Bone marrow aspiration and biopsy
    D. Bone marrow transplant

12. A 21-year-old 22 weeks pregnant female presents with recurrent episodes of giddiness. Her initial workup indicates a pancytopenia which is following a 7-day history of fevers joint pains and a macular skin rash. On her clinical examination, there appears to be a nonhomogeneous discoloration of her right cheek. Her most likely diagnosis is:
    A. Aplastic anemia
    B. Parvovirus B19 infection
    C. Anemia of pregnancy
    D. Myelophthisic anemia with myelofibrosis

13. In the patient mentioned in Question 12, a fetal ultrasound reveals fetal distress with a heart rate of 180 bpm. Her best therapeutic option is:
    A. Medical termination of pregnancy
    B. IV immunoglobulins for 5 days
    C. IV acyclovir for 5 days
    D. Intrauterine fetal blood transfusion

14. In pregnant patients undergoing treatment for active tuberculosis, when a diagnosis of retroviral disease is made, antiretroviral therapy should be initiated in:
    A. ART is ideal only in third trimester
    B. ART is indicated after completion of anti-tubercular therapy
    C. ART is indicated after patient has delivered
    D. ART should be started in first trimester

15. In toxoplasmosis and pregnancy:
    A. Asymptomatic patients need not be evaluated or treated
    B. Intrauterine growth retardation is not a feature
    C. Lymphadenopathy should be evaluated vigorously to initiate potential treatment
    D. Termination of pregnancy is always indicated

16. A 54-year-old male presents with a fourth event of Salmonella bacteremia in one calendar year, associated with 7 kg weight loss. He has now oral thrush and signs of cerebral irritation. The likeliest reason for his recurrent salmonellosis is:
    A. Incorrect treatment
    B. Drug-resistant infection
    C. Patient is a carrier state for *Salmonella*
    D. AIDS-defining illness

17. A 56-year-old professional pet trainer presents to emergency room (ER) with abdominal bloating, vomiting, and fever. Her initial bloods show transaminitis and an initial USG abdomen is labeled peliosis hepatis. Her likeliest diagnosis is:
    A. *Bartonella henselae* infection
    B. Hepatitis B
    C. Hepatitis C
    D. Chronic granulomatous disease

18. A 77-year-old man has a 7-day history of a febrile illness 3 weeks ago for which he took no treatment. He now presents with altered sensorium, pain abdomen and orthopnea. A CT scan of the chest shows pulmonary hemorrhages and in the workup a real-time polymerase chain reaction (PCR) is positive for leptospirosis. The treatment of choice is:
    A. Doxycycline
    B. Crystalline penicillin
    C. Clarithromycin
    D. Levofloxacin

19. The most likely surgical emergency in infectious mononucleosis (IM) is:
    A. Suppurative tonsillitis
    B. Spinal abscess and cord compression
    C. Catastrophic gastrointestinal bleed
    D. Spontaneous rupture of spleen

20. A 20-year-old female presents with seizures, arthralgia and palpitation for 3 days. There is a history of travel to rain forests of Southeast Asia 2 months ago, longest duration being in Vietnam. Family also describes a rash that appears to be migratory in nature. Once samples are collected for routine tests, cultures and serology, the next best step is:
    A. Lumbar puncture and MRI brain
    B. EEG

C. Commence treatment with ceftriaxone and crystalline penicillin
D. Await serology for Lyme disease

21. A 55-year-old male with a clinical diagnosis of filariasis presents to emergency with hemodynamic collapse and shock. He has taken a single dose of diethylcarbamazine (DEC) 2 hours before this event. This event is:
    A. Septicemia and shock
    B. Myocarditis and complete heart block
    C. Encephalitis due to microfilariae
    D. Mazzotti reactions

22. A post-cerebral malaria and acute respiratory distress syndrome (ARDS)-affected patient recovering in ICU goes into pancytopenia, and is comatose with a Glasgow Coma Scale (GCS) score of 3 within 2 hours. There is no obvious cause of bleeding and a peripheral smear shows fragmented and dyskaryotic cell lines which is confirmed on bone marrow. The likeliest diagnosis is:
    A. Myelodysplastic syndrome
    B. Acute myeloid leukemia
    C. Bone marrow suppression secondary to malaria
    D. Hemophagocytic syndrome

23. In the same patient as in Question 22, the treatment of choice is:
    A. Intravenous immunoglobulin G (IVIG)
    B. Quinine plus sulfadiazine/pyrimethamine
    C. Dexamethasone and etoposide
    D. Bone marrow transplant

24. A 22-year-old female presents with a history of fever, a seventh nerve palsy, and cervical lymphadenopathy. Additionally she has a morbilliform rash that presented after a single dose of Augmentin. She now has a seventh nerve palsy and worsening urinary incontinence. An IgM for infectious mononucleosis is negative on two occasions 2 weeks apart. Her likeliest diagnosis is:
    A. Infectious mononucleosis
    B. T-cell lymphoma
    C. Transverse myelitis
    D. Staphylococcal shock syndrome

25. A 17-year-old boy is discharged from hospital after recovering from bronchopneumonia and ARDS. This is his ninth chest infection in 2 years and on six occasions *Streptococcus pneumoniae* was isolated from sputum and blood cultures. The most likely reason is:
    A. A hyper-IgM syndrome
    B. Lack of pneumococcal neutralizing antibodies
    C. Hypereosinophilia
    D. Complement deficiency

26. A 54-year-old male with a history of recurrent gut infections has grown *Shigella* and *Campylobacter* repeatedly in a background of dermatomyositis and is on azathioprine maintenance. His best investigation would be:
    A. Muscle biopsy and myonecrosis
    B. Bone marrow for aplastic anemia
    C. Colonoscopy for colon cancer
    D. HLA-DR link association for muscle atrophy

27. A 47-year-old male on azathioprine for rheumatoid arthritis presents with urosepsis and septic shock. A lymphocyte enumeration shows T- and B-cell population to be below 5%. The duration of antibiotic cover based on T-cell population recovery will be:
    A. 7 days
    B. 48 hours
    C. 4 months
    D. 3 weeks

28. A 33-year-old male postrenal transplant presents with an acute myocardial infarction. In his workup he has pancytopenia, a creatinine of 7.3 mg/dL, and a ninefold normal transaminitis. A CT coronary angiogram while on continuous venovenous hemodialysis (CVVHD) shows diffuse atherosclerotic changes of coronary and renal arteries and aorta. His most likely diagnosis is:
    A. Cytomegalovirus infection
    B. Polyangiitis overlap syndrome
    C. Vaso-occlusive disease
    D. Drug-induced bone marrow depression

29. A 23-year-old female with retroviral infection has a 3-week history of painful dysphagia and altered bowel movements. Her last CD4 counts 5 days ago were 54 cells/mm^3. Three stool cultures are negative for microorganisms. She now has hematemesis and undergoes upper and lower GI endoscopy showing multiple varied sized ulcers throughout the GI tract. She is likeliest to have:
    A. *Helicobacter pylori* disseminated disease
    B. B-cell lymphoma of HIV
    C. Cytomegalovirus infection
    D. Ulcerative esophagitis and inflammatory bowel disease

30. A 57-year-old female diagnosed with dengue both on NS1 antigen and IgM for dengue is hospitalized with fevers. Her platelet count is 46,000/mm^3. In 24 hours, it falls to 31,000/mm^3.
    She is given six units of random donor platelets (RDPs). On the fourth day, she develops a left hemiparesis and a noncontrast CT shows a large intracerebral bleed. In the absence of other hematological evaluation, the most likely reason for the bleed is:
    A. Hypertensive stroke

B. Autoantibodies and antiplatelet antibodies
C. Disseminated intravascular coagulation (DIC)
D. Dengue-induced encephalopathy

31. A 56-year-old female with chronic hepatitis C has a flare with transaminitis × 10-fold after she has discontinued her medications 4 months ago. She now has a wet gangrene involving her right foot and a lobar pneumonia. Her Coombs' test workup is positive. Her last viral load is 383,790 copies/mm^3. She has:
    A. Thromboembolic disease
    B. Cold agglutinin disease associated with *Mycoplasma*
    C. Varicose veins of hepatitis C
    D. Primary vasculitis

32. The biggest risk factor for systemic complications of hepatitis E virus (HEV) infection is:
    A. Hepatorenal syndrome
    B. Intravenous drug use (IVDU)
    C. Paracetamol ingestion
    D. Pregnancy

33. A 38-year-old bone marrow transplant recipient presents with fever, generalized weakness and dyspnea of 5 days duration. On clinical examination, she has hepatosplenomegaly, palpable lymph nodes in her neck, axilla, and groin. Her post-transplant immunosuppression has been altered after a recent pancytopenia. She has a childhood history of infectious mononucleosis that resolved completely. Her likeliest diagnosis is:
    A. Epstein–Barr-associated post-transplant lymphoproliferative disease (PTLD)
    B. Disseminated CMV
    C. Drug-induced pancytopenia
    D. Burkitt lymphoma

34. A 27-year-old male presents with acute dyspnea of 3 days duration. He has immunodeficiency of retroviral illness and is stable on highly active antiretroviral therapy (HAART) with a CD4 count of 210 cells/mm^3. He works on a shop that feeds pigeons daily. In his evaluation, his CT chest and pulmonary function test (PFT) show restrictive airways disease with fine reticular shadows. He is likely to have:
    A. HIV-associated lymphocytic pneumonia
    B. Allergic bronchopulmonary aspergillosis
    C. Bird fancier's lung—hypersensitivity alveolitis
    D. *Pneumocystis jirovecii* pneumonia

35. A 48-year-old male on HAART with nevirapine plus lamivudine and efavirenz is diagnosed with tuberculous lymphadenitis and commenced on [streptomycin (S), isoniazid (H), rifampicin (R) and pyrazinamide (Z) SHRZ]. His last CD4 count was 388/mm^3 and viral load is undetectable. He now presents with seizures and an space occupying lesion (SOL) which is being evaluated. His CD4 count is 21/mm^3 and viral load is 317,000 copies. This is because:
    A. He is a treatment defaulter
    B. Spurious medications
    C. He is required to take all medications on empty stomach
    D. Rifampicin reduces drug levels of HAART

36. In treatment of *Pneumocystis Jirovecii* in immunocompromised with trimethoprim–sulfamethoxazole patients:
    A. Duration of treatment is 5 days
    B. Prophylaxis is lifelong
    C. Patients are best monitored as outpatients
    D. Patients will need steroid cover to prepare for initial worsening

37. A 63-year-old female with post-chikungunya arthritis is on hydroxychloroquine and prednisone with worsening joint disability. She is put on infliximab and has immediate relief. Six weeks later she presents with progressive loss of vision. Evaluation reveals a scleral abscess that requires drainage and there is growth of *Mycobacterium chelonae*. This is due to:
    A. Association of chikungunya and mycobacteria
    B. Contaminant
    C. Steroid-induced growth
    D. Infliximab-associated flare of mycobacteria

38. A 36-year-old female is brought to emergency in a comatose condition. Her examination reveals multiple crusting skin lesions on trunk and arms, and her left breast has a crimson red appearance. On further evaluation her cerebrospinal fluid (CSF) shows evidence of meningitis, a left shoulder and right hip osteomyelitis and multiple pockets of abscess in her chest and abdomen. Her only significant medical history is a left breast implant surgery 6 weeks ago. She has:
    A. Bacteroides septicemia
    B. Collagen vascular disease with suppuration
    C. Gram-positive bacteremia
    D. *Mycobacteria fortuitum*

39. A family of four have repeated presentations to hospital with suppurative lymphadenitis and respiratory tract infections. The family are of

farmers and have been investigated extensively, including HIV serology which is negative. On various occasions a *Mycobacterium avium* complex (MAC) growth has been identified in lungs. In absence of immunodeficiency, the likeliest reason for this presentation is:

A. Inadequately controlled tubercular infection
B. Dysfunctional interferon and tumor-necrosis factor (TNF) pathways
C. Pandrug-resistant MAC infection
D. Natural killer cell deficiency

40. A 27-year-old girl presents with a degloving injury of her face after being in contact with an undomesticated cat. She has presented 10 hours after injury. In her treatment, the most effective regimen is:

A. Tetanus toxoid (TT) and surgical opinion
B. TT, rabies immunoglobulin, antirabies vaccine, and surgery of cheek
C. Only antirabies vaccine
D. Surgical repair and observation for 10 days. Cats do not transmit rabies

ANSWERS WITH EXPLANATIONS

1. **Ans. D**
The most common sites of infection are the respiratory apparatus (lungs and sinuses).
Chronic pulmonary aspergillosis (CPA) is a long-term *Aspergillus* infection of the lung and *Aspergillus fumigatus* is almost always the species responsible for this illness. Patients fall into several groups as listed below:
- Aspergilloma in a single lung cavity
- *Aspergillus* nodule
- Chronic fibrosing pulmonary aspergillosis

Ref:
1. Denning DW, Riniotis K, Dobrashian R, Sambatakou H. Chronic cavitary and fibrosing pulmonary and pleural aspergillosis: case series, proposed nomenclature change, and review. Clin Infect Dis. 2003;37(Suppl 3): S265-80.

2. **Ans. B**
Chest radiography is an initial examination of choice in patients with respiratory symptoms or suspected pulmonary disease.
Features of ABPA on CT are nondiagnostic but, the features of the demonstration of bronchial dilatation, wall thickening, and centrilobular nodules are highly suggestive of the diagnosis.
Mobile mass within a cavity on supine and prone scans is virtually diagnostic of a mycetoma.
Computed tomography scan findings in angioinvasive aspergillosis are more specific and the presence of nodules with a halo of ground-glass attenuation in the appropriate clinical setting allows confident diagnosis.
Ref:
1. Medscape. Infectious Diseases. [online] Available from: https://www.medscape.com/infectiousdiseases [Last accessed February, 2020].

3. **Ans. B**
Ref:
1. Medscape. Infectious Diseases. [online] Available from: https://www.medscape.com/infectiousdiseases [Last accessed February, 2020].

4. **Ans. A**
A study by Glover and Larsen is the most significant study that underscores the coexistence of candida with normal vaginal flora. The majority of women who have vaginal yeast also carry the organism in the gut.
Ref:
1. Ohm JM, Galask RP. Bacterial flora of the cervix from 100 prehysterectomy patients. Am J Obstet Gynecol. 1975;122(6):683-7.
2. Tashjian JH, Coulam CB, Washington JA 2nd. Vaginal flora in asymptomatic women. Mayo Clin Proc. 1976;51(9):557-61.

5. **Ans. A**
Immune system suppression or dysfunction is a major risk factor in molds becoming systemic infections. Enucleation rates were much higher in mold cases.
Ref:
1. Medscape. Infectious Diseases. [online] Available from: https://www.medscape.com/infectiousdiseases [Last accessed February, 2020].

6. **Ans. C**
Most individuals with histoplasmosis are asymptomatic. Most patients are immunocompromised. Histoplasmosis is often reactivated through cell-mediated immunity.
These are the established categories of presentation—asymptomatic pulmonary histoplasmosis, symptomatic pulmonary histoplasmosis, acute diffuse pulmonary histoplasmosis, chronic pulmonary histoplasmosis, acute respiratory distress syndrome,

disseminated histoplasmosis, broncholithiasis, mediastinal granuloma, fibrosing mediastinitis, endobronchial histoplasmosis, and lung nodules.
Ref:
1. Medscape (2019). Histoplasmosis Treatment and Management. [online] Available from: https://emedicine.medscape.com/article/299054-treatment [Last accessed February, 2020].

7. **Ans. C**

The CD4:CD8 ratio acts as a surrogate marker of T-cell compartment balance: CD4 T-cell recovery and CD8 T-cell expansion.

Successful antiretroviral therapy (ART) restores balance to minimize opportunist infections. In long-term treated patients, the progressive correction of the CD4:CD8 ratio is solely a result of CD4 recovery, as CD8 T-cell counts remains constant. Early ART initiation is indicated.
Ref:
1. Serrano-Villar S, Pérez-Elias MJ, Dronda F, Casado JL, Moreno A, Royuela A, et al. Increased risk of serious non-AIDS-related events in HIV-infected subjects on antiretroviral therapy associated with a low CD4/CD8 ratio. PLoS One. 2014;9(1):e85798.
2. Mudd JC, Lederman MM. CD8 T cell persistence in treated HIV infection. Curr Opin HIV AIDS. 2014; 9(5):500-5.

8. **Ans. A**

In immunocompromised individuals, symptomatic disease usually manifests as a mononucleosis syndrome. Symptomatic CMV disease can affect almost every organ of the body. Rarely can manifest Guillain–Barré syndrome.

Retinitis is the most common manifestation of CMV disease in patients who are HIV positive.
Ref:
1. Medscape. Cytomegalovirus. [online] Available from: https://www.medscape.com/infectiousdiseases [Last accessed February, 2020].

9. **Ans. D**

High-risk asymptomatic patients in close contact with infected ones are treated with home quarantine without antiviral therapy unless they begin to show symptoms of infection.
Ref:
1. WHO (2009). Avian Influenza recommendations, National Centre for Disaster Control (NCDC) National guidelines. [online] Available from: https://www.who.int/influenza/resources/documents/guidelinestopics/en/ [Last accessed February, 2020].

10. **Ans. C**

Scedosporium typically occurs in trauma leading to subcutaneous lesions arising from injury following *Scedosporium* (disseminated) "traumatic implantation" of the agent via contaminated splinters. Most infections are localized.

Response to antifungal therapy is variable. Disseminated infections carry a high mortality.

Resistant infections may respond to a combination of voriconazole and terbinafine, and also to a combination of posaconazole, miltefosine, and albaconazole.
Ref:
1. Cortez KJ, Roilides E, Quiroz-Telles F, Meletiadis J, Antachopoulos C, Knudsen T, et al. Infections caused by Scedosporium spp. Clin Microbiol Rev. 2008;21(1): 157-97.
2. Elad D. Infections caused by fungi of the Scedosporium/Pseudallescheria complex in veterinary species. Vet J. 2011;187(1):33-41.

11. **Ans. B**

Thrombocytopenia: Seroconversion from HIV-negative status to HIV-positive status is often characterized by a flu-like syndrome and western blot may require repeat samples at 3 months duration before it is clearly positive.

Thrombocytopenia may be a feature at any stage of HIV illness but especially in early seroconversion part. The etiology may include immune-mediated destruction, thrombotic thrombocytopenic purpura, impaired hematopoiesis, and toxic effects of medications.
Ref:
1. Zon LI, Groopman JE. Hematologic manifestations of the human immune deficiency virus (HIV). Semin Hematol. 1988;25(3):208-18.
2. Spivak JL, Barnes DC, Fuchs E, Quinn TC. Serum immunoreactive erythropoietin in HIV-infected patients. JAMA. 1989;261(21):3104-7.

12. **Ans. B**

Fifth disease or erythema infectiosum is only one of several expressions of Parvovirus B19. Any age may be affected, although it is most common in children aged 6–10 years. Incubation period is 4–14 days. Fever, malaise, nausea, and diarrhea are most common presentations.
Ref:
1. Servey JT, Reamy BV, Hodge J. Clinical presentations of Parvovirus B19 infection. Am Fam Physician. 2007;75(3):373-6.

13. **Ans. D**

Severe anemia in fetus is suggested by sonographic signs, such as fetal skin edema, ascites, or pleural or pericardial effusions. Intrauterine transfusion of RBCs is indicated to prevent fetal death from severe anemia.
Ref:
1. Von Kaisenberg CS, Jonat W. Fetal Parvovirus B19 infection. Ultrasound Obstet Gynecol. 2001;18(3):280-8.

14. **Ans. A**

Pregnant patients: All HIV-infected pregnant women with active TB should be started on ART as early as feasible, both for treatment of maternal HIV infection and to prevent perinatal transmission of HIV (AIII). The choice of ART should be based on efficacy and safety

in pregnancy and should take into account potential drug-drug interactions between antiretrovirals (ARVs) and rifamycins (AIII: Strong recommendation for the statement based on expert opinion) (see Perinatal Guidelines for more detailed discussions).
Ref:
1. World Health Organization (2015). Global Tuberculosis Report 2015. [online] Available from: http://apps.who.int/iris/bitstream/10665/191102/1/9789241565059_eng.pdf?ua=1 [Last accessed February, 2020].
2. Lawn SD, Harries AD, Williams BG, Chaisson RE, Losina E, De Cock KM, et al. Antiretroviral therapy and the control of HIV-associated tuberculosis. Will ART do it? Int J Tuberc Lung Dis. 2011;15(5):571-81.
3. Moore DL, Allen UD. HIV in pregnancy: identification of intrapartum and perinatal HIV exposures. Paediatrics & Child Health. 2019;24(1):42-5.

15. **Ans. C**
Congenital toxoplasmosis is the consequence of transplacental hematogenous fetal infection by *Toxoplasma gondii* during primary infection in pregnant women. Primary infection in an otherwise healthy pregnant woman is asymptomatic in 60% of cases. Symptoms during pregnancy are frequently mild. The most common manifestations are fatigue, malaise, low-grade fever, lymphadenopathy, and myalgias. Latent *Toxoplasma* infection with reactivation during pregnancy may lead to congenital infection only in immunocompromised women (most commonly, those with AIDS).

The classic triad of chorioretinitis, hydrocephalus, and intracranial calcifications cannot be used as a strict diagnostic criterion for congenital toxoplasmosis because a large number of cases would be missed.

When clinically recognized in the neonate, congenital toxoplasmosis, spontaneous abortions, prematurity, or stillbirth may result.
Ref:
1. Medscape. Infectious Diseases. [online] Available from: https://www.medscape.com/infectiousdiseases [Last accessed February, 2020].

16. **Ans. D**
Salmonella septicemia is a condition wherein the presence of *Salmonella* bacteria in the blood triggers a potentially life-threatening, whole-body inflammatory response. Recurrent *Salmonella* septicemia is classified as an AIDS-defining condition by the US Centers for Disease Control and Prevention (CDC).
Ref:
1. Centers for Disease Control and Prevention. Diagnoses of HIV Infection in the United States and Dependent Areas, 2016. HIV Surveillance Report, 2016; Vol. 28.

17. **Ans. A**
Cat-scratch Disease (Bartonella henselae): The disease occurs most frequently in children under 15 years of age. Cats can harbor infected fleas that carry *Bartonella* bacteria. These bacteria can be transmitted from a cat to a person during a scratch.

Ticks may carry some species of *Bartonella* bacteria
Ref:
1. Baranowski K, Huang B. Cat Scratch Disease; 2020. In: StatPearls [Internet]. Treasure Island (FL): StatPearls Publishing; 2020. PMID: 29489252.

18. **Ans. B**
Oral doxycycline in uncomplicated infections has been shown to decrease duration of fever and most symptoms. In hospitalized patients, intravenous penicillin G has been the treatment of choice.
Ref:
1. Haake DA, Levett PN. Leptospirosis in humans. Curr Top Microbiol Immunol. 2015;387:65-97. doi:10.1007/978-3-662-45059-8_5

19. **Ans. D**
Fatality secondary to infectious mononucleosis (IM) is most often are the result of splenic rupture. Other causes are secondary bacterial infection, hepatic failure, and myocarditis.

Airway obstruction can occur due to massive edema of the Waldeyer's ring.

Evidence also exists to suggest Epstein–Barr virus (EBV) infection in an adult and is a risk factor for the development of multiple sclerosis.

Hematologic complications can include development of autoimmune hemolytic anemia, pancytopenia, red cell aplasia, severe thrombocytopenia, or agranulocytopenia.
Ref:
1. Medscape. Infectious Diseases. [online] Available from: https://www.medscape.com/infectiousdiseases [Last accessed February, 2020].

20. **Ans. C**
Empiric treatment is indicated in endemic areas. Diagnosis requires two-step test done with ELISA and PCR, false positives are known to be reported.

First-line agents include doxycycline, penicillin, cefuroxime, and ceftriaxone; however, doxycycline is contraindicated in patients younger than 8 years and in pregnant women.
Ref:
1. Ross Russell AL, Dryden MS, Pinto AA, Lovett JK. Lyme disease: diagnosis and management. Pract Neurol. 2018;18(6):455-464. doi: 10.1136/practneurol-2018-001998. Epub 2018 Oct 3. PMID: 30282764.

21. **Ans. D**
Treatment of loiasis involves chemotherapy or, in some cases, surgical removal of adult worms followed by systemic treatment. Drug of choice is DEC and ivermectin.

In patients with high microfilaria load, albendazole is drug of choice to prevent systemic complications.

Mazzotti reactions can be life-threatening and are characterized by fever, urticaria, swollen and tender lymph nodes, tachycardia, hypotension, arthralgia, edema, and abdominal pain that occur within 7 days of treatment of microfilariasis.

Ref:
1. Ottesen EA. Description, mechanisms and control of reactions to treatment in the human filariases. Ciba Found Symp. 1987;127:265-83. doi: 10.1002/9780470513446.ch18.

22. **Ans. D**

Hemophagocytic lymphohistiocytosis (HLH) is a rapidly progressive, life-threatening syndrome of excessive immune activation. Most patients with HLH are acutely ill with multiorgan involvement, cytopenias, liver function abnormalities, and neurologic symptoms. HLH may also occur in the setting of infections due to bacteria, parasites (e.g., leishmaniasis, malaria), and fungi.

Ref:
1. Ramos-Casals M, Brito-Zerón P, López-Guillermo A, Khamashta MA, Bosch X. Adult haemophagocytic syndrome. Lancet. 2014;383(9927):1503-16.

23. **Ans. C**

Ref:
1. Henderson LA, Cron RQ. Macrophage activation syndrome and secondary hemophagocytic lymphohistiocytosis in childhood inflammatory disorders: diagnosis and management. Paediatr Drugs. 2020;22(1):29-44. doi:10.1007/s40272-019-00367-1.

24. **Ans. A**

Epstein–Barr virus infection induces specific antibodies to EBV and various unrelated non-EBV heterophile antibodies.

Paul-Bunnell test is diagnostic but can be false-negative up to 2 weeks after infection. PCR-based assays are done in reference laboratories. The latex agglutination assay, which is the basis of the Monospot test using horse RBCs, is highly specific. Sensitivity is 85% and specificity is 100%.

Ref:
1. Medscape. Infectious Diseases. [online] Available from: https://www.medscape.com/infectiousdiseases [Last accessed February, 2020].

25. **Ans. D**

Deficiencies of complement proteins may be acquired or inherited. Acquired complement deficiencies are relatively common and may occur as a result of decreased synthesis, increased protein loss, or increased consumption. The liver is the most important organ for the synthesis of several complement proteins, and therefore, low complement levels are often seen in persons with advanced liver disease. Decreased levels of C3, C4, and CH50 have association with pneumonia caused by *S. pneumoniae* and septicemia with *Staphylococcus aureus* and *Escherichia coli*.

Ref:
1. Audemard-Verger A, Descloux E, Ponard D, Deroux A, Fantin B, Fieschi C, et al. Infections Revealing Complement Deficiency in Adults: A French Nationwide Study Enrolling 41 Patients. Medicine (Baltimore). 2016;95(19):e3548.

26. **Ans. C**

Cancer risk
- Risk is highest within the first year of diagnosis
- In those with polymyositis, the risk falls to expected rates 5 years after diagnosis
- In those with dermatomyositis, the risk does not fall to expected rates
    - Ovarian, pancreatic, lung remain high up to 5 years
    - Pancreatic and colorectal cancer risks remain elevated past 5 years

Ref:
1. Hill CL, Zhang Y, Sigurgeirsson B, Pukkala E, Mellemkjaer L, Airio A, et al. Frequency of specific cancer types in dermatomyositis and polymyositis: a population-based study. Lancet. 2001;357(9250): 96-100.

27. **Ans. D**

While the biological half-life of azathioprine is usually 8–10 hours after dosing, the presence of active metabolites in circulation may persist for up to 3 weeks after discontinuation of the last dose and impact on both T-cell and B-cell function.

Ref:
1. Mohammadi O, Kassim TA. Azathioprine [Updated 2020 May 7]. In: StatPearls [Internet]. Treasure Island (FL): StatPearls Publishing; 2020. [online] Available from: https://www.ncbi.nlm.nih.gov/books/NBK542190/.

28. **Ans. A**

Cytomegalovirus infection may cause direct or indirect effects. Direct effects include bone marrow suppression, pneumonia, myocarditis, GI disease, hepatitis, pancreatitis, nephritis, retinitis, and encephalitis, among others. The main indirect effects include acute and chronic graft rejection, accelerated atherosclerosis (heart transplants), secondary bacterial or fungal infections, EBV-associated post-transplant lymphoproliferative disease (PTLD), and decreased graft and patient survival.

Ref:
1. Azevedo LS, Pierrotti LC, Abdala E, et al. Cytomegalovirus infection in transplant recipients. Clinics (Sao Paulo). 2015;70(7):515-23.
2. Griffiths P, Baraniak I, Reeves M. The pathogenesis of human cytomegalovirus. J Pathol. 2015;235(2):288-97. doi: 10.1002/path.4437. PMID: 25205255

29. Ans. C

In patients with HIV infection, CMV involves the entire GI tract. In the upper GI tract, CMV has been isolated from esophageal ulcers, gastric ulcers, and duodenal ulcers. Patients with upper GI tract esophageal disease can present with painful dysphagia. Patients with CMV disease of the lower GI tract may present with diarrhea (colitis). CMV colitis frequently affects only the right colon, necessitating full colonoscopy and multiple biopsies for accurate diagnosis. Diagnosis of CMV GI disease depends on a biopsy specimen demonstrating the typical CMV intranuclear inclusions.

Ref:
1. *Serlin MH, Dieterich D. Gastrointestinal Disorders in HIV. Global HIV/AIDS Medicine; 2008. pp. 251-60.*
2. *Dupont L, Reeves MB. Cytomegalovirus latency and reactivation: recent insights into an age old problem. Rev Med Virol. 2016;26(2):75-89. doi: 10.1002/rmv.1862. Epub 2015 Nov 17. PMID: 26572645; PMCID: PMC5458136.*

30. Ans. B

Dengue virus infection causes intense immune activation. Aberrant immune responses such as CD4/CD8 ratio inversion not only impair the ability of the immune system to clear the virus, but also cause overproduction of cytokines that can affect monocytes, endothelial cells, and hepatocytes. The rate of viral replication is increased, and a vicious cycle is amplified. Virions expand dramatically. On this basis, both antibody-dependent enhancement and virus virulence theories can be explained. Viral load becomes the common denominator of both theories. Secondary infection by different serotypes of dengue virus produces a higher viral load and a stronger immune deviation than does primary infection. At defervescence of dengue virus infection, endothelial cells are damaged by either direct virus cytopathy or immune-mediated pathology. Plasma leakage is observed clinically because of structural alterations in endothelial cells. Hemoconcentration results from hypovotemic loss. Ptatelets are destroyed by crossreactive anti-platelet autoantibodies. Titers of anti-platelet or anti-endothelial cell antibodies are higher in DHF/DSS than in DF because of high affinity antibody or immune memory on antibody production

Over- production of IL-6 might play a crucial role in the enhanced production of anti-platelet autoantibodies, elevated levels of tPA, and the deficiency of coagulation factor XII in the intrinsic pathway.

Ref:
1. *Lin CF, Wan SW, Cheng HJ, Lei HY, Lin YS. Autoimmune pathogenesis in dengue virus infection. Viral Immunol. 2006;19(2):127-32.*
2. *Lei HY, Yeh TM, Liu HS, Lin YS, Chen SH, Liu CC. Immunopathogenesis of dengue virus infection. J Biomed Sci. 2001;8(5):377-88. doi: 10.1007/BF02255946. PMID: 11549879.*

31. Ans. B

Cold antibody hemolytic anemia (CAHA) is classified as primary (idiopathic) or secondary. In most cases, CAHA is a primary disorder that typically becomes apparent at 50–60 years of age. Cold antibody hemolytic anemia may also occur as a secondary disorder in association with a number of different underlying disorders, such as certain infectious diseases (e.g., *Mycoplasma* infection and infectious mononucleosis) and lymphoproliferative diseases (e.g., non-Hodgkin's lymphoma and chronic lymphocytic leukemia).

Extrapulmonary complications may present before, during, after, or in the absence of pulmonary signs. An increase in cold agglutinin titers is frequently observed during *Mycoplasma pneumoniae* infection; it has been reported that 50–60% of these patients had cold agglutinins, which appear 1 week after the onset of the illness and decline toward undetectable levels after 2–6 weeks. Cold agglutinins appear to be more specific for I antigen of the red blood cell surface and often result in mild, subclinical hemolysis and mild reticulocytosis. Severe hemolytic anemia is rare and is usually associated with marked pulmonary involvement. In 90% of such patients, cold agglutinin disease is mediated by an IgM molecule.

The induction of cold agglutinins may be triggered by the formation of *Mycoplasma*-receptor complexes in which the lipid-rich *Mycoplasma* surface plays the role of an adjuvant.

The phagocytic and other destructive cells of the immune system do not have receptors for IgM as they do for IgG and IgA. Thus, since cold agglutinins are usually IgM, destruction of RBCs is primarily complement-mediated, occurring either by direct destruction of the membrane (direct lysis) or immunoadherence mediated by target-bound components (indirect lysis). Both of these processes are relatively inefficient in the absence of exposure to cold.

Typical laboratory features common to all forms of extravascular hemolysis include indirect hyperbilirubinemia and increased concentration of lactate dehydrogenase, whereas the hallmarks of intravascular hemolysis include a decrease in the serum level of haptoglobin and an increase in plasma-free hemoglobin. The coincidence of elevated serum levels of lactate dehydrogenase and bilirubin with low levels of haptoglobin is common in hemolytic anemia caused by cold agglutinins. Our patient showed both features of extra- and intravascular hemolysis.

Clues to the diagnosis of cold agglutinin disease include acrocyanosis and Raynaud's phenomenon. Moreover, autoagglutination on the peripheral blood film, which disappears on warming the blood sample, suggests a cold antibody.

Diagnosis of CAHA is based on a positive direct Coombs' test in the presence of cold agglutinins.

Ref:
1. Clyde WA Jr. Clinical overview of typical Mycoplasma pneumoniae infections. Clin Infect Dis. 1993;17:(Suppl 1):S32-6.
2. Foy HM. Infections caused by Mycoplasma pneumoniae and possible carrier state in different populations of patients. Clin Infect Dis. 1993;17(Suppl 1):S37-6.
3. Waites KB, Talkington DF. Mycoplasma pneumoniae and its role as a human pathogen. Clin Microbiol Rev. 2004;17(4):697-728.

32. Ans. D

Hepatitis E infection with genotype 1 during the third trimester can lead to maternal mortality in 15–25% of cases. Most of the studies showing high maternal mortality are from India, where infection occurs in epidemics. There is a very high risk of vertical transmission of HEV from the mother to the fetus. During a Delhi epidemic, a hospital-based study revealed that HEV infection during pregnancy was associated with miscarriage, stillbirth, or neonatal death in 56% of infants. One recent study highlights that HEV infection might be responsible for 2,400–3,000 stillbirths each year in developing countries, with many additional fetal deaths linked to antenatal maternal deaths. There is a very high risk of preterm delivery in pregnant women with HEV infection, with poor neonatal survival rates. In two separate studies from India, 15–50% of live-born infants of mothers with HEV infection died within 1 week of birth. During an outbreak in Sudan in 2010–2011, among 39 pregnant women with HEV infection there were 14 intrauterine deaths and 9 premature deliveries.

Ref:
1. Rein DB, Stevens GA, Theaker J, Wittenborn JS, Wiersma ST. The global burden of hepatitis E virus genotypes 1 and 2 in 2005. Hepatology. 2012;55(4):988-97.
2. Khuroo MS. Discovery of hepatitis E: the epidemic non-A, non-B hepatitis 30 years down the memory lane. Virus Res. 2011;161(1):3-14.
3. Aggarwal R, Gandhi S. The global prevalence of hepatitis E virus infection and susceptibility: a systematic review. Geneva, Switzerland: World Health Organization; 2010.
4. Xia H, Wahlberg N, Belák S, Meng XJ, Liu L. The emergence of genotypes 3 and 4 hepatitis E virus in swine and humans: a phylogenetic perspective. Arch Virol. 2011;156(1):121-4.

33. Ans. A

Diseases caused by the EBV are of great significance among organ transplant recipients. One of these diseases, PTLD, is a major complication among organ transplant recipients. Management of this entity is problematic due to the difficulties with laboratory surveillance, diagnosis, prevention and treatment. A group of Canadian and American experts was assembled to discuss these aspects of EBV diseases in Canadian organ transplant recipients. This report summarizes the relevant background literature and levels of evidence in relation to the outcomes of the deliberations and recommendations by the expert panel.

The EBV is recognized primarily for its etiological role in infectious mononucleosis, a usually benign lymphoproliferative disorder most prevalent in adolescents and young adults. Under conditions of severe T-cell immunosuppression, which prevail in patients with AIDS and transplant recipients, EBV-infected B cells may expand unchecked, resulting in malignant lymphoproliferation. In this context, the virus is able to transform and immortalize B lymphocytes, leading to their uncontrolled proliferation. This is particularly likely in settings where the host lacks adequate cytotoxic T-lymphocyte surveillance. One such setting occurs when transplant recipients experience primary EBV infection.

Ref:
1. Pope JH, Horne MK, Scott W. Transformation of foetal human leukocytes in vitro by filtrates of a human leukemic cell line containing herpes-like virus. Int J Cancer. 1968;3(6):857-66.
2. Hanto DW, Frizzera G, Gajl-Peczalska KJ, Sakamoto K, Purtilo DT, Balfour HH Jr, et al. Epstein-Barr virus (EBV) induced B-cell lymphoma after renal transplantation. N Engl J Med. 1982;306(15):913-8.
3. Starzl TE, Nalesnik MA, Porter KA, Ho M, Iwatsuki S, Griffith BP, et al. Reversibility of lymphomas and lymphoproliferative lesions developing under cyclosporin-steroid therapy. Lancet. 1984;1(8377):583-7.
4. Shapiro RS, McClain K, Frizzera G, Gajl-Peczalska KJ, Kersey JH, Blazar BR, et al. Epstein-Barr virus-associated B cell lymphoproliferative disorders following bone marrow transplantation. Blood. 1988;71(5):1234-43.
5. Nalesnik MA, Jaffe R, Starzl TE, Demetris AJ, Porter K, Burnham JA, et al. The pathology of posttransplant lymphoproliferative disorders occurring in the setting of cyclosporine A-prednisone immunosuppression. Am J Pathol. 1988;133(1):173-92.

34. Ans. C

Ref:
1. Chopra V, Joshi JL, Mrigpuri P, Chahal AS. Pigeon fancier's lung—an under-diagnosed cause of severely debilitating and chronic breathlessness. Egyptian Journal of Chest Diseases and Tuberculosis. 2017;66(3):557-9.
2. Chan AL, Juarez MM, Leslie KO, Ismail HA, Albertson TE. Bird fancier's lung: a state-of-the-art review. Clin Rev Allergy Immunol. 2012;43(1-2):69-83. doi: 10.1007/s12016-011-8282-y. PMID: 21870048.

35. Ans. D

The ratio of nevirapine AUC (0–12) to the AUC (0–12) of its 12-hydroxy metabolite was significantly lower in the presence of antitubercular therapy, consistent with induced metabolism.

Nevirapine concentrations were significantly decreased by concomitant rifampicin-based antitubercular therapy and a high proportion of patients had subtherapeutic plasma concentrations.

Ref:
1. Corbett EL, Marston B, Churchyard GJ, De Cock KM. Tuberculosis in sub-Saharan Africa: opportunities, challenges, and change in the era of antiretroviral treatment. Lancet. 2006;367(9514):926-37.
2. Erickson DA, Mather G, Trager WF, Levy RH, Keirns JJ, et al. Characterization of the in vitro biotransformation of the HIV-1 reverse transcriptase inhibitor nevirapine by human hepatic cytochromes P-450. Drug Metab Dispos. 1999;27(12):1488-95.

36. **Ans. D**

Ref:
1. Truong J, Ashurst JV. Pneumocystis Jiroveci Pneumonia. [Updated 2020 Aug 10]. In: StatPearls [Internet]. Treasure Island (FL): StatPearls Publishing; 2020. Available from: https://www.ncbi.nlm.nih.gov/books/NBK482370/.

37. **Ans. D**

Ref:
1. Wang Q, Wen Z, Cao Q. Risk of tuberculosis during infliximab therapy for inflammatory bowel disease, rheumatoid arthritis, and spondyloarthropathy: a meta-analysis. Exp Ther Med. 2016;12(3):1693-704. doi: 10.3892/etm.2016.3548.

38. **Ans. D**

Ref:
1. Kothavade RJ, Dhurat RS, Mishra SN, Kothavade UR. Clinical and laboratory aspects of the diagnosis and management of cutaneous and subcutaneous infections caused by rapidly growing mycobacteria. Eur J Clin Microbiol Infect Dis. 2013;32(2):161-88.

39. **Ans. B**

Mycobacterium avium complex is transmitted via inhalation into the respiratory tract and ingestion into the GI tract. It then translocates across mucosal epithelium, infects the resting macrophages in the lamina propria and spreads into the submucosal tissue. MAC is then carried to the local lymph nodes by lymphatics. In immunocompromised hosts, such as those with AIDS, the bacteria subsequently spread hematogenously to the liver, spleen, bone marrow, and other sites.

Disseminated MAC (DMAC) infection usually develops in patients with AIDS and/or lymphomas whose CD4 count has fallen below 50 cells/μL. In patients with AIDS, colonization of the GI or respiratory tract has been associated with an increased risk of developing MAC bacteremia. Approximately 60% of patients with MAC colonization in one series developed bacteremia; however, screening cultures from the respiratory or GI tract is not useful because most patients who develop bacteremia are not colonized prior to developing disseminated disease.

The most important risk factor for MAC infection in patients without HIV infection is underlying lung disease. Pulmonary disease is the most common manifestation of MAC infection in these patients. It can also cause lymphadenitis in children. MAC has surpassed *Mycobacterium scrofulaceum* as the most common cause of cervical adenitis in developed countries.

Both TNF-α and interferon gamma (IFN-γ) play important roles in defending against mycobacterial infections. Like other mycobacteria, MAC can cause disseminated infection in multiple family members who have a deficiency of IFN-γ receptor expression or IFN-γ production due to genetic defects.

Ref:
1. Ramirez-Alejo N, Santos-Argumedo L. Innate defects of the IL-12/IFN-γ axis in susceptibility to infections by Mycobacteria and Salmonella. J Interferon Cytokine Res. 2014;34(5):307-17.
2. Cavalcanti YVN, Brelaz MCA, Neves JK de AL, Ferraz JC, Pereira VRA. Role of TNF-alpha, IFN-gamma, and IL-10 in the development of pulmonary tuberculosis. Pulmonary Medicine. 2012 Nov 28;2012:745483.

40. **Ans. B**

Types of contact are:

Category I: Touching or feeding animals, licks on the skin

Category II: Nibbling of uncovered skin, minor scratches or abrasions without bleeding, licks on broken skin

Category III: Single or multiple transdermal bites or scratches, contamination of mucous membrane with saliva from licks; exposure to bat bites or scratches

For category I no treatment is required, whereas for category II immediate vaccination and for category III immediate vaccination and administration of rabies immunoglobulin are recommended in addition to immediate washing and flushing of all bite wounds and scratches. Depending on vaccine type, the postexposure schedule prescribes intramuscular doses of 1 mL or 0.5 mL given as 4–5 doses over 4 weeks. For rabies-exposed patients who have previously undergone complete pre-exposure vaccination or postexposure treatment with cell-derived rabies vaccines, two intramuscular doses of a cell-derived vaccine separated by 3 days are sufficient. Rabies immunoglobulin treatment is not necessary in such cases. The same rules apply to persons vaccinated against rabies who have demonstrated neutralizing antibody titers of at least 0.5 IU/mL.

Ref:
1. Rabies Vaccines and Immunoglobulins: WHO Position April 2018.

CHAPTER 2

Gram-negative Crisis

Pradip Kumar Bhattacharya

1. A 47-year-old man with alcoholic liver cirrhosis and ascites is admitted to hospital. He is febrile with abdominal pain and delirium. Routine blood tests show increased white blood cell (WBC) and C-reactive protein (CRP) with normal electrolytes and renal function. An ascitic tap shows 500 WBCs/μL and organisms visible on microscopy.
   What is the most likely organism?

   A. *Klebsiella pneumoniae*
   B. *Escherichia coli*
   C. Enterobacteriaceae
   D. *Streptococcus pneumoniae*
   E. *Staphylococcus aureus*

2. A 64-year-old woman has been in the intensive care unit (ICU) for 12 days. She was initially admitted from the operation theater after an emergency laparotomy for colonic perforation and fecal peritonitis. She is currently sedated, ventilated, and requires hemodynamic support and hemofiltration. Results of a blood culture from 2 days ago show a gram-negative bacilli. Which of the following newer antibacterial agents is likely to be the most effective against a gram-negative bacillus?

   A. Teicoplanin   B. Ertapenem
   C. Tigecycline   D. Daptomycin
   E. Linezolid

3. A 79-year-old nursing home patient presents with fever, confusion, productive cough, and shortness of breath. He has diabetes, hypertension, and dementia. He takes insulin, metoprolol, and aspirin. He is allergic to eggs, sulpha, and angiotensin-converting enzyme inhibitors. He is diagnosed with a left lower lobe healthcare-associated pneumonia (HAP). On admission, he is given linezolid, meropenem, and levofloxacin. His condition improves markedly, and on the fifth hospital day, he is ready to be discharged back to his nursing home. His sputum and blood cultures grow *K. pneumoniae*. It is resistant to ampicillin and cefazolin but susceptible to ceftriaxone, piperacillin/tazobactam, meropenem, ciprofloxacin, and trimethoprim (TMP)/sulfamethoxazole (SMX).
   Which of the following statements regarding discharge antibiotics is correct?

   A. Discharge the patient on the same intravenous antibiotics since his condition improved on them
   B. Discharge the patient on oral TMP/SMX
   C. Discharge the patient on oral amoxicillin
   D. Discharge the patient on oral ciprofloxacin
   E. Discharge the patient on intravenous piperacillin/tazobactam

4. Burn patients are at risk for multiple infections. What is the most common organism to cause infection in burn patients?

   A. *S. aureus*   B. *S. pyogenes*
   C. *S. agalactiae*   D. *P. aeruginosa*
   E. *Candida albicans*

5. A 56-year-old woman comes to the outpatient clinic for a postoperative visit 1 week after open fixation of an ankle fracture and complains of pain and swelling in her foot. She states that she first noticed a patch of redness and some pain near the surgical incision last night but woke up to find it had spread to encompass her entire foot. She reports that she "just does not feel well," and chills overnight. On physical examination, her temperature is 101°F (38.3°C), blood pressure 118/78 mm Hg, and heart rate (HR) 86 beats per minute (bpm). The right foot is edematous, erythematous, warm, and tender to the touch with no crepitus or fluctuance present. The incision site is intact, and no purulent material is noted. Which of the following infectious organisms should be suspected in this patient?

   A. Group A hemolytic streptococci
   B. *P. aeruginosa*
   C. *S. aureus*
   D. *E. coli* and other gram-negative species
   E. All except B

6. A 72-year-old woman saw her general practitioner with a 2-week history of general malaise. She mentioned that over the last 3 years, she occasionally leaked urine when coughing, laughing, or lifting things, but had never suffered from urgency of micturition, dysuria, or hematuria. Examination of her abdominal, cardiac, and respiratory systems

were normal. There was no lymphadenopathy. She was on no medication. Dipstick testing of her urine was positive for nitrites only. 3 days later, the following normal test results were seen: Full blood count (FBC), urea and electrolytes (U&E), serum calcium, liver and thyroid function. Urine culture showed >100,000 colony-forming units/mL of *E. coli*. What is the next most appropriate step in her management?

- A. Advise pelvic floor exercises
- B. External vaginal examination
- C. Nothing more needs to be done
- D. Refer to the continence adviser
- E. Treat with antibiotics

7. A 59-year-old man undergoes coronary bypass surgery. He receives vancomycin prophylactically for 24 hours. On the ninth postoperative day, he develops a fever of 39.8°C (103°F) with an HR of 115 bpm and a blood pressure of 105/65 mm Hg. The surgical site is healing well with no redness or discharge. His white blood cell count is 14,000/mm³ and urinalysis reveals many white blood cells per high-power field. Blood and urine cultures grow a nonlactose-fermenting oxidase-positive gram-negative rod. Which of the following antibiotics is most appropriate to treat this infection?

- A. Moxifloxacin
- B. Ceftriaxone
- C. Imipenem
- D. TMP-SMX
- E. Tigecycline

8. A 36-year-old man with history of acute myelogenous leukemia is admitted to the ICU with neutropenic fever and low blood pressure that requires norepinephrine drip. The patient finished his first cycle of chemotherapy 10 days ago. He denies respiratory, gastrointestinal, or urinary symptoms. Complete blood count (CBC) reveals mild thrombocytopenia and an absolute neutrophil count of 100/µL. Urinalysis is within normal limits and chest X-ray (CXR) does not show any infiltrate. Awaiting culture results, which of the following antibiotic regimens is most appropriate?

- A. Imipenem
- B. Vancomycin
- C. Vancomycin, piperacillin/tazobactam, and tobramycin
- D. Cefepime, levofloxacin, and amphotericin B
- E. Continue supportive measures awaiting culture results

9. A 70-year-old ICU patient complains of fever and shaking chills. The patient develops hypotension, and blood cultures are positive for gram-negative bacilli. The patient begins bleeding from venipuncture sites and around his Foley catheter. Laboratory studies are as follows:

- Hematocrit (Hct): 38%
- WBC: 15,000/µL
- Platelet count: 40,000/µL (normal 150,000–400,000)
- Peripheral blood smear: Fragmented RBCs
- Prothrombin time (PT): Elevated
- Partial thromboplastin time (PTT): Elevated
- Plasma fibrinogen: 70 mg/dL (normal 200–400)

Which of the following is the best course of therapy in this patient?

- A. Begin heparin
- B. Treat underlying disease
- C. Begin plasmapheresis
- D. Give vitamin K
- E. Begin red blood cell transfusion

10. A 30-year-old man has developed fever, chills, and neck stiffness. Cerebrospinal fluid (CSF) shows gram-negative diplococci. He has had a past episode of sepsis with meningococcemia.

The most likely immunologic deficiency is:

- A. Complement deficiency C5-C9
- B. Postsplenectomy
- C. Drug-induced agranulocytosis
- D. Interleukin-12 receptor deficit
- E. Hyper-IgE (Job) syndrome
- F. Adenosine deaminase deficiency

11. A 43-year-old undomiciled man is brought to the emergency department (ED) after being found intoxicated on the street. He is currently rousable and expresses a request to be left alone. Initial vitals include an HR of 92 bpm, a BP of 125/80 mm Hg, and a respiratory rate (RR) of 14 breaths/min with an oxygen saturation of 93% on room air. His rectal temperature is 101.2°F. A chest radiograph shows infiltrates involving the right lower lobe. Given this clinical presentation, what initial antibiotic coverage is most appropriate for this patient?

- A. Gram-negative coverage only
- B. Gram-positive coverage only
- C. Broad-spectrum with anaerobic coverage
- D. *Pneumocystis carinii* pneumonia (PCP) coverage
- E. Antifungal therapy

12. A 48-year-old man with a past medical history of hepatitis C and cirrhosis presents to the ED complaining of acute-onset abdominal pain and chills. His BP is 118/75 mm Hg, HR is 105 bpm, RR is 16 breaths/min, temperature is 101.2°F rectally, and oxygen saturation is 97% on room air. His abdomen is distended and diffusely tender.

You decide to perform a paracentesis and retrieve 1 L of cloudy fluid. Laboratory analysis of the fluid shows a neutrophil count of 550 cells/mm^3. Which of the following is the most appropriate choice of treatment?

A. Metronidazole
B. Vancomycin
C. SMX/TMP
D. Neomycin and lactulose
E. Cefotaxime

13. A 59-year-old woman presents to the ED complaining of worsening lower abdominal pain over the previous 3 days. She describes feeling constipated recently and some burning when she urinates. Her BP is 135/75 mm Hg, HR is 89 bpm, temperature is 101.2°F, and her RR is 18 breaths/min. Her abdomen is mildly distended, tender in the left lower quadrant, and positive for rebound tenderness. CT scan is consistent with diverticulitis with a 7 cm abscess. Which of the following is the most appropriate management for this condition?

A. Reserve the operating room (OR) for emergent laparotomy
B. Start treatment with ciprofloxacin and metronidazole and plan for CT-guided draining of the abscess
C. Give an IV dose of ciprofloxacin and make the patient follow-up with her primary physician
D. Start treatment with ciprofloxacin and metronidazole and plan for an emergent barium enema
E. Start treatment with ciprofloxacin and metronidazole and prepare for an emergent colonoscopy

14. Which of the following statements is true regarding pertussis infection?

A. Infection is more severe in adults than children
B. The organism is identified in routine sputum culture
C. Treatment is with a macrolide antibiotic
D. Antibiotics do not alter the course of illness
E. The first phase of illness involves paroxysms of cough

15. Regarding febrile neutropenia in cancer patients, which of the following is true?

A. Gram-negative enteric bacteria currently account for 60–70% of microbiologically confirmed infections
B. *S. epidermidis* cultured in the blood is usually not a contaminant
C. Indwelling vascular catheters should immediately be removed if no other source of infection is found on initial examination
D. *Pseudomonas* is the most common pathogen

16. An 18-year-old male has presented to the ED with a rapid-onset febrile illness associated with myalgia. You consider meningococcemia as a potential diagnosis. Which of the following is incorrect regarding meningococcemia?

A. The rash of meningococcemia may be urticarial, macular, or maculopapular
B. Carriers have some immunity against invasive disease
C. Serogroup B causes most of the diseases in India
D. The mortality of a patient with meningococcal meningitis is higher than that of patients with invasive meningococcal disease

17. A patient presents with cellulitis of the lower limb. Which of the following is true regarding cellulitis?

A. *Aeromonas* species are implicated in infections associated with fresh water
B. Mild-to-moderate chronic diabetic foot infections should be treated with amoxicillin-clavulanate 875/125 mg orally bd or ciprofloxacin 500 mg bd in penicillin-allergic patients
C. Laboratory tests can accurately differentiate between cellulitis and deep venous thrombosis (DVT) of the lower limb
D. Previous venous harvest is not a risk factor for cellulitis

18. A 25-year-old man is evaluated in the ED for fever, headache, and mental status changes of 4 hours' duration. He underwent a cadaveric kidney transplantation 10 months ago, and his immunosuppressive regimen includes prednisone and azathioprine. He has no allergies. On physical examination, his temperature is 38°C (101.6°F), HR is 115 bpm, RR is 25 breaths/min, and blood pressure is 100/60 mm Hg. He is oriented as to the year and his name but cannot recall the month. His neck is supple, and Kernig and Brudzinski signs are absent. The neurologic examination is normal. His peripheral leukocyte count is 20,000/mm^3. A CT scan of the head shows no sign of hemorrhage, hydrocephalus, mass effect, or midline shift. An lumbar puncture (LP) is performed and examination of the CSF shows leukocyte count 2,000/mm^3 (60% neutrophils, 40% lymphocytes), glucose 25 mg/dL, protein 150 mg/dL, and a negative Gram stain. The opening spinal pressure is normal. Results of blood, urine, and CSF cultures are pending. Which of the following is the most appropriate empiric antibiotic therapy?

A. Ampicillin and ceftriaxone
B. Ampicillin, ceftriaxone, and vancomycin
C. Ceftriaxone and moxifloxacin

D. Ceftriaxone and vancomycin
E. Moxifloxacin

19. A 65-year-old man with a history of hepatitis C and progressive liver disease presents to the hospital with increasing low-grade fever, abdominal pain, and distension. He is currently on furosemide, spironolactone, and nadolol. On physical examination, his temperature is 37.5°C (99.5°F), and blood pressure is 100/50 mm Hg. Abdominal examination reveals distended abdomen and marked ascites. The abdomen is mildly tender upon palpation. Creatinine is 0.8 mg/dL and total bilirubin is 2.1 mg/dL.

    Abdominal ultrasound is consistent with cirrhosis, splenomegaly, and large volume of ascites. Diagnostic paracentesis is scheduled. The most appropriate initial treatment is:

    A. Cefotaxime
    B. Cefotaxime and albumin
    C. Furosemide and spironolactone
    D. Large-volume paracentesis

20. A 66-year-old woman presents with a chief complaint of fever, nausea, and vomiting. On physical examination, she appears ill. Her temperature is 39.9°C, blood pressure is 127/878, and pulse rate is 120/min. Laboratory studies reveal a leukocyte count of 23,000 with 87% neutrophils. Urinalysis demonstrates >68 leukocytes/hpf and has a positive leukocyte esterase. Gram-negative rods are seen upon microscopic examination. She is admitted to the hospital with a diagnosis of probable urinary tract infection. On the second day of her hospitalization, her urine and blood cultures are positive for *E. coli*, susceptible to piperacillin/tazobactam, ciprofloxacin, imipenem, ampicillin, and ceftriaxone.

    Which of the following is the most appropriate management?

    A. Continue piperacillin/tazobactam
    B. Discontinue piperacillin/tazobactam and begin ampicillin
    C. Discontinue piperacillin/tazobactam and begin ciprofloxacin
    D. Discontinue piperacillin/tazobactam and begin ceftriaxone

21. A 35-year-old man underwent a heart transplant 5 days ago. He is receiving immunosuppressive therapy with methylprednisolone, cyclosporine, and azathioprine. Today, he develops a temperature of 102°F. *Physical examination*: Ill-appearing man on the ventilator since surgery, BP 130/50 mm Hg, temperature 102°F, RR 30 breaths/min, and pulse rate 100/min. *Significant findings*: Chest—crackles and rhonchi heard over the right lung fields. *Laboratory*: Tracheal secretions are now yellow. FiO$_2$ requirements have increased from 35 to 50%. Pulmonary artery wedge pressure is 15 mm Hg (normal 6–12). *WBC*: 17,000/mm^3 with 90% neutrophils. *CXR*: Dense consolidation in right middle and lower lobes.

    Which of the following is most likely the etiology for his pneumonia?

    A. *Legionella pneumoniae*
    B. *Pneumocystis jiroveci*
    C. Cytomegalovirus (CMV)
    D. *P. aeruginosa*
    E. *Cryptococcus neoformans*

22. A 60-year-old woman who has been on mechanical ventilation for 1 week due to ARDS from a pneumococcal pneumonia is slowly being weaned. Clinically, she is doing well and you are pleased with her progress. *Medications*: Day 8 of ceftriaxone. *Physical examination*: Head, eyes, ears, nose, and throat (HEENT) examination—pupils responsive and equal. Mild thrush of her oral mucosa. *Neck*: Supple, no masses. *Heart*: RRR without murmurs, rubs, or gallops. *Lungs*: Still with basilar crackles right greater than left. *Abdomen*: Positive bowel sounds, tolerating tube feeds well; no masses. *Extremities*: No cyanosis, clubbing, or edema. *Laboratory*: CBC shows a mild increase in WBC to 11,000 from 9,500 yesterday with 80% lymph. Tracheal aspirate culture from 2 days ago returns today and shows *P. aeruginosa* sensitive only to amikacin, piperacillin/tazobactam, and ceftazidime. Aspartate transaminase (AST) 25, alanine transaminase (ALT) 26, bilirubin 0.2 mg/dL, creatinine 0.5 mg/dL, blood urea nitrogen (BUN) 10 mg/dL, *CXR*: Slow improvement from admission; no new infiltrates.

    Based on clinical evaluation and laboratory results, which of the following is the most appropriate next step?

    A. Switch antibiotic coverage to piperacillin/tazobactam alone
    B. Add amikacin to ceftriaxone
    C. Switch antibiotics to piperacillin/tazobactam + amikacin
    D. Perform bronchoscopy and then start piperacillin/tazobactam + amikacin
    E. Continue current therapy

23. A 24-year-old woman presents with persistent cough for 4 weeks. She had upper respiratory infection (URI)-like symptoms 2 weeks earlier and then developed a persistent cough for the next month.

She states she has had coughing fits many times during the day and "could not stop coughing" for almost a minute when she started. Which of the following is true regarding this patient?

A. The disease is caused by a gram-negative *Coccobacillus*
B. Antibiotic therapy should eliminate the symptoms within a few days
C. Bacterial culture is indicated to confirm the diagnosis
D. The disease is not contagious
E. Mortality is close to 30%

24. Pulmonary infections with which of the following may be transmitted from person to person?

    A. *Coxiella burnetii*
    B. *Yersinia pestis*
    C. *Histoplasma capsulatum*
    D. *Francisella tularensis*
    E. *Bacillus anthracis*

25. A 26-year-old G2P2 presents to the ED 3 days after spontaneous vaginal delivery of a healthy male infant with a chief complaint of crampy low abdominal pain and a foul-smelling vaginal discharge. On examination, she has a fever of 102°F and a tender uterus on bimanual pelvic examination. Which of the following is true?

    A. This condition is more common after vaginal delivery than cesarean section
    B. She has postpartum pelvic inflammatory disease
    C. *Chlamydia* and *Mycoplasma* are the most common etiologic agents
    D. Premature rupture of membranes (PROM) is a risk factor for her condition
    E. All of the above

26. A 20-year-old man presents with a painful, ulcerated lesion on his penis. He noticed it 3 days before and the pain became progressively worse. Examination shows a tender, 1 cm ulcerated lesion at the base of his penis with a single, large, tender inguinal lymph node. Gram stain of the ulcer shows gram-negative bacilli. Which of the following is the most likely cause?

    A. Herpes simplex virus
    B. *Chlamydia trachomatis*
    C. *S. epidermidis*
    D. *H. ducreyi*
    E. *Treponema pallidum*

27. Which of the following findings is seen in most patients with meningococcemia?

    A. Bilateral adrenal infarction
    B. Skin lesions
    C. Hypothermia
    D. Seizure
    E. Arthritis

28. Which of the following is most useful in differentiating a patient with acute cholangitis from a patient with acute cholecystitis?

    A. Jaundice
    B. Fever
    C. Abdominal tenderness
    D. Leukocytosis
    E. Murphy's sign

29. Which of the following is the most common organism isolated in SBP?

    A. *E. coli*
    B. *S. aureus*
    C. *S. pneumoniae*
    D. *K. pneumoniae*
    E. Anaerobic species

30. Oroya fever is caused by:

    A. *Agrobacterium tumefaciens*
    B. *Bartonella quintana*
    C. *Rochalimaea quintana*
    D. *B. bacilliformis*

31. Risk factors for multidrug-resistant enterobacteriaceae (MDRE) infection and colonization with carbapenemase and/or extended-spectrum β-lactamase (ESBL)-producing bacteria are all, *except*:

    A. Prior and recent antibiotic (especially fluoroquinolone) use
    B. Long-term use of steroid
    C. Healthcare-associated risks including residence in long-term acute-care facilities, presence of feeding tubes, mechanical ventilation, or a central venous catheter
    D. Obstructive uropathy
    E. Organ and stem cell transplantation

32. Which of the following hand hygiene agent is best against gram-negative bacteria?

    A. Chlorhexidine
    B. Chloroxylenol
    C. Hexachlorophene
    D. Quaternary ammonium
    E. Iodophors

33. According to the American Thoracic Society (ATS) guidelines for treatment of nosocomial pneumonia "core pathogens" include all, *except*:

    A. *S. aureus*
    B. Pneumococcus
    C. *P. aeruginosa*
    D. *E. coli*

34. Necrotic pancreas becomes secondarily infected with:

    A. Gram-positive bacteria of alimentary origin

B. Gram-negative bacteria of alimentary origin
C. Gram-positive bacteria of hematogenous origin
D. Gram-negative bacteria of hematogenous origin

35. **Limulus amebocyte lysate assay in CSF is diagnostic of:**
    A. Gram-negative bacterial meningitis
    B. Fungal meningitis
    C. Tuberculous meningitis
    D. Carcinomatous meningitis

36. **The spectrum for etiology of a pneumonia changes with patient's age. Which are probable pneumonia-causing agents in neonates?**
    A. Group B *streptococci*
    B. *L. monocytogenes*
    C. Enteric gram-negative bacilli
    D. *Chlamydia*
    E. Viral: Rubella, CMV, and herpes

37. **The most common bacterial superinfection in association with *Aspergillus* pneumonia is caused by:**
    A. Gram-positive cocci
    B. Gram-negative cocci
    C. Gram-positive bacilli
    D. Gram-negative rods

38. **Epiglottitis is most commonly caused by:**
    A. *S. pyogenes*
    B. *Pneumococcus*
    C. *S. aureus*
    D. *H. influenza*

39. **Which of the following is responsible for pneumonia from cooling systems?**
    A. *Listeria*
    B. *Mycoplasma*
    C. *Legionella*
    D. *Chlamydia*

40. **Which of the following organism is responsible for bones and joint infections in children <4 years?**
    A. *C. burnetii*
    B. *Shigella flexneri*
    C. *B. fragilis*
    D. *Kingella kingae*

ANSWERS WITH EXPLANATIONS

1. **Ans. B**
   Spontaneous bacterial peritonitis (SBP) is typical of liver cirrhosis with ascites. It represents 10–30% of every bacterial disease in patients with cirrhosis and is there in around 10% of all cirrhotic inpatients. Earlier SBP had a death rate of 90%; however, this has enormously improved to roughly 20% for the first incidence. One-year mortality after the first incidence of SBP is somewhere in the range from 30 to 90% and thus should trigger an assessment for liver transplantation. Bacteria from the gut are the causative organisms of SBP. Patients with cirrhosis have expanded bacterial numbers in their gut because of diminished motility, decreased pancreatic secretions, and modified pH. Patients with cirrhosis also have expanded intestinal permeability and decreased immunological capacity. These variables increase the danger of bacterial translocation.

   The most common causative organism is *E. coli*, which is found in over 40% of cases. Others are gram-negative bacilli, *Klebsiella* and *Enterobacteriaceae* species. Some gram-positive creatures are known to cause SBP, especially streptococcal and enterococcal species.

   Treatment of SBP should begin following a positive ascitic tap and should not be delayed for microbiological culture results. 60% of SBP have no bacteria that are recognized in ascitic liquid. Wide range of anti-infection agents are prescribed. Third- and fourth-age cephalosporins, carbapenems, and penicillins, e.g., piperacillin/tazobactam, are conceivable treatments. Nephrotoxic anti-infection agents should be avoided initially.

2. **Ans. B**
   Ertapenem is a carbapenem, a class of drugs that has good activity against gram-negative organisms. All of the other agents are newer antibacterials with predominantly gram-positive activity. Gram-negative organisms are common causes of infection in the ICU, many of which are resistant to various common antibiotics. In particular, *Acinetobacter baumannii*, *Pseudomonas aeruginosa*, and *Enterobacter* species are widely drug resistant, forming part of the "ESKAPE" group of pathogens (also including *Enterococcus faecium*, *S. aureus*, and *K. pneumoniae*). The ESKAPE pathogens have been identified as one of the main current challenges in the battle against multidrug-resistant bacteria. Newer drugs that have been licensed and widely used in the past 15 years include linezolid, ertapenem, daptomycin, tigecycline, and doripenem. The majority of these agents have a particular activity against gram-positive organisms, possibly in response to the rise of methicillin-resistant *Staphylococcus aureus* (*MRSA*) over the same time period. The carbapenems are a class of drugs with good activity against both gram-positive and gram-negative organisms, although resistance to carbapenems is on the increase. More recent agents include telavancin and ceftaroline fosamil along with combinations of antibacterial drugs

with beta-lactamase inhibitors. Most of the new drugs are in the same class as existing agents with similar actions and a risk of cross-resistance; drugs with novel mechanisms of action are few and far between.

3. **Ans. D**
The patient has HAP. He was started on broad-spectrum antibiotics to cover likely pathogens, which include MRSA and resistant gram-negative bacteria such as *P. aeruginosa*. His condition improved markedly and the culprit bacterium in his case was not as resistant as feared. Furthermore, his pneumonia was not complicated by cavitation or empyema, and he did not have vomiting or diarrhea to preclude finishing his antibiotic course orally. This case represents an opportunity for antibiotic de-escalation, which involves the practice of starting with a broad-spectrum empiric antibiotic regimen (designed to avoid inadequate therapy) combined with a commitment to change from broad- to narrow-spectrum therapy and from multiple agents to fewer medications. Continuing all of the empirically chosen antibiotics puts this patient at risk for drug-drug interaction and *Clostridium difficile* infection and is not justifiable given the susceptible culprit isolated. De-escalation is an example of antimicrobial stewardship, a coordinated effort that aims at optimizing clinical outcomes while minimizing antibiotic toxicity, cost, and resistant bacteria selection. Discharging the patient on meropenem or piperacillin/tazobactam would have been an appropriate choice had this been a mixed infection (e.g., aspiration pneumonia). TMP/SMX is an inappropriate choice, given the reported sulfa allergy. This patient's *Klebsiella* is resistant to ampicillin and cefazolin.

4. **Ans. D**
Infections in burn patients can be problematic for multiple reasons. It may delay wound healing, encourages scarring, and can result in bacteremia which may lead to sepsis. *P. aeruginosa* is a gram-negative bacillus and is considered to be the most common cause of infections in burn patients. (A) MRSA is also commonly seen in burn patients and is difficult to treat due to a large number of virulence factors. (B) *S. pyogenes* is more of a concern in pediatric burn patients because they may have colonization of *S. pyogenes* in their oropharynx. (C) *S. agalactiae* is not an organism thought to infect burn patients. This organism can colonize the genitourinary tract and be transmitted to the neonate during birth which may result in bacteremia, pneumonia, or meningitis. Fungal infections tend to occur in burn patients during the later stages of recovery because by this time the majority of bacteria have been eliminated by the use of antibiotics. The most common cause of fungal infection in burn patients is by (E) *C. albicans*.

5. **Ans. E**
This patient has cellulitis that she developed after a surgical procedure. The defect in the skin barrier and any metal hardware implanted during the procedure are risks for developing this type of infection. She has the classic findings of edema, erythema, warmth, and pain. The lack of crepitus and fluctuance is reassuring that this infection is not necrotizing fasciitis or an abscess. Common pathogens for cellulitis include group A β-hemolytic streptococci and *S. aureus* species; however, this patient is also at risk for *E. coli* and gram-negative infection because the wound is below the waist. Thus initial antibiotic coverage should have activity against these pathogens and can be adjusted later if the pathogen(s) can be identified.

6. **Ans. B**
She has asymptomatic bacteriuria (clinically significant bacteriuria without symptoms related to the urinary tract), which does not require antibiotic treatment. This occurs in approximately 20% of females at this age. *Antibiotic treatment risks*: Bacterial resistance, candidiasis, and *C. difficile*. Asymptomatic bacteriuria may be associated with urge incontinence, but not stress incontinence (which she has had for several years anyway). Before referral to the continence adviser, who might well advise pelvic floor exercises, an external pelvic floor examination needs to be performed to exclude a cystocele or vaginal prolapse.

7. **Ans. C**
The patient has a healthcare-associated urinary tract infection (UTI) complicated by gram-negative bacteremia. The complete identification of gram-negative rods might take 48 hours. Knowing the ability of the growing bacteria to ferment lactose might help in the early prediction of the likely pathogen at hand. Among lactose-fermenting gram-negative rods, Enterobacteriaceae such as *E. coli* are most common. Among nonlactose-fermenting oxidase positive gram-negative bacteria, *P. aeruginosa* is the most common. Ceftriaxone, imipenem, and TMP/SMX can be used to treat UTIs while moxifloxacin and tigecycline do not achieve high enough concentration in urine to be used for this indication. Of the listed antibiotics, imipenem, which is a carbapenem beta-lactam antibiotic, is the only one with antipseudomonal activity. Antibiotics with antipseudomonal activity include certain penicillins (piperacillin/tazobactam and ticarcillin/clavulanate), cephalosporins (ceftazidime and cefepime), carbapenems (imipenem, meropenem, and doripenem), fluoroquinolones (ciprofloxacin and levofloxacin), and aminoglycosides (gentamicin, tobramycin, and amikacin).

8. **Ans. C**

Neutropenic fever is a medical emergency. Infections, most commonly caused by gram-negative bacteria such as *P. aeruginosa*, are responsible for most cases. Prompt empiric antibiotic therapy with two antibiotics from two different antibiotic classes (double coverage) that have antipseudomonal activity is most appropriate. Adding an antibiotic with anti-MRSA activity to the initial antibiotic regimen is indicated if the patient was on antibiotic prophylaxis before the onset of the neutropenic fever or if he has any of the following conditions: Skin infection, moderate-to-severe mucositis, central venous catheter, or shock (as in this case). Imipenem alone is not enough because it lacks anti-MRSA activity. Vancomycin does not provide gram-negative coverage and should never be used alone in the treatment of neutropenic fever. Awaiting culture results without initiating empirical antibiotic coverage is inappropriate because it increases the patient's mortality risk. Antifungal therapy is often added in the subsequent days if the patient fails to respond to broad-spectrum antibiotics.

9. **Ans. B**

This patient with gram-negative bacteremia has developed disseminated intravascular coagulation (DIC), as evidenced by multiple-site bleeding, thrombocytopenia, fragmented red blood cells on peripheral smear, prolonged PT and PTT, and reduced fibrinogen levels from depletion of coagulation proteins. Initial treatment is directed at correcting the underlying disorder—in this case, infection. Although heparin was formerly recommended for the treatment of DIC, it is now used rarely and only in unusual circumstances (such as acute promyelocytic leukemia). For the patient who continues to bleed, supplementation of platelets and clotting factors (with fresh frozen plasma or cryoprecipitate) may help control life-threatening bleeding. Red cell fragmentation and low platelet count can be seen in microangiopathic disorders such as thrombotic thrombocytopenic purpura (TTP), but in these disorders the coagulation pathway is not activated. Therefore, in TTP the PT, PTT, and plasma fibrinogen levels will be normal. Plasmapheresis, vitamin K therapy, and RBC transfusion will not correct the underlying cause.

10. **Ans. A**

Patients who have a deficiency of one of the terminal components of complement have a remarkable susceptibility to disseminated *Neisseria* infection, particularly meningococcal disease. This association with meningococcal disease is related to the host inability to assemble the membrane attack complex a single molecule of complement components that creates a discontinuity in the bacteria's membrane lipid bilayer. The complement deficiency results in inability to express complement-dependent bactericidal activity. The pneumococcus is the most important cause of postsplenectomy sepsis, making up about 67% of all cases (*Haemophilus influenzae* is the second most common organism). The spleen serves a variety of immunologic functions, but as it is the main production site for opsonizing antibody, it is specially important for the clearance of encapsulated bacteria from the bloodstream. A polysaccharide capsule surrounds all invasive pneumococci, and a deficiency in opsonizing antibody postsplenectomy can result in overwhelming sepsis with pneumonia, bacteremia, meningitis, and death. Drug-induced agranulocytosis causes acute pharyngitis ("agranulocytic angina"), fever, and sepsis. Absolute neutrophil count is close to 0; recovery occurs 7–10 days after withdrawal of the offending drug. Antibiotics, antithyroid, or antiepileptic drugs are the common offenders. Interleukin-12 receptor deficiency impairs production of interferon-gamma, leading to disseminated mycobacterial infection, often with nontuberculous species. The hyper-IgE syndrome causes recurrent staphylococcal abscesses, sometimes leading to pneumatoceles in the lung. The genetics of this syndrome is not well understood. Adenine deaminase deficiency accounts for 50% of cases of autosomal recessive severe combined immunodeficiency (SCID). Accumulation of purine metabolites leads to rapid apoptosis of both T- and B- cells.

11. **Ans. C**

Aspiration pneumonia occurs secondary to the aspiration of either oropharyngeal or gastric contents into the lower airways. Aspiration of gastric juices may cause a pulmonary inflammatory response. This type of mechanism of acquiring pneumonia is commonly seen in those with *swallowing difficulties* or *a relaxed lower esophageal sphincte*r because of *alcohol*. Given these factors, this patient is in a high-risk category for aspiration pneumonia. The small degree of angulation of the right mainstem bronchus makes the right lung at higher risk. Most particles easily travel down this route, ending up in the *right middle or lower lobe* of the lung. *Antibiotic coverage* should be *broad*, covering for both *gram-positive* and *gram-negative organisms including anaerobes*, which are commonly present in the mouth. Given the severity, these patients may go on to develop acute respiratory distress syndrome (ARDS), an inflammatory response to infection, and, subsequently, respiratory failure. (A) Gram-negative organisms, such as *H. influenzae, P. aeruginosa, K. pneumoniae,* and *E. coli,* are the most frequent causes of nosocomial pneumonia. (B) Gram-positive organisms such as *S. pneumoniae* and *S. aureus* are most commonly associated with community acquired pneumonia. (D) *PCP* is found in immunocompromised patients, such as those with AIDS, or those receiving immunosuppressants secondary to organ transplantation. They are also at risk for fungal pneumonias (E); however, treatment should not be initiated unless there is high clinical suspicion.

12. **Ans. E**

    Analysis of abdominal fluid and clinical presentation are consistent with *SBP*. It is recommended to start antibiotic treatment for SBP if the neutrophil count is >250 cells/mm^3. Causative organisms include gram-negative Bacteriaceae such as *E coli* and *Klebsiella*, as well as *Streptococcus* sp, and *S. pneumoniae*. Therefore, the most appropriate antibiotic for treatment is *a third-generation cephalosporin* such as *cefotaxime*.

13. **Ans. B**

    Management for *complicated acute diverticulitis* involves *admission* and *antibiotic treatment*. Treatment is directed against both anaerobic and gram-negative bacteria. Intra-abdominal *abscess* formation secondary to diverticulitis requires prompt surgical consultation and should be *drained* using CT or ultrasound-guided percutaneous draining. Abscesses < 5 cm in diameter may be treated with antibiotics alone. The patient's vital signs are stable and there is no evidence for peritonitis; therefore, she does not require an emergent laparotomy (A). The patient should not be discharged from the hospital (C). Because of the risk for bowel perforation, barium enema and colonoscopy are contraindicated (D and E); however, once the diverticulitis is controlled, the patient should undergo one of the procedures to look for other pathology and exclude complications, such as fistula formation.

14. **Ans. C**

    Bordetella pertussis is a gram-negative bacillus, which causes a respiratory illness most commonly in the summer and fall months. Over time, immunity conferred by the vaccine loses its effectiveness and as a result, we have seen a resurgence of this infection recently.

    There are *three stages* of illness: (1) catarrhal—characterized by sneezing, rhinorrhea, and coughing; (2) paroxysmal—frequent coughing episodes followed by an inspiratory "whop," post-tussive emesis; and (3) convalescent—chronic cough lasting several months. Treatment is with *macrolides*, preferably erythromycin for 14 days. Azithromycin, an TMP/SMX, may also be used. Pertussis infections in the adult population (A) are less severe than that in infants and children. The organism is not easily identified on routine sputum culture (B) and requires nasopharyngeal swab and culture, which takes about 1 week to grow. Antibiotics (D) impact the course of illness but only when they are prescribed early. After 2 weeks of infection, the role of antibiotics is primarily to decrease transmission to others. As mentioned earlier, the first phase of illness (E) is the catarrhal phase. The paroxysms of cough occur in phase 2.

15. **Ans. B**

    Approximately 85% of the initial pathogens are bacterial. Gram-negative bacilli, particularly *P. aeruginosa*, used to be the most common pathogens found in the blood of febrile neutropenic patients until the 1980s. However, the administration of prophylactic antibiotics primarily active against gram-negative pathogens during chemotherapy, the widespread use of indwelling intravascular devices, and newer chemotherapy regimens have led to an increase in gram-positive pathogens and currently gram-positive bacteria account for 60–70% of microbiologically confirmed infections in these patients. *S. aureus*, *S. epidermidis* and *S. epidermidis* are the predominant gram-positive organisms. Once believed to be a contaminant, S. epidermidis has arisen as a major pathogen. *E. coli*, *P. aeruginosa*, and *K. pneumoniae* remain the most common gram-negative pathogens. Fungal, viral, and parasitic infections are also important primary and secondary complications. Vascular access can be challenging in patients receiving chemotherapy. Therefore, indwelling vascular catheters should be retained as far as possible. Even when catheter infection is suspected, the infection can be successfully treated in most cases without removing the catheter. The collection of a blood culture from vascular catheter lumen in addition to peripheral blood cultures may further assist in the diagnosis of clinically relevant catheter-related blood stream infections (CRBSI) by allowing the time necessary for blood culture from the peripheral vein to become positive to be compared with the time until blood culture from a central venous catheter becomes positive. A differential time to positivity of ≥120 minutes has been shown to be predictive of CRBSI. This approach is particularly useful in patients in whom catheter retention is desirable. Removal of the line is indicated in the context of tunnel infections, persistent bacteremia despite adequate treatment, atypical mycobacteria infection, and candidemia. Vancomycin should be added when infection of the line is suspected and should be administered through the line when possible.

16. **Ans. D**

    Neisseria meningitidis, a gram-negative intracellular diplococcus, is classified into serogroups according to their capsular polysaccharides. Group A is the most common serotype in India. Cases occur when organisms are transmitted to a susceptible individual from the nasopharynx of a carrier, who often have some immunity from invasive disease caused by the organisms they carry. Clinical disease typically takes the form of meningitis or meningococcemia; the two may coexist. Meningococcal disease has a wide spectrum of presentation including nausea, vomiting, myalgias, abdominal pain, leg or joint pain, pharyngitis, septic shock, pneumonia, myopericarditis, and DIC. The rash associated with meningococcal infection may be petechial or purpuric, but also may be urticarial, macular or maculopapular, particularly early in the disease. Patients with meningococcemia without meningitis have a greater mortality than those with meningitis.

17. **Ans. A**

Predisposing factors for cellulitis are:
- Arterial or venous disease/harvest
- Diabetes
- Previous significant fracture
- Dermatological conditions including eczema and dry skin
- Trauma, bites, and clenched fist injuries.

The majority of cellulites are caused by gram-positive bacteria, of which the most common pathogens are β-hemolytic streptococci, *S. pyogenes*, *S. aureus* and gram-negative aerobic bacilli. *Aeromonas* species are associated with fresh water exposure, whereas *Vibrio* species are seen in salt water-associated infections. *Pseudomonas* is seen in infected burns, and mixed gram-negative and gram-positive aerobes and anaerobes are seen in diabetic foot infections. Most uncomplicated cases can be managed with outpatient antibiotics and supportive care including elevation of the affected part and addressing underlying causes; patient education is important. Certain patients should be treated aggressively including surgical debridement where needed; such patients include those with clenched fist injuries, orbital cellulitis, and diabetic foot infections. Patients with diabetic foot infections will require anaerobic as well as aerobic cover. Suggested antibiotic regimes for mild-to-moderate diabetic foot infections include amoxicillin + clavulanic acid 875/125 mg PO bd plus metronidazole 400 mg bd. For patients with penicillin hypersensitivity, ciprofloxacin 500 mg bd plus clindamycin 600 mg tds can be given orally. Often it is difficult to distinguish clinically between cellulitis and deep vein thrombosis (DVT), especially when the erythema overlaps the path of the deep veins in the leg. Additionally, laboratory tests may not be specific enough to help differentiate between the two disease entities; there are no diagnostic laboratory tests for DVT and the white cell count may be normal or elevated in both conditions. An ultrasound is therefore indicated if any doubt exists regarding the diagnosis.

18. **Ans. B**

Risk factors for *Listeria meningitis* include immunosuppression, neonatal status, or age >50 years, alcoholism, malignancy, diabetes mellitus, hepatic failure, renal failure, iron overload, CVDs, and HIV infection. The most appropriate empiric therapy is ampicillin (the drug of choice for *Listeria*), with ceftriaxone and/or vancomycin. The CSF fluid supports a diagnosis of meningitis. Empiric vancomycin and ceftriaxone are recommended for the treatment of meningitis in patients 2–50 years of age. This covers *S. pneumoniae* and *N. meningitidis*, the most common organisms responsible for meningitis in this age group. The analysis of CSF in patients with *L. meningitis* often fails to reveal typical gram-positive rods with characteristic "tumbling motility" in wet mount preparations, but often shows pleocytosis and may demonstrate a significant number of lymphocytes in addition to neutrophils. Patients usually have increased CSF protein levels; decreased CSF glucose levels are found less commonly and less profoundly with *L. meningitis*. The fluoroquinolones may be effective but do not penetrate the CNS well. Gentamicin is synergistic with ampicillin, despite poor CNS penetration.

19. **Ans. A**

Spontaneous bacterial peritonitis is a common complication of end-stage liver disease. Initial treatment consists of antibiotics that have coverage of gram-negative bacteria. Common isolates are *E. coli* and *K. pneumonia*. There is no evidence that large-volume paracentesis improves outcomes in patients with SBP. Diagnostic paracentesis should be undertaken to confirm the diagnosis. SBP is confirmed when a WBC count of >250/µL is found. Additional paracentesis can be considered to determine the efficacy of treatment or to relieve symptoms.

20. **Ans. B**

In this patient, broad-spectrum antibiotics on presentation are indicated. However, once the specific organism is isolated and sensitivities are known, it is beneficial to de-escalate therapy to a limited-spectrum antibiotic. De-escalation strategies involve not only changing antibiotics but can reduce dosage as well. This may present as a challenge in a situation where a patient has responded well to a broad-spectrum antibiotic. However, failure to do so places the patient at additional risk for antibiotic-induced complications. Ciprofloxacin may be considered, but it provides unnecessarily broad-spectrum coverage. Studies have shown that appropriate de-escalation improves outcomes in cases of sepsis and ventilator-related pneumonia.

21. **Ans. D**

    Note: He is only 5 days out from his transplant. The most common organisms to cause problems this early are hospital-acquired infections, particularly with gram-negative bacteria such as *Pseudomonas* or gram-positive bacteria such as *S. aureus*. CMV and *Pneumocystis* are likely 1–4 months out. *Cryptococcus* is a problem more often at 4 or more months out. *Legionella* does not have much more increased incidence, unless there were something wrong with the processing of water in the hospital.

22. **Ans. E**

    Clinically, she is doing well. You are weaning her off the vent; her physical examination is stable; her laboratory is stable (*never base antibiotic therapy on a minor bump in WBC*). The sputum results are not unusual for a patient in the ICU; they will frequently become colonized with gram-negative organisms, particularly *Pseudomonas*. Never change therapy based on just a tracheal aspirate; you must have some other change in examination or laboratory that is significant for you to consider treating the organism found on a tracheal aspirate. Recognize that sputum results from a tracheal aspirate are rarely useful.

23. **Ans. A**

    The patient has evidence of whooping cough caused by *B. pertussis*, a gram-negative *Coccobacillus* (like *H. influenzae*). The disease occurs in three phases—the catarrhal phase, a nonspecific URI-like syndrome lasting 1–2 weeks; the paroxysmal phase lasting up to 1 month, with paroxysms of coughing fits; and the convalescent phase lasting up to several months, with a chronic, intermittent cough. Antibiotic therapy with macrolides is usually only effective in the catarrhal phase, but should be given to patients to reduce the high degree of contagiousness. Corticosteroids and β-agonist nebulizers may be useful as adjunctive therapy. Cultures are useful only in the catarrhal phase, and have low sensitivity during the paroxysmal phase. Mortality is low.

24. **Ans. B**

    Yersinia. pestis, the etiologic agent of bubonic plague, is a gram-negative Coccobacillus which can cause a number of different clinical syndromes. In this country, it is endemic in the southwestern United States but it has gained notoriety along with anthrax and tularemia because of its potential use as a possible biologic weapon. Pneumonic plague is caused by the inhalation of infective droplets from animals or *persons*. Rodents are the natural hosts but pets can "bring the disease home." After an incubation period of 1–6 days, pneumonic plague is an aggressive disease and many patients progress rapidly to septic shock and death without early treatment. Initially, patients may complain of typical symptoms of pneumonia, and their CXRs frequently show alveolar infiltrates. CXRs may also demonstrate an ARDS-like picture with diffuse patchy bilateral infiltrates and cavitation. None of the other agents demonstrate person-to-person transmission.

25. **Ans. D**

    This patient has endometritis, which is the most common puerperal infection. The primary risk factor for endometritis is cesarean section, although young age, low socioeconomic status, prolonged stage 2 of labor, prolonged ruptured membranes, and multiple vaginal examinations are also risk factors. Patients typically present 2–3 days after delivery with fever, abdominal pain, and foul-smelling lochia. Infections are polymicrobial and most commonly caused by gram-negative enteric pathogens as well as *Bacteroides* and *Prevotella* species. *Chlamydia* is rarely responsible and may cause late-onset puerperal infection.

26. **Ans. D**

    The patient has evidence of chancroid, caused by *H. ducreyi*, a gram-negative bacillus. A painful chancre-like lesion combined with a solitary tender unilateral lymph node which may also ulcerate is classic. Chancroid, unlike syphilis (caused by *T. pallidum*), is painful and tender. Treatment of chancroid is with azithromycin or ceftriaxone. Herpes simplex virus can cause ulcerated or vesicular lesions, but these are usually grouped and Gram stain of the lesions will be negative. *C. trachomatis*, a spirochete, may cause lymphogranuloma venereum, which is manifested by a painless ulcer combined with significant lymphadenopathy with a negative Gram stain. *S. epidermidis* may cause skin lesions in the genital region but Gram stain would show gram-positive cocci.

27. **Answer is B**

    Meningococcemia refers to systemic infection with *N. meningitidis*, a gram-negative *Diplococcus*. Mortality is as high as 50%, due to multiorgan failure from septic shock which can occur within hours. Fever and rash occur in most patients. About 50% of patients present with true petechiae, and another 20–30% exhibit a maculopapular rash which later turns into petechiae or purpura. Bilateral adrenal infarction, part of a constellation of signs known as the *Waterhouse-Friderichsen syndrome*, occurs in approximately 10% of cases. Hypothermia, seizure, and arthritis each occurs <10% of the time. Laboratory studies may demonstrate a significant leukocytosis (although leukopenia, when present, is a poor prognostic indicator), thrombocytopenia, and DIC. Treatment is with a third-generation cephalosporin and aggressive management of shock (fluids, vasoactive agents, and ICU monitoring).

28. Ans. A

There is considerable overlap in the clinical presentation of patients with acute cholecystitis and acute cholangitis. However, patients with acute cholecystitis rarely exhibit jaundice and tend to be less toxic-appearing. Although the cystic duct is usually blocked in acute cholecystitis, the hepatic and common bile ducts are patent and free of infection and inflammation. Charcot's triad (fever, right upper quadrant pain, and jaundice) is the hallmark of acute cholangitis. Fever is nearly universal, present in 95% of patients, right upper quadrant tenderness in 90% and jaundice in 80%. Hypotension and altered mental status are present in 15% of patients and suggest gram-negative sepsis. When present in concert with Charcot's triad, these findings are known as *Reynolds' pentad*. Although mildly elevated bilirubin levels may be present in patients with acute cholecystitis, these levels rarely rise above 4 mg/dL.

29. Ans. A

Escherichia coli is isolated in 47–55% of the cases of SBP and gram-negative organisms are the most common etiologic agents as a group. *K. pneumoniae* is the second most commonly isolated organism. This is followed by *S. pneumoniae*, and other *Streptococcus* and *Staphylococcus* species. Although there have been isolated reports of anaerobic and polymicrobial infections in SBP, they are generally not considered to be causes of SBP. Fever or abdominal pain in a patient with ascites should raise the suspicion of infection and prompt a paracentesis. The presentation of SBP may be subtle, however, and include only mental status changes without abdominal pain or tenderness upon examination. All patients with an ascitic fluid neutrophil count ≥ 250/mm^3 and a clinical picture consistent with infection should be treated with antibiotic therapy.

30. Ans. D

The disease is restricted to the Andean cordillera in Peru, Ecuador, and Colombia with sporadic cases being reported in Bolivia, Chile, and Guatemala. This focality is mainly due to the characteristics of its putative principal sand-fly vector, Lutzomyia verrucarum, which has a weak, hopping flight and is intolerant of extreme temperatures. Young children under the age of 10 years are the most affected age group in endemic communities, partly because of a predominantly younger population but also due to the presumed protective immunity that develops with repeated infection. There are two well-described phases of the illness. The initial acute phase, known as Oroya fever, occurs typically around 2–6 weeks after inoculation of the microorganism by the bite of an infected sandfly. It is characterized by fever, pallor, malaise, joint pain, headache, and anorexia. In severe cases, with high parasitemia, this progresses to severe hemolytic anemia. High-mortality rates of 44–88% have been reported in untreated individuals.

31. Ans. B

Risk factors for MDRE infection and colonization with carbapenemase and/or ESBL-producing bacteria are as follows: (1) Prior and recent antibiotic (especially fluoroquinolone) use; (2) healthcare-associated risks including residence in long-term acute-care facilities, presence of feeding tubes, mechanical ventilation, or a central venous catheter; (3) obstructive uropathy; (4) increased age; (5) receiving healthcare in, or travel to, endemic areas; and (6) organ and stem cell transplantation. The patient presented in this case possesses many of these risk factors; steroid is amongst the lowest-risk factor for MDRE.

32. Ans. E

Quaternary ammonium compounds, hexachlorophene, and chloroxylenol are minimally effective against gram-negative bacteria. Chlorhexidine is moderately effective whereas iodophors and alcohols are best effective.

33. Ans. B

The pathogens that are most frequently involved in HAP are aerobic gram-negative bacilli (*P. aeruginosa*, *E. coli*, *K. pneumoniae*, *Acinetobacter* spp., etc.) and *S. aureus*. These bacteria can be considered the "core" pathogens in HAP along with *S. pneumoniae*. The role of a polymicrobial etiology of HAP has been proposed in ~50% of cases.

34. Ans. B

Infection occurs as a complication in 20% of patients with necrotizing pancreatitis and is thought to result from bacterial translocation from the gut to adjacent necrotic pancreatic parenchyma. The most common bacterial organisms include *E. coli*, *S. aureus*, and *E. faecalis*, although several other organisms may be found. Infection can occur at any time during the course of the disease, but most commonly occurs 2–4 weeks after presentation.

35. Ans. A

Limulus amebocyte lysate test was a simple and cost-effective means to screen CSF for gram-negative agents of meningitis.

36. Ans. C

Pneumonia contributes to between 750,000 and 1.2 million neonatal deaths and an unknown number of stillbirths each year worldwide. The etiology depends on the time of onset. Gram-negative bacilli predominate in the first week of life, and gram-positive bacteria after that.

37. **Ans. D**

    Superinfections are frequent in patients with documented invasive aspergillosis, and clinicians must be on the alert to detect these. In one series, nearly half of patients with documented aspergillosis had coinfections. In some cases, the other infection was present concomitantly with the aspergillosis diagnosis, underscoring the importance of bronchoscopic evaluation at the outset, even if the serum galactomannan is positive. Bacterial coinfections are most frequent, as with our patient, with three-fourths due to gram-negative rods. Viral copathogens are next in frequency with CMV and respiratory viruses being the most common. A small percentage may become coinfected by other fungi or mycobacteria.

38. **Ans. D**

    A bacterial infection is the most common cause of epiglottitis. Bacteria can enter your body when you breathe it in. It can then infect your epiglottis. The most common strain of bacteria that causes this condition is *H. influenzae* type b, also known as Hib.

39. **Ans. D**

    Legionella pneumophila usually causes sporadic cases of pneumonia but does occur in outbreaks, classically when an air-conditioning system's water supply becomes contaminated, particularly if this occurs in a public or highly populated building. *L. pneumophila* tends to affect males twice as often as females and has a preponderance for smokers. Point-source outbreaks occur when a group of people is exposed to the organism in aerosols from contaminated cooling systems or air-conditioning. Immunocompromised patients are particularly vulnerable to developing *Legionella* pneumonia.

40. **Ans. D**

    Kingella kingae is a species of gram-negative facultative anaerobic β-hemolytic coccobacilli. First isolated in 1960 by Elizabeth O King, it was not recognized as a significant cause of infection in young children until the 1990s, when culture techniques had improved enough for it to be recognized. *K. kingae* is a common etiology of pediatric bacteremia and the leading agent of osteomyelitis and septic arthritis in children aged 6–36 months. This gram-negative bacterium is carried asymptomatically in the oropharynx and disseminates by close interpersonal contact. The colonized epithelium is the source of bloodstream invasion and dissemination to distant sites, and certain clones show significant association with bacteremia, osteoarthritis, or endocarditis.

    Ref:
    1. Kasper DL, Fauci AS, Hauser SL, Longo DL, Fauci A, Loscalzo J. Harrison's Principles and Practice of Medicine, 19th edition. New York, United States: McGraw Hill Education; 2015

CHAPTER 3

Emerging Fungal Infections in Non-neutropenic Patients

Ketan Kargirwar, Mayur Patel, Darshana Rathod, Mehul Shah, Vivek Kumar

1. **Aspergillosis is recognized in tissue by the presence of:**
   A. Pseudohyphae
   B. Metachromatic granules
   C. Dichotomous and septate hyphae
   D. Budding cells

2. **Which of the following diseases show halo sign in radiological imaging?**

   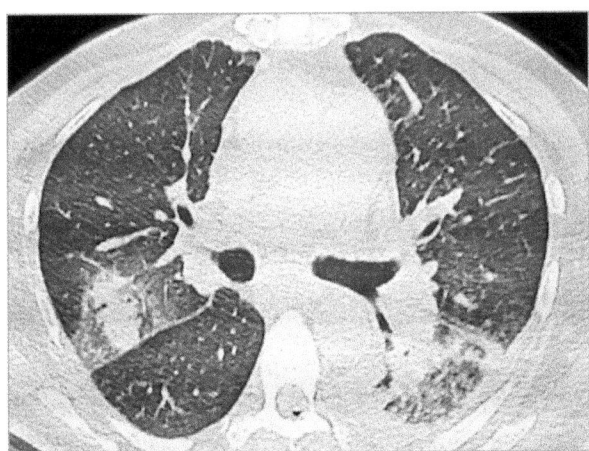

   A. Pulmonary zygomycosis
   B. Invasive pulmonary aspergillosis (IPA)
   C. Chronic aspergillosis (colonizing aspergillosis)
   D. Rhino cerebral zygomycosis

3. **Which of the following is used for primary treatment of invasive aspergillosis?**
   A. Caspofungin
   B. Micafungin
   C. Fluconazole
   D. Voriconazole

4. A 73-year-old male, hypertensive, chronic obstructive pulmonary disease (COPD) on steroids, underwent off-pump coronary artery bypass grafting (CABG). During the first 48 hours patient had hypotension requiring vasopressor support. Perioperative myocardial infarction was ruled out. Antibiotics (meropenem + teicoplanin) were escalated and antifungal (caspofungin) was added empirically. All cultures and serum procalcitonin were negative. CT chest revealed bilateral infiltrates. Since endotracheal (ET) cultures were negative and cause of sepsis could not be ascertained, bronchoalveolar lavage (BAL) was done. BAL was positive for galactomannan (GM) assay suggestive of *Aspergillus fumigatus* and voriconazole was added. In spite of all aggressive measures patient remained in profound shock and eventually died.
   Regarding aspergillosis, the rate of mortality is high in patients suffering from:
   A. IPA
   B. Allergic bronchopulmonary aspergillosis
   C. Chronic pulmonary aspergillosis
   D. *Aspergillus* sinusitis

5. A 42-year-old man having acquired immunodeficiency syndrome (AIDS) presents to his physician with progressively increasing dyspnea over the past 3 weeks. He also complains of a dry, painful cough, fatigue, and low-grade fever. CD4+ cell count 180 per mm^3. A chest X-ray reveals bilateral symmetrical interstitial and alveolar infiltration. **Which of the following agents is the most likely cause of the above?**

   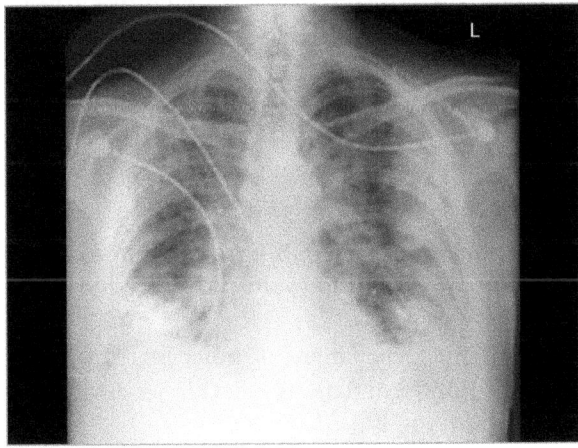

   A. *Cryptosporidium parvum*
   B. *Toxoplasma gondii*
   C. *Pneumocystis jirovecii* pneumonia (PJP)
   D. *Histoplasma capsulatum*
   E. *Cryptococcus neoformans*

6. A 68-year-old male, with history of diabetes mellitus, ischemic heart disease, and diabetic nephropathy was admitted with acute onset breathlessness, cough with expectoration, and fever for 3 days. Chest X-ray revealed right lower zone pneumonia. Laboratories revealed leukocytosis. He was intubated in view of acute respiratory failure. He was treated with intravenous (IV) antibiotics and showed signs of recovery. He was extubated after 5 days from admission. ET culture on fifth day revealed *Candida albicans* with colony count 10^4. What are the options of treatment?
   A. Oral fluconazole
   B. Oral voriconazole
   C. Caspofungin
   D. No addition of antifungals

7. A 55-year-old female following renal transplantation was found to have an invasive fungal infection (IFI) with *Candida glabrata*. Which antifungal is best suited to treat this infection?
   A. Voriconazole
   B. Amphotericin B
   C. Fluconazole
   D. Meropenem
   E. Caspofungin

8. A 35-year-old woman is receiving total parenteral nutrition (TPN) therapy post-Hartmann procedure for carcinoma colon. She is being admitted to the surgical ICU and clinically appears septic. The team wishes to cover likely fungal pathogens in addition to broad spectrum antibiotics and asks your advice. Which one of the following drugs is best to recommend for this patient's empiric antifungal therapy?
   A. Caspofungin
   B. Amphotericin B
   C. Amphotericin B lipid complex
   D. Fluconazole

9. Lipid amphotericin B formulation has advantage over traditional amphotericin B deoxycholate, which is:
   A. Lipid formulations are much less expensive
   B. Lipid formulations have higher clinical efficacy with candidiasis infections
   C. Lipid formulations are better suited to treat urinary tract fungal infections
   D. Lipid formulations are less renal toxic

10. A 36-year-old man after allogeneic hematopoietic stem cell transplant was admitted in transplant ICU on high-flow oxygen and receiving voriconazole 4 mg/kg intravenously twice daily for invasive *Aspergillus* infection. His oxygenation has not been improving, so the infectious disease specialist ordered a voriconazole levels. On day 5 of therapy, voriconazole trough concentration is 1.2 mg/L. The ICU team asks for recommendations on how to interpret this concentration and adjust his voriconazole dose. At this time the patient's clinical condition has not improved and he is close to needing invasive ventilation due to worsening hypoxia. He is not displaying any signs of voriconazole toxicity. What would be the best intervention?
    A. Change IV voriconazole to IV amphotericin B, watch and for clinical response
    B. Increase the dose of voriconazole 4 mg/kg to 6 mg/kg and watch for toxicity
    C. Look for any other cause of worsening respiratory condition
    D. Wait and watch, and repeat the voriconazole level after 7 days of therapy

11. Which one of the following would be best indicator to predict efficacy of voriconazole in a patient being treated for invasive aspergillosis?
    A. Voriconazole peak concentrations
    B. Voriconazole trough concentrations
    C. GM
    D. Voriconazole minimum inhibitory concentration (MIC)

12. A 67-year-old man with a history of COPD, hypertension, and chronic renal failure on hemodialysis with right subclavian Permcath catheter is admitted to the ICU with sepsis. His treatment includes broad-spectrum antibiotics, corticosteroids, and inhaled β2 stimulants. Due to a severe ileus and gastric intolerance, TPN is commenced. The patient's temperature normalizes after the third day in ICU and his oxygenation improves. However, on the ninth day in ICU he develops fever with an increase in the peripheral leukocyte count. Blood and sputum cultures are done. *C. krusei* is isolated from a single peripheral blood culture. Which of the following is the most appropriate next step in the management of this patient?
    A. Remove, culture, and replace Permcath catheter
    B. Remove, culture, and replace Permcath catheter and begin IV fluconazole
    C. Remove, culture, and replace Permcath catheter and begin IV amphotericin B
    D. Repeat the blood and urine cultures and observe the patient

13. All the statements regarding mechanism of actions of antifungal agents are true, *except*:
    A. Amphotericin B binds irreversibly to sterol component, ergosterol of cell membrane causing fungal cell death
    B. Fluconazole inhibits 14α-demethylase
    C. Caspofungin inhibits catalytic subunit of beta-(1,3)-D-glucan synthase
    D. Fluconazole is active against *C. krusei*

14. A 55-year-old with type 2 diabetes mellitus and invasive zygomycosis has been admitted in ICU with severe sepsis due to necrotizing soft-tissue infection. Initial treatment should include all of the following, *except*:
    A. Surgical debridement
    B. Vasopressor support and resuscitation with fluids
    C. Amphotericin B or equivalent liposomal formulation
    D. An echinocandin as monotherapy
    E. Broad spectrum antibiotics

15. A 65-year-old man with a history of hypertension, diabetes, COPD, and benign prostatic hyperplasia is postoperative day 3 after right hepatectomy and cholecystectomy complicated by significant blood loss. He was extubated today and weaned off vasopressors this morning. He is afebrile. On the morning round the ICU registrar notes that the urine in the indwelling catheter collection bag is cloudy. Urinalysis demonstrates budding yeasts, and urine culture demonstrates *Candida* species. Which of the following is the most appropriate next step?
    A. Start fluconazole
    B. Obtain blood cultures and drain cultures
    C. Obtain an ophthalmologic examination
    D. Replace the indwelling urinary catheter

16. A 55 years human immunodeficiency virus (HIV) positive male admitted with altered sensorium and seizures. On evaluation, cerebrospinal fluid (CSF) studies were positive for cryptococcal meningitis. Which antifungal has excellent CSF penetration for treatment of cryptococcal meningitis?
    A. Caspofungin
    B. Fluconazole
    C. Itraconazole
    D. Ketoconazole

17. A 70-year-old, HIV positive male patient, on regular antiretroviral treatment after a recent travel to Africa, presents with persistent headache since a month, with low-grade fever and cough. He has skin lesions like Erythema multiforme with patch in the lung for which he was treated with broad-spectrum antibiotic and fluconazole. However, because of persistent headache and fever, CSF study was done which revealed eosinophilia, lymphocytosis, and mildly low glucose. Sputum examination revealed fungi elements. Most likely diagnosis is?
    A. Blastomycosis
    B. *Cryptococcus*
    C. Coccidioidomycosis (CM)
    D. Aspergillosis

18. A 45-year-old banker presents with worsening weakness in all four limbs and altered sensorium. He was diagnosed to have acute demyelinating encephalomyelitis disease for which he was treated with steroids, immunosuppressant therapy, and subsequently plasmapheresis. During the course of his illness, he had persistent fever for which he was treated with broad spectrum antibiotics and fluconazole. The blood culture after 7 days revealed *Candida auris*. Which of the following regimen is appropriate for the treatment of *C. auris*?
    A. Continue fluconazole
    B. Combination of echinocandins and azoles
    C. Combination of echinocandin and liposomal amphotericin B
    D. Posaconazole

19. A 68-year-old man undergoes total colectomy due to severe pseudomembranous colitis. He was started postoperatively on oral vancomycin, IV metronidazole and piperacillin/tazobactam. Postoperatively, he develops fever, tachycardia, and leukocytosis. His urine culture and central with peripheral blood cultures are done. Other laboratory findings include hemoglobin 9.7 g/dL and serum creatinine 1.8 mg/dL. White blood cell count 18,000/µL. Also his drain culture was send within 24 hours postoperatively which grew *C. albicans* while other cultures were negative. What is the significance of *Candida* growth from an intra-abdominal drain sample?
    A. It is a marker of IC if sample is within 24 hours of drain insertion
    B. It is a marker of drain colonization
    C. It is marker of multidrug resistant bacterial colonization
    D. It warrants antifungal therapy

20. A 49-year-old woman who has metastatic breast cancer is admitted for shortness of breath, fever,

and chills. She is undergoing chemotherapy through a tunneled CVC; her last chemo cycle was 5 days ago. Blood cultures are drawn and she is started empirically on IV imipenem, teicoplanin, and fluconazole. Her vital signs showed temperature 39.4°C (102.9°F), heart rate 121 beats/min, blood pressure 78/42 mm Hg, and respiratory rate 30 breaths/min. Chest radiography reveals pulmonary infiltrates. CVC line and arterial line was inserted. Which of the following have the strongest association with nonalbicans *Candida* infection?

A. CVC use
B. Treatment with aminopenicillins, carbapenems, and glycopeptides
C. Chemotherapy
D. Previous surgery

21. A 50-year-old woman who has received chemotherapy preoperatively undergoes cytoreductive surgery for metastatic carcinoma of ovaries with peritoneal metastasis. She was started postoperatively on IV metronidazole, cefoperazone/sulbactam, and TPN. On day 5, she develops new onset fever, tachycardia, and leukocytosis and her antibiotics were escalated to meropenem. Her urine culture, drain, and central with peripheral blood cultures are done. Other laboratory findings include hemoglobin 9.0 g/dL, serum creatinine 1.2 mg/dL, and white blood cell count to 16,000/μL. What would have been the ideal time to start antifungal therapy in this patient?

A. At time of presentation to hospital
B. Immediately postoperatively
C. At time of postoperative deterioration
D. After 48 hours of revised antibiotic therapy following postoperative deterioration
E. After receiving a positive tissue culture

22. Which one of the following is not a risk factor for intra-abdominal fungal infections?

A. Recent abdominal surgery
B. Presence of CVC
C. Use of TPN
D. Anastomotic leaks
E. Age

23. A 70-year-old male, a known case of type 2 diabetes mellitus presented to the hospital with history of periumbilical pain of 5 days duration worsening after meals. Clinical examination and laboratories were unremarkable. Abdominal arterial Doppler showed a thrombus in proximal superior mesenteric artery. Contrast-enhanced computed tomography (CECT) abdomen with oral contrast showed bowel wall thickening with thrombus in proximal superior mesenteric artery.

He was managed on broad-spectrum antibiotics (beta-lactam + beta-lactamase inhibitor) and unfractionated heparin. He underwent an exploratory laparotomy which revealed an ischemic bowel segment requiring resection with end-to-end anastomosis. Postoperatively he was started on TPN. He developed acute kidney injury requiring continuous renal replacement therapy (CRRT). Blood, urine, and tracheal cultures were sent and antibiotic cover was escalated to include carbapenems with glycopeptides. There was no significant improvement after 48 hours of antibiotic cover. Intraoperative tissue cultures revealed growth of *C. glabrata*. Blood culture sent postoperatively also grew *C. glabrata*. The patient was started on IV anidulafungin. He showed a gradual improvement over the next 10 days. What is the appropriate management of intra-abdominal *Candida* infection?

A. Source control
B. Antifungal
C. Source control + antifungal × 2 weeks
D. Source control + antifungal × 4 weeks
E. Source control + antifungal × 2 weeks after last negative fungal culture

24. A 72-year-old female patient with diabetes mellitus and chronic backache presented with headache, word finding difficulty, mild fevers, nausea, and vomiting. She had undergone multiple procedure including epidural steroid injections in the past for chronic backache. She had been worked up in another institute with meningeal enhancement on the neuroimaging for which a CSF done was suggestive of lymphocytic cytology, low glucose, and elevated proteins. CSF culture and PCR were negative; however, she improved on voriconazole. Similar reports of other patients with postepidural steroids were reported likely secondary to drug contamination with *Exserohilum rostratum*, a dematiaceous (pigmented) mold. How does one evaluate the progress of the clearance of these fungi in CSF?

A. Serial CFS lactate
B. Serial CSF β-glucan
C. Serial CSF fungal culture
D. Serial CSF proteins

25. A 42-year-old lady, postlung transplant patient on tacrolimus, mycophenolate mofetil, and prednisolone was admitted with respiratory failure requiring intubation and ventilation. BAL revealed

acute-angle branching hyphae. She was started on IV voriconazole, doses of which of her medication should be reduced?

A. Mycophenolate mofetil
B. Voriconazole
C. Tacrolimus
D. Prednisolone

26. Invasive candidiasis is a spectrum of syndromes and includes the following:
    A. BSI or candidemia
    B. Deep-seated *Candida* infections in the presence of BSI
    C. Deep-seated infections without BSI
    D. All of the above
    E. Both A and B

27. A 58-year-old farmer with bronchiectasis develops headache, malaise, fever, and chronic fatigue symptoms. His chest X-ray revealed bilateral pulmonary nodules. He was suspected to have histoplasmosis. List the test that can be done for immediate diagnosis of the same?
    A. PCR
    B. Culture
    C. Microscopy
    D. Antigen detection

28. Which antifungal drug is associated with "shake and bake" adverse effects?
    A. Griseofulvin
    B. Caspofungin
    C. Amphotericin B
    D. Micafungin

29. A 60-year-old male farmer with COPD had recently come back from vacation at east coast of United States, presented with fever with chills, chest pain, dry cough, shortness of breath, and muscle aches. Laboratories were unremarkable including respiratory BioFire. X-ray chest revealed bilateral pulmonary infiltrates. He was intubated in view of acute respiratory failure. High-resolution computed tomography (HRCT) chest revealed miliary pulmonary infiltration, cavitation formation, and significant hilar lymph node as shown in the below CT image. He was treated with broad spectrum antibiotics. ET aspirate culture was negative, but BAL culture was positive for *H. capsulatum*.

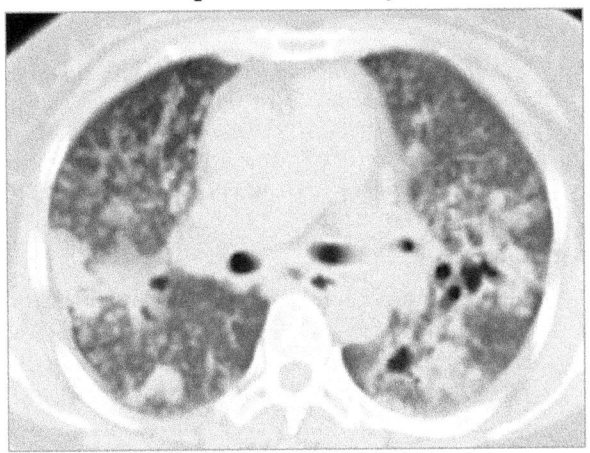

The initial treatment recommendation for acute severe pulmonary manifestations of histoplasmosis in adults is:

A. Amphotericin B
B. Itraconazole
C. Amphotericin B+ steroids for 1-2 weeks followed by itraconazole
D. Voriconazole

30. All the following statements are true regarding *Candida auris*, except:
    A. *C. auris* spreads easily in healthcare setting causing nosocomial outbreak
    B. Fluconazole is sensitive against *C. auris*
    C. Mutation in *ERG11* gene is responsible for drug resistance in *C. auris*
    D. Echinocandins are used as front-line therapy for infection

ANSWERS WITH EXPLANATIONS

1. **Ans. C**
   Aspergillosis is caused by a fungus (mold) *Aspergillus fumigatus*. In infected tissues, it appears as septate hyphae with acute angle branching. In tissues *Candida* appear as mats of yeasts (budding yeast cells often present) intermingled with pseudohyphae (also referred to as filaments). Metachromatic granules (also known as volutin granules) are intracytoplasmic storage form of inorganic polyphosphate present in *Corynebacterium diphtheriae*.

   Ref:
   1. Segal BH. Aspergillosis. N Engl J Med. 2009;360:1870-84.
   2. Alexopoulos CJ, Mims CW. Introductory Mycology, 3rd edition. New York: Wiley; 1979.

2. **Ans. B**
   Classical CT findings of angioinvasive aspergillosis include macronodule(s) >1 cm, which may be surrounded by a halo of ground-glass attenuation, pleural based wedge-shaped areas of consolidation, alveolar consolidations, masses especially in solid

organ transplant (SOT) recipients, cavity or air-crescent sign (delayed finding), ground glass opacities, and pleural effusion. It should be noted that the halo sign is mostly found in neutropenic patients, while relevant findings of non-neutropenic patients are nonspecific.
Ref:
1. Desoubeaux G, Bailly E, Chandenier J. Diagnosis of invasive pulmonary aspergillosis: updates and recommendations. Med Mal Infect. 2014;44:89-101.
2. Bruno C, Minniti S, Vassanelli A, Pozzi-Mucelli R. Comparison of CT features of Aspergillus and bacterial pneumonia in severely neutropenic patients. J Thorac Imag. 2007;22:160-5.

3. **Ans. D**
Although amphotericin B deoxycholate had historically been the "gold standard" for the treatment of invasive aspergillosis, most seasoned clinicians and the most recent Infectious Diseases Society of America (IDSA) guidelines recommend voriconazole as the primary treatment option.
Ref:
1. Limper AH, Knox KS, Sarosi GA, Ampel NM, Bennett JE, Catanzaro A, et al. An official American Thoracic Society statement: Treatment of Fungal Infections in Adult Pulmonary and Critical Care patients. Am J Respir Crit Care Med. 2011;183:96-128.
2. Desoubeaux G, Bailly E, Chandenier J. Diagnosis of invasive pulmonary aspergillosis: updates and recommendations. Med Mal Infect. 2014;44:89-101.

4. **Ans. A**
Mortality rates in IPA range from 40 to 90% in high-risk populations and are dependent on factors such as host immune status, the site of infection, and the treatment regimen applied. Intensive care unit (ICU) patients colonized with *Aspergillus* also tend to do poorly, because almost half of these patients have numerous sources of *Aspergillus* species in the ICU. Aerosolized spores may become a potential source of infection through improperly cleaned ventilation systems, water systems, or even computer consoles. The lungs and sinuses are implicated in 90% of these cases as colonization source. GM detection in fluids (especially BAL) is more sensitive than culture for diagnosis of IPA. It is estimated that 4% of nonhematological ICU patients develop IPA.
Ref:
1. Sun K-S, Tsai C-F, Chen SC-C, Huang W-C. Clinical outcome and prognostic factors associated with invasive pulmonary aspergillosis: an 11-year follow-up report from Taiwan. PLoS One. 2017;12(10):e0186422.
2. Meersseman W, Lagrou K, Maertens J, Wilmer A, Hermans G, Vanderschueren S, et al. Galactomannan in bronchoalveolar lavage fluid: a tool for diagnosing aspergillosis in intensive care unit patients. Am J Respir Crit Care Med. 2008;177:27-34.
3. Lin SJ, Schranz J, Teutsch SM. Aspergillosis case-fatality rate: systematic review of the literature. Clin Infect Dis. 2001;32:358-66.

5. **Ans. C**
The classic presentation of PJP includes nonproductive cough, shortness of breath, fever, and bilateral interstitial infiltrates with or without hypoxemia. The radiological features suggestive of PJP are small pneumatoceles, subpleural blebs, fine reticular interstitial changes predominantly perihilar in distribution, and ground glass pattern. Also, pneumothorax is seen in some cases. There are times when a definitive diagnosis cannot be made due to a low burden of organisms and/or the inability to obtain the necessary specimen. Clinical and radiographic findings can be highly suggestive of a diagnosis of PJP in patients with risk factors for PJP. The definitive diagnosis of PJP requires identification of the organism either by tinctorial (dye-based) staining, fluorescent antibody staining, or polymerase chain reaction (PCR)-based assays of respiratory specimen. Bronchoscopy with BAL should be performed. Lung biopsy with tissue stains and PCR has excellent sensitivity.
Ref:
1. Thomas CF Jr, Limper AH. Pneumocystis pneumonia. N Engl J Med. 2004;350:2487-98.
2. Thomas CF Jr, Limper AH. Current insights into the biology and pathogenesis of Pneumocystis pneumonia. Nat Rev Microbiol. 2007;5:298-308.

6. **Ans. D**
Candida species are normally found in the mouth, throat, vagina, and gastrointestinal tract. By comparison, isolation of *C. albicans* and other *Candida* species from ET aspirates is common, but usually represents colonization of the airways, rather than pneumonia in immunocompetent patients, and rarely requires treatment with antifungal therapy. Moreover, cultures from nonsterile sites, although not useful for establishing a diagnosis, may be useful for initiating antifungal therapy in patients with fever that is unresponsive to broad-spectrum antimicrobials.
Ref:
1. Ferreira D, Grenouillet F, Blasco G, Samain E, Hénon T, et al. Outcomes associated with routine systemic antifungal therapy in critically ill patients with Candida colonization. Int Care Med. 2015;41:1077-88.
2. American Thoracic Society; Infectious Diseases Society of America. Guidelines for the management of adults with hospital-acquired, ventilator-associated, and healthcare-associated pneumonia. Am J Respir Crit Care Med. 2005;171:388-416.

7. **Ans. E**
The risk of IFI is increases in patients after a SOT and is associated with decreased survival. *Candida* and *Aspergillus* species are the most common organisms, with nonalbicans species increasing in frequency. Historically amphotericin B was the antifungal of choice, but it is associated with significant liver and renal toxicity. Newer liposomal formulations have decreased these risks. However, because of

their clinical efficacy, a broad spectrum of activity, and favorable side effect profile, echinocandins are becoming the antifungal of choice in many patient populations.

Echinocandins include caspofungin, micafungin, and anidulafungin. Comparisons of caspofungin to amphotericin B have shown equivalent efficacy and a more favorable side effect profile of the former. In SOT recipients, caspofungin was found to be effective as both a first and second line treatment, with success in 87% of candidal and 74% of *Aspergillus* infections.

In vitro studies have found efficacy against non-albicans species such as *Candida glabrata*, *C. krusei*, *C. parapsilosis*, and *C. tropicalis*, as well as fluconazole-resistant albicans isolates. The echinocandins also have the benefit of fewer drug-drug interactions in transplant patients. Specifically, unlike the azoles, they are not inhibitors of cytochrome P450 and are unlikely to alter pharmacodynamics of the calcineurin inhibitors used for immunosuppression.

In general, guidelines for fungal treatment and prophylaxis recommend posaconazole for prophylaxis in bone marrow transplant patients, caspofungin in confirmed or suspected candidal invasive fungal infection in neutropenic and non-neutropenic patients and for febrile neutropenia, and voriconazole in invasive aspergillosis. Liposomal preparation of amphotericin B should be considered a second-line agent for IFI.

Ref:
1. Farmakiotis D, Kontoyiannis DP. Emerging issues with diagnosis and management of fungal infections in solid organ transplant recipients. Am J Transplant. 2015;15:1141-7.
2. Winkler M, Pratschke J, Schulz U, Zheng S, Zhang M, Li W, et al. Caspofungin for post solid organ transplant invasive fungal disease: results of a retrospective observational study. Transpl Infect Dis. 2010;12:230-7.

8. **Ans. D**

Invasive candidiasis (IC) has a known mortality of >50%. Risk factors include neutropenia, central venous catheters (CVCs), known colonization, hemodialysis, parenteral nutrition, broad-spectrum antibiotic exposure, trauma, and recent abdominal surgery. Meta-analyses have shown that prophylaxis with fluconazole in non-neutropenic critically ill patients with risk factors for candidiasis reduces IFIs and improves mortality.

Ref:
1. Koehler P, Cornely OA. Contemporary strategies in the prevention and management of fungal infections. Infect Dis Clin North Am. 2016;30:265-75.
2. Cortegiani A, Russotto V, Maggiore A, Attanasio M, Naro AR, Raineri SM, et al. Antifungal agents for preventing fungal infections in non-neutropenic critically ill patients. Cochrane Database Syst Rev. 2018;16:CD004920.
3. Playford GE, Webster EC, Sorrell TC, Craig JC. Antifungal agents for preventing fungal infections in non-neutropenic critically ill and surgical patients: systematic review and meta-analysis of randomized clinical trials. J Antimicr Chem. 2006;57:628-63.

9. **Ans. D**

Amphotericin B is a member of the polyene antibiotic family along with nystatin and natamycin. Polyene antibiotics bind to ergosterol, the fungal version of cholesterol, in the fungal cell membrane. As a result of this binding, fungal cell membrane permeability increases and the cell dies. Amphotericin B comes in two broad types: lipid based and traditional. There are three distinct lipid formulae: liposomal amphotericin B, amphotericin B lipid complex, and amphotericin B cholesteryl sulfate complex.

The most important advantage of the lipid formulations over amphotericin B deoxycholate is less renal toxicity. Amphotericin B deoxycholate has been found to cause acute kidney injury in up to 50% of patients. Lipid formulations, in general, are more expensive. There are no comparative studies to support lipid amphotericin B for *Candida* infections with regards to clinical efficacy. Amphotericin B deoxycholate is metabolized in the liver and eliminated from the body via excretion in the urine. Lipid formulations undergo less renal elimination than nonlipid amphotericin and therefore are not ideal for treating urinary fungal infections.

Ref:
1. Walsh TJ, Finberg RW, Arndt C, Hiemenz J, Schwartz C, Bodensteiner D, et al. Liposomal amphotericin B for empirical therapy in patients with persistent fever and neutropenia. National Institute of Allergy and Infectious Diseases Mycoses Study Group. N Engl J Med. 1999;340:764-71.
2. Ostrosky-Zeichner L, Marr KA, Rex JH, Cohen SH. Amphotericin B: Time for a new "gold standard". Clin Infect Dis. 2003;37:415-25.
3. Adler-Moore JP, Proffitt RT. Amphotericin B lipid preparations: what are the differences? Clin Microb Infect. 2008;14:25-36.

10. **Ans. B**

The British Society for Medical Mycology recommends that a voriconazole trough concentration more than 1 mg/L taken within 7 days of treatment is an adequate serum concentration for treatment of IFIs. Therefore, this level taken on day 5 of therapy should be representative of a therapeutic steady state concentration.

However, because of the nonlinear pharmacokinetics and lack of data strongly correlating drug concentration and clinical outcome, it is important to interpret this level also based on the clinical picture of the patient. The reasons for this patient to have concentrations on the lower side of therapeutic levels, include a genetic polymorphism of CYP2C19 and his history of hematopoietic stem cell transplant (this population tends to have lower concentrations than healthy volunteers). There is evidence to suggest that trough concentrations less than 2 mg/L may be associated with clinical failure in patients with invasive aspergillosis. Therefore, it would be reasonable to increase the dosage to 6 mg/kg IV twice daily and monitor for signs of toxicity. It would also be reasonable to repeat another trough concentration in 5–7 days because of the nonlinear kinetics. If the clinical picture worsens significantly, it may be time to consider alternate or combination therapy for this patient. Concentrations less than 2 mg/L may be associated with clinical failure in patients with invasive aspergillosis.

Ref:
1. Andes D, Pascual A, Marchetti O. Antifungal therapeutic drug monitoring: established and emerging indications. Antimicrob Agents Chemother. 2009;53:24-34.
2. Ashbee HR, Barnes RA, Johnson EM, Richardson MD, Gorton R, Hope WW. Therapeutic drug monitoring of antifungal agents: guidelines from the British Society of Medical Mycology. J Antimicrob Chemother 2014;69:1162-76.
3. Smith J. Voriconazole therapeutic drug monitoring. Antimicrob Agents Chemother. 2006;50:1570-2.

11. Ans. B

Voriconazole is a first-line agent for the treatment of invasive aspergillosis and IC caused by *Candida* species with reduced susceptibility to fluconazole.

Voriconazole exhibits classical Michaelis-Menten (nonlinear) pharmacokinetics in adults that are related to saturable clearance mechanisms. This has important implications for dosage adjustment because of unanticipated and unpredictable changes in drug level. Voriconazole has high oral bioavailability, with current estimates of—80–86% in children and adults, although estimates as low as 60% have recently been reported, hence therapeutic drug monitoring is especially important in this setting.

Voriconazole is metabolized via oxidative mechanisms. The predominant cytochrome P450 isoenzymes involved in this process are CYP3A4, CYP2C19, and CYP2C9. CYP2C19 exhibits a number of clinically relevant polymorphisms that have been associated with differing rates of enzyme activity and therefore clearance of voriconazole. Voriconazole toxicity may manifest as visual disturbances (photopsia), liver dysfunction, skin reactions, and neurotoxicity (confusion and visual hallucinations). Trough concentrations that are associated with greater probability of toxicity vary from study to study, and include a serum level of 4–6 mg/L. As per British mycology guideline active dosage adjustment should be done to keep serum trough concentrations <5.5 mg/L to prevents voriconazole-related toxicity.

Ref:
1. Johnson LB, Kauffman CA. Voriconazole: a new triazole antifungal agent. Clin Infect Dis. 2003;36:630-7.
2. Denning DW, Ribaud P, Milpied N, Caillot D, Herbrecht R, Thiel E, et al. Efficacy and safety of voriconazole in the treatment of acute invasive aspergillosis. Clin Infect Dis. 2002;34:563-71.
3. Ashbee HR. Therapeutic drug monitoring of antifungal agents: guidelines from the British Society of Medical Mycology. J Antimicrob. 2014;69:1162-76.

12. Ans. C

The risk factors for *Candida* intravascular infection include use of broad-spectrum antibiotics, TPN, and immunosuppressive therapy. Because a single positive blood culture is highly predictive of systemic *Candida* infection, it should never be considered a contaminant. The initial treatment of *Candida* infections includes removal of all possible foci of infection, including removal of intravascular lines. Candidemia may resolve spontaneously after removal of intravascular catheters. However, increasing evidence suggests that metastatic foci of infection may develop in some patients even after catheter removal and may manifest as endophthalmitis, endocarditis, arthritis, or meningitis. Therefore, all critically ill patients with candidemia should be regarded as having systemic infection and should be treated accordingly.

Fluconazole and amphotericin B demonstrate similar effectiveness in treating candidemia in patients without neutropenia and without major immunodeficiency. However, both in vitro and clinical data have demonstrated *C. krusei* to be intrinsically resistant to fluconazole.

Ref:
1. Rex JH, Bennett JE, Sugar AM, Pappas PG, van der Horst CM, Edwards JE, et al. A randomized trial comparing fluconazole with amphotericin B for the treatment of candidemia in patients without neutropenia. N Engl J Med. 1994;331:1325-30.
2. Rex JH, Pfaller MA, Barry AL, Webb CD. Antifungal susceptibility testing of isolates from a randomized, multicenter trial of fluconazole versus amphotericin B as treatment of nonneutropenic patients with candidemia. NIAID Mycoses Study Group and the Candidemia Study Group. Antimicrob Agents Chemother. 1995;39:40-4.
3. Pappas PG1, Kauffman CA, Andes D, Benjamin DK Jr, Calandra TF, Edwards JE Jr, et al. Clinical practice guidelines for the management of candidiasis: 2009 update by the Infectious Diseases Society of America. Clin Infect Dis. 2009;48:503-35.

13. Ans. D

The active ingredient of amphotericin B, acts by binding to the sterol component, ergosterol, of the cell membrane of susceptible fungi. It forms transmembrane channels leading to alterations in cell permeability through which monovalent ions (Na^+, K^+,

H⁺, and Cl⁻) leak out of the cell, resulting in cell death. While amphotericin B has a higher affinity for the ergosterol component of the fungal cell membrane, it can also bind to the cholesterol component of the mammalian cell, leading to cytotoxicity.

Ergosterol serves as a bioregulator of membrane fluidity and asymmetry and consequently of membrane integrity in fungal cells. Integrity of the cell membrane requires that inserted sterols lack C-4 methyl groups. Inhibition of 14α-demethylase leads to depletion of ergosterol and accumulation of sterol precursors, including 14α-methylated sterols (lanosterol, 4,14-dimethylzymosterol, and 24-methylenedihydrolanosterol), resulting in the formation of a plasma membrane with altered structure and function.

The echinocandins act as noncompetitive inhibitors of beta-(1,3)-D-glucan synthase, an essential component of the fungal cell wall that is not present in mammals. Inability of the organism to synthesize beta-(1,3)-D-glucan leads to osmotic instability and cell death.

Ref:
1. *Lewis RE. Current concepts in antifungal pharmacology. Mayo Clin Proc. 2011;86:805-17.*
2. *Hamilton-Miller JM. Chemistry and biology of the polyene macrolide antibiotics. Bacteriol Rev. 1973;37:166-96.*
3. *Wiederhold NP, Lewis RE. The echinocandin antifungals: an overview of the pharmacology, spectrum and clinical efficacy. Expert Opin Investig Drugs. 2003;12:1313-33.*

14. **Ans. D**

    When invasive zygomycosis has been demonstrated, amphotericin B or equivalent liposomal formulation should be initiated, along with surgical debridement and appropriate supportive care with fluids and vasopressors. The liposomal formulation allows higher dosing with less nephrotoxicity. Echinocandins have no in vitro activity against zygomycetes and should be avoided. Broad-spectrum antibiotics are started empirically and then tapered once the causative organism(s) is identified.

    Ref:
    1. *Spellberg B, Walsh TJ, Kontoyiannis DP, Edwards J Jr, Ibrahim AS. Recent advances in the management of mucormycosis: from bench to bedside. Clin Infect Dis. 2009;48:1743-51.*
    2. *Austin CL, Finley PJ, Mikkelson DR, Tibbs B. Mucormycosis: a rare fungal infection in tornado victims. J Burn Care Res. 2014;35:e164-71.*
    3. *Prasanna Kumar S, Ravikumar A, Somu L. Fungal necrotizing fasciitis of the head and neck in 3 patients with uncontrolled diabetes. Ear Nose Throat J. 2014;93:E18-21.*

15. **Ans. D**

    Candiduria is common in hospitalized patients and is usually benign. Risk factors for candiduria include immunosuppression, diabetes, use of broad-spectrum antibacterial agents, use of CVCs, malignancy, receipt of parenteral nutrition, urinary tract abnormalities and obstruction, recent urologic procedure, and presence of urinary tract devices.

    In this case, the candiduria represents contamination or colonization. Colonization is difficult to differentiate from infection based on urinalysis and culture alone, and the patient's clinical history must be considered. Patients who are symptomatic or who have concerning systemic signs or symptoms (flank pain, hypotension, etc.) should be treated with an antifungal and evaluated for disseminated infection with blood cultures. Usually observation without treatment is all that is required if no predisposing factor is identified. If there is a predisposing factor, then managing that factor, such as removing or replacing the urinary catheter, may be sufficient to eliminate the candiduria, without antifungal therapy. Patients with candidemia should have an ophthalmological examination, regardless of ocular symptoms, to evaluate for endophthalmitis and chorioretinitis.

    Ref:
    1. *Kauffman CA, Fisher JF, Sobel JD, Newman CA. Candida urinary tract infections—diagnosis. Clin Infect Dis. 2011;52:S452-6.*
    2. *Pappas PG, Kauffman CA, Andes D, Benjamin DK Jr, Calandra TF, Edwards JE Jr, et al. Clinical practice guidelines for the management of candidiasis: 2009 update by the Infectious Diseases Society of America. Clin Infect Dis. 2009;48:503-35.*
    3. *Au L, Guduru K, Lipscomb G, Kelly SP. Candida endophthalmitis: a critical diagnosis in the critically ill. Clin Ophthalmol. 2007;1:551-4.*

16. **Ans. B**

    The Fluconazole, the most widely used of the azoles, has excellent activity against *Cryptococcus* meningitis. It has a great bioavailability and can easily penetrate the CSF. Fluconazole can be used in central nervous system (CNS) infection including those caused by *Cryptococcus* species. IDSA and World Health Organization (WHO) guidelines recommend high-dose fluconazole monotherapy at 1,200 mg/day for 10–12 weeks, if amphotericin B and flucytosine are not available.

    Ref:
    1. *Abassi M, Boulware DR, Rhein J. Cryptococcal meningitis: diagnosis and management update. Curr Trop Med Rep. 2015;1:90-9.*
    2. *Menichetti F, Fiorio M, Tosti A, Gatti G, Bruna Pasticci M, Miletich F, et al. High-dose fluconazole therapy for cryptococcal meningitis in patients with AIDS. Clin Infect Dis. 1996;22:838-40.*
    3. *World Health Organization (2011). Rapid advice: Diagnosis, prevention and management of cryptococcal disease in HIV-infected adults, adolescents and children. [online] Available from http://www.who.*

int/hiv/pub/cryptococcal_disease2011 [Last accessed February 2020].
4. Perfect JR, Dismukes WE, Dromer F, Goldman DL, Graybill JR, Hamill RJ, et al. Clinical practice guidelines for the management of cryptococcal disease: 2010 update by the Infectious Diseases Society of America. Clin Infect Dis. 2010;50:291-322.

17. Ans. C

The second most common cause of CNS fungal infections is *Coccidioides immitis*. It is a dimorphic organism. In nature, it is a mold and inhalation of the arthroconidia may result in asymptomatic infection, limited infection, or disseminated disease. Involvement of the meninges is considered disseminated disease. There may be meningeal involvement alone or with pulmonary, cutaneous, and osseous findings. Disseminated disease is commonly seen in immunosuppressed states such as HIV, organ transplant, chronic corticosteroid use, pregnancy, and the use of α-tumor necrosis factor (α-TNF) antagonists.

The key to diagnosing CM is suspicion. The travel history is extremely important for visitation or residence in the endemic areas. The CSF parameters are much the same as those for cryptococcal meningitis; however, coccidioidal meningitis may have a number of eosinophils in the CSF.

Tests available for the diagnosis of CM are: Enzyme-immunoassay methods are very sensitive and commonly used. The immunodiffusion (ID) assay detects immunoglobulin M (IgM) and is positive early in the infection. But it is the complement fixation (CF) IgG antibody testing of the CSF that is time honored in the diagnosing of meningitis. CSF titers are also followed during treatment to measure response. In some areas, PCR may be available if *Coccidioides* is present in other organ systems, it may be diagnosed by microscopic examination of tissue samples or pus. If the disease is diagnosed by microscopy and/or serology, then culture should not be performed.
Ref:
1. Galgiani JN, Ampel NM, Blair JE, Catanzaro A, Johnson RH, Stevens DA, et al. Coccidioidomycosis. Infect Dis. 2005;41:1217-23.
2. Pappagianis D, Zimmer BL. Serology of coccidioidomycosis. Microbiol Rev. 1990;3:247-68.
3. Vucicevic D, Blair JE, Binnicker MJ, McCullough AE, Kusne S, Vikram HR, et al. The utility of Coccidioides polymerase chain reaction testing in the clinical setting. Mycopathologia. 2010;170:345-51.

18. Ans. C

The recommended initial therapy for clinically relevant infections with *C. auris* in adults is an echinocandin at standard dosing, despite its multidrug-resistant nature. The most *C. auris* isolates to date have been susceptible to echinocandins. Patients should be monitored closely for resolution of infection given that resistance to echinocandins has been documented and because resistance has emerged on serial isolates from a single patient after exposure to the drug. Adding liposomal amphotericin B (5 mg/kg daily) could be considered if the patient is clinically unresponsive to echinocandin treatment or has candidemia for >5 days.
Ref:
1. Tsay S, Kallen A, Jackson BR, Chiller TM, Vallabhaneni S. Approach to the investigation and management of patients with Candida auris, an emerging multidrug-resistant yeast. Clin Infect Dis. 2018;66:306-11.

19. Ans. A

A growth of *Candida* from an intra-abdominal drain could represent true infection, drain colonization, and sample contamination. The predictive value for a true *Candida* infection is maximum with growth from a normally sterile intra-abdominal specimen taken intraoperatively or an intra-abdominal drain in place for less than 24 hours. Growth from swabs taken from superficial wounds and from intra-abdominal catheters that have been in place for more than 24 hours lack predictive value and should not be sampled.
Ref:
1. Pappas PG, Kauffman CA, Andes DR, Clancy CJ, Marr KA, Ostrosky-Zeichner L, et al. Clinical Practice Guideline for the Management of Candidiasis: 2016 Update by the Infectious Diseases Society of America. Clin Infect Dis. 2016;62:e1-50.

20. Ans. A

The CVC use, previous use of fluconazole, treatment with aminopenicillins, carbapenems and glycopeptides, chemotherapy, previous surgery, and neutropenia, are all risk factors for nonalbicans *Candida* bloodstream infections (BSIs). However, in multiple logistic regression analysis only CVC and previous use of fluconazole are statistically significant.
Ref:
1. Chow JK, Golan Y, Ruthazer R, Karchmer AW, Carmeli Y, Lichtenberg D, et al. Factors associated with candidemia caused by non-albicans Candida species versus Candida albicans in the intensive care unit. Clin Infect Dis. 2008;46:1206-13.

21. Ans. B

The presence of risk factors for fungal infection warrants initiation of antifungal therapy at the time of suspicion of infection. A prophylactic approach is recommended for patients with risk factors for IC and also high risk for candida infection (high risk ≥5%). There is a significant difference in number needed to treat (9 for high risk and 188 for low risk) when prophylactic antifungal therapy is used. Prophylactic therapy is associated with a small mortality benefit. Empiric antifungal therapy should be considered for patients with clinical evidence of intra-abdominal infection and significant risk factors. This patient has high risk for fungal infections. She is an ideal

candidate for prophylactic antifungal therapy to be started in immediate postoperative period. Also, there are no well-validated rapid diagnostic tests for IC. The sensitivity and specificity of serum beta-D-glucan for IC is 75–80% and 80%, respectively. Blood cultures are usually negative. Hence, definitive antibiotic therapy in high-risk cases invariably results in delayed therapy and poor outcomes.
Ref:
1. Pappas PG, Kauffman CA, Andes DR, Clancy CJ, Marr KA, Ostrosky-Zeichner L, et al. Clinical Practice Guideline for the Management of Candidiasis: 2016 Update by the Infectious Diseases Society of America. Clin Infect Dis. 2016;62:e1-50.

22. **Ans. E**
Recent gastrointestinal surgery, presence of a CVC, use of TPN, anastomotic leaks, recurrent gastroduodenal perforation, and necrotizing pancreatitis are risk factors for IC. The presentation of IC may include peritonitis, abdominal abscess, purulent or necrotic infection at sites of gastrointestinal perforation, or an anastomotic leak. The incidence of IC is as high as 40% in cases of secondary or tertiary peritonitis. Most infections are polymicrobial with fungus involved in 20% cases and in 40% of those with recent gastroduodenal perforation.
Ref:
1. Pappas PG, Kauffman CA, Andes DR, Clancy CJ, Marr KA, Ostrosky-Zeichner L, et al. Clinical Practice Guideline for the Management of Candidiasis: 2016 Update by the Infectious Diseases Society of America. Clin Infect Dis. 2016;62:e1-50.

23. **Ans. E**
The management of intra-abdominal fungal infection involves source control with adequate drainage or debridement along with appropriate and adequate antifungal therapy. Initial drug therapy should consider hemodynamic stability, organ involvement, comorbid illness, history of recent azole or echinocandin exposure, the dominant *Candida* species, and current antifungal sensitivity patterns.

Echinocandins are the drugs of choice for initial therapy in critically ill or hemodynamically unstable patient. Fluconazole is an acceptable alternative to an echinocandin as initial therapy in selected patients, including those who are not critically ill and who are considered unlikely to have a fluconazole-resistant *Candida* species. Testing for azole susceptibility is recommended for all bloodstream and other clinically relevant *Candida* isolates.

Testing for echinocandin susceptibility should be considered in patients who have had prior treatment with an echinocandin and among those who have infection with *C. glabrata* or *C. parapsilosis*. Transition from an echinocandin to fluconazole (usually within 5–7 days) is recommended for patients who are clinically stable, have isolates that are susceptible to fluconazole, and have negative repeat blood cultures following initiation of antifungal therapy.

For infection due to *C. glabrata*, transition to higher dose fluconazole 800 mg (12 mg/kg) daily or voriconazole 200–300 (3–4 mg/kg) twice daily should only be considered among patients with susceptible isolates. Among patients with suspected azole- and echinocandin-resistant *Candida* infections, lipid formulation of amphotericin B is recommended. Duration of antifungal therapy is dictated by adequacy of source control and clinical response.
Ref:
1. Kollef M, Micek S, Hampton N, Doherty JA, Kumar A. Septic shock attributed to Candida infection: importance of empiric therapy and source control. Clin Infect Dis. 2012;54:1739-46.
2. Pappas PG, Kauffman CA, Andes DR, Clancy CJ, Marr KA, Ostrosky-Zeichner L, et al. Clinical Practice Guideline for the Management of Candidiasis: 2016 Update by the Infectious Diseases Society of America. Clin Infect Dis. 2016;62:e1-50.

24. **Ans. B**
Interest and attention in these infections spiked in 2012–2013 with the nationwide outbreak of fungal meningitis due to three lots of contaminated methylprednisolone. The methylprednisolone was used in epidural spinal injection for relief of back pain. Approximately, 753 patients were identified with CNS infections in this outbreak with 64 deaths. The organism most commonly recovered was *Exserohilum rostratum*, a dematiaceous (pigmented) mold. CNS infections with this organism had not been previously reported. Dematiaceous organisms are common causes of chronic fungal sinusitis, but the one dematiaceous organism that may rarely reach the CNS is *Cladosporium bantiana*.

The types of infections seen with the multistate outbreak included:
- Meningitis only
- Meningitis plus paraspinal infection
- Stroke only
- Paraspinal infection only
- Paraspinal plus peripheral joint infection

These patients had abnormal CSF findings, which included increased white blood cell counts (predominately lymphocytes) ranging from 26–1200 per mL^3, elevated protein, and mildly low CSF glucose. MRI findings included enhancement of the meninges, evidence for arachnoiditis and in a few cases, stroke. The latter finding is most likely due to the angioinvasive nature of the organism.

Perhaps the most exciting new clinical application learned was measuring the levels of beta-D-glucan in the CSF. This was important in managing these patients, as cultures and PCR were not always positive.

The downward trend of serial beta-D-glucan levels correlated with improvement and eventual cure.

Although sporadic cases of meningitis due to *Exserohilum* or other dematiaceous fungi will most likely only occur very rarely, it will be important to include in the history of patients with signs and symptoms of meningitis exposure to epidural injections.

Ref:
1. *Kerkering TM, Grifasi ML, Baffoe-Bonnie AW, Bansal E, Garner DC, Smith JA, et al. Early clinical observations in prospectively followed patients with fungal meningitis related to contaminated epidural steroid injections. Ann Intern Med. 2013;158: 154-61.*
2. *Litvintseva AP, Lindsley MD, Gade L, Smith R, Chiller T, Lyons JL, et al. Utility of (1–3)-β-D-glucan testing for diagnostics and monitoring response to treatment during the multistate outbreak of fungal meningitis and other infections. Infect Dis. 2014;58:622-30.*
3. *Centers for Disease Control and Prevention (2012). Meningitis and stroke associated with potentially contaminated product. [online] Available from https://www.cdc.gov/hai/pdfs/outbreaks/han-advisory_meningitis_and_stroke_associated_with_potentially_contaminated_product-10-4-12.pdf [Last accessed February, 2020].*
4. *Centers for Disease Control and Prevention (2012). Notice to clinicians: Continued vigilance urged for fungal infections among patients who received contaminated steroid injections. [online] Available from https://emergency.cdc.gov/HAN/han00342.asp [Last accessed February, 2020].*
5. *Revankar SG, Sutton DA, Rinaldi MG. Primary central nervous system phaeohyphomycosis: a review of 101 cases. Infect Dis. 2004;38:206-16.*

25. Ans. C

Voriconazole, class of "azole" is known inhibitor of cytochrome 3A4. Tacrolimus is cleared through cytochrome P450-3A4. When both medications are given simultaneously, tacrolimus will accumulate resulting in high serum levels. Therefore, tacrolimus dose is to be reduced.

Ref:
1. *Venkataramanan R, Zang S, Gayowski T, Singh N. Voriconazole inhibition of the metabolism of tacrolimus in a liver transplant recipient and in human liver microsomes. Antimicrob Agents Chemother. 2002;46:3091-3.*

26. Ans. D

Invasive candidiasis is distinct from localized, mucocutaneous candidiasis, is a prevalent and burdensome infection of particular importance to ICU physicians. Candidemia is the most common means by which IC is diagnosed clinically. It should be borne in mind that organ involvement can take on many forms, including peritoneal, ocular, pulmonary, and CNS manifestations. IC is a spectrum of syndromes, including BSI or candidemia, deep-seated *Candida* infections in the presence of BSI, and deep-seated infections without BSI, each contributing of almost a third of ICU IC. Recognition and, therefore, treatment of this infection is frequently delayed, with dramatic clinical deterioration and death often preceding the detection of *Candida* in blood cultures.

Ref:
1. *Ostrosky-Zeichner L, Al-Obaidi M. Invasive fungal infections in the intensive care unit. Infect Dis Clin N Am. 2017;31:475-87.*
2. *Epelbaum O, Chasan R. Candidemia in the intensive care unit. Clin Chest Med. 2017;38:493-509.*

27. Ans. D

Histoplasma antigen detection in urine and/or serum is the most widely used and most sensitive method for diagnosing disseminated histoplasmosis and acute pulmonary histoplasmosis following exposure to a large inoculum. Other methods include antibody tests, culture, and microscopy.

Antigen detection: Enzyme immunoassay (EIA) is typically performed on urine and/or serum, but can also be used on CSF or BAL fluid.

Antibody tests: Because development of antibodies to Histoplasma can take 2–6 weeks, antibody tests are not as useful as antigen detection tests in diagnosing acute histoplasmosis or in immunosuppressed persons, who may not mount a strong immune response.

Immunodiffusion: Tests for the presence of H (indicates chronic or severe acute infection) and M (develops within weeks of acute infection and can persist for months to years after the infection has resolved) precipitin bands; ~80% sensitivity.

Complement fixation: Complement-fixing antibodies may take up to 6 weeks to appear after infection. CF is more sensitive but less specific than ID.

Culture: It can be performed on tissue, blood, and other body fluids, but may take up to 6 weeks to become positive; most useful in the diagnosis of the severe forms of histoplasmosis. A commercially available deoxyribonucleic acid (DNA) probe (AccuProbe, GenProbe Inc.) can be used to confirm.

Microscopy: For detection of budding yeast in tissue or body fluids, low sensitivity, but can provide a quick proven diagnosis if positive.

Polymerase chain reaction: PCR for detection of Histoplasma directly from clinical specimens is still experimental, but promising.

Ref:
1. *Azar MM, Hage CA. Laboratory diagnostics for histoplasmosis. J Clin Microbiol. 2017;55:1612-20.*
2. *Scheel CM, Gómez BL. Diagnostic methods for histoplasmosis: focus on endemic countries with variable infrastructure levels. Curr Trop Med Rep. 2014;1:129-37.*

28. Ans. C

It is also called "amphoterrible" in medical slang. Amphotericin B is known for its severe and potentially lethal side effects. A serious acute reaction after the infusion (1–3 hours later) is noted, consisting of high fever, shaking chills, hypotension, anorexia, nausea, vomiting, headache, dyspnea and tachypnea, and generalized weakness. This reaction sometimes subsides with later applications of the drug and may in part be due to histamine release. An increase in prostaglandin synthesis may also play a role. This nearly universal febrile response necessitates a critical (and diagnostically difficult) professional determination as to whether the onset of high fever is a novel symptom of a fast-progressing disease or merely the induced effect of the drug.

Ref:
1. Hartsel SC. Studies on Amphotericin B. [online] Available from www.chem.uwec.edu/chem491_w09/ambliposomereview.pdf [Last accessed February, 2020].
2. Lowe D (2012). Nasty Drug Molecules: Amphotericin B. [online] Available from https://blogs.sciencemag.org/pipeline/archives/2012/10/08/nasty_drug_molecules_amphotericin_b [Last accessed February, 2020].

29. Ans. C

Histoplasmosis disease is caused by the fungus *H. capsulatum*. Most people with histoplasmosis have no symptoms. However, *Histoplasma* can cause acute or chronic lung disease and progressive disseminated histoplasmosis affecting a number of organs. It can be fatal if left untreated.

Histoplasma occurs in many people living in areas where the fungus is common, such as the eastern and central United States. Infants, young children, and older persons, those with chronic lung disease, are at increased risk for severe disease. Disseminated disease is more frequently seen in people with cancer or AIDS or those on drugs that suppress the immune system or steroids.

Incubation period is 3–17 days after exposure; the average being 10 days.

Histopathology using stains for fungi, cultures, antigen detection, and serologic tests for *Histoplasma*-specific antibodies can all help to make the diagnosis of pulmonary histoplasmosis.

Treatment includes itraconazole which is generally preferred for mild-to-moderate histoplasmosis, and amphotericin B has a role in the treatment of moderately severe and severe infections. *H. capsulatum* is highly susceptible in vitro to posaconazole and has been used successfully as salvage therapy in patients who had failed other regimens. The addition of methylprednisolone (0.5–1.0 mg/kg/day intravenously) for 1–2 weeks has been used in some patients with clinical benefit; the IDSA guidelines for treatment of histoplasmosis suggest that corticosteroids be considered for severe acute pulmonary histoplasmosis.

Ref:
1. Wheat LJ, Freifeld AG, Kleiman MB, Baddley JW, McKinsey DS, Loyd JE, et al. Clinical practice guidelines for the management of patients with histoplasmosis: 2007 update by the Infectious Diseases Society of America. Clin Infect Dis. 2007;45:807-25.
2. Wheat LJ, Conces D, Allen SD, Blue-Hnidy D, Loyd J. Pulmonary histoplasmosis syndromes: recognition, diagnosis, and management. Semin Respir Crit Care Med. 2004;25:129-44.
3. Hage CA, Davis TE, Fuller D, Egan L, Witt JR 3rd, Wheat LJ, et al. Diagnosis of histoplasmosis by antigen detection in BAL fluid. Chest. 2010;137:623-8.
4. Wheat J, French ML, Kohler RB, Zimmerman SE, Smith WR, Norton JA, et al. The diagnostic laboratory tests for histoplasmosis: analysis of experience in a large urban outbreak. Ann Intern Med. 1982;97:680-5.

30. Ans. B

Candida auris is a public health concern worldwide. The global emergence, its ability to cause nosocomial outbreaks in healthcare settings, its innate and emerging resistance to multiple antifungal drugs has made *C. auris* challenging fungal infection. Because of the varying susceptibility of *C. auris* to azoles and amphotericin B, public health recommendations have led to the use of echinocandins as front-line therapy for infection. Increasing mutation of *ERG11* gene has recently been suggested as a mechanism of drug resistance to azole in *C. auris*. Currently there are no established breakpoints for antifungal susceptibility in *C. auris*. It is generally accepted that most isolates are multidrug resistant, based on applying *C. albicans* breakpoints [both Clinical Laboratory Standards Institute (CLSI) and European Committee on Antimicrobial Susceptibility Testing (EUCAST)]. Also, the infection control measures such as Standard Precautions and Contact Precautions along with isolation in a private room with daily and terminal cleaning with a disinfectant agent is recommended.

Ref:
1. Saris K, Meis JF, Voss A. Candida auris. Curr Opin Infect Dis. 2018;31:334-40.
2. Muñoz JF, Gade L, Chow NA, Loparev VN, Juieng P, Berkow EL, et al. Genomic insights into multidrug-resistance, mating and virulence in Candida auris and related emerging species. Nat Commun. 2018;9:5346.
3. Chowdhary A, Sharma C, Meis JF. Candida auris: a rapidly emerging cause of hospital-acquired multidrug-resistant fungal infections globally. PLoS Pathog. 2017;13:e1006290.
4. Healey KR, Kordalewska M, Jimenez-Ortigosa C, Singh A, Berrío I, Chowdhary A, et al. Limited ERG11 mutations identified in isolates of Candida auris directly contribute to reduced azole susceptibility. Antimicrob Agents Chemother. 2018;1062:e01427-18.

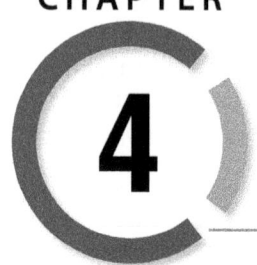

CHAPTER 4

Fungal Infections in Neutropenia

Vasant C Nagvekar

1. What do we know about *Candida auris*?
   A. It is a sensitive Candida
   B. It is not a yeast
   C. It is a multidrug-resistant *Candida*
   D. It is not relevant

2. Which is the first-line treatment in suspected or Confirmed *C. auris*?
   A. Echinocandins
   B. Polyenes
   C. Voriconazole
   D. Fluconazole

3. When would you suspect *C. auris* in laboratory?
   A. *C. haemulonii*
   B. *C. tropicalis*
   C. *C. krusei*
   D. *C. glabrata*

4. Which IPC precautions are necessary for patients colonized or infected with *C. auris*?
   A. No recommendations
   B. Contact precautions only
   C. Standard precautions is good
   D. Both contact and standard precautions

5. For how long should the contact precautions continue for a patient who is having infection or colonization?
   A. No need
   B. Up to 7 days after starting treatment
   C. Up to 14 days of completion of treatment
   D. Till the length of stay in hospital

6. A 77-year-old female undergone double (D)-J stenting for repeated UTI, abdominal pain and mild-to-moderate hydronephrosis are found. 20 days later again admitted with abdominal pain with following:
   - 12300
   - Blood and urine culture both *C. auris*
   - Source is DJ
   Which are the antifungals which have good penetration in urine?
   A. Echinocandins
   B. Liposomal amphotericin B
   C. Voriconazole
   D. 5 flucytosine (5FC)

7. What is the sensitivity of *C. auris* and which is the most sensitive of all antifungals?
   A. Azoles
   B. Polyenes
   C. Echinocandins
   D. 5 flucytosine

8. (1-3)-β-D-Glucan (BG) is positive in all, *except*:
   A. PCP
   B. *Mucor*
   C. *Aspergillus*
   D. Candida

9. What is the A1 antifungal recommendation for treatment of invasive aspergillosis?
   A. Echinocandins
   B. Fluconazole
   C. Voriconazole
   D. Polyenes

10. What is the antifungal prophylaxis of choice in induction chemotherapy for acute myeloid leukemia for prevention of molds?
    A. Fluconazole
    B. Voriconazole
    C. Posaconazole
    D. Echinocandins

11. What is the AII recommendation for treatment of mucormycosis?
    A. Diagnosis important
    B. Polyenes
    C. Surgery
    D. Control of underlying factors
    E. All of above

12. For Fusarium mold infection, drug of choice is:
    A. Liposomal amphotericin B
    B. Voriconazole
    C. Echinocandins
    D. Combination with liposomal amphotericin B with voriconazole until susceptibility available

13. A ring enhancing lesion which is a mold usually seen in immunocompetent hosts is?
    A. *Fusarium*
    B. Aspergillosis
    C. *Cladophialophora bantania*
    D. Cryptococcoma

14. A 13-year-old ALF postviral hepatitis (1 month post-liver transplant) presented with following results:
    - Fever with cough
    - No weight loss
    - BAL galactomannan: 2.32
    - Cultures: Negative
    - AFB stain and culture: Negative
    - TB Gene Xpert: Negative

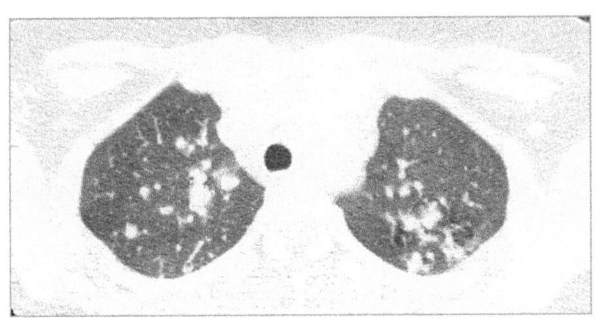

What treatment would you start on?
A. Voriconazole
B. Anti-Tb treatment
C. Both
D. Do not know

15. A 56-year-old living donor kidney transplantation (LDKT) (July 2010), has the following features:
    - On tacrolimus 1 mg bd, MMF 500 mg 2 tds, prednisolone 10 mg with serum creatinine of 1.73 admitted with on 12 June 2017
    - Fever, headache, vomiting
    - Hb: 12.1 g/dL, TLC: 11560/mm^3, PLT: 2.24/mm^3
    - MRI mild leptomeningeal enhancement
    - CSF: CSF on 12/06/17
    - Sugar: 26
    - Proteins: 84.4
    - WBC: 100, Lymphocytes: 88%
    - CSF cryptococcal antigen: Positive
    - India ink: Positive
    - CSF biofire: Positive
    - Tacrolimus was reduced

    Which is the correct statement of severity of meningitis?
    A. Cryptococcal antigen titer > 256
    B. Titer of > 512
    C. It does not matter
    D. Titer of >1,024

16. Which of the following is the correct?
    A. Lower CSF cell count suggest poor prognosis in Cryptococcal meningitis
    B. No correlation
    C. High cell count poor prognosis

17. Choice of antifungal treatment in cryptococcal meningitis:
    A. Echinocandins
    B. Liposomal amphotericin B with 5 flucytosine
    C. Fluconazole
    D. Fluconazole with 5 flucytosine

18. While identifying a relapse or persistence in cryptococcal meningitis, which is wrong?
    A. Development of new clinical signs and symptoms
    B. Repeat positive cultures
    C. Cryptococcal antigen positive

19. Following tests will favor mucormycosis, *except:*
    A. Calcofluor white staining to rapidly distinguish septated versus aseptate hyphae
    B. Negative galactomannan
    C. Positive Beta-D-Glucan

20. Management of mucormycosis involves which of the following steps?
    A. Liposomal amphotericin B (LAMB) alone good
    B. Surgical intervention and LAMB
    C. Surgical intervention and LAMB and rapid diagnosis
    D. Surgical intervention and LAMB and Rapid diagnosis and modification of metabolic factors and immunosuppression

21. Which one is not an endemic fungal infection?
    A. Coccidioidomycosis
    B. Histoplasmosis
    C. Aspergillosis
    D. Penicilliosis

22. Which of the following is not a dimorphic fungus?
    A. Histoplasmosis
    B. Talaromyces
    C. Paracoccidioidomycosis
    D. Mucormycosis

23. *Candida krusei* **is inherently resistant to:**
    A. Voriconazole
    B. Fluconazole
    C. Echinocandins
    D. Posaconazole

24. Which Candida species has more predilection for vascular catheters?
    A. *Candida albicans*
    B. *Candida tropicalis*
    C. *Candida parapsilosis*
    D. *Candida krusei*

25. Ostrosky validation of a clinical prediction has more:
    A. More specificity and less sensitivity with negative predictive value
    B. Equal specificity and sensitivity
    C. More sensitivity than specificity

26. A 27-year-old male undergoes laparotomy for small bowel fistula with jejunum resection in a case of Crohn's disease. The following are observed:
    - Febrile postoperative and receives Piperacillin-Tazobactam
    - Post day 4 fever shifted to ICU
    - BP 90/60, 112/min
    - WBC 17,600; platelets 1.43
    - Blood cultures are obtained
    - Vancomycin and Fluconazole 400 mg added
    - Hemodynamics stable but fever persists
    - Postoperative day 6: Blood cultures grew *C. glabrata*

What is the best therapy?
A. Increase fluconazole to 800 mg
B. Start voriconazole
C. Start an echinocandin (Anidulafungin, Caspofungin, Micafungin)
D. Start liposomal Amp B
E. Echinocandin plus fluconazole

27. Is there any role of prophylaxis in medical or surgical ICU?
A. Yes
B. No
C. Not sure

28. A diabetic 67-year-old male being treated for acute pancreatitis at day 16 starts with new onset fever and following history:
- Antibiotics: Meropenem and teicoplanin
- Central line catheterization
- Foley catheterization
- X-ray: Normal
- HR 120/min, BP 90/60 mm Hg

If you suspect invasive candidiasis what would be the choice of antifungal?
A. Voriconazole
B. Fluconazole
C. Amphotericin B
D. Echinocandins

29. What is the criterion for switching from echinocandin to fluconazole or voriconazole?
A. 3 days
B. Not to switch
C. 5-7 days
D. Not sure

30. A 54-year-old male undergone renal transplant 6 months back, admitted with breathlessness with hypoxia and following history:
- HRCT chest suggestive of bilateral ground glass opacity with peripheral sparing
- Immunosuppressants were Tacrolimus, Mycophenolate and Prednisolone
- Room air saturation was 80% and PaO_2 of 48
- Differential were CMV versus PCP

What investigation below may favor *Pneumocystis jirovecii* (PCP)?
A. Galactomannan
B. Beta-D-Glucan
C. Procalcitonin

31. Treatment of PCP with Trimethoprim-Sulfamethoxazole (TMP-SMX) is:
A. 5 mg/kg of TMP
B. 10 mg/kg of TMP
C. 15-20 mg/kg of TMP

32. Criteria for starting steroids in PCP is:
A. All patients should be treated
B. PaO_2 less than 70
C. PaO_2 less than 80

33. Prophylaxis for PCP in HIV with TMP-SMX is:
A. TMP-SMX DS (double strength) once a week
B. Daily TMP-SMX
C. Alternate day TMP-SMX

34. G6PD patient detected to have PCP positive on PCR and GMS stain:
A. Treat with primaquine and clindamycin
B. Caspofungin with clindamycin
C. Dapsone

ANSWERS WITH EXPLANATIONS

1. **Ans. C**
   Candida auris is a multidrug resistant *Candida* seen in nosocomial settings and usually resistant to many of the commonly used antifungals. It has a great propensity to spread and important to have strict infection control practices.

2. **Ans. A**
   An echinocandin is recommended as first-line treatment. Amphotericin B deoxycholate is an alternative agent in settings where echinocandins are unavailable and is recommended for central nervous system, urinary tract or eye infections.
   Azole antifungal agents such as fluconazole and voriconazole are not recommended as initial treatment for suspected or confirmed *C. auris* invasive disease. In many centers, reduced susceptibility or high-level resistance has been demonstrated to these agents. Posaconazole takes 5-7 days to reach a therapeutic level and so to be considered only with specialized consultation.
   C. auris requires specialized methods for identification and it could therefore be misidentified as another yeast when using traditional biochemical methods.
   Nearly all *C. auris* isolates have had high minimum inhibitory concentrations (MICs) for fluconazole, suggesting that they are fluconazole-resistant.
   More than half of isolates have had high MICs for voriconazole, and a lower proportion for amphotericin B and echinocandins.

Some isolates have had elevated MICs for all three major antifungal classes (azoles, polyenes, echinocandins). Mortality rates are high, approaching 70% during candidemia.
Ref:
1. CDC (2016). Global Emergence of Invasive Infections Caused by the Multidrug-Resistant Yeast Candida auris. [online] Available from: http://www.cdc.gov/fungal/diseases/candidiasis/candida-auris-alert.html. [Last accessed on February, 2020].

3. **Ans. A**

A comprehensive study from India investigated *C. auris* prevalence among 102 clinical isolates previously identified as *C. haemulonii* or *C. famata* with the VITEK system and found that 88.2% of the isolates were *C. auris*, as confirmed by ITS sequencing.
Ref:
1. Chowdhary A, Sharma C, Meis JF. Candida auris: a rapidly emerging cause of hospital-acquired multidrug-resistant fungal infections globally. PLoS Pathog. 2017;13(5):e1006290.

4. **Ans. D**

Both sets of precautions are recommended. *Standard precautions:* These apply to all patients and in all situations and are designed to reduce the risk of transmission of microorganisms from both recognizes and unrecognized sources of infection in healthcare settings and also very important is contact transmission-based precautions for patients known to be colonized or infected with *C. auris*. These are designed to prevent transmission of *C. auris* based on the contact route of transmission.

5. **Ans. D**

Contact precautions should be implemented for the length of stay in an acute care healthcare facility owing to prolonged colonization, probable shedding of *C. auris* into the environment and no known effective methods for decolonization. Patients known to be colonized or infected with *C. auris* should ideally have contact precautions implemented when readmitted to a healthcare facility.

6. **Ans. A**

	Suscepti-bility	Blood	Urine	Cidal	Biofilm in UT
Fluconazole	?	√	√		
Voriconazole	?	√			
AmB d	√	√	√	√	
L AmB	√	√		√	
Echinocandin	√	√		√	
5FC	√	√	√	√	

7. **Ans. C**

Causes invasive infections, predominantly fungemia Multidrug resistant:
- 93% resistant to fluconazole
- 54% resistant to voriconazole
- >50% resistant to amphotericin B
- 7% resistant to echinocandins
- 4% resistant to azoles, amphotericin B, and echinocandins
- Requires molecular methods to distinguish from other *Candida species* phenotypically similar to *C. haemulonii*

Ref:
1. Satoh K, Makimura K, Hasumi Y, Nishiyama Y, Uchida K, Yamaguchi H. Candida auris sp. nov., a novel ascomycetous yeast isolated from the external ear canal of an inpatient in a Japanese hospital. Microbiol Immunol. 2009;53:41-4.

8. **Ans. B**

The assay did not detect elevated levels of BG in subjects infected with *Mucor*, *Rhizopus*, or *Cryptococcus* species. The explanation for this is that Zygomycetes do not produce BG, and the BG produced by encapsulated *Cryptococcus* species is at low levels in infection.

9. **Ans. C**

We recommend primary treatment with voriconazole (strong recommendation; high-quality evidence).

Early initiation of antifungal therapy in patients with strongly suspected IPA is warranted while a diagnostic evaluation is conducted (strong recommendation; high-quality evidence).

Alternative therapies include liposomal AmB (strong recommendation; moderate-quality evidence), isavuconazole (strong recommendation; moderate-quality evidence), or other lipid formulations of AmB (weak recommendation; low-quality evidence).
Ref:
1. Ledoux M, Toussaint E, Denis J, Herbrecht R. New pharmacological opportunities for the treatment of invasive mould diseases. Journal of Antimicrobial Chemotherapy. 2017;72:(1)i48-i58.

10. **Ans. C**

Recommend prophylaxis with posaconazole (strong recommendation; high-quality evidence), voriconazole (strong recommendation; moderate-quality evidence), and/or micafungin (weak recommendation; low-quality evidence) during prolonged neutropenia for those who are at high risk for IA (strong recommendation; high-quality evidence). Prophylaxis with caspofungin is also probably effective (weak recommendation; low-quality evidence).

Ref:
1. Patterson TF, Thompson GR 3rd, Denning DW et al. Executive Summary: Practice Guidelines for the Diagnosis and Management of Aspergillosis: 2016 update by the Infectious Diseases Society of America. Clin Infect Dis. 2016;63:433-42.
2. Patterson TF, Thompson GR 3rd, Denning DW et al. Practice Guidelines for the Diagnosis and Management of Aspergillosis: 2016 update by the Infectious Diseases Society of America. Clin Infect Dis. 2016;63:e1-60.

11. Ans. E

In the treatment of mucormycosis, diagnosis, early surgery, antifungal therapy especially polyenes and control of immunosuppression and metabolic factors are recommended.

12. Ans. D

In *Fusarium*, until sensitivity not available, treat with Voriconazole and Amphotericin B.
Ref:
1. Al-Hatmi AMS, Curfs-Breuker I, de Hoog GS, Meis JF, Verweij PE. Antifungal susceptibility testing of Fusarium: a practical approach. J Fungi (Basel). 2017;3(2):19. Published 2017 Apr 26.

13. Ans. C

Dematiaceous fungi are a group of molds characterized by the presence of melanin-like pigment within cell wall that is pale brown to black. The mold infections of the CNS caused by *C. bantania* are manifested as a slowly expanding space occupying lesion causing headache, seizure, and localizing neurologic signs that simulate a brain tumor and usually seen in young immunocompetent hosts.

14. Ans. D

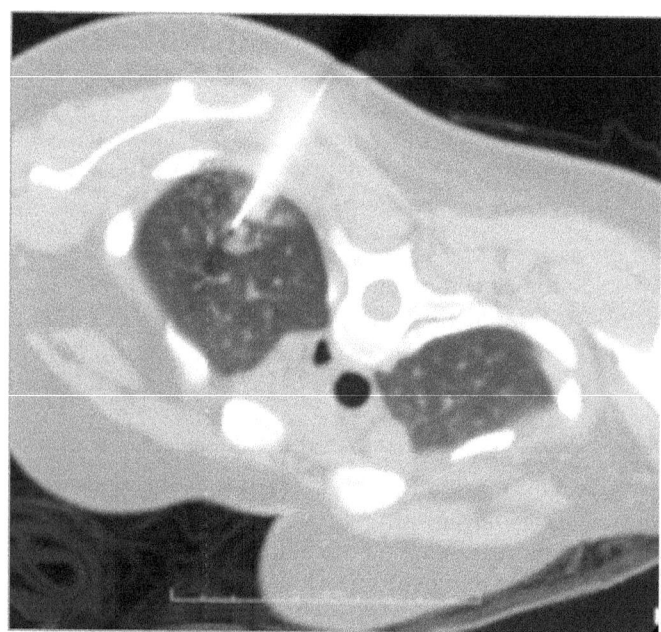 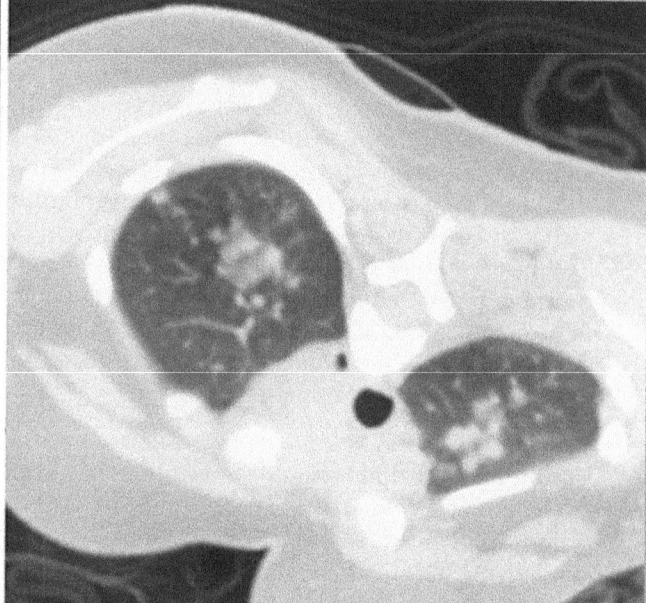

Histpathology–granulomatous disease
Culture–positive for mycobacterial tuberculosis

Lesson learnt:
- Do not rely completely on biomarkers and serology
- Gold standard is histopathology.

15. Ans. D

Initial high titers (≥1:1,024) demonstrate a high burden of yeasts in the host, poor host immunity, and a greater chance of therapeutic failure.
Ref:
1. Powderly WG, Cloud GA, Dismukes WE, Saag MS. Measurement of cryptococcal antigen in serum and cerebrospinal fluid: value in the management of AIDS-associated cryptococcal meningitis. Clin Infect Dis. 1994;18:789-92.

16. Ans. A

Three major prognostic findings: (1) Burden of yeasts at presentation, (2) Poor inflammatory response, and (3) Level of the patient's sensorium at presentation. For example, a poor prognosis is indicated by a strongly positive India ink examination, a high polysaccharide antigen titer (≥1:1,024), and a poor inflammatory response in the CSF (<20 cells/μL).

17. Ans. B

Amphotericin B remains the cornerstone of therapy for cryptococcal meningitis, and from the early studies when it was used alone to its use in combinations.

The combination of amphotericin B and flucytosine has become the standard therapy for meningitis, and in patients without AIDS it usually sterilizes CSF after 2 weeks of therapy. In fact, it clears CSF yeast counts significantly faster than amphotericin B alone, amphotericin B plus fluconazole, or all three agents together.

Patients without AIDS can be given either a 4-week induction phase regimen of amphotericin B.
Ref:
1. van der Horst CM, Saag MS, Cloud GA, Hamill RJ, Graybill JR, Sobel JD, et al. Treatment of cryptococcal meningitis associated with the acquired immunodeficiency syndrome. N Engl J Med. 1997;337: 15-21.
2. Pappas PG, Chetchotisakd P, Larsen RA, Manosuthi W, Morris MI, Anekthananon T, et al. A phase II randomized trial of amphotericin B alone or combined with fluconazole in the treatment of HIV-associated cryptococcal meningitis. Clin Infect Dis. 2009;48:1775-83.

18. Ans. C

Identifying a relapse or persistence can be difficult in patients with cryptococcal infections. The two clearest signs of relapse after at least 4 weeks of an established antifungal regimen that suggest a change in management are: (1) Development of new clinical signs and symptoms, and (2) Repeat positive cultures. The persistence of a positive India ink examination or changing versus fixed polysaccharide antigen titers are not precise indications of relapse.
Ref:
1. Katial RK, Brandt BL, Moran EE, Marks S, Agnello V, Zollinger WD. Immunogenicity and safety testing of a group B intranasal meningococcal native outer membrane vesicle vaccine. Infect Immun. 2002;35: 128-33.

19. Ans. C

Differentiation of mucormycosis from aspergillosis could be improved by using a three-step analysis approach for biopsy specimens: (1) Calcofluor white staining to rapidly distinguish septated versus aseptate hyphae, (2) *Aspergillus* galactomannan and PCR testing for rapid identification, and (3) Negative beta-D-Glucan.

Galactomannan is positive in *Aspergillus* and beta-D-Glucan is positive in *Candida*, *Aspergillus* and *Pneumocystis* and negative in mucormycosis.

20. Ans. D

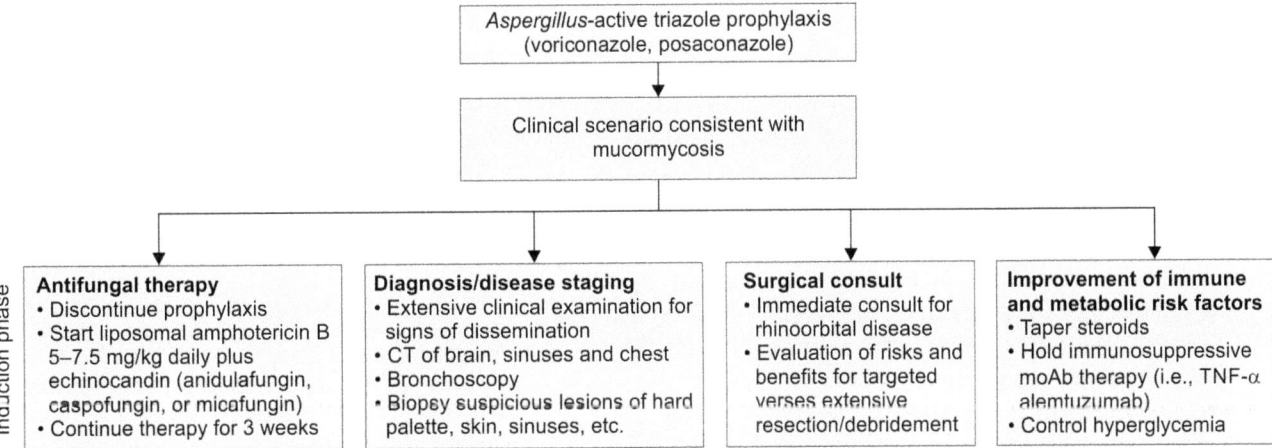

21. Ans. C

Aspergillosis is an opportunistic Fungi and not an Endemic Fungi seen in hematological and transplant patients worldwide whereas Coccidioidomycosis is seen in some states of United States of America; Histoplasmosis seen again in Northeast part of India, USA and Penicilliosis seen in Northeast India and Southeast Asian countries.

22. Ans. D

Dimorphic fungi are fungi that can exist in the form of both mold and yeast. This is usually brought about by change in temperature and the fungi are also described as *thermally dimorphic fungi*. Mucormycosis is not a dimorphic fungi.

23. Ans. B

Candida krusei is 100% inherently resistant to fluconazole.

24. Ans. C

Candida species	Risk factor
Candida tropicalis	Neutropenia and bone marrow transplantation
Candida krusei	• Fluconazole use • Neutropenia and bone marrow transplantation
Candidata glabrata	• Fluconazole use • Surgery • Vascular catheters • Cancer • Older age
Candida parapsilosis	• Parenteral nutrition and hyperalimentation • Vascular catheters • Being neonate
Candida lusitaniae and Candida guilliermondii	Previous polyene use
Candida rugosa	Burns

25. Ans. A

- *Mandatory*: Systemic antibiotics and presence of a CVC
- *Two additional risk factors*: TPN, dialysis, steroid use, major surgery, pancreatitis, other immuno-suppressants
- Sensitivity 34%, specificity 90%, negative predictive value 97%

Ref:
1. Ostrosky-Zeichner L, Sable C, Sobel J, Alexander BD, Donowitz G, Kan V, et al. Multicenter retrospective development and validation of a clinical prediction rule for nosocomial invasive candidiasis in the intensive care setting. Eur J Clin Microbiol Infect Dis. 2007;26:271.

26. Ans. C

Species	Fluconazole	Itraconazole	Voriconazole	Posaconazole	Flucytosine	Amphotericin B	Candins
Candida albicans	S	S	S	S	S	S	S
Candida tropicalis	S	S	S	S	S	S	S
Candida parapsilosis	S	S	S	S	S	S	S to R
Candida glabrata	S-DD to R	S-DD to R	S-DD to R	S-DD to R	S	S to I	S
Candida krusei	S	S-DD to R	S	S	I to R	S to I	S
Candida lusitaniae	S	S	S	S	S	S to R	S

27. Ans. B

- Randomized ICU patients who had fever on broad spectrum antibiotics to fluconazole 800 mg daily for 14 days or placebo
- Success rates 36% versus 38%
- So no role for routine empiric therapy

Ref:
1. Schuster MG, Edwards JE Jr, Sobel JD, Darouiche RO, Karchmer AW, Hadley S, et al. Empirical fluconazole versus placebo for intensive care unit patients: a randomized trial. Ann Intern Med. 2008;149:83.

28. Ans. D

An echinocandin (caspofungin: loading dose 70 mg, then 50 mg daily; micafungin: 100 mg daily; anidulafungin: loading dose 200 mg, then 100 mg daily) is recommended as initial therapy (strong recommendation; high-quality evidence).

Fluconazole, intravenous or oral, 800 mg (12 mg/kg) loading dose, then 400 mg (6 mg/kg) daily is an acceptable alternative to an echinocandin as initial therapy in selected patients, including those who are not critically ill and who are considered unlikely to have a fluconazole-resistant *Candida* species (strong recommendation; high-quality evidence).

Ref:
1. Pappas PG, Kauffman CA, Andes DR, et al. Clinical Practice Guideline for the Management of Candidiasis: 2016 Update by the Infectious Diseases Society of America. Clin Infect Dis. 2016;62(4):e1-e50.

29. Ans. C

Transition from an echinocandin to fluconazole (usually within 5–7 days) is recommended for patients who are clinically stable, have isolates that are susceptible to fluconazole (e.g., *C. albicans*), and have negative repeat blood cultures following initiation of antifungal therapy (strong recommendation; moderate-quality evidence).

Ref:
1. Pappas PG, Kauffman CA, Andes DR, et al. Clinical Practice Guideline for the Management of Candidiasis: 2016 Update by the Infectious Diseases Society of America. Clin Infect Dis. 2016;62(4):e1-e50.

30. Ans. B

Galactomannan favors Aspergillosis. Beta-D-Glucan comes from cell wall polysaccharide of pneumocystis and other fungi. It can detect in serum with chromogenic quantitative immunoassay. Pooled sensitivity and specificity of 95% and 86% only. Negative predictive value of over 95%.

Ref:
1. Karageorgopoulos DE, Qu JM, Korbila IP, Zhu YG, Vasileiou VA, Falagas ME. Accuracy of β-D-glucan for the diagnosis of Pneumocystis jirovecii pneumonia: a meta-analysis. Clin Micro Infect. 2013;19:39.

31. Ans. C

Dosage for treatment for PCP is 15–20 mg/kg in three or four divided doses.

Ref:
1. Castro JG, Morrison-Bryant M. Management of Pneumocystis jirovecii pneumonia in HIV infected patients: current options, challenges and future directions. HIV AIDS (Auckl). 2010;2:123-34.

32. Ans. B

A PaO_2 of greater than 70 mm Hg (while breathing room air) indicates mild PCP, and less than 70 mm Hg indicates severe disease. When expressed as the alveolar-arterial oxygen gradient, PCP can be classified as mild (<35 mm Hg), moderate (35–45 mm Hg), and severe (>45 mm Hg).

Patients with mild PCP may be treated as outpatients under close supervision of the clinician. Patients with moderate to severe PCP should be treated with IV therapy and adjunctive corticosteroids.

33. **Ans. C**

TMP-SMX is the drug of choice for chemoprophylaxis. Three oral TMP-SMX regimens have similar rates of efficacy; however, single strength (SS) TMP-SMX may have fewer adverse reactions than double-strength (DS) TMP-SMX.

34. **Ans. B**

In view of G6PD deficiency, we cannot use TMP-SMX or Primaquine or Dapsone and so caspofungin plus clindamycin will be the choice.

Ref:
1. *Korraa H, Saadeh C. Options in the management of pneumonia caused by Pneumocystis carinii in patients with acquired immune deficiency syndrome and intolerance to trimethoprim/sulfamethoxazole. South Med J. 1996;89(3):272-7.*

CHAPTER 5

Infection-related Malignancies

Pritam Kataria

1. **The ideal time of giving the inactivated influenza vaccine is:**
   A. 2 weeks before chemotherapy
   B. 1 week before chemotherapy
   C. Between chemotherapy cycles
   D. Not to be given at all

2. **Which of the following for *Legionella* infection is correct?**
   A. One way to differentiate from pneumococcal infection is to look for clinical features such as diarrhea, rhabdomyolysis, and lack of response to beta lactam antibiotics
   B. *Legionella maltophilia* serogroup 1 is responsible for 80% infection
   C. Drugs of choice (DOC) are azithromycin or fluoroquinolone
   D. All of the above

3. **Which of the following is/are correct regarding the neutropenic enterocolitis?**
   A. Most commonly observed in case of neutropenia observed with leukemia
   B. *Clostridial* species are most common anaerobes
   C. The investigation of choice is CT scan
   D. All of the above

4. **Trimethoprim-sulfamethoxazole (TMP–SMX) prophylaxis is indicated in patients undergoing chemotherapy if:**
   A. Risk of *Pneumocystis carinii* pneumonia (PCP) is >3.5% with chemotherapy
   B. Prednisolone ≥20 mg use for ≥1 month
   C. Patient on purine analogs
   D. All of the above

5. **Which of the following with regards to influenza vaccination is correct?**
   A. Yearly influenza vaccination with inactivated quadrivalent vaccine is recommended
   B. Must be taken >7 days after the last treatment or >2 weeks before chemotherapy starts
   C. All family and household contacts and healthcare providers
   D. All of the above

6. **Diagnosis of central line-associated bloodstream infection (CLABSI) is suggestive in following indication:**
   A. Multiple positive blood culture results
   B. Isolation of the same organism from quantitative catheter cultures and percutaneous blood cultures
   C. A differential growth time of >2 hours for cultures of blood samples obtained through the CVC, compared with cultures of peripheral blood samples
   D. All of the above

7. **Which of the following regarding antifungal prophylaxis is recommended?**
   A. Population level risk of *Candida* infection >3% and a mold-active triazole when the population level risk of aspergillosis is >3%
   B. Population level risk of *Candida* infection >8% and a mold-active triazole when the population level risk of aspergillosis is >8%
   C. Population level risk of *Candida* infection >10% and a mold-active triazole when the population level risk of aspergillosis is >6%
   D. None of the above

8. **Risk of febrile neutropenia is higher with regimens at following doses, *except*:**
   A. Anthracyclines ≥90 mg/m^2
   B. Cisplatin ≥100 mg/m^2
   C. Ifosfamide ≥9 mg/m^2
   D. Etoposide ≥100 mg/m^2

9. **What is the indication of quinolone prophylaxis in the patient?**
   A. Neutropenia >7 days
   B. Neutropenia <7 days
   C. Not indicated
   D. All patients

10. **Which antifungal agent has shown survival benefit as a preventive modality in aspergillosis?**
    A. Posaconazole   B. Voriconazole
    C. Amphotericin B   D. Caspofungin

11. **Indication of prophylactic PCP:**
    A. Prednisolone 20 mg daily for >1 month

B. Chronic lymphocytic leukemia (CLL) receiving fludarabine
C. Gliomas receiving concurrent temozolomide (TMZ) and radiation
D. All of the above

12. **Prophylactic agents for PCP prophylaxis:**
    A. Trimethoprim/sulfamethoxazole (TMP/SMX) double strength 2 atb/day twice in a week
    B. Dapsone 50 mg BD
    C. Pentamidine 300 mg every 4 weeks
    D. All of the above

13. **Rituximab has been associated with following infections:**
    A. Hepatitis B virus (HBV) reactivation
    B. JC encephalopathy
    C. *Cytomegalovirus* (CMV) disease
    D. All of the above

14. **Prophylactic nucleoside analogs in HBsAg patients have been advised for what duration?**
    A. 3 months
    B. 6 months
    C. 9 months
    D. 12 months

15. **Risk stratification in neutropenic fever by MASCC, low risk has been defined as:**
    A. >5
    B. >10
    C. >15
    D. >21

16. **Which lymphoma is associated with *Helicobacter pylori*?**
    A. Mucosa-associated lymphoid tissue (MALT) lymphoma
    B. Diffuse large B-cell lymphoma
    C. Chronic lymphocytic lymphoma
    D. Follicular lymphoma

17. **Immunoproliferative small intestinal disease (IPSID) has been associated epidemiologically with enteric infection possibly due to:**
    A. *Vibrio cholerae*
    B. *Salmonella typhi*
    C. *Escherichia coli*
    D. *Shigella* infection

18. **Febrile neutropenia (FN) patient—high risk of classification:**
    A. If duration of neutropenia >7
    B. Score ≥21
    C. ANC <100
    D. All of the above

19. **Empirical antifungal in low risk FN:**
    A. In all patients
    B. Persistent fever of unidentified cause following 4–7 days of antibiotic treatment
    C. In case of documented fungal infection only
    D. Neutropenia that is expected to last >7 days

20. **Treatment in neutropenic fever is necessary until the patient is:**
    A. Afebrile for at least 48 hours
    B. Clinically stable with resolution of neutropenia (ANC of at least 500 cells/µL)
    C. Negative blood cultures
    D. All of the above

21. **Severe mucositis is a risk factor for:**
    A. *Viridans* group of streptococci
    B. *Staphylococci*
    C. *Enterococci*
    D. *Clostridia*

22. **The risk of infection with steroids increases:**
    A. If steroids are administered 20 mg/day for 4–6 weeks
    B. Steroids of any dose but >15 days
    C. Steroids of any duration but >10 mg/day
    D. None of the above

23. **The microorganisms most commonly associated with peripheral vascular and central venous catheter (CVC) infection are:**
    A. Coagulase-negative staphylococci (CoNS), *Staphylococcus aureus*, different species of aerobic gram-negative bacilli, and *Candida albicans*
    B. Coagulase-positive staphylococci
    C. Gram-positive bacilli
    D. *Pseudomonas aeruginosa*

24. **High dose cytosar is associated with increased risk of which infection?**
    A. Gram-positive streptococcal infection
    B. Gram-positive staphylococcal infection
    C. *Pseudomonas* infection
    D. *Aspergillus* infection

25. **Which of the following of *Candida* infection is not correct?**
    A. *Candida* is the most common infection
    B. *Candida krusei* is resistant to fluconazole
    C. *Candida tropicalis* is highly virulent in the neutropenic patient
    D. *Candida albicans* is mostly associated with the catheters

26. **Drug of choice in patient on azole developing breakthrough candidemia is:**
    A. Echinocandins
    B. Voriconazole
    C. Amphotericin B
    D. None of the above

48 Infection-related Malignancies

27. Treatment of choice in treatment of invasive candidiasis in pregnant patients is:
A. Fluconazole
B. Amphotericin B
C. Voriconazole
D. Posaconazole

28. CT scan features of invasive aspergillosis in neutropenic patients is:
A. One or more well-circumscribed nodules
B. Halo sign—haziness around the nodule representing the alveolar hemorrhage
C. Crescent sign—cavitation coinciding with neutrophil recovery
D. All of the above

29. β-D-glucan assay does not detect which of the following fungal infection?
A. Candidiasis
B. Fusariosis
C. Aspergillosis
D. Mucormycosis

30. Which one of the following is not correct?
A. Bronchoalveolar lavage (BAL) has 50% sensitivity in focal aspergillosis
B. *Aspergillus* galactomannan and β-D-glucan have been accepted as diagnostic adjuncts by European Organization for the Research and Treatment of Cancer (EORTC) group
C. Serum β-D-glucan does not detect mucormycosis
D. All of the above

ANSWERS WITH EXPLANATIONS

1. Ans. A

The ideal time to vaccinate with influenza vaccine is 2 weeks before initiation of chemotherapy, 1 month after completion of chemotherapy or after the peripheral WBC count recovers to greater than 1,000 cells/mm^3, and 2 months after completion of chemotherapy.
Ref:
1. Arrowood JR, Hayney MS. Immunization recommendations for adults with cancer. Ann Pharmacother. 2002;36:1219-29.

2. Ans. D

In the cancer population, patients at highest risk include those receiving high-dose corticosteroids, T-cell depleting agents, and allogeneic HSCT. There are no clinical or radiologic criteria that reliably distinguish legionellosis from pneumococcal pneumonia, although diarrhea, rhabdomyolysis, and lack of response to β-lactam antibiotics have been proposed as suggestive of the diagnosis. A combination of culture (special culture medium required) and urinary antigen test is the optimal diagnostic combination in most situations. Azithromycin or fluoroquinolones (e.g., levofloxacin, moxifloxacin) are standard therapy for legionellosis.
Ref:
1. Murdoch DR. Diagnosis of Legionella infection. Clin Infect Dis. 2003;36(1):64-9.
2. Watkins RR, Lemonovich TL. Diagnosis and management of community-acquired pneumonia in adults. Am Fam Physician. 2011;83(11):1299-306.

3. Ans. D

Results from a combination of neutropenia and defects in the bowel mucosa related to cytotoxic chemotherapy. Typhlitis is characterized by ulceration and necrosis of the bowel wall, hemorrhage, and masses of organisms. Typhlitis ("inflammation of the cecum") results from a combination of neutropenia and defects in the bowel mucosa related to cytotoxic chemotherapy. Patients receiving chemotherapy for acute leukemia are at highest risk. Positive CT scan findings are present in about 80% of cases of typhlitis.
Ref:
1. Rodrigues FG, Dasilva G, Wexner SD. Neutropenic enterocolitis. World J Gastroenterol. 2017;23(1):42-7.

4. Ans. D

The panel recommends that prophylaxis with TMP-SMX only be used if the risk for PCP is >3.5% (e.g., patients administered regimens with ≥20 mg of prednisone equivalents daily for ≥1 month or those based on purine analogs).
Ref:
1. Flowers CR, Seidenfeld J, Bow EJ, Karten C, Gleason C, Hawley DK, et al. Antimicrobial prophylaxis and outpatient management of fever and neutropenia in adults treated for malignancy: American Society of Clinical Oncology clinical practice guideline. J Clin Oncol. 2013;31(6):794-810.

5. Ans. D

As per the recommendations, influenza vaccine should be taken once yearly. It must be taken ideally >7 days after the last treatment or >2 weeks before chemotherapy starts. It is also recommended in patients with age older than 65 years. It is also indicated in those patients with all family members and household contacts and healthcare providers.
Ref:
1. Taplitz RA, Kennedy EB, Bow EJ, Crews J, Gleason C, Hawley DK, et al. Antimicrobial prophylaxis for adult patients with cancer-related immunosuppression: ASCO and IDSA Clinical Practice Guideline Update. J Clin Oncol. 2018;36(30):3043-54.

6. Ans. D

Diagnosis of CLABSI is suggestive of following indication in case of multiple positive blood culture reports.

Ref:
1. *Mermel LA, Farr BM, Sherertz RJ, Raad II, O'Grady N, Harris JS, et al. Guidelines for the management of intravascular catheter-related infections. Clin Infect Dis. 2001;32(9):1249-72.*

7. Ans. C

Antifungal prophylaxis with an oral triazole or parenteral echinocandin in the case of a population level risk of *Candida* infection >10% and a mold-active triazole when the population level risk of aspergillosis is >6%.

Ref:
1. *Flowers CR, Seidenfeld J, Bow EJ, Karten C, Gleason C, Hawley DK, et al. Antimicrobial prophylaxis and outpatient management of fever and neutropenia in adults treated for malignancy: American Society of Clinical Oncology clinical practice guideline. J Clin Oncol. 2013;31(6):794-810.*

8. Ans. D

French ELYPSE study demonstrated high incidence of neutropenic fever with following drugs with respective drug dosages: Anthracyclines ≥90 mg/m^2, Cisplatin ≥100 mg/m^2, Ifosfamide ≥9 mg/m^2, Etoposide ≥100 mg/m^2.

Ref:
1. *Bachelot T, Ray-Coquard I, Menetrier-Caux C, Rastkha M, Duc A, Blay JY. Prognostic value of serum levels of interleukin 6 and of serum and plasma levels of vascular endothelial growth factor in hormone-refractory metastatic breast cancer patients. Br J Cancer. 2003;88(11):1721-6.*

9. Ans. A

Quinolone prophylaxis for patients has been indicated at high risk such as patients with hematologic malignancies or HSCT recipients in whom profound neutropenia (absolute for more than 7 days) is present.

Ref:
1. *Tomblyn M, Chiller T, Einsele H, Gress R, Sepkowitz K, Storek J, et al. Guidelines for preventing infectious complications among hematopoietic cell transplantation recipients: a global perspective. Biol Blood Marrow Transplant. 2009;15(10):1143-238.*
2. *Freifeld AG, Bow EJ, Sepkowitz KA, Boeckh MJ, Ito JI, Mullen CA, et al. Clinical practice guideline for the use of antimicrobial agents in neutropenic patients with cancer: 2010 update by the Infectious Diseases Society of America. Clin Infect Dis. 2011;52(4):e56-93.*

10. Ans. A

Prevention of aspergillosis with posaconazole has been associated with survival benefit.

Ref:
1. *Cornely OA, Maertens J, Winston DJ, Perfect J, Ullmann AJ, Walsh TJ, et al. Posaconazole vs. fluconazole or itraconazole prophylaxis in patients with neutropenia. N Engl J Med. 2007;356(4):348-59.*

11. Ans. D

Pneumocystis carinii pneumonia prophylaxis should be considered in patients with cancer who receive prolonged high-dose steroids (i.e., equivalent of prednisone 20 mg daily for ≥1 month). Other candidates for prophylaxis include alemtuzumab recipients (package insert recommends prophylaxis until at least 2 months after completion of alemtuzumab and CD4 count ≥200/μL, whichever occurs later), patients with CLL receiving fludarabine, and patients with gliomas receiving TMZ and radiation or corticosteroids.

Ref:
1. *©Therapeutic Guidelines Ltd (eTG June 2019). Therapeutic Guidelines: Antibiotics.*

12. Ans. D

The most effective agent is TMP/SMX. A variety of dosages seem to be effective (from one double-strength tablet daily, to one double-strength tablet twice daily 2 days per week). When TMP/SMX cannot be administered because of marrow intolerance or hypersensitivity reaction, second-line agents include dapsone (50 mg twice daily or 100 mg orally daily), inhaled pentamidine (300 mg every 4 weeks), and atovaquone (1,500 mg daily). All second-line agents are less effective than TMP/SMX, with the difference increasing with the degree of immune compromise.

Ref:
1. *Martin SI, Fishman JA; AST Infectious Diseases Community of Practice. Pneumocystis pneumonia in solid organ transplantation. Am J Transplant. 2013;13(Suppl 4):272-9.*

13. Ans. D

Rituximab has been associated with HBV reactivation leading to a black box warning regarding the same. Also, rituximab has also been associated with progressive multifocal leukoencephalopathy also known as JC encephalopathy caused by JC virus activation acquired during infancy. Other rare infection associated with the use of rituximab includes enteroviral meningoencephalitis, CMV disease, disseminated varicella zoster virus (VZV), refractory babesiosis, Parvovirus B19, and nocardiosis.

Ref:
1. *Ozurus R, Ar C, Onguren S, Mete B, Tabak F, Mert A, et al. Acute hepatitis B despite a previous high titer of anti-HBs. Hepatol Int. 2010;4(2):530-2.*
2. *Carson KR, Evens AM, Richey EA, Habermann TM, Focosi D, Seymour JF, et al. Progressive multifocal leukoencephalopathy after rituximab therapy in HIV-negative patients: a report of 57 cases from the Research on Adverse Drug Events and Reports project. Blood. 2009;113(20):4834-40.*

14. Ans. D

HBsAg-positive patients, regardless of their HBV DNA level, should be treated with lamivudine or some other of the nucleoside/nucleotide analogs currently available during the duration of chemotherapy and for up to 12 months thereafter.

Ref:
1. *European Association for the Study of the Liver. EASL clinical practice guidelines: management of chronic hepatitis B virus infection. J Hepatol. 2012;57(1):167-85.*

15. Ans. D

The MASCC index was designed as a tool to identify adult patients at low risk of complications. To obtain a MASCC score, points are allocated and added up. Points are given for burden of illness {no or mild symptoms (5), moderate symptoms (3), severe symptoms (0)}, absence of hypotension (5), absence of chronic obstructive pulmonary disease (4), solid tumor or no previous fungal infection (4), absence of dehydration (3), outpatient status (3), and age <60 years (2). The points are added up, and patients with a score of ≥21 points (of 26 possible) are "low risk" and can be considered for oral therapy.

Ref:
1. *Klastersky J, Paesmans M, Rubenstein EB, Boyer M, Elting L, Feld R, et al. The Multinational Association for Supportive Care in Cancer risk index: A multinational scoring system for identifying low-risk febrile neutropenic cancer patients. J Clin Oncol. 2000;18(16):3038-51.*

16. Ans. A

Gastric lymphoma of MALT type is closely related to *H. pylori* infection. In vitro studies have demonstrated *H. pylori*-induced B cell proliferation to be strain dependent. High prevalences of CagA protein and FldA protein have been reported in strains obtained from patients with gastric lymphoma of MALT type.

Ref:
1. *Delchier JC, Lamarque D, Levy M, Tkoub EM, Copie-Bergman C, Deforges L, et al. Helicobacter pylori and gastric lymphoma: high seroprevalence of CagA in diffuse large B-cell lymphoma but not in low-grade lymphoma of mucosa-associated lymphoid tissue type. Am J Gastroenterol. 2001;96:2324-8.*

17. Ans. A

Disease known as "immunoproliferative small intestinal disease (IPSID)" has been associated epidemiologically with enteric infection possibly due to *Vibrio cholerae*, primarily in developing countries.

Ref:
1. *Isaacson PG. Gastrointestinal lymphoma. Hum Pathol. 1994;25:1020-9.*

18. Ans. D

High risk FN is described by following features:
- ANC less than 100 cells/mm^3
- Absolute monocyte count < 100 cells/mm^3
- Duration of neutropenia >1 week
- Expected resolution of neutropenia >10 days.

Ref:
1. *Sylvester RK. Pharmacotherapy Self-Assessment Program: Infections in Patient with Cancer, 5th edition; 2005. p. 148.*

19. Ans. D

In patients whose expected duration of neutropenia is >7 days and who do not respond to first-line antibacterial treatment, specifically in the absence of mold-active antifungal prophylaxis, further therapy should be directed also against fungi, in particular *Aspergillus* species.

Ref:
1. *Heinz WJ, Buchheidt D, Christopeit M, von Lilienfeld-Toal M, Cornely OA, Einsele H, et al. Diagnosis and empirical treatment of fever of unknown origin (FUO) in adult neutropenic patients: guidelines of the Infectious Diseases Working Party (AGIHO) of the German Society of Hematology and Medical Oncology (DGHO). Ann Hematol. 2017;96:1775-92.*

20. Ans. D

Treatment is necessary until the patient is afebrile for at least 48 hours, clinically stable with resolution of neutropenia (ANC of at least 500 cells/µL), and has negative blood cultures.

Ref:
1. *Freifeld AG, Bow EJ, Sepkowitz KA, Boeckh MJ, Ito JI, Mullen CA, et al. Clinical practice guideline for the use of antimicrobial agents in neutropenic patients with cancer: 2010 update by the Infectious Diseases Society of America. Clin Infect Dis. 2011;52:e56-93.*
2. *National Comprehensive Cancer Network (2017). NCCN Clinical Practice Guidelines in Oncology. Prevention and Treatment of Cancer Related Infections, version 2. 2017. [online] Available from https://www.nccn.org/professionals/physician_gls/default.aspx#site [Last accessed March, 2020]*
3. *Govidan R. Devitta, Hellman, and Rosenberg's Cancer: Principles and Practice of Oncology Review, 3rd edition. Philadelphia, PA: Lippincott Williams and Wilkins; 2012. pp. 1931-59.*

21. Ans. A

Oral mucositis is a strong predictor of oral *viridans streptococci* (OVS), *Streptococcus viridans* bacteremia and simultaneously coagulase-negative staphylococci (CoNS) bacteremia is clearly associated with mucositis.

Ref:
1. *Blijlevens NM, Donnelly JP, de Pauw BE. Empirical therapy of febrile neutropenic patients with mucositis: challenge of risk-based therapy. Clin Microbiol Infect. 2001;7(Suppl 4):47-52.*
2. *Govidan R. Devita, Hellman, and Rosenberg's Cancer: Principles and Practice of Oncology Review, 3rd edition. Philadelphia, PA: Lippincott Williams and Wilkins; 2012. pp. 1931-59.*

22. Ans. A

Ref:
1. *Youssef J, Novosad SA, Winthrop KL. Infection Risk and Safety of Corticosteroid Use. Rheum Dis Clin North Am. 2016;42(1):157-76, ix-x.*

23. Ans. A

Coagulase-negative staphylococci, *S. aureus*, different species of aerobic gram-negative bacilli, and *C. albicans*

24. Ans. A

High dose cytosar is associated with increased risk of Gram-positive streptococcal infection.

Ref:
1. *Gamis AS, Howells WB, DeSwarte-Wallace J, Feusner JH, Buckley JD, Woods WG. Alpha hemolytic streptococcal infection during intensive treatment for acute myeloid leukemia: a report from the Children's cancer group study CCG-2891. J Clin Oncol. 2000;18(9): 1845-55.*

25. Ans. D

Candida albicans is the most common and it is usually susceptible to fluconazole, but the proportion of nonalbicans *Candida* has been increasing. *C. tropicalis* is highly virulent in neutropenic hosts but is susceptible to most agents. *C. krusei* is always resistant to fluconazole, and *C. glabrata* has variable susceptibility. *C. parapsilosis* is mostly associated with vascular catheters and is usually susceptible to fluconazole but relatively resistant to echinocandins.

Ref:
1. *Trofa D, Gácser A, Nosanchuk JD. Candida parapsilosis, an emerging fungal pathogen. Clin Microbiol Rev. 2008;21(4):606-25.*

26. Ans. A

Patient on azoles developing breakthrough candidemia the drug of choice is echinocandins.

Ref:
1. *Govidan R. Devitta, Hellman, and Rosenberg's Cancer: Principles and Practice of Oncology Review, 3rd edition. Philadelphia, PA: Lippincott Williams and Wilkins; 2012.*

27. Ans. B

Amphotericin B is the treatment of choice for invasive candidiasis in pregnant women.

Ref:
1. *Moudgal VV, Sobel JD. Antifungal drugs in pregnancy: a review. Expert Opin Drug Saf. 2003;2:475-83.*

28. Ans. D

The most common finding on chest CT in early invasive pulmonary aspergillosis in patients with neutropenia and hematopoietic stem cell transplant (HSCT) recipients is the presence of one or more well-circumscribed nodules. These may be in apparent on chest radiographs. Other characteristic findings include the "halo sign," a haziness surrounding a nodule or infiltrate representing the alveolar hemorrhage, and the "crescent sign" (cavitation that usually coincides with neutrophil recovery). These signs reflect different stages of hemorrhagic infarction secondary to angioinvasive organisms.

Ref:
1. *Collins J. CT signs and patterns of lung disease. Radiol Clin North Am. 2001;39:1115-35.*
2. *Walker CM, Abbott GF, Greene RE, Shepard JA, Vummidi D, Digumarthy SR. Imaging pulmonary infection: classic signs and patterns. Am J Roentgenol. 2014;202:479-92.*

29. Ans. D

The serum β-D-glucan assay has recently received FDA approval as a diagnostic adjunct. In patients with acute myeloid leukemia and myelodysplastic syndrome, the assay was highly sensitive and specific in detecting early invasive fungal infections, including candidiasis, fusariosis, trichosporonosis, and aspergillosis. It does not detect mucormycosis.

Ref:
1. *Lamoth F, Cruciani M, Mengoli C, Castagnola E, Lortholary O, Richardson M, et al. β-Glucan antigenemia assay for the diagnosis of invasive fungal infections in patients with hematological malignancies: a systematic review and meta-analysis of cohort studies from the Third European Conference on Infections in Leukemia (ECIL-3). Clin Infect Dis. 2012;54:633-43.*

30. Ans. D

Bronchoalveolar lavage cultures have approximately 50% sensitivity in focal pulmonary lesions, and definitive diagnosis often requires an invasive procedure and is usually made only when the disease is advanced. Both the serum *Aspergillus* galactomannan and β-D-glucan assays, immunoassays that detect fungal antigens in peripheral blood, have been accepted as diagnostic adjuncts of invasive fungal infections in the revised European Organization for the Research and Treatment of Cancer/Mycosis Study Group consensus criteria. False negative results can occur with piperacillin-tazobactam and few other antibiotics.

Ref:
1. *Maertens J, Maertens V, Theunissen K, Meersseman W, Meersseman P, Meers S, et al. Bronchoalveolar lavage fluid galactomannan for the diagnosis of invasive pulmonary aspergillosis in patients with hematologic diseases. Clin Infect Dis. 2009;49:1688-93.*
2. *Zou M, Tang L, Zhao S, Zhao Z, Chen L, Chen P, et al. Systematic review and meta-analysis of detecting galactomannan in bronchoalveolar lavage fluid for diagnosing invasive aspergillosis. PLoS One. 2012; 7:e43347.*
3. *Leeflang MM, Debets-Ossenkopp YJ, Visser CE, Scholten RJ, Hooft L, Bijlmer HA, et al. Galactomannan detection for invasive aspergillosis in immunocompromised patients. Cochrane Database Syst Rev. 2008;(4):CD007394.*
4. *Lamoth F, Cruciani M, Mengoli C, Castagnola E, Lortholary O, Richardson M, et al. β-Glucan antigenemia assay for the diagnosis of invasive fungal infections in patients with hematological malignancies: a systematic review and meta-analysis of cohort studies from the Third European Conference on Infections in Leukemia (ECIL-3). Clin Infect Dis. 2012;54:633-43.*

Ref:
1. *Maki DG, Mermel LA. Infections due to Infusion Therapy. In: Bennett JV, Brachman PS (Eds). Hospital Infections. Philadelphia: Lippincott-Raven; 1998. pp. 689-724.*

CHAPTER 6

Fever in Non-infection Settings

Reena Sharma

1. A 33-year-old woman presents with low-grade fever, more often in the evening hours a malar rash that is exacerbated by sun exposure. She has experienced episodes of myalgia, pleural effusion, pericarditis, and arthralgia without joint deformity over the course of several years. She has a history of hematuria and no history of drug intake prior to the onset of these symptoms. The best screening test for her disease would be:
   A. Antinuclear antibody
   B. Anti-ds-DNA antibody
   C. TB quantifier on gold test
   D. Anti-histone antibody

2. In the above case, what would be the most specific test to confirm the diagnosis?
   A. Anti-ds-DNA
   B. Anti-Ssa
   C. Anti SM-RNP
   D. Anti-histone

3. A 35-year-old male, with a known case of asthma for the last 4 years, presented with a 2-month history of fever off and on and numbness in the right upper and left lower limbs. Examination revealed asymmetric neuropathy and palpable purpura over the lower limbs. Investigations revealed eosinophilia. What is the likely diagnosis?
   A. Systemic lupus erythematosus
   B. Polyarteritis nodosa (PAN)
   C. Giant cell arteritis (GCA)
   D. Churg-Strauss syndrome

4. Which of the following statements about EGPA/Churg-Strauss syndrome is not correct?
   A. It is a rare systemic necrotizing vasculitis
   B. It affects medium-to-large sized vessels
   C. It is associated with severe asthma and blood and tissue eosinophilia
   D. It is an antineutrophil cytoplasmic antibody (ANCA)-associated vasculitides

5. A 3-year-old boy presents with fever and conjunctivitis. Physical examination is significant for oral erythema and fissuring along with a generalized maculopapular rash and cervical lymphadenopathy. What is the most likely diagnosis?
   A. Henoch-Schönlein purpura
   B. Polyarteritis nodosa
   C. Kawasaki disease
   D. Takayasu's arteritis

6. A 37-year-old female complained of fever high grade for 3 days followed by development of pain and swelling in both wrists and knees since 3 months. There is increased stiffness in the hands early in the morning, which lasts for about an hour. On examination, the metacarpophalangeal joints and wrists are warm and tender. There are no other joint abnormalities. There is no alopecia, photosensitivity, kidney disease, or rash. No history of fever episodes after the first one. What is the most likely diagnosis in this patient?
   A. Rheumatoid arthritis
   B. Polymyalgia rheumatica
   C. Gouty arthritis
   D. Osteoarthritis

7. A 35-year-old man presents with fever, bilateral conductive deafness, palpable purpura on the legs, and hemoptysis. A radiograph of the chest shows a thin-walled cavity in the left lower zone. Investigations reveal red cell casts in the urine and an elevated serum creatinine level (3 mg/dL). What is the most probable diagnosis?
   A. Henoch-Schönlein purpura
   B. Polyarteritis nodosa
   C. Granulomatosis with polyangiitis
   D. Disseminated tuberculosis

8. A 7-year-old girl has had hectic fevers for the past 5 days, a diffuse morbilliform rash on his trunk, swollen hands and feet, erythematous oral mucosa with no exudates, cracked lips, and red eyes. He has diffuse lymphadenopathy and slight hepatomegaly. He is very irritable.
   Laboratory data include:
   ESR: 80 mm/h
   RBC: Mild anemia
   Hgb: 1.1 g/dL
   WBC: 17,000/mm^3
   Platelet count: 450,000/mm^3
   Urinalysis: Some WBCs but no bacteria or proteinuria
   Echocardiography: Normal
   Spinal fluid analysis: A few lymphocytes but no organisms on Gram stain

Which of the following is the most appropriate treatment?
A. IVIG 2 g/kg over 12 hours
B. Aspirin 325 mg/day
C. Prednisone 2 mg/kg/day
D. Ibuprofen 40 mg/kg/day
E. Infliximab 5 mg/kg single dose

9. A 64-year-old woman who has had deforming RA for the past 20 years now has persistent neutropenia. She has been living in an old age home for the past 2 years. Despite bilateral knee replacements, her mobility and ability to live independently have been progressively impaired by arthritis of her ankles, feet, wrists, and hands. Past therapies have included parenteral gold, penicillamine, hydroxychloroquine, methotrexate, and etanercept. At the time of admission to the facility, she had low grade fever and her WBC was 3,200/mm³ and her physician chose to maintain her on prednisone 7.5 mg alone for her RA. Her only infection was a urinary tract infection 3 months ago treated with oral ciprofloxacin. Other than the 10-day course of ciprofloxacin, she has not been on any new medications for the past 12 months.
WBC: 1,800/mm³ (25% neutrophils, 65% lymphocytes)
Hgb: 10.3 g/dL
Peripheral smear: Paucity of neutrophils, occasional large lymphocyte with pale blue cytoplasm, and azurophilic granules.
Which of the following studies is most likely to establish the diagnosis?
A. Abdominal ultrasonography to measure spleen size
B. Flow cytometry of peripheral blood
C. Test for cyclic citrullinated peptide (CCP) antibodies
D. Granulocyte antibody test
E. Test for antinuclear antibodies (ANA)

10. An 80-year-old man was brought to the hospital with a 2-day history of a swollen, red, warm, and tender elbow. He has a temperature of 100.9°F (38.27°C). On admission, WBC was 12,500/mm³ with 60% PMN, and chest radiograph showed mild right lower lobe atelectasis. His elbow was aspirated and 4 cc of cloudy fluid was obtained. Synovial fluid analysis showed cloudy fluid with a WBC of 95,000/mm³. Gram stain was negative, and the fluid was sent for culture. The patient was started on an intravenous antibiotic to cover gram-positive bacteria for presumed septic arthritis.
His elbow is held in a flexed position and is slightly swollen in the area between the olecranon and lateral epicondyle. It is minimally erythematous, warm, and tender. He resists any attempt to move the elbow. Findings on examination of the other joints are normal. CBC now has a WBC of 10,000/mm³. Radiograph of the elbow shows only soft tissue swelling. His synovial fluid and blood cultures have no growth. Sputum Gram stain shows a few gram-positive cocci in pairs but grows out mixed flora. Which of the following is the most appropriate next step in management?
A. Surgical open drainage of the joint
B. Continue present antibiotic regimen
C. Aspirate the elbow and look for crystals
D. Add another antibiotic to cover gram-negative organisms

11. An 8-year-old boy has high grade fevers for the past 5 days, a diffuse evanescent rash on his trunk and polyarthralgia. He has diffuse lymphadenopathy and slight hepatomegaly.
Laboratory data include:
ESR: 80 mm/h
RBC: Mild anemia
Hgb: 8.8 g/dL
WBC: 17,000/mm³
Platelet count: 650,000/mm³
Urinalysis: Some WBCs but no bacteria or proteinuria
Which of the following is the most appropriate diagnosis?
A. Kawasaki's disease
B. Juvenile idiopathic arthritis
C. Juvenile SLE
D. Acute rheumatic fever
E. Still's disease

12. What is the best diagnostic test for confirming the diagnosis in the above case?
A. Rheumatoid factor
B. ANA
C. Serum ferritin
D. C-reactive protein (CRP)

13. A 52-year-old man is evaluated in the emergency department for a 2-week history of progressive fever and malaise with gradual onset of shortness of breath, pleuritic chest pain, myalgia, arthralgia, and rash. He reports no cough. He has a 15-year history of RA, which is well controlled with methotrexate and etanercept; his last flare was 1 year ago. Other medications are naproxen and folic acid.
On physical examination, temperature is 39.0°C (102.2°F), blood pressure is 148/94 mm Hg, pulse rate is 90 beats/min, and respiration rate is 22 breaths/min. Cardiac examination is normal. Pulmonary examination reveals a left pleural friction rub. There is synovial thickening of the

wrists and metacarpophalangeal and proximal interphalangeal joints bilaterally as well as small bilateral knee effusions. A nonblanching purpuric rash is noted over the distal lower extremities. Investigations are suggestive of pancytopenia with raised ESR, and chest radiograph reveals blunted costophrenic angles bilaterally without infiltrate. Blood and urine culture results are pending.

Which of the following is the most appropriate diagnostic test to perform next?

A. Antinuclear antibody and anti-double-stranded DNA antibody assay
B. Bone marrow aspiration and biopsy
C. CT of the chest, abdomen, and pelvis
D. Rheumatoid factor and anti-cyclic citrullinated peptide antibody assay

14. A 71-year-old man was recently admitted to the emergency room for management of congestive heart failure. While hospitalized, he experienced acute and spontaneous onset of right knee pain and swelling with spike in temperature.
He has a longstanding history of seronegative nodular RA that has been refractory to disease-modifying anti-rheumatic drugs (DMARDs), including hydroxychloroquine and methotrexate, but responsive to brief courses of prednisone.
On physical examination, his fingers are deformed with nodules at the proximal but not distal IP joints (see figure below). He has bilateral, cool olecranon bursa. His right knee is visibly swollen, erythematous, and warm to the touch and has a ballotable effusion.

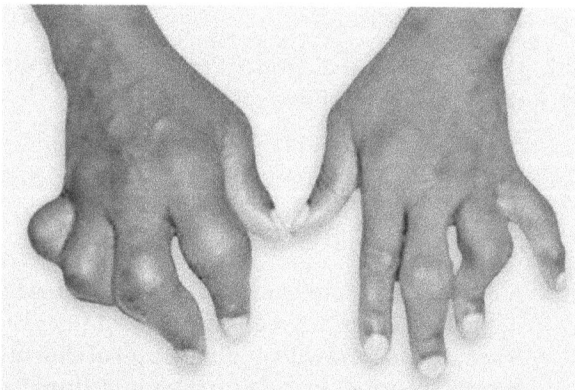

Which of the following is the most appropriate course of action?

A. Obtain a radiograph of the inflamed knee
B. Perform arthrocentesis on the inflamed knee
C. Start a nonsteroidal anti-inflammatory drug (NSAID)
D. Start "pulse" corticosteroids

15. A 52-year-old woman with longstanding lupus treated with low-dose corticosteroids and hydroxychloroquine has been doing well for many years apart from occasional spikes in temperature with polyarthralgia lasting for 3–4 days at 2–3 months intervals. She presented at age 18 with severe Raynaud's phenomenon and finger necrosis that was treated with IV cyclophosphamide. Other manifestations included chronic thrombocytopenia and pulmonary embolus secondary to antiphospholipid antibodies. She has never had cardiac or kidney involvement. The patient would like to stop taking hydroxychloroquine because she has been doing so well and finds the yearly eye examinations inconvenient.

Which of the following is most appropriate advice to the patient at this time?

A. Stop the annual eye examinations
B. Discontinue the hydroxychloroquine
C. Continue the hydroxychloroquine
D. Discontinue visual field testing at her annual eye examinations
E. Increase the dose of corticosteroids

16. A 38-year-old woman has had a 4-month history of low-grade fever, oral ulcers, and recurring confluent erythematous macules over the sun-exposed areas of the forearms, anterior torso, face, and neck that are occasionally associated with superficial ulceration. She has not had associated sicca symptoms, xerostomia, or joint problems. Evaluation at the time her symptoms began was remarkable only for the rash and an otherwise very fair complexion; serology studies were notable for positive ANA at a titer of 1:640 (speckled pattern) and anti-SSA/Ro antibodies in a significant elevated titer. She was initially advised to use a high SPF sunscreen and was prescribed hydroxychloroquine 400 mg daily and prednisone 40 mg daily. The rash promptly responded to corticosteroids but has flared each time the prednisone is tapered below 20 mg/day. Other than persistent leukopenia (WBC 2,200/mm^3), other blood counts, chemistry profile, and urinalysis have been repeatedly normal.

Which of the following is the most appropriate recommendation at this time?

A. Add pulse intravenous cyclophosphamide 750 mg/m^2
B. Add azathioprine 2 mg/kg/day
C. Add dapsone 50 mg/day
D. Add quinacrine 100 mg/day
E. Add thalidomide 50 mg/day

17. A 35-year-old male patient is undergoing evaluation following diagnosis with hepatitis C infection and RA. Which of these drugs is most appropriate for treatment of this patient's RA?

A. Etanercept
B. Adalimumab
C. Certolizumab pegol
D. Infliximab
E. Golimumab

18. Which of these adverse events is uncommon in a patient with psoriatic arthritis (PsA) who is taking apremilast?
    A. Diarrhea
    B. Fever
    C. Nausea
    D. Headache
    E. Insomnia

19. Which of these statements regarding serologic testing for patients with suspected Lyme disease is true?
    A. Western blot testing should be performed first
    B. Enzyme immunoassay (EIA) is an option for second-tier testing
    C. Serologic tests are insensitive during the initial infection
    D. Results of IgM testing are sufficient for diagnosis

20. Which of these statements regarding Whipple disease is true?
    A. It is diagnosed via small-bowel biopsy
    B. It is characterized by arthralgia alone
    C. Doxycycline and hydroxychloroquine for 1 month is recommended
    D. Patients should have treatment as needed for re-infections

21. A 25-year-old male patient is undergoing evaluation because of migratory arthritis. 3 weeks ago, he reports he had fever with sore throat which was diagnosed with "strep throat." Poststreptococcal reactive arthritis (PSReA) is suspected. Which of these statements regarding PSReA is true?
    A. It generally occurs within 10 days of the infection
    B. It is responsive to NSAIDs
    C. Cardiac involvement is common
    D. Extra-articular manifestations are common

22. Your 57-year-old male patient is undergoing evaluation because of skin eruptions, myalgia, and polyarthralgia. He also has a 3-day history of fever, chills, and aching joints. 15 years ago, he underwent gastric bypass surgery. Bowel-associated dermatosis-arthritis syndrome (BADAS) is suspected. Which of these laboratory results is most likely in this patient?
    A. Elevated rheumatoid factor (RF) levels
    B. Elevated anti-nuclear antibody levels
    C. Elevated uric acid levels
    D. Presence of cryoglobulins in the serum

23. A patient with established RA continues to have high disease activity while receiving combination disease-modifying antirheumatic drug (DMARD) therapy. The addition of an anti-TNF biologic agent is being considered. Which of these is the most appropriate approach for latent tuberculosis testing in this patient prior to initiating anti-TNF therapy?
    A. Screening following a positive chest X-ray only
    B. Screening following identification of a risk factor only
    C. Screening following identification of a prior BCG vaccination only
    D. Screening regardless of additional factors

24. A patient with RA is undergoing evaluation because of the recent onset of skin abnormalities, unintentional weight loss, and fever. The presence of which of these findings in this patient is most likely to be a distinguishing marker of rheumatoid vasculitis?
    A. Perivascular infiltrates that do not involve the vessel wall
    B. Nail fold infarcts
    C. Inflammation of >3 cell layers of the vessel
    D. Capillaritis documented by histopathology

25. A 32-year-old woman presents to her GP complaining of fatigue, joint stiffness and pain, mouth ulcers, and hair loss. She first noticed fatigue about 6 months ago, and at that time, complete blood count and thyroid function tests were normal. Since then, she feels like her symptoms are getting progressively worse. For the past 1 month, she has had an area of hair loss on her scalp associated with a raised scaly rash. During this time, she intermittently developed painful mouth ulcerations that would spontaneously resolve. She also reports a severe "sunburn" on her face, upper neck, and back that occurred after <1 hour of sun exposure and which was unusual for her. On physical examination, the vital signs are: temperature—39.6°C, blood pressure—136/82 mm Hg, heart rate—98 beats/min, respiratory rate—19 breaths/min, and SaO$_2$—98% on room air. The oropharynx shows a single 2-mm aphthous ulceration on the buccal mucosa. Both wrists and knee were inflamed. Other system examinations are normal. Laboratory studies show the following: White blood cell count—2,300/L; Hemoglobin—8.9 g/dL; Platelets—98,000/L; and the differential is 80% polymorphonuclear cells, 12% lymphocytes, 7% monocytes, 1% eosinophils, and 1% basophils. ANA is positive at a titer of 1:640. Antibodies to double-stranded DNA are negative, and anti-Smith antibodies are positive at a titer of 1:160. The rheumatoid factor level is 37 IU/L. What is the most likely diagnosis?
    A. Behçet's disease
    B. Discoid lupus erythematosus
    C. Rheumatoid arthritis
    D. Sarcoidosis
    E. Systemic lupus erythematosus

26. A 26-year-old woman is evaluated for a 2-month history of pain and swelling in the hands and daily morning stiffness that lasts for 3 to 4 hours. She is 4 months postpartum, and her pregnancy was without complications. She has no history of rash and is otherwise well. Her only medication is ibuprofen, which has not sufficiently relieved her symptoms. On physical examination, temperature is 100°C, blood pressure is 110/68 mm Hg, pulse rate is 92 beats/min, and respiration rate is 20 breaths/min. The second and third proximal interphalangeal and metacarpophalangeal joints and the wrists are tender and swollen bilaterally. Laboratory studies show an erythrocyte sedimentation rate of 67 mm/h and titers of IgM antibodies against Parvovirus B19 are negative. Which of the following is the most likely diagnosis?

   A. Gout
   B. Osteoarthritis
   C. Parvovirus B19 infection
   D. Rheumatoid arthritis

27. A 42-year-old Turkish man presents to his physician complaining of recurring ulcers in the mouth and on his penis. He states that the ulcers are painful and last for about 2 weeks before spontaneously resolving. In addition, he intermittently gets skin lesions that he describes as painful nodules on his lower extremities associated with low-grade fever. You suspect that he has Behçet's syndrome. A pathergy test is performed. What response would you expect after injecting 0.3 mL of sterile saline under the skin?

   A. Development of 10 mm of induration with overlying erythema after 72 hours
   B. Development of a 2- to 3-mm papule at the site of insertion in 2–3 days
   C. Development of granulomatous inflammation 4–6 weeks after the injection
   D. Development of an urticarial reaction within 15 minutes
   E. No reaction

28. A 53-year-old man is evaluated in the emergency department for a 2-day history of acute swelling and pain in the right knee. He also has had fever up to 38.3°C (101.0°F). 3 weeks ago, he was evaluated in the emergency department for cellulitis. Medical history is significant for chronic tophaceous gout and hypertension. Medications are allopurinol, atenolol, and enalapril. He has a monogamous sexual relationship with his wife of 30 years. On physical examination, temperature is 38.1°C (100.5°F), blood pressure is 124/90 mm Hg, and pulse rate is 98 beats/min. Cardiopulmonary examination is normal. Tophi are present on both elbows. The right fourth proximal interphalangeal joint and left third metacarpophalangeal joint have soft-tissue swelling but no warmth or erythema. The right knee is markedly swollen and has overlying warmth and erythema. Palpation of this joint elicits pain. Laboratory studies reveal a leukocyte count of 15,000/μL (15 × 10⁹/L). Arthrocentesis is performed. The synovial fluid leukocyte count is 110,000/μL (95% neutrophils). Polarized light microscopy of the fluid reveals negatively birefringent monosodium urate crystals. Gram stain of the aspirated fluid is negative. Culture results are pending. Which of the following is the most appropriate treatment for this patient?

   A. Ciprofloxacin
   B. Intra-articular corticosteroids
   C. Prednisone
   D. Vancomycin

29. A 24-year-old woman is evaluated for a 2-week history of persistent pain and swelling in the right foot and knee and the left heel. One month ago, she developed an episode of conjunctivitis that resolved spontaneously. She also had an episode of severe diarrhea with high grade fever which lasted for 3 days, 1 month ago while that was successfully treated with a 3-day course of ciprofloxacin and loperamide. She has not had other infections of the gastrointestinal or genitourinary tract, rash, or oral ulcerations. Her weight has been stable, and she has not had abdominal pain, blood in the stool, or changes in her bowel habits. Musculoskeletal examination reveals swelling, warmth, and tenderness of the right knee and ankle. There is tenderness to palpation at the insertion site of the left Achilles tendon. Which of the following is the most likely diagnosis?

   A. Enteropathic arthritis   B. Psoriatic arthritis
   C. Reactive arthritis   D. Rheumatoid arthritis

30. A 63-year-old woman is evaluated during a follow-up visit for a 4-week history of fatigue; pain in the proximal interphalangeal joints, knees, and hips; and low-grade fever. She has not had joint swelling, chest pain, or shortness of breath. Over the past 4 years, she has had progressive dryness of the eyes and mouth. She has a 5-month history of Raynaud phenomenon, which has been less symptomatic since beginning nifedipine 4 months ago. On physical examination, temperature is 38.2°C (100.8°F), blood pressure is 125/72 mm Hg, pulse rate is 74 beats/min, and respiration rate is 18 breaths/min. Cardiac examination is normal, and the lungs are clear. She has bilateral parotid gland enlargement, a firm 4-cm left axillary lymph node, and a shotty 0.3-cm

left anterior cervical lymph node. Musculoskeletal examination reveals bilateral crepitus of the knees. There is no joint swelling. Laboratory studies: Hemoglobin—11.6 g/dL (116 g/L); Leukocyte count—3,400/μL (3.4 × 10^9/L); Platelet count—120,000/μL (120 × 10^9/L); Rheumatoid factor—76 U/mL (76 kU/L); Antinuclear antibodies—positive; Anti-Ro/SSA antibodies—positive; Anti-La/SSB antibodies—positive; Urinalysis—normal; Blood cultures—no growth; and a chest radiograph and mammogram are normal.

Which of the following is the next best step in this?

A. Excisional axillary lymph node biopsy
B. Minor salivary gland biopsy
C. Prednisone
D. Transthoracic echocardiography

ANSWERS WITH EXPLANATIONS

1. **Ans. A**

A malar rash with arthralgia, serositis, and hematuria in a female of childbearing age suggests the possibility of systemic lupus erythematosus (SLE). However, an SLE-like picture may be seen in drug-induced lupus and mixed connective tissue disorder. Antinuclear antibody is the most sensitive test to screen for SLE. Its repeated absence virtually rules out the possibility of SLE. Anti-ds-DNA (and anti-Sm) antibodies have high specificity and are used to confirm the diagnosis of SLE; however, because of their poor sensitivity, they are not used as screening tests. Anti-histone antibody is seen in drug-induced lupus (which is unlikely, as there is no history of drug intake prior to the onset of symptoms).

Ref:
1. *Rahman A, Isenberg DA. Systemic lupus erythematosus and related disorders. In: Warrell DA, Cox TM, Firth JD (Eds). Oxford Textbook of Medicine, 5th edition. Oxford: Oxford University Press; 2010.*
2. *Hahn B. Systemic lupus erythematosus. In: Longo DL, Fauci AS, Kasper DL, Hauser SL, Jameson J, Loscalzo J (Eds). Harrison's Principles of Internal Medicine, 18th edition. New York: McGraw Hill Professional; 2011.*

2. **Ans. A**

As described in Answer 1.

3. **Ans. D**

Peripheral neuropathy is broadly divided into mononeuritis simplex, mononeuritis multiplex, and polyneuropathy. This patient has asymmetric neuropathy or mononeuritis multiplex. Common causes of mononeuritis multiplex are vasculitic syndromes, infectious diseases such as HIV or leprosy, and other conditions such as diabetes. A vasculitic neuropathy (palpable purpura) with asthma and eosinophilia favors the diagnosis of Churg-Strauss syndrome or as is called the eosinophilic granulomatous polyangiitis. Asthma and eosinophilia are not seen in conditions such as SLE, GCA, or PAN.

Ref:
1. *Langford CA, Fauci AS. The Vasculitis Syndromes. In: Longo DL, Fauci AS, Kasper DL, Hauser SL, Jameson J, Loscalzo J (Eds). Harrison's Principles of Internal Medicine, 18th edition. New York: McGraw Hill Professional; 2011.*
2. *Wells AU, M. du Bois R. The lung in vasculitis. In: Warrell DA, Cox TM, Firth JD (Eds). Oxford Textbook of Medicine, 5th edition. Oxford: Oxford University Press; 2010.*

4. **Ans. B**

Eosinophilic granulomatosis with polyangiitis (EGPA), or as it was traditionally termed, Churg–Strauss syndrome, is a rare systemic necrotizing vasculitis that affects small-to-medium-sized vessels and is associated with severe asthma and blood and tissue eosinophilia. Like granulomatosis with polyangiitis (Wegener granulomatosis) and the microscopic form of periarteritis (i.e., microscopic polyangiitis), EGPA is an ANCA-associated vasculitides. In 1951, Churg and Strauss first described the syndrome in 13 patients who had asthma, eosinophilia, granulomatous inflammation, necrotizing systemic vasculitis, and necrotizing glomerulonephritis.

Ref:
1. *Lowe ST. Eosinophilic granulomatosis with polyangiitis (Churg-Strauss Syndrome). [online] Available from: https://emedicine.medscape.com/article/333492-treatment [Last accessed February, 2020].*

5. **Ans. C**

Symptoms of vasculitis vary greatly and depend upon the organs affected and the severity of the disease. The involvement of large vessels (giant cell arteritis, Takayasu's disease) frequently results in limb claudication, asymmetric blood pressure in the limbs, and the absence of pulses. The involvement of medium vessels (polyarteritis nodosa, Kawasaki disease) results in cutaneous nodules, livedo reticularis, microaneurysms, and mononeuritis multiplex. The involvement of small vessels

(ANCA-associated vasculitis, Henoch–Schönlein purpura) results in glomerulonephritis, purpura, and alveolar hemorrhage. Kawasaki disease often begins with fever that is not very responsive to paracetamol. Bilateral conjunctival injection usually begins shortly after the onset of fever. It is not purulent, and it is not painful. Oral manifestations of this disease include erythematous and swollen lips and "strawberry tongue." Cervical lymphadenopathy is seen in about three-fourths of patients, which are usually nontender and nonsuppurative. Henoch–Schönlein purpura presents with abdominal pain, rashes, palpable purpura, and arthritis. Polyarteritis nodosa and Takayasu's arteritis have distinct presentations and are unlikely at this age.

Ref:
1. Langford CA, Fauci AS. The vasculitis syndromes. In: Longo DL, Fauci AS, Kasper DL, Hauser SL, Jameson J, Loscalzo J (Eds). Harrison's Principles of Internal Medicine, 18th edition. New York: McGraw Hill Professional; 2011.
2. Kawasaki T. Acute febrile mucocutaneous syndrome with lymphoid involvement with specific desquamation of the fingers and toes in children. Arerugi. 1967;16(3):178-222.

6. **Ans. A**

Among articular disorders, gout and the spondyloarthropathies are more common in men, whereas rheumatoid arthritis (RA) and lupus are more frequent in women. This female patient has symmetrical arthritis with early morning stiffness and involvement of the wrist and metacarpophalangeal joints. All of them are characteristic features of RA. Osteoarthritis is seen in elderly patients and is noninflammatory arthritis. Gout is common in males or postmenopausal females. Its most common presentation is acute mono-articular arthritis, frequently involving the first metatarsophalangeal joint. Swelling and tenderness of the metacarpophalangeal joints and wrists suggests articular disorder and hence rules out polymyalgia rheumatica.

Ref:
1. Maini RN. Rheumatoid arthritis. In: Warrell DA, Cox TM, Firth JD (Eds). Oxford Textbook of Medicine, 5th edition. Oxford: Oxford University Press; 2010.
2. Shah A, St. Clair E. Rheumatoid arthritis. In: Longo DL, Fauci AS, Kasper DL, Hauser SL, Jameson J, Loscalzo J (Eds). Harrison's Principles of Internal Medicine, 18th edition. New York: McGraw Hill Professional; 2011.

7. **Ans. C**

With vasculitis, lung involvement is commonly seen with granulomatosis with polyangiitis, microscopic PAN, Churg-Strauss disease, and Takayasu's arteritis. PAN and Henoch–Schönlein purpura rarely show lung involvement. A triad of upper respiratory tract diseases (including rhinitis, sinusitis, and otitis media), lower respiratory disease (including pulmonary nodules, cavities, and hemoptysis), and glomerulonephritis (red cell cast, raised creatinine) characterizes granulomatosis with polyangiitis (Wegner's granulomatosis). Polyarteritis nodosa is not associated with glomerulonephritis (red cell casts) and Henoch–Schönlein purpura typically presents in children between 4 and 7 years of age. Disseminated tuberculosis is often associated with features such as fever, anorexia, and weight loss. In addition, a history of exposure to another patient with tuberculosis or a history of HIV infection is frequently elicited.

Ref:
1. Langford CA, Fauci AS. The vasculitis syndromes. In: Longo DL, Fauci AS, Kasper DL, Hauser SL, Jameson J, Loscalzo J (Eds). Harrison's Principles of Internal Medicine, 18th edition. New York: McGraw Hill Professional; 2011.
2. Wells AU, du Bois RM. The lung in vasculitis. In: Warrell DA, Cox TM, Firth JD (Eds). Oxford Textbook of Medicine, 5th edition. Oxford: Oxford University Press; 2010.

8. **Ans. A**

The clinical description is classic for Kawasaki disease. Although staphylococcal toxic shock syndrome and EBV and CMV infections can sometimes present in a similar way, echocardiographic changes are often later in the course.

When there is a clinical index of suspicion for Kawasaki disease, the recommended treatment is high dose IVIG over 12 hours. This is most effective early in the course, before periungual desquamation or echocardiographic changes have occurred. Corticosteroids may be used if IVIG has failed; aspirin (not ibuprofen) is recommended as an antiplatelet agent. Studies are ongoing to determine effectiveness of anti-TNF agents in Kawasaki disease; their effectiveness in treatment is not yet established.

9. **Ans. B**

The leading diagnostic considerations for this patient are Felty's syndrome and large granular lymphocyte (LGL) syndrome. The LGL syndrome is a clonal disorder of cytotoxic T-lymphocytes and has been classified as leukemia, even though it usually has an indolent clinical course. About 25% of patients with LGL syndrome have RA. The demonstration of a clonal population of CD3+, CD8+, CD16+, CD57+ T cells with flow cytometry of the peripheral blood would serve to establish the diagnosis of LGL syndrome. Splenomegaly and granulocyte antibodies are common to both disorders. The histopathology of the bone marrow does not usually differentiate the two.

10. **Ans. C**

    Calcium pyrophosphate dihydrate (CPPD) crystals can elicit an intense inflammatory response in a single joint that may mimic septic arthritis. It is appropriate to start antibiotics in this clinical setting, but when cultures are negative, one should suspect a crystal-induced process. Open drainage is appropriate in septic arthritis, if the joint effusion cannot be controlled by percutaneous aspiration.

11. **Ans. E**

    Still's disease/Systemic-onset juvenile idiopathic arthritis is marked by the severity of the extra-articular manifestations (fever, cutaneous eruptions) and by an equal sex ratio.

    It represents 10-11% of cases of juvenile idiopathic arthritis (JIA). The prevalence has been estimated at 1-10 in 30,000 children with an annual incidence of 1-20 in 900,000 children.

    Onset usually occurs between 3 and 5 years of age. The clinical signs include fever with oscillating temperatures over a 24-hour period and peaks of over 39°C or more. These fever peaks are associated with transient cutaneous eruptions and diffuse erythematosis or urticarial-like lesions. The presence of arthritis is essential for diagnosis but may appear later in the disease course. The number of sites affected is variable (mono-, oligo- or polyarthritis) affecting both the small and large joints in a nearly symmetrical manner. This characteristic diagnostic triad may also be associated with an adenopathy and hepatosplenomegaly. Visceral complications (pericarditis, pleural effusion or serous peritonitis with abdominal pain) may be present. There are no specific biological signs but the inflammatory disease is severe with a large increase in the level of ferritin and a decrease in the percentage of glycosylated ferritin.

12. **Ans. C**

    As described in Answer 11.

13. **Ans. A**

    Testing for ANA, as well as anti-double-stranded DNA antibodies and complement levels, is indicated for this patient with suspected drug-induced lupus erythematosus (DILE) caused by the tumor necrosis factor (TNF)-α inhibitor etanercept. He has new-onset fever, arthralgia, myalgia, nonblanching purpuric rash, pleuritis, pancytopenia, and proteinuria with active urine sediment, all of which are suggestive of a clinical diagnosis of SLE. Although these findings might also be compatible with an infection, he has no focal symptoms or findings to suggest sepsis and has been appropriately tested with blood and urine cultures. Most patients with DILE caused by TNF-α inhibitors have fever, rash, arthritis, and hematologic abnormalities in the presence of positive ANA as well as anti-double-stranded DNA antibodies. This clinical and serologic profile is in contrast to DILE induced by other medications, which is characterized by positive ANA, anti-histone antibodies, and anti-single-stranded DNA antibodies. Nephritis is not common but has been reported in patients with DILE caused by TNF-α inhibitors.

    If DILE and infection are both ruled out, bone marrow aspiration and biopsy to evaluate for the presence of a primary hematologic diagnosis or CT of the chest, abdomen, and pelvis to evaluate for lymphadenopathy suggestive of underlying lymphoma would be indicated.

    Testing of rheumatoid factor and anti-CCP antibodies is not appropriate because the patient has had a clear diagnosis of RA, and, even if a flare were present, rheumatoid factor and anti-CCP antibodies would not necessarily increase.

14. **Ans. B**

    Although the patient carries the diagnosis of "nodular rheumatoid arthritis" and is already being treated with disease-modifying agents, a patient with rheumatoid nodules would be expected to be seropositive for rheumatoid factor. This merits a reassessment of his diagnosis and management.

    The most appropriate course of action is to perform arthrocentesis to assist in both re-evaluating the underlying diagnosis and in determining why this joint is flaring out of proportion to the other joints in what is normally a symmetric polyarthritis–rheumatoid arthritis.

    Radiography would be useful in ruling out a bony injury if there were a history of trauma. Instead, the patient's symptoms developed spontaneously and only after admission. NSAIDs and/or pulse corticosteroids are effective interventions for the acute management of many inflammatory arthritis, but their salt- and fluid-retentive effects could be deleterious to the patient because he has congestive heart failure.

15. **Ans. C**

    Hydroxychloroquine is a useful treatment for the cutaneous and musculoskeletal manifestations of lupus. Irreversible retinal toxicity is rare but occurs with greater frequency the longer the drug is used. The permanent visual damage results from binding of the drug to melanin. The recommended dose is 5 mg/kg. Discontinuation of hydroxychloroquine has been associated with an increased risk of flares.

Eye examinations should be continued while the patient takes antimalarial medications, especially if the patient has been taking them for many years. A full visual field and color test is required to optimally track the retinal effects of hydroxychloroquine. Increasing steroids in lieu of taking hydroxychloroquine increases the likelihood of corticosteroid-related complications; corticosteroid use should be kept at a minimum.

16. **Ans. D**

    Cutaneous manifestations of lupus are quite variable, manifesting as erythematous macular or maculopapular rashes, discoid plaques, bullous lesions, or vasculitis manifest as nonblanching purpura, cutaneous ulcers, or urticarial lesions. While antimalarials are effective for suppressing many of the cutaneous manifestations of lupus and corticosteroids in sufficient dose will usually affect resolution of cutaneous flares, other immunomodulating therapies are often required to suppress cutaneous manifestations of lupus to avoid the toxicity associated with long-term corticosteroid use.

    Intravenous pulse cyclophosphamide is effective in managing severe manifestations of SLE but is typically reserved for severe lupus nephritis, severe CNS manifestations, or refractory severe immune-mediated cytopenias, with other less toxic options employed to manage active skin disease. Azathioprine is often effective as a corticosteroid-sparing therapy for a variety of lupus manifestations, including skin disease. However, concurrent leukopenia as is present in this patient may preclude use of azathioprine in doses sufficient to effectively manage skin disease. In the setting of leukopenia, mycophenolate mofetil might also be considered as an alternative to azathioprine as a corticosteroid-sparing therapy because it impacts predominantly lymphocyte proliferation with minimal impact on granulopoiesis, but the efficacy of mycophenolate in managing cutaneous manifestations of lupus is not well established.

    Other alternatives that do not impact granulopoiesis, such as dapsone, addition of a second antimalarial, or thalidomide, are often quite effective in managing cutaneous manifestations of lupus. Dapsone has been shown to be particularly useful in managing cutaneous ulcers in SLE caused by small vessel vasculitis or bullous disease. Persistent maculopapular eruptions that are not adequately suppressed with hydroxychloroquine often will respond to addition of a second antimalarial such as quinacrine. If this option is used, combined use of these two antimalarials is more effective than either alone and the concurrent use of both is recommended rather than discontinuing hydroxychloroquine and adding quinacrine.

    Quinacrine is usually well tolerated although patients with a fair complexion may find it objectionable because of predictable yellow discoloration of the skin with prolonged use. Thalidomide is highly effective in managing mucocutaneous ulcers, as well as refractory erythematous rashes, including the eruption associated with subacute cutaneous lupus, a variant associated with elevated titers of anti-SSA/Ro antibodies.

17. **Ans. A**

    The American College of Rheumatology's panel on RA recommends etanercept for the treatment of RA patients with hepatitis C.
    Ref:
    1. Singh JA, Furst DE, Bharat A, Bharat A, Curtis JR, Kavanaugh AF, et al. 2012 update of the 2008 American College of Rheumatology recommendations for the use of disease-modifying antirheumatic drugs and biologic agents in the treatment of rheumatoid arthritis. Arthritis Care Res. 2012;64(5):625-39.

18. **Ans. B**

    Fever has not been reported in patients taking apremilast. However, nasopharyngitis and URTI occurred in 2.6% and 3.9% of patients, respectively, with up to 112 days of treatment with apremilast. Diarrhea, nausea, and vomiting occurred in more than 5% of patients in clinical trials and were the most common adverse events leading to discontinuation of apremilast.
    Ref:
    1. Celgene Corporation. OTEZLA® (apremilast) tablets, for oral use (2014). [online] Available from: https://media2.celgene.com/content/uploads/otezla-pi.pdf [Last accessed February, 2020].

19. **Ans. C**

    During the initial phase, patients with an erythema migrans rash may be diagnosed clinically. A two-tier testing protocol is recommended for serologic testing for Lyme disease—EIA or immunofluorescence assay tests performed first and followed by Western blot if they are positive or equivocal. Positive IgM results alone are not sufficient to diagnose current Lyme disease; therefore, only IgG testing should be performed in persons with illness >1 month.
    Ref:
    1. US Department of Health and Human Services (2014). Tickborne Diseases of the United States: A Reference Manual for Health Care Providers, 2nd edition.

20. **Ans. A**

    Whipple disease is caused by *Tropheryma whipplei* and is characterized by arthralgia and diarrhea. The disease is diagnosed by the histological involvement seen in small-bowel biopsy. A 1-year treatment with doxycycline and hydroxychloroquine is recommended,

and patients should have lifelong treatment with doxycycline to prevent re-infections.
Ref:
1. Lagier JC, Fenollar F, Lepidi H, Giorgi R, Million M, Raoult D. Treatment of classic Whipple's disease: from in vitro results to clinical outcome. J Antimicrob Chemother. 2014;69(1):219-27.

21. **Ans. D**

Poststreptococcal reactive arthritis presents on average 21 days after infection. It is unresponsive to aspirin or other NSAIDs. Cardiac involvement is not common, but extra-articular manifestations, such as tenosynovitis, are often seen.
Ref:
1. Grover V, Dibner R. Polyarthritis following a streptococcal infection, a doctor's dilemma in treatment: a case report. Cases J. 2009;2:9140.

22. **Ans. D**

Rheumatoid factor, anti-nuclear antibody, immunoglobulin, and uric acid levels are usually within normal limits in patients with BADAS. However, cryoglobulins have been reported in the serum during symptomatic periods.
Ref:
1. Patton T, Jukic D, Juhas E. Atypical histopathology in bowel-associated dermatosis-arthritis syndrome: a case report. Dermatol Online J. 2009;15(3):3.

23. **Ans. D**

Screening to identify latent tuberculosis infection is recommended for all patients with RA who are being considered for therapy with biologic agents.
Ref:
1. Singh JA, Furst DE, Bharat A, Bharat A, Curtis JR, Kavanaugh AF, et al. 2012 update of the 2008 American College of Rheumatology recommendations for the use of disease-modifying antirheumatic drugs and biologic agents in the treatment of rheumatoid arthritis. Arthritis Care Res. 2012;64(5):625-639.

24. **Ans. C**

This is considered to be a sensitive and specific finding to determine the presence of vasculitis in RA. The other conditions can be seen in RA without vasculitis.
Ref:
1. Bartels CM, Bridges AJ. Rheumatoid vasculitis: vanishing menace or target for new treatments? Curr Rheumatol Rep. 2010;12(6):414-9.

25. **Ans. E**

Systemic lupus erythematosus is an autoimmune disease. It can affect the skin, joints, kidneys, brain, and other organs. Symptoms vary from person to person, and may come and go. Everyone with SLE has joint pain and swelling at some time. Some develop arthritis. SLE often affects the joints of the fingers, hands, wrists, and knees. Other common symptoms include chest pain when taking a deep breath, fatigue, fever with no other cause, general discomfort, uneasiness, or ill feeling (malaise), hair loss, weight loss, mouth sores, sensitivity to sunlight, and skin rash. A "butterfly" rash develops in about half the people with SLE. The rash is mostly seen over the cheeks and bridge of the nose. It can be widespread. It gets worse in sunlight. Diagnostic tests include antinuclear antibody, complement components (C3 and C4), and antibodies to double-stranded DNA.
Ref:
1. MedlinePlus. Systemic lupus erythematosus. [online] Available from: https://medlineplus.gov/ency/article/000435.htm [Last accessed February, 2020].

26. **Ans. D**

The 2010 ACR/EULAR classification criteria for RA are designed to identify patients with unexplained inflammatory arthritis in at least one peripheral joint and a short duration of symptoms who would benefit from early therapeutic intervention. According to the ACR/EULAR criteria, patients who should be tested are those—(1) who have at least one joint with definite clinical synovitis and (2) whose synovitis is not better explained by another disease (e.g., lupus, psoriatic arthritis, or gout). The ACR/EULAR classification system is a score-based algorithm for RA that incorporates the following four factors: Joint involvement, serology test results, acute-phase reactant test results, and patient self-reporting of the duration of signs and symptoms. The maximum number of points possible is 10. A classification of definitive RA requires a score of 6/10 or higher. This patient fits into the criteria for RA.

27. **Ans. B**

Pathergy test (PT) is an easy to perform skin test to look for the pathergy phenomenon. This test is used as a criterion in most diagnostic criteria for Behçet's disease.

Clinical evaluation: Readings are taken after 48 hours of the needle prick. A 1-2 mm papule that is usually felt by palpation and which is surrounded by an erythematous halo is formed on the skin. The papule may remain as a papule or transform into a 1-5 mm pustule. The pustule becomes prominent in 24 hours, becomes maximum in size in 48 hours, and disappears in 45 days. Erythema without induration is interpreted as a negative result.

28. **Ans. B**

Several different therapies, including systemic and intra-articular glucocorticoids, NSAIDs, and colchicine, are each effective for the treatment of the gout flare; there is no single best agent for all patients experiencing a flare. The availability of multiple classes of agents and approaches likely to provide treatment benefit permits the opportunity to choose therapy, based upon an assessment of specific features of the individual patient and the flare history, is most likely to achieve benefit and minimize the risk of adverse therapeutic consequences. Arthrocentesis is suggested in patients with joint fluid aspiration and intra-articular injection of glucocorticoids for patients with gout who have only one or two actively inflamed joints or are unable to take oral medications, and (in either situation) for whom the likelihood of infection is judged remote.

29. **Ans. C**

Reactive arthritis is joint pain and swelling triggered by an infection in another part of your body—most often your intestines, genitals or urinary tract. Reactive arthritis usually targets your knees and the joints of ankles and feet. Inflammation also can affect your eyes, skin, and urethra. The signs and symptoms of reactive arthritis generally start 1-4 weeks after exposure to a triggering infection.

30. **Ans. B**

The Sjögren's syndrome (SS) is an autoimmune exocrine disorder with signs and symptoms of dry mouth and keratoconjunctivitis sicca, which may sometimes display a wide range of systemic, nonglandular alterations. The prevalence of this syndrome has been estimated to range between 0.5 and 1%, with a female:male ratio of about 9 : 1.

Histopathology in minor salivary gland (presence of focal lymphocytic sialadenitis with a focus score ≥1) is one out of the six diagnostic criteria set in the revised international classification for Sjögren's syndrome for diagnosis of SS. It has recently become more important because of the consensus in considering only objective criteria to define an SS case, which has to meet at least two of the following three findings—(1) Positivity serum anti-SSA and/or SSB; (2) Ocular staining score >3; and (3) Presence of focal lymphocytic sialadenitis with a focus score >1 per 4 mm^2 of glandular tissue.

CHAPTER 7

Immune Dysfunction and Infections

Om Shrivastav

1. A 26-year-old female has laryngeal edema along with edema in all four limbs following a pneumonia caused by *Acinetobacter baumannii*. In her subsequent investigations, her antinuclear antibody (ANA) is weakly positive, C1 is normal, and CH50 is 3 (units). Her working diagnosis is:
   A. Hereditary angioedema
   B. Infection-induced hypocomplementemia
   C. Small vessel vasculitis
   D. Adenocarcinoma of lung

2. In the same patient in Question 1, the most definitive treatment is:
   A. Bone marrow transplant
   B. Chronic glucocorticoid therapy
   C. Monthly immunoglobulins
   D. Steroids + biologicals

3. The same patient in Question 1 is reluctant to take vaccines and agrees for any one vaccine. The most important vaccine for her is:
   A. Human papillomavirus vaccine (HPV vaccine)
   B. Hepatitis C vaccine
   C. Pneumococcal conjugated 13 followed pneumococcal 23 strained vaccine
   D. Hepatitis A vaccine

4. A 21-year-old male has dengue and chikungunya testing positive by polymerase chain reaction (PCR). He is discharged after 2 weeks' stay in hospital. In his follow-up, he complains of low-grade fevers and joint pains involving shoulder, ankle, and spine with small joints of both hands. The best investigation would be:
   A. Positron emission tomography computed tomography (PET-CT)
   B. Blood cultures
   C. Magnetic resonance imaging (MRI) of spine
   D. Bone scan

5. In the patient in Question 4, the fever and joint pain is most likely due to:
   A. Persistent chikungunya
   B. Paraneoplastic syndrome
   C. Postinfectious inflammatory sequelae
   D. Acute on chronic rheumatoid arthritis (RA)

6. In the same patient in Question 4, the most accurate laboratorial investigation to monitor recovery is:
   A. T-cell markers, CD4, CD8 counts
   B. Tumor necrosis factor α (TNF-α)
   C. B cell and natural killer cell markers
   D. Ig quantitative

7. In the same patient in Question 4, the bone pain and limitations of movement have worsened over 2 months of treatment with nonsteroidal anti-inflammatory drugs (NSAIDs), this patient now complains of crippling arthritis. The next best evidence-based treatment in postinfectious inflammatory arthritis is:
   A. Joint replacement
   B. Steroids + etanercept
   C. Etanercept + infliximab
   D. IV β-lactam + aminoglycoside for 6 weeks

8. This patient is commenced on etanercept with low-dose prednisolone in 2 weeks, he presents now with worsening fever and no appetite. CT abdomen demonstrates noncaseating abdominal lymphadenopathy at multiple sites.

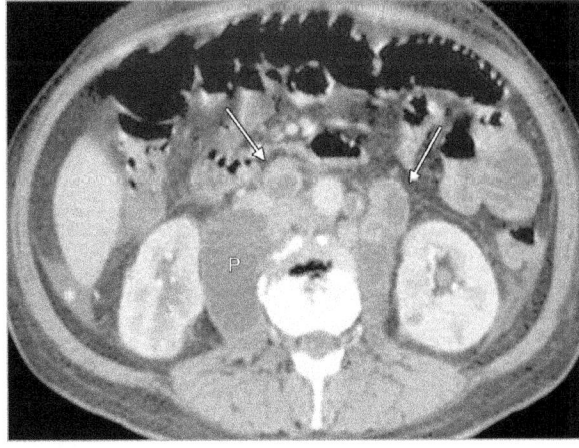

Source: da Rocha EL, Pedrassa BC, Bormann RL, Kierszenbaum ML, Torres LR, D'Ippolito G. Abdominal tuberculosis: a radiological review with emphasis on computed tomography and magnetic resonance imaging findings. Radiol Bras. 2015;48(3):181-91.

The most likely approach to give diagnosis is?
A. Bone marrow examination
B. Fine-needle aspiration
C. PET-CT
D. Abdominal laparoscopy

9. A 56-year-old woman presents to emergency with severe dyspnea and circulatory collapse. She is on aspirin and beta blockers for cardiomyopathy and azathioprine for inflammatory bowel disease. She is stabilized in intensive care unit (ICU) after discontinuation of her immunosuppression. During her stay, she contracts multiorgan infections and in spite of appropriate antibiotics; she is poorly responsive to treatment. The most likely cause for this is:
   A. Therapeutic monitoring is not done
   B. Inappropriate antibiotic use
   C. Severely impaired cell-mediated immunity (CMI)
   D. Poor complement function

10. In the same patient in Question 9, the reason for impaired CMI is:
    A. Bone marrow aplasia
    B. Cytokine storm secondary to infection
    C. Azathioprine has long half-life
    D. Clinical asplenia

11. In the same patient in Question 9, in addition to antibiotics, vasopressors, and ventilatory support, the best benefit would come from:
    A. Immunoglobulins 400 mg/kg for 5–7 days
    B. Low-dose hydrocortisone
    C. Bone marrow transplant
    D. Aspirin + plasmapheresis

12. A 27-year-old female is diagnosed with septic arthritis in a background of asplenia. She is advised knee washout after appropriate antibiotic therapy in preparation for surgery, the most important step would be:
    A. Concentrated 20% albumin for 3 weeks
    B. Appropriate antibiotic therapy for 2 weeks
    C. Quadrivalent influenza vaccine and conjugated pneumococcal vaccine
    D. PET-CT for other sites of infection

13. A 44-year-old breast cancer patient presents with fever, skin rash, cervical lymphadenopathy, and 11 kg weight loss over the last 3 months. She has presence of Hickman catheter and undergoes biopsy that grows a *Fusarium* species. The growth of such infections in this kind of patients is as a result of:
    A. Hyperstimulated TNF-α
    B. Dysfunctional T-cell response
    C. Uncontrolled cytokine response due to CA breast
    D. Macrophage inactivation and dysfunction

14. In deciding the immune response to a fungal septicemia, the most important mechanism is:
    A. Neutrophil activation
    B. Interleukin (IL)-1 and IL-6 activation cascade
    C. IgM response to infection
    D. Dectin receptors dectin-1

15. A 37-year-old female presents with progressively worsening dyspnea over 3 days. She has a low white cell count and metabolic acidosis on blood gas. Her chest X-ray shows rapidly progressive peripheral reticular shadowing that is diagnosed as aspergillosis. A bronchoscopy and bronchoalveolar lavage (BAL) was done which confirmed *Aspergillus fumigatus*. In spite of treatment with voriconazole, her immune system demonstrates progressively worsening CD4, CD8, and CD16 counts. The most likely reason for this is:
    A. Mycotoxins, especially gliotoxin, leading to progressive immune suppression
    B. Immunosuppression due to human immunodeficiency virus (HIV)
    C. Dysfunctional cytokine responses
    D. Coinfection with other fungi

16. A 37-year-old female presents to emergency with a painful forearm without a history of trauma. She has associated palpitations over the last 5 days. Her X-ray demonstrates osteopenia and a 2D ECHO reveals dilated cardiomyopathy. She has tested positive for chikungunya and dengue over the last 2 weeks (IgM and PCR both positive for both infections). The most likely diagnosis in her is:
    A. Hormone imbalance-induced osteoporosis
    B. Postchikungunya cardiomyopathy and pathological fracture
    C. Rheumatic valvular heart disease and dengue-induced bone crisis
    D. Systemic cytomegalovirus (CMV) infection

17. In the same patient in Question 16, to assess the severity of this condition, the best diagnostic test is:
    A. Endomyocardial biopsy
    B. Bone biopsy
    C. Erythrocyte sedimentation rate (ESR), high-sensitivity C-reactive protein (hs-CRP), and TNF-α
    D. Complement studies

18. In the same patient in Question 16, her stay in hospital is a stormy one, her fracture is treated by an external fixature and the cardiomyopathy is treated with angiotensin-2 receptor antagonists, β-blockers,

and aspirin. In the 6 weeks following discharge, her laboratory reports are as follows:

	2 weeks	4 weeks	6 weeks
ESR	40	66	80
hs-CRP	70	74	92
TNF-α	96	128	156

She is on a progressively increasing dose of NSAIDs and steroids, but complains of having very little relief. She now has inability to use the small joints of both hands and feet. The next step in her treatment would be:

A. Intravenous immunoglobulin (IVIg) for 7 days
B. Anti-CD20 antibodies (MabThera)
C. Increased bone marrow stimulation support commence granulocyte colony-stimulating factor (GCSF)
D. Trial of soluble TNF-α receptor antagonist

19. A 16-year-old girl tests positive for dengue and has persistent thrombocytopenia and immunoglobulin G (IgG) and IgM positive for dengue on four samples over 6 months. Her lowest platelet count was 38,000 3 months ago for which she received eight bags of single donor platelets during her stay. After giving her single-donor platelet components (SDPs), her immature platelet fraction is persistently 4% in sequential analysis. What is the most likely cause for the thrombocytopenia?

A. Immune complex disease following platelet transfusion
B. Myelodysplastic syndrome following dengue
C. Myelofibrosis of uncertainty origin
D. Thrombocytopenia due to hypersplenism

20. In the same patient in Question 19, the reason for persistence of IgM for dengue is because of:

A. Persistent dengue infection due to immune complexes
B. Laboratory error
C. IgM for dengue can persist for up to 12 months after the resolution of infection
D. DEN II and DEN IV may lead to subclinical infection

21. In viral infections, viruses evade immune mechanisms for detection so that they cannot be detected and therefore destroyed. The most common mechanism for immune system cells to see the presence of viral particles inside them is:

A. Natural killer (NK) cell signaling
B. Major histocompatibility complex (MHC) proteins class I
C. Complement-activated pathways
D. IL-1 and IL-12 program killing

22. A 61-year-old HIV positive female is having CMV involving her eye, lungs, and kidneys. She has commenced on valganciclovir with the satisfactory response. She undergoes an interferon assay and is commenced on monthly IVIg following a diagnosis of T-cell dysfunction (CD4 count—38 cells/mm^3; CD4:CD8—0.1; CD4%—2.8%). The role of IVIg is:

A. Boost the IgG%
B. Prevent recurrent infections in T-cell deficiency
C. Enhance mechanical barriers of gut and respiratory mucosa
D. Bone marrow stimulation

23. A 16-year-old girl presents with high-grade fever, cervical lymphadenopathy, and severe dysphagia. She gives a history of physical intimacy preceding these symptoms. A throat swab is negative for infectious pathology as is her IgM for infectious mononucleosis. The IgM is repeat for 5 days and 10 days of symptoms is negative each times, the reason for this test being negative is:

A. She has diphtheria
B. Serology for infectious mononucleosis can be negative for up to 2 weeks after the onset of infection
C. Diagnostic laboratory error
D. Cervical T-cell lymphoma

24. Worsening of infectious mononucleosis symptoms is most commonly due to:

A. Depletion of T-cells
B. Inactivated Ig response
C. Myeloproliferation
D. Depleted natural killer cells

25. In the same patient at 6 weeks in Question 23, she complains of severe abdominal pain requiring admission in emergency, a clinical assessment of an acute abdomen requiring imaging and surgical exploration is made. The most likely diagnosis is:

A. Spontaneous rupture of spleen
B. Peptic ulcer disease
C. Emphysematous and gangrenous gallbladder (GB)
D. Acute pancreatitis with septic shock

26. A 21-year-old female is exposed to an unvaccinated dog bite at multiple sites. She delays her treatment for 2 weeks after which she presents to emergency with aerophobia. She undergoes cerebrospinal fluid (CSF) studies and work-up for rabies. The most likely tissue biopsy to give result is:

A. The site of bite closest to brain
B. Nuchal and buccal biopsy
C. Immunohistochemistry in blood
D. Brain biopsy

27. In the above said scenario in Question 26, the best treatment option in this patient is:
    A. Plasmapheresis
    B. Methylprednisolone 1 g/day for 5 days
    C. Antirabies Ig with rabies vaccine
    D. Rabies vaccine alone

28. A 26-year-old female having the HIV infection, follows up in the outpatient department of your hospital regularly by last 5 years. Her CD4+ counts for last 5 years have been in the range of 600–650 cells/mm^3, without treatment. This clinical scenario is because of:
    A. Patient has hyperstimulatory T-cell function
    B. Patient has poor cytokine responses to HIV
    C. Patient carries a CC-chemokine receptor 5 (CCR-5) or C-X-C chemokine receptor type 4 (CXCR-4) mutation
    D. Patients viral load is suppressed due to human T-lymphocyte virus (HTLV) infection

29. A 30-year-old pregnant woman having an uncomplicated 34 weeks' pregnancy presented with new-onset pancytopenia, fever, and facial rash of 10 days' duration.

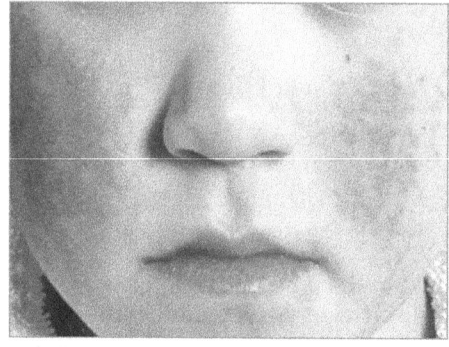

Her hemoglobin remains persistently around 4–6 g% and now has the features of fetal distress. Her ANA is strongly positive. The most likely diagnosis is:
    A. Systemic lupus erythematosus (SLE)
    B. Tuberculosis involving bone marrow
    C. Fifth disease
    D. Non-Hodgkin lymphoma (NHL)

30. In the same patient in Question 29, the features of fetal distress continue to worsen. Her fetal ultrasound reveals ascites, large bilateral pleural effusion, and pericardial effusion in the fetus.

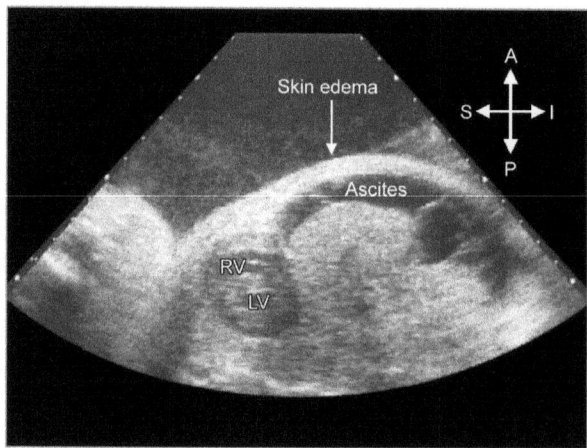

This condition is:
    A. Hypoalbuminemia and impending marasmus
    B. Hydrops fetalis
    C. Intrauterine liver failure with right-sided heart failure
    D. Maternal malnutrition leading to hypoproteinemia

Immune Dysfunction and Infections

ANSWERS WITH EXPLANATIONS

1. **Ans. B**

   Complement dysfunction may be masked in various events, even in adulthood, most importantly infections. This patient has complement deficiency, which will lead to peripheral and laryngeal edema.

   Ref:
   1. Farkas H. Management of upper airway edema caused by hereditary angioedema. Allergy Asthma Clin Immunol. 2010;6(1):19.

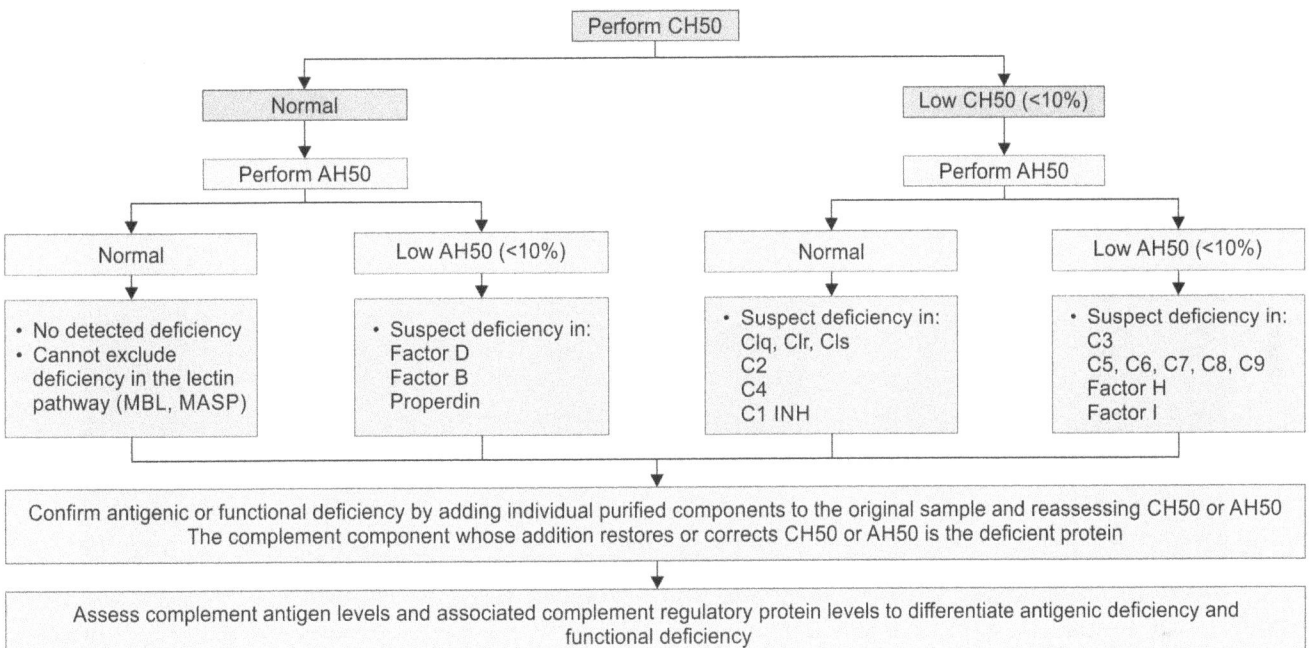

(MBL: mannose-binding lectin; MASP: mannose-binding lectin-associated serine proteases)
Source: Shih AR, Murali MR. Laboratory tests for disorders of complement and complement regulatory proteins. Am J Hematol. 2015;90(12):1180-6.

2. **Ans. B**

   The most effective treatment is unclear in complement deficiency as per current evidence-based medicine. The importance of low-dose steroids has been shown to be of marginal benefit; the remaining options are still investigational.
   Ref:
   1. Laitman RS, Glicklich D, Sablay LB, Grayzel AI, Barland P, Bank N. Effect of long-term normalization of serum complement levels on the course of lupus nephritis. Am J Med. 1989;87(2):132-8.

3. **Ans. C**

   Complement deficiencies have a strong association with infections with encapsulated bacteria. Pneumococcal vaccines are lifesaving with these disorders.
   Ref:
   1. Vinuesa CG, de Lucas C, Cook MC. Clinical implications of the specialised B cell response to polysaccharide encapsulated pathogens. Postgrad Med J. 2001;77(911):562-9.

4. **Ans. D**
   Ref:
   1. Steven J Baccei. Imaging techniques for evaluation of the painful joint. In: UpToDate, Post TW (Ed), UpToDate, Waltham, MA; 2020.

5. **Ans. C**
   Ref:
   1. Krutikov M, Manson J. Chikungunya virus infection: an update on joint manifestations and management. Rambam Maimonides Med J. 2016;7(4):e0033.

6. **Ans. B**

   Tumor necrosis factor-α is the most sensitive marker in chronic slow resolving postinfectious inflammatory conditions.
   Ref:
   1. Popa C, Netea MG, van Riel PL, van der Meer JW, Stalenhoef AF. The role of TNF-alpha in chronic inflammatory conditions, intermediary metabolism, and cardiovascular risk. J Lipid Res. 2007;48(4):751-62.

7. **Ans. B**

   Inflammatory arthropathy following infections having failed with first-line therapy with NSAIDs will benefit from steroids with soluble TNF-receptor antagonists such as etanercept.
   Ref:
   1. Schulz M, Dotzlaw H, Neeck G. Ankylosing spondylitis and rheumatoid arthritis: Serum levels of TNF-α and its soluble receptors during the course of therapy with etanercept and infliximab. Biomed Res Int. 2014;2014:675108.

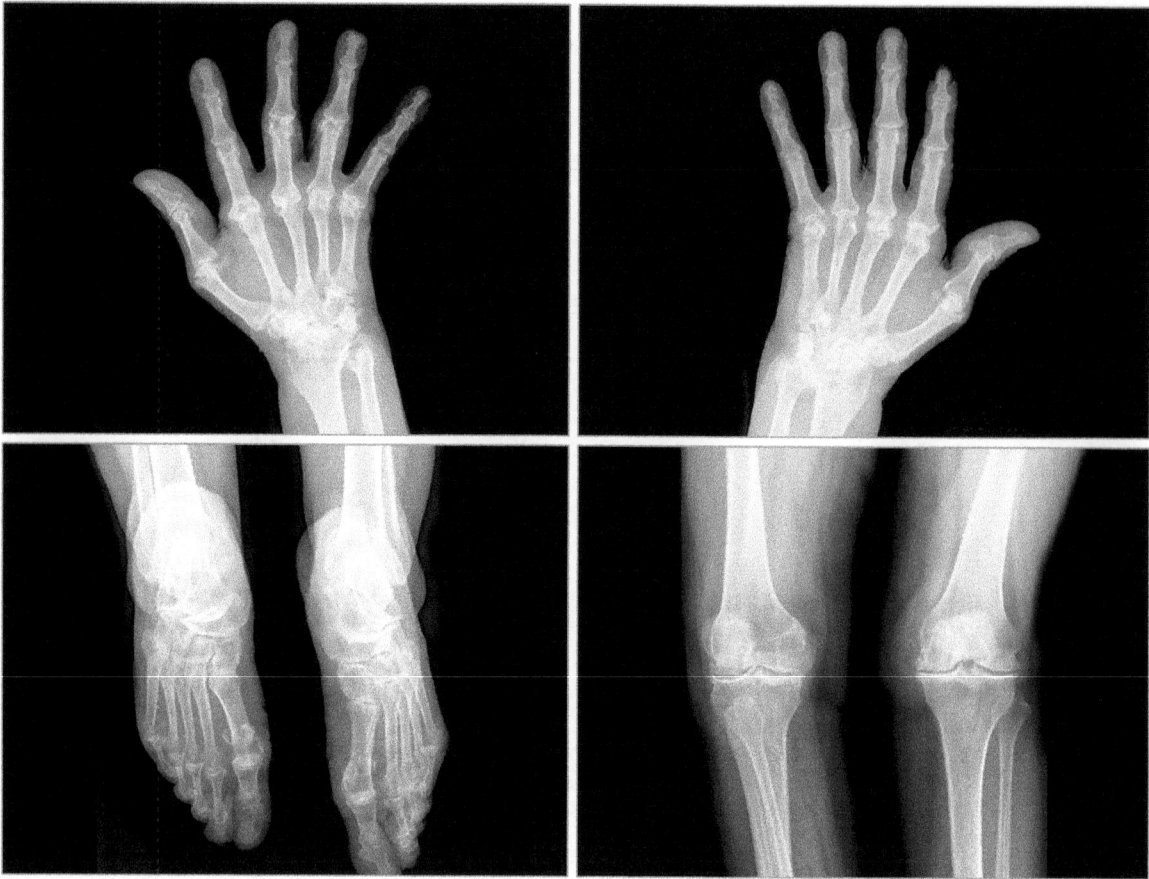

Source: Liddle AD, Rodríguez-Merchán EC. Inflammatory arthropathy of the knee. In: Rodríguez-Merchán E, Oussedik S, (Eds). Total Knee Arthroplasty. Switzerland: Springer; 2015. pp. 39-49.

8. **Ans. B**

   Fine needle aspiration with GeneXpert.
   Ref:
   1. *Robert L Ferrer. Evaluation of peripheral lymphadenopathy in adults. In: UpToDate, Post TW (Ed), UpToDate, Waltham, MA; 2019.*

9. **Ans. C**

   In patients who are receiving immunosuppression, CMI is impaired leading to poor responses to infectious agents.
   Ref:
   1. *Human Immunodeficiency Virus (HIV). British Society for Immunology. [online] Available from https://www.immunology.org/public-information/bitesized-immunology/pathogens-and-disease/human-immunodeficiency-virus-hiv [Last accessed December, 2020].*

10. **Ans. C**

    While the biological half-life of azathioprine can vary from 5 to 8 hours, presence of its metabolites may be circulating in patient's system for up to 3 weeks.
    Ref:
    1. *https://www.accessdata.fda.gov/drugsatfda_docs/label/2011/016324s034s035lbl.pdf [Last accessed December, 2020].*

11. **Ans. A**

    Patients in whom CMI is impaired are most likely to benefit from immunoglobulins to help clear immune complexes until the impaired CMI recovers.
    Ref:
    1. *Klaesson S, Ringdén O, Markling L, Remberger M, Lundkvist I. Immune modulatory effects of immunoglobulins on cell-mediated immune responses in vitro. Scand J Immunol. 1993;38(5):477-84.*

12. **Ans. C**

    Risk of encapsulated bacteria and viruses is significant in patients with such conditions. Vaccines should be given at least 3 weeks before surgical procedure to enable production antibodies.
    Ref:
    1. *Bonanni P, Grazzini M, Niccolai G, Paolini D, Varone O, Bartoloni A, et al. Recommended vaccinations for asplenic and hyposplenic adult patients. Hum Vaccin Immunother. 2017;13(2):359-68.*

13. **Ans. D**

    Macrophage dysfunction is an important mechanism for the growth of fungi such as *Fusarium*.

    This type of reaction is common for species such as *Fusarium*.

Ref:
1. *Immune responses to fungal pathogens. British Society for Immunology. [online] Available from https://www.immunology.org/public-information/bitesized-immunology/pathogens-and-disease/immune-responses-fungal-pathogens [Last accessed December, 2020].*

14. **Ans. D**

Dectin-1 are also called c-type dectin receptors which are important in activating the Th1 response.

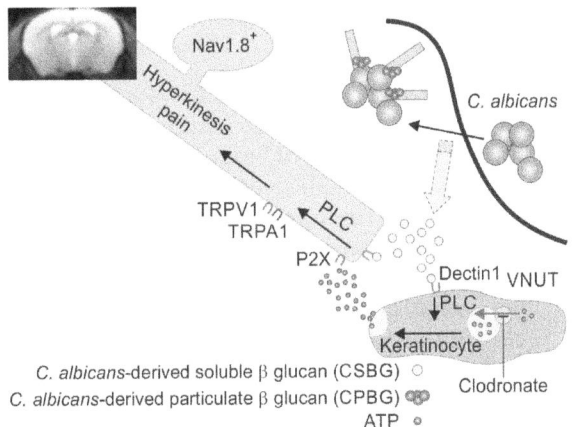

Source: Osaka University. [online] Available from: https://www.osaka-u.ac.jp/en. [Last accessed February, 2020].

Ref:
1. *Takano T, Motozono C, Imai T, Sonoda K-H, Nakanishi Y, Yamasaki S. Dectin-1 intracellular domain determines species-specific ligand spectrum by modulating receptor sensitivity; 2017. doi:10.1074/jbc.M117.800847.*

15. **Ans. A**

Mycotoxins such as gliotoxins are known to produce immune complexes that weaken the immune system further. The treatment requires combination of antifungals in strict isolation facilities.

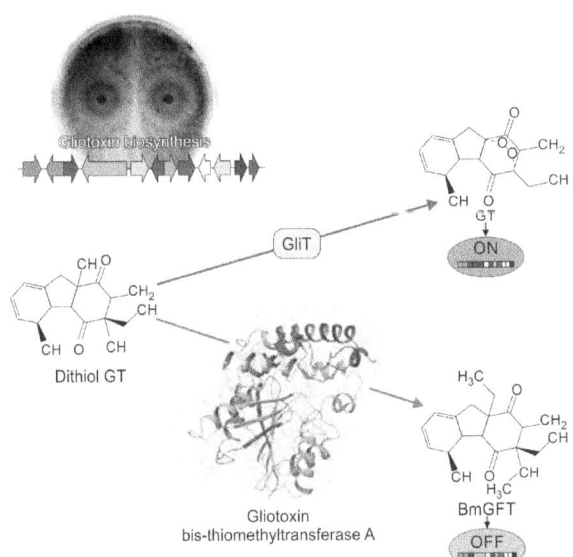

Source: Dolan SK, Owens RA, O'Keeffe G, Hammel S, Fitzpatrick DA, Jones GW, et al. Regulation of nonribosomal peptide synthesis: bis-thiomethylation attenuates gliotoxin biosynthesis in *Aspergillus fumigatus*. Chem Biol. 2014;21(8):999-1012.

Ref:
1. *Koenig S, Pace S, Pein H, Heinekamp T, Kramer J, Romp E, et al. Gliotoxin from Aspergillus fumigatus Abrogates leukotriene B4 formation through inhibition of leukotriene a4 hydrolase. Cell Chemical Biology, 2019;26(4):524-34.e5.*

16. **Ans. B**

Unregulated immune response postchikungunya is known to cause several systemic complications, especially of heart and bone.

Ref:
1. *Clinical Evaluation & Disease; Chikungunya virus; CDC. [online] Available from https://www.cdc.gov/chikungunya/hc/clinicalevaluation.html [Last accessed December, 2020].*

17. **Ans. C**

In clinically active chikungunya, hs-CRP and TNF-α usually have elevated values sometimes exceeding 10 times normal. These are often used as markers to assess indications for treatment and response to treatment.

Ref:
1. *Hoarau JJ, Jaffar Bandjee MC, Trotot PK, Das T, Li-Pat-Yuen G, Dassa B, et al. Persistent chronic inflammation and infection by Chikungunya arthritogenic alphavirus in spite of a robust host immune response. J Immunol. 2010;184(10):5914-27.*

18. **Ans. D**

In patients, failing first- and second-line treatments of pain relief by NSAIDs and steroids, and soluble TNF-α receptor antagonist, such as etanercept, along with immunomodulators should be considered as third-line therapy. This patient responded to two cycles of etanercept therapy.

Ref:
1. *Suhrbier A. Rheumatic manifestations of chikungunya: emerging concepts and interventions. Nat Rev Rheumatol. 2019;15(10):597-611.*

19. **Ans. A**

In patients where platelets are given without presence of bleeding, patients rapidly develop antiplatelet antibodies. These antibodies are often detrimental to the formation and circulation of new platelets. Immature platelet fraction between 1 and 5% suggests that new platelets are been formed in the absence of active bleeding.

Platelets should be reserved.

Ref:
1. *Kantharaj A. Role of red cell and platelet indices as a predictive tool for transfusions in dengue. Glob J Transfus Med. 2018;3:103-8.*

20. **Ans. C**

Ref:
1. *Chien YW, Liu ZH, Tseng FC, Ho TC, Guo HR, Ko NY, et al. Prolonged persistence of IgM against dengue virus detected by commonly used commercial assays. BMC Infect Dis. 2018;18(1):156.*

21. Ans. B

When a virus infects a person (host), it invades the cells of its host in order to survive and replicate. Once inside, the cells of the immune system cannot "see" the virus and therefore do not know that the host cell is infected. To overcome this, cells employ a system that allows them to show other cells what is inside them—they use molecules called class I MHC proteins (or MHC class I, for short) to display pieces of protein from inside the cell upon the cell surface.

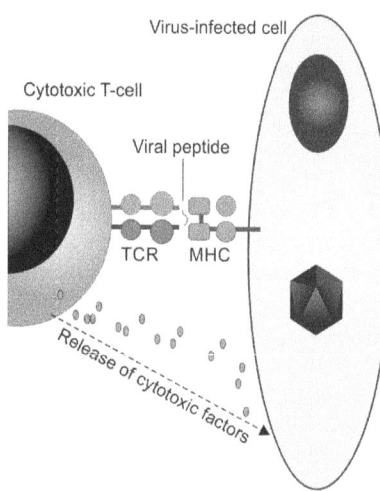

Source: British Immunological Society [Last accessed December, 2019].

22. Ans. B
Ref:
1. Mark Ballow. Overview of intravenous immune globulin (IVIG) therapy. In: UpToDate, Post TW (Ed), UpToDate, Waltham, MA; 2020.

23. Ans. B
Ref:
1. Mark D Aronson. Infectious mononucleosis. In: UpToDate, Post TW (Ed), UpToDate, Waltham, MA; 2019.

24. Ans. D
Ref:
1. Chijioke O, Müller A, Feederle R, Barros MH, Krieg C, Emmel V, et al. Human natural killer cells prevent infectious mononucleosis features by targeting lytic Epstein-Barr virus infection. Cell Reports. 2013;5(6):1489-98.

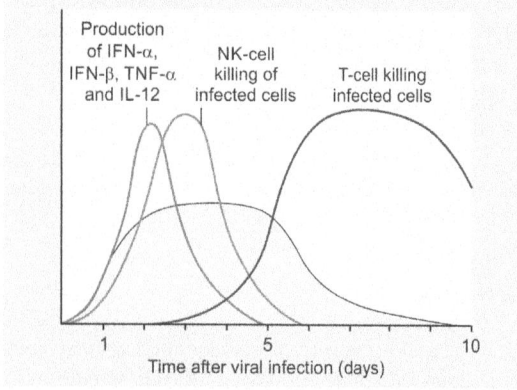

(IFN: interferon; NK: natural killer)

25. Ans. A
Ref:
1. Mark D Aronson. Infectious mononucleosis. In: UpToDate, Post TW (Ed), UpToDate, Waltham, MA; 2019.

26. Ans. B
The response after exposure to a cytopathic virus such as rabies is best elicited by examining the buccal mucosa and full thickness nuchal biopsy.
Ref:
1. DeMaria A. Clinical manifestations and diagnosis of rabies. In: UpToDate, Post TW (Ed), UpToDate, Waltham, MA, 2020.

27. Ans. C
The incubation period of rabies vaccine varies from 9 days to 19 years. Once the virus begins to attach itself to the specific areas of brain, the process of recovery can be poorly responsive. Cytopathic viruses, such as rabies require strategies for complete elimination since otherwise the outcome is uniformly fatal. In this case, for vaccines to start making antibodies would take between 10 and 14 days and immunoglobulins helping clearing virus-induced immune complexes.
Ref:
1. Catherine M Brown. Rabies immune globulin and vaccine. In: UpToDate, Post TW (Ed), UpToDate, Waltham, MA; 2019.

28. Ans. C
Patients expressing CCR-5 or CXCR-4 mutations of T-cell receptors are called slow progressors of the HIV infection. Such patients lose 15–40 CD4 cells per year as against 80–150 CD4 cells lost in the patients who do not express this mutation.
Ref:
1. Chaudhuri RP, Neogi U, Rao SD, Shet A. Genetic factors associated with slow progression of HIV among perinatally-infected Indian children. Indian Pediatr. 2014;51(10):801-3.
2. Cohen OJ, Paolucci S, Bende SM, Daucher M, Moriuchi H, Moriuchi M, et al. CXCR4 and CCR5 genetic polymorphisms in long-term non progressive human immunodeficiency virus infection: Lack of association with mutations other than CCR5-D32. J Virol. 1998;72(7):6215-7.

29. Ans. C
Erythema infectiosum or Parvovirus B19 infection: The features are classically described as slapped-cheek appearance and are often associated with anemia and pancytopenia. The treatment is mostly supportive.
Ref:
1. Jeanne A Jordan. Clinical manifestations and diagnosis of parvovirus B19 infection. In: UpToDate, Post TW (Ed), UpToDate, Waltham, MA; 2019.

30. Ans. B
Hydrops fetalis is a potentially fatal complication of parvovirus that leads to edema of two or more compartments in the fetus. The condition requires to be treated as an emergency with blood transfusions, immunoglobulins, and circulatory support for mother.
Ref:
1. Charles J Lockwood. Nonimmune hydrops fetalis. In: UpToDate, Post TW (Ed), UpToDate, Waltham, MA; 2020.

CHAPTER 8

Approach to Cutaneous and Soft-tissue Infections

Om Shrivastav

1. A 37-year-old male having renal transplant 13 years ago, stable on immunosuppression receives interferon alpha 6 weeks ago, presents with multiple painful skin lesions with copious serous ooze. Series of oral antibiotics do not resolve this condition. He is commenced on oral fluconazole that leads to flair of lesion. Commenced interferon for recently diagnosed hepatitis B. The most likely diagnosis is:

   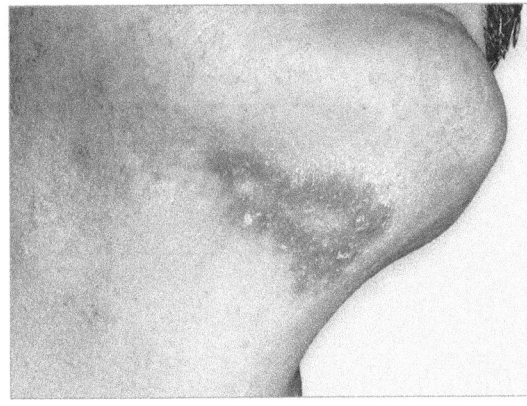

   Source: Science Photo Library Limited; 2019.

   A. Histoplasmosis
   B. Leishmaniasis
   C. Cutaneous mycobacterial infection
   D. Sezary syndrome cutaneous T-cell lymphoma

2. A 5-year-old child is brought with rash (images). What is the cause of this condition?

   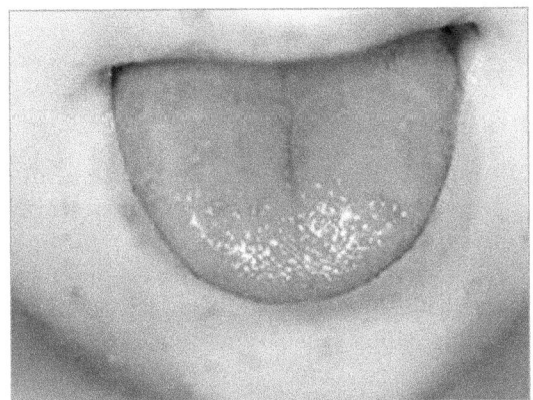

   Source: Dr P Marazzi, Science Photo Library; 2019.

   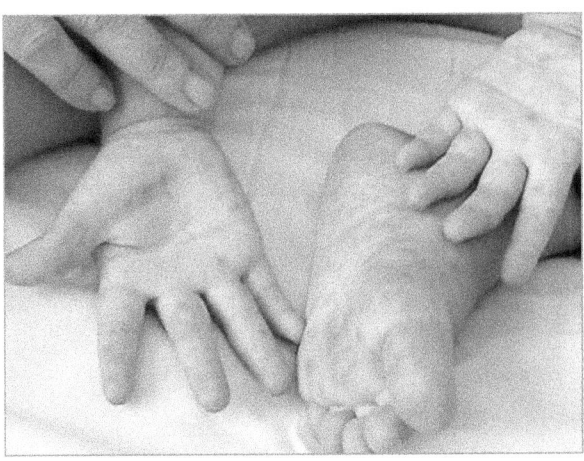

   Source: El Universal; 2019.

   A. Human herpesvirus 7
   B. Poxvirus
   C. Molluscum contagiosum
   D. Coxsackievirus

3. A 41-year-old male presents with fever and headache since 4 days. On examination, rash over legs are appreciated (image). What is the diagnosis?

   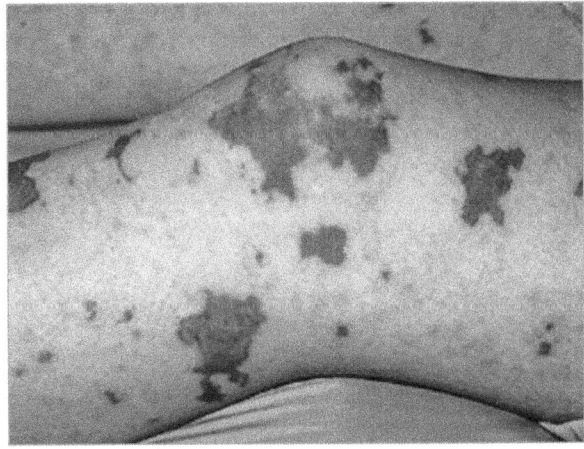

   Source: Meningitis Research Foundation of Canada; 2019.

   A. Dengue hemorrhagic fever
   B. Enteric fever
   C. Meningococcemia
   D. Scrub typhus

4. Which of the following skin infection is commonly seen in children, and is characterized by single or multiple pearly white skin coloured smooth dome-shaped papules with central pitting?

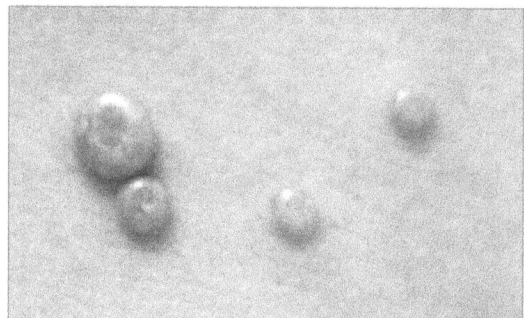

Source: Centers for Disease Control and Prevention; 2019.

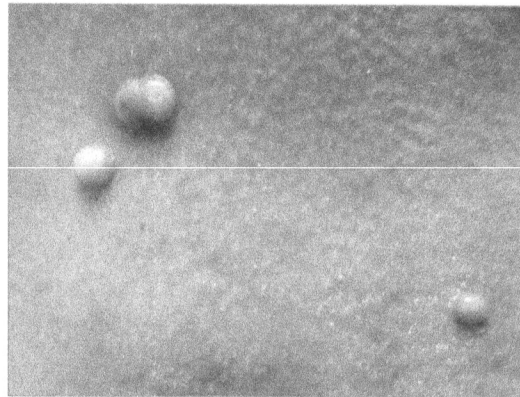

Source: 2013 Decision Support in Medicine, LLC; 2019.

A. Molluscum contagiosum   B. Chicken pox
C. Herpes zoster   D. Verruca vulgaris

5. A 30-year-old female, hospitalized with the complaining of right thigh pain, provisionally diagnosed as cellulitis was treated with oxacillin IV. The next day she develops septic shock with systolic blood pressure (BP) < 90 mm Hg, acute renal failure, and disseminated intravascular coagulation (DIC). CT scan of the right thigh is shown in image. What is further line of medical management along with the surgical intervention?

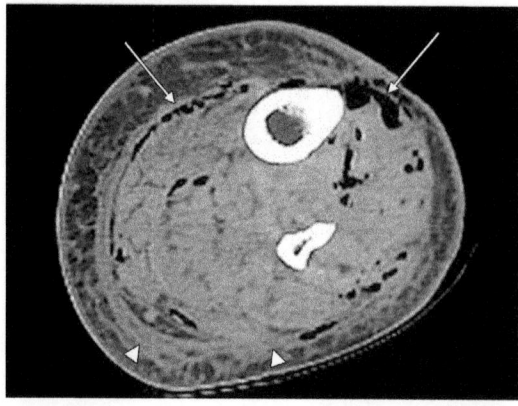

Source: Chaudhry AA, Baker KS, Gould ES, Gupta R. Necrotizing Fasciitis and its mimics: what radiologists need to know. Am J Roentgenol. 2015;204(1):128-39.

A. Add clindamycin
B. Replace with piperacillin-tazobactam and vancomycin
C. Add clindamycin with gentamicin
D. Replace with vancomycin, clindamycin, and gentamicin

6. A young male, presents with genital ulcers developed since 8–10 days, which he complains are tender with occasional bleeding tendency. On clinical examination, the lesions are extremely tender and soft on palpation. What is the diagnosis?

A. *Treponema pallidum*
B. Herpes simplex virus
C. Human immunodeficiency virus (HIV)
D. *Haemophilus ducreyi*

7. A 32-year-old male presented with generalized body ache and rash. What is the causative organism for the following rash (image)?

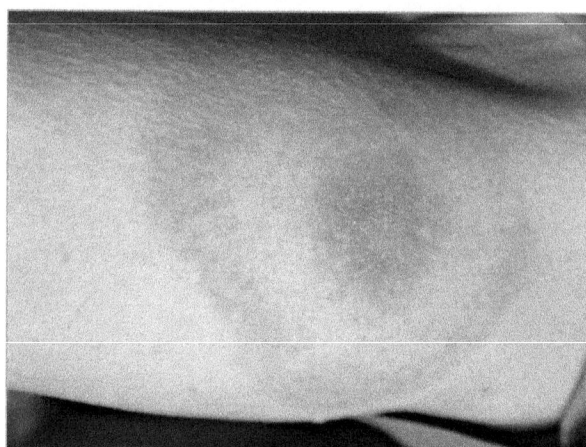

Source: Centers for Disease Control and Prevention (2018). Lyme disease rashes and look-alikes. [online] Available from https://www.cdc.gov/lyme/signs_symptoms/rashes.html [Last accessed February, 2020].

A. *Rickettsia rickettsii*
B. *Ehrlichia chaffeensis*
C. *Borrelia burgdorferi*
D. *Bartonella henselae*

8. A college student presents with painless non-pruritic rash over trunk since 10 days. He elaborates and gives history of unprotected sexual intercourse followed by occurrence of painless papule on penis, which had healed spontaneously following which he had developed rash. What should be the treatment for him?

A. Benzathine penicillin G 2.4 MU intramuscular (IM) single dose
B. Penicillin G 18–24 MU per day IV for 14 days
C. Azithromycin 1 g oral single dose
D. Doxycycline 100 mg oral BD for 14 days

9. In the patient discussed in Question 8, the primary complaint after 10 years is difficulty in breathing, his two-dimensional (2D) echo and CT chest reveal cardiomyopathy and aortitis and clinically he now has multiple ulceration in the soft palate and collapse of bridge of nose. The most likely diagnosis is:
   A. HIV with multisystem involvement
   B. Takayasu arteritis
   C. Syphilitic aortitis
   D. Mixed connective tissue disorder

10. In the patient discussed in Questions 8 and 9, the most sensitive serology for diagnosing syphilis is:
    A. *Treponema pallidum* hemagglutination assay (TPHA)
    B. Rapid plasma reagin (RPR)
    C. Punch biopsy from affected tissue
    D. Fluorescent treponema antigen absorption (FTA-ABS) assay

11. In penicillin allergy, the drug of choice for treatment of syphilis is:
    A. Meropenem + sulbactam
    B. Cefazolin
    C. Amikacin + moxifloxacin
    D. Ceftriaxone

12. A 37-year-old seropositive woman newly commenced on lopinavir/ritonavir, abacavir, and nevirapine breaks into a skin rash 2 weeks into her treatment. Her doctor discontinues all medications and subsequently commences lamivudine, abacavir, and dolutegravir. On day 3, patient is admitted to intensive care unit (ICU) with acute pancreatitis, respiratory failure, and lactic acidosis. The likeliest cause is?
    A. Mitochondrial encephalopathy, lactic acidosis, and stroke-like episodes (MELAS) syndrome
    B. HIV-induced pancreatitis
    C. Drug hypersensitivity to abacavir
    D. Lamivudine-induced metabolic shock

13. In an endemic area, *Borrelia burgdorferi* serology test is indicated in which of the following scenario?
    A. Young female with second episode of inflammation involving her knee and ankle
    B. Young male presenting with erythema migrans lesion at the site of tick bite
    C. Old female presenting with fever, myalgia, and arthralgia
    D. Old male presenting with fever, malaise, and migratory arthralgia with erythema migrans lesions.

14. A 36-year-old male presented with non-itchy and patchy discoloration on his back. Which of the following not appropriate treatment of the following?

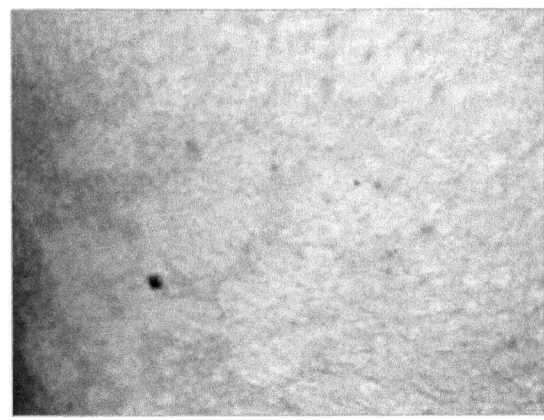

Source: Dr P Marazzi, Science Photo Library; 2019.

A. Griseofulvin B. Topical ketoconazole
C. Terbinafine   D. Selenium sulfide

15. A 30-year-old male presents to you with this rash. He elaborates that it has been there 2 weeks from now and over his palms and soles without itching sensation. Which of the following is the likely cause?

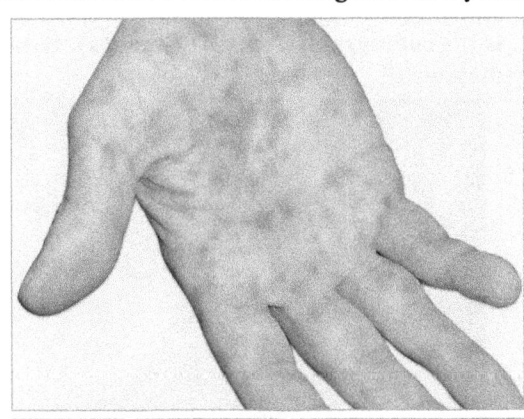

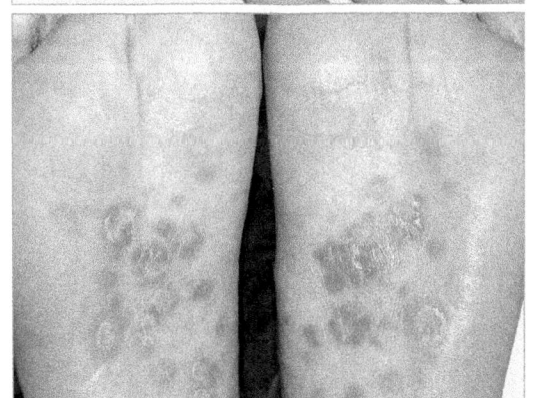

Source: Lamb CA, Mary Lamb El, Mansfield JC, Sankar KN. Sexually transmitted infections manifesting as proctitis. Frontline Gastroenterol. 2013;4:32-40.

A. Measles   B. Parvovirus B19
C. *Treponema pallidum* D. Coxsackie A

16. **Which of the following is true in case of pityriasis rosea (PR)?**
    A. Caused by dermatophytes
    B. Self-limiting infection
    C. Chronic and relapsing infection
    D. Life-threatening

17. **What is the likely cause of the following (image)?**

    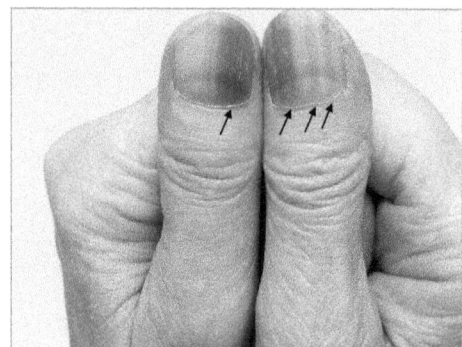

    Source: NEJM; 2020.

    A. Minocycline   B. Zidovudine
    C. Doxorubicin   D. All of the above

18. **An old-aged man was on long-term prophylaxis with voriconazole, she presents with bilateral hand swelling and generalized body ache. Following is his radiograph and MRI (images). What is the diagnosis?**

    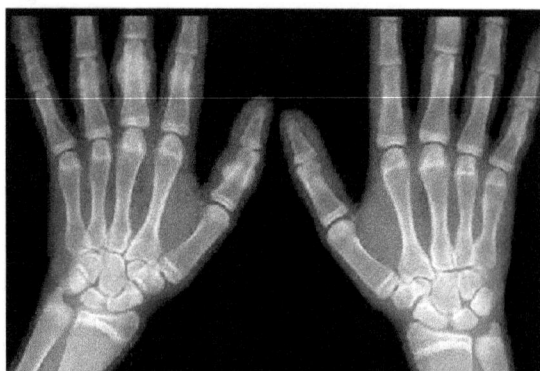

    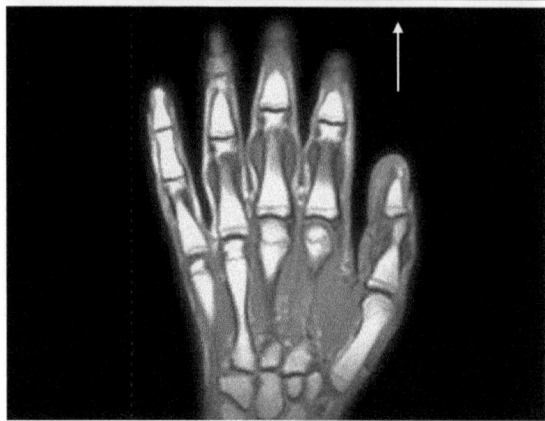

    Source: Ladak K, Rubin L. Voriconazole-induced periostitis deformans: a mimicker of hypertrophic pulmonary osteoarthropathy. Clin Med Res. 2017;15:19-20.

    A. Rheumatoid arthritis
    B. Periostitis
    C. Seronegative osteoarthropathy
    D. Reactive arthritis secondary to respiratory infection

19. **A 38-year-old commercial sex worker presents with the non-pruritic lesions (image). What is the diagnosis?**

    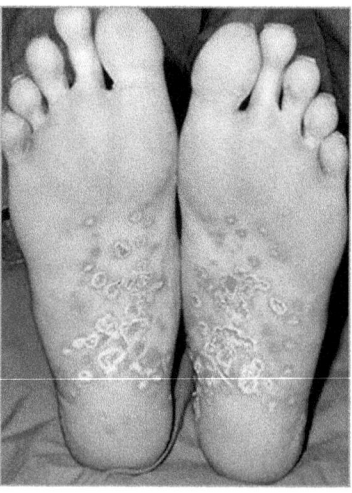

    Source: Tonna I, Laing RBS. Images in clinical medicine. Keratoderma blennorrhagica. N Engl J Med. 2008;358:2160.

    A. Lichen planus
    B. Psoriasis
    C. Dermatopathia pigmentosa reticularis
    D. Keratoderma blennorrhagicum

20. **A 26-year-old male shepherd presents with lesion on his palm (image), what is the likely diagnosis?**

    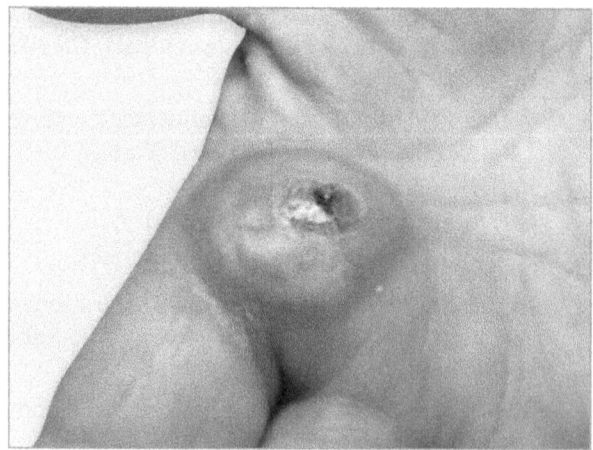

    Source: Bass J (2012). Human Orf Virus Infection From Household Exposures. [online] Available from https://www.medscape.com/viewarticle/767315 [Last accessed February, 2020].

    A. Furuncle
    B. Orf
    C. Cutaneous anthrax
    D. Sporotrichosis

21. A 46-year-old woman presents with swollen finger, no history of trauma. Physical examination—soft-tissue swelling, erythema, warm on touch, which involves proximal, and distal interphalangeal joints (image). What is the cause?

    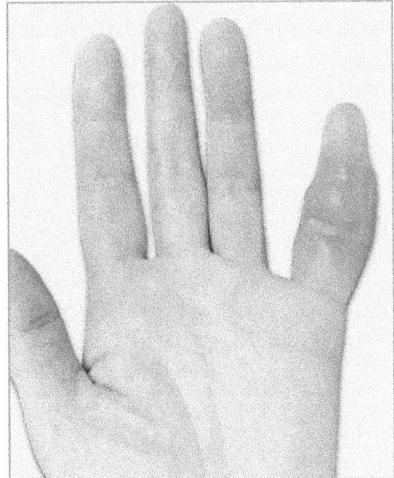

    Source: Mandal J, Margaretten M. Tuberculosis of the finger. N Engl J Med. 2018;379:1161.

    A. Acute gout
    B. Septic arthritis
    C. Osteoarthritis
    D. Extrapulmonary TB

22. A 55-year-old male admitted in the hospital and was immobilized for a long course, has developed pressure sore (bed sore) (image). What should be the further line of management?

    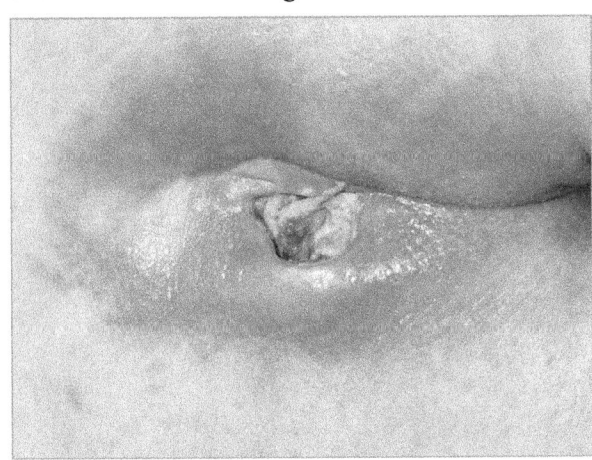

    Source: Dr P Marazzi, Science Photo Library; 2019.

    A. Cefazolin
    B. Clindamycin
    C. Aminoglycoside
    D. Both B and C

23. In the patient discussed in Question 22, supportive care should include:

    A. Removal of devitalized tissue
    B. Wound care in the form of cleansing with normal saline, keeping the surface free of moisture
    C. Appropriate positioning of the patient
    D. All of the above

24. A 54-year-old patient with known case of diabetes presents with an ulcer (images) and fever. What should be the appropriate antibiotic therapy?

    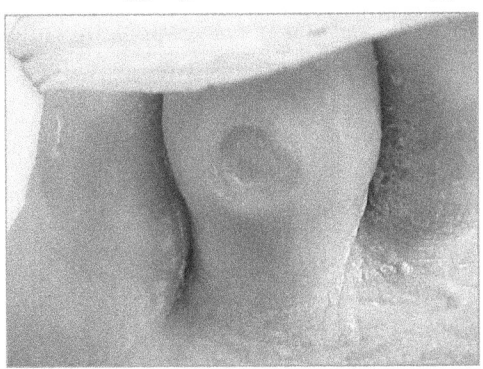

    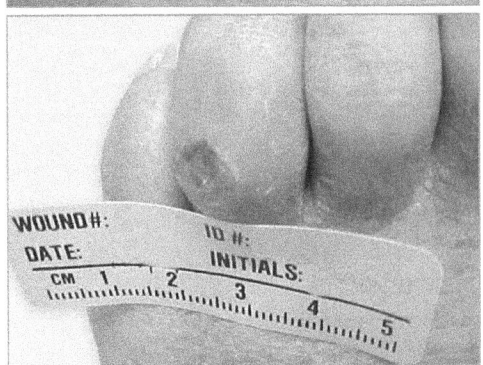

    Source: Medscape, Vincent Lopez Rowe; 2019.

    A. Amikacin
    B. Penicillin
    C. Erythromycin
    D. Amoxicillin-clavulanic acid

25. In the patient discussed in Question 24, what is the probable cause?

    A. *Staphylococcus aureus*   B. Streptococci
    C. *Bacteroides fragilis*   D. All of the above

26. A 43-year-old aged man with known case of diabetes develops erysipelas (image). What is the likely cause?

    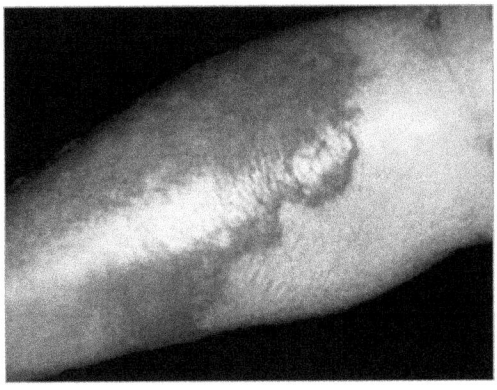

    Source: Springer Science + Business Media; 2019.

A. Group A beta-hemolytic *Streptococcus*
B. *Streptococcus pyogenes*
C. *Staphylococcus aureus*
D. Both A and B

27. A 33-year-old male presents with impetigo (image). He gives previous history of penicillin allergy. What should be the appropriate management?

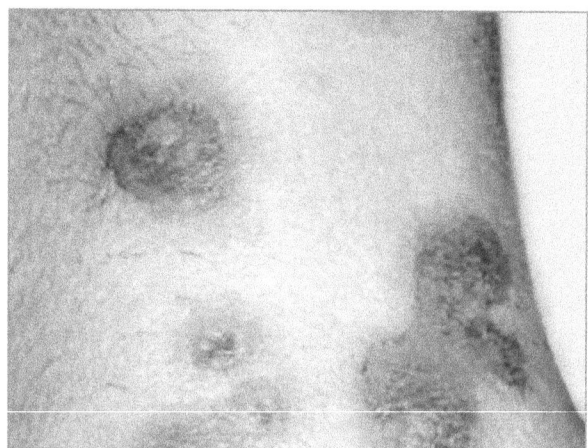

Source: Åsa Thörn; 2011.

A. Topical ozenoxacin
B. Mupirocin
C. Erythromycin
D. All of the above

28. A 44-year-old poorly controlled diabetic presents with cellulitis (image) and fever. What is the causative organism of the following?

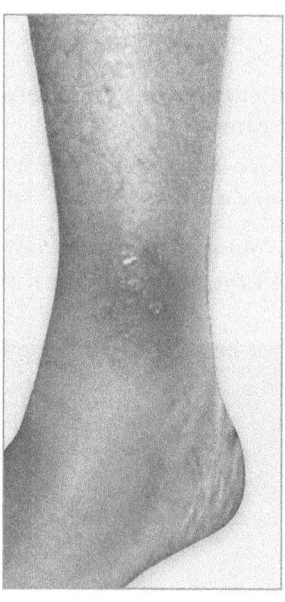

Source: Texas Department of Public Health; 2019.

A. *Staphylococcus aureus*
B. *Streptococcus pyogenes*
C. Group A streptococci
D. *Staphylococcus epidermidis*
E. All of the above

29. A 29-year-old male presented with furuncle (image), mild pain at the site without history of fever. What is the initial management for the following?

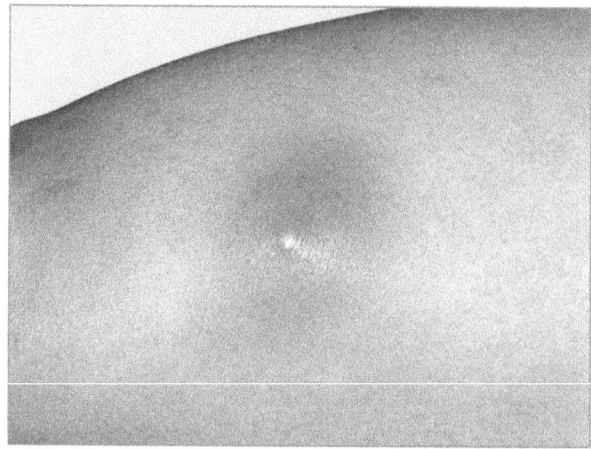

Source: Jere Mammino, American Osteopathic College of Dermatology; 2019.

A. Topical mupirocin   B. Clindamycin
C. Erythromycin   D. Moist heat

30. An opinion with regards to rule out infection is given. The patient is post-renal transplant and had developed necrotic ulcers (image). What is the likely cause?

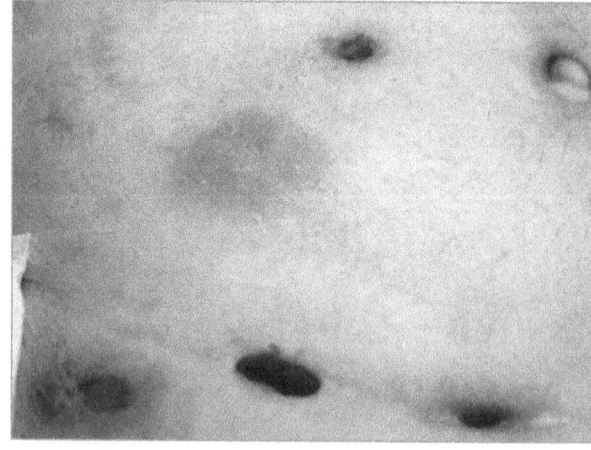

Source: Mina Yassaee Kingsbery, Medscape; 2018.

A. *Staphylococcus aureus*
B. *Pseudomonas aeruginosa*
C. Methicillin-resistant *Staphylococcus epidermidis*
D. Both B and C

ANSWERS WITH EXPLANATIONS

1. **Ans. C**

   While the patient of renal transplant on immunosuppression is at high risk of this condition the interferon therapy is known to provoke latent tuberculosis (TB) or initiate a new infection. A diagnosis was established after biopsy. Patient responded to therapy for extrapulmonary mycobacterial infection.

   Cutaneous lesions are relatively uncommon manifestations of TB, occurring in only 1–2% of infected patients. The clinical findings vary—inflammatory papules, verrucous plaques, suppurative nodules, chronic ulcers, or other lesions may be seen. Factors such as the pathway of bacterial entry into the skin, the host's immune status, and the presence or absence of host sensitization to *Mycobacterium tuberculosis* influence the morphologic presentation of TB in the skin.
   Ref:
   1. Handog EB, Enriquez-Macarayo MJ (2018). Cutaneous manifestations of tuberculosis. [online] Available from https://www.uptodate.com/contents/cutaneous-manifestations-of-tuberculosis [Last accessed February, 2020].

2. **Ans. D**

   The images suggest vesicular eruptions over the tongue and also over the palm. Since there is involvement of oropharynx, palm, and soles, it is the feature of hand-foot-mouth disease. The causative organism is coxsackievirus A16. These lesions are sometimes painful and take 2–4 weeks to heal.
   Ref:
   1. Kasper DL, Fauci AS, Hauser SL, Longo DL, Fauci A, Loscalzo J. Harrison's Principles and Practice of Medicine, 19th edition. New York, United States: McGraw Hill Education; 2015.
   2. Nervi SJ, Schwartz RA, Kapila R (2018). Hand-Foot-and-Mouth Disease (HFMD). [online] Available from https://emedicine.medscape.com/article/218402-overview [Last accessed February, 2020].

3. **Ans. C**

   There is persistent fever with rash which is stellate purpura with central gray hue suggestive of meningococcal rash. The recommended treatment for meningococcemia is ceftriaxone 2 g intravenous (IV) daily or cefotaxime 2 g IV QID for 7–10 days. Alternatively ampicillin and moxifloxacin can be used.
   Ref:
   1. Kasper DL, Fauci AS, Hauser SL, Longo DL, Fauci A, Loscalzo J. Harrison's Principles and Practice of Medicine, 19th edition. New York, United States: McGraw Hill Education; 2015.
   2. Javid MH (2019). Meningococcemia Clinical Presentation. [online] Available from https://emedicine.medscape.com/article/221473-clinical [Last accessed February, 2020].

4. **Ans. A**

   Molluscum contagiosum caused by deoxyribonucleic acid (DNA) virus. Skin lesions may be single or multiple, rounded, dome-shaped pink-colored waxy papules measuring 2–5 mm in size. They can be discrete, non-tender, skin-colored, and dome-shaped papules which show central umbilication, which is more apparent when lesion is frosted with liquid nitrogen.
   Ref:
   1. Banyameen IM, Atul JK, Tushar KJ. Molluscum contagiosum. Med J DY Patil Univ. 2015;8:54-6

5. **Ans. D**

   The CT scan demonstrates collection of fluid and gas in the deep fascia of right thigh, suggestive of necrotizing fasciitis. Necrotizing fasciitis leads to extensive necrosis of subcutaneous tissue and fascia, caused by Group A streptococci and facultative anaerobic flora. Risk factors include diabetes mellitus, peripheral vascular diseases, and IV drug usage. This infection is life-threatening with mortality rate from 30 to 70% and 100% if surgical debridement is not intervened. Treatment of choice is IV vancomycin, gentamicin, and clindamycin; 30 mg/kg/day, 1,800 mg/day, and 15 mg/kg/day, respectively.
   Ref:
   1. Roje Z, Roje Z, Matić D, Librenjak D, Dokuzović S, Varvodić J. Necrotizing fasciitis: literature review of contemporary strategies for diagnosing and management with three case reports: torso, abdominal wall, upper and lower limbs. World J Emerg Surg. 2011;6(1):46.

6. **Ans. D**

   Genital ulceration causes syphilis, herpes simplex virus, and chancroid. *Haemophilus ducreyi* is causative organism for chancroid in which there are multiple ulcers which initiates as pustules, soft, and extremely tender.
   Ref:
   1. Lewis, DA. Chancroid: Clinical manifestations, diagnosis, and management. Sexually Transmitted Infections. 2003;79:68-71.
   2. Stephen A. Morse. Chancroid and Haemophilus ducreyi. Clinical Microbiology Reviews. 1989;2(2):137-57.

7. **Ans. C**

   The image shows rash of erythema migrans which is typically seen in Lyme disease. The causative organism is *Borrelia burgdorferi*. Erythema migrans occurs at the site of tick bite usually within 1 week to 1 month of bite. Initially, the lesion occurs as red macule or papule and progresses to form classic bull's eye appearance with outer ring of bright red color central region of erythema with clearing in between.
   Ref:
   1. Shapiro ED. Lyme disease. N Engl J Med. 2014;371(7): 684.

8. **Ans. A**

   A nonpruritic, diffuse, symmetrical, maculopapular rash on the trunk, palms, and soles is characteristic of secondary syphilis. Treatment is penicillin G benzathine 2.4 million units IM as a single dose.
   Ref:
   1. *Kasper DL, Fauci AS, Hauser SL, Longo DL, Fauci A, Loscalzo J. Harrison's Principles and Practice of Medicine, 19th edition. New York, United States: McGraw Hill Education; 2015.*

9. **Ans. C**

   Secondary or late syphilis often presents after long intervals following primary exposure. The collapse of bridge of nose and oral ulcerate are consistent with this stage of syphilis. Benzathine carries 40% failure rate.
   Ref:
   1. *Kasper DL, Fauci AS, Hauser SL, Longo DL, Fauci A, Loscalzo J. Harrison's Principles and Practice of Medicine, 19th edition. New York, United States: McGraw Hill Education; 2015.*

10. **Ans. B**

    In patients with syphilis, TPHA may remain positive for 5 years after resolution of infection. The FTA-ABS is a non-sensitive assay for active infection. Demonstration of RPR especially climbing titers in blood is a sensitive marker for active disease.
    Ref:
    1. *Morshed MG, Singh AE. Recent trends in the serologic diagnosis of syphilis. Clin Vaccine Immunol. 2015;22(2):137-47.*

11. **Ans. D**

    Regimens used in penicillin allergy for syphilis are doxycycline 100 mg orally twice daily for 14 days, tetracycline (500 mg four times daily for 14 days), ceftriaxone (1-2 g daily either IM or IV for 10-14 days), and azithromycin as a single 2-g oral dose (in few cases) are effective. However, use of alternative regimens to penicillin for treatment of primary and secondary syphilis are limited.
    Ref:
    1. *Ghanem KG, Erbelding EJ, Cheng WW, et al. Doxycycline compared with benzathine penicillin for the treatment of early syphilis. Clin Infect Dis. 2006;42:e45-e49.*
    2. *Wong T, Singh AE, De P. Primary syphilis: serological treatment response to doxycycline/tetracycline versus benzathine penicillin. Am J Med. 2008;121:903-8.*
    3. *Hook EW 3rd, Roddy RE, Handsfield HH. Ceftriaxone therapy for incubating and early syphilis. J Infect Dis. 1988;158:881-4.*
    4. *Riedner G, Rusizoka M, Todd J, et al. Single-dose azithromycin versus penicillin G benzathine for the treatment of early syphilis. N Engl J Med. 2005;353:1236-44.*
    5. *Hook EW 3rd, Behets F, Van Damme K, et al. A phase III equivalence trial of azithromycin versus benzathine penicillin for treatment of early syphilis. J Infect Dis. 2010;201:1729-35.*

12. **Ans. C**

    Suspected hypersensitivity to abacavir is a clear for rechallenge therapy in a patient, the human leukocyte antigen (HLA) association with HIV can be tested before commencing treatment with abacavir and should not be attempted even if genotype resistance testing does not show a resistance pattern.
    Ref:
    1. *Mounzer K, Hsu R, Fusco JS, et al. HLA-B*57:01 screening and hypersensitivity reaction to abacavir between 1999 and 2016 in the OPERA® observational database: a cohort study. AIDS Res Ther. 2019;16(1):1.*

13. **Ans. A**

    Lyme diseases can also be present in chronic form.
    Ref:
    1. *Arvikar SL, Steere AC. Diagnosis and treatment of Lyme arthritis. Infect Dis Clin North Am. 2015;29(2):269-80.*
    2. *Bockenstedt LK, Wormser GP. Review: unraveling Lyme disease. Arthritis Rheumatol. 2014;66(9):2313-23.*

14. **Ans. A**

    This condition is more likely pityriasis versicolor, also known as tinea versicolor, is chronic cutaneous fungal infection caused by proliferation of lipophilic yeast which is caused by *Malassezia* species (*M. globosa, M. sympodialis,* and *M. furfur*) in the stratum corneum. It is one of the most common superficial fungal infections, which is particularly seen in tropical climates. Diagnosis is confirmed by microscopy through skin scrapings from the borders of lesions and Wood's light examination where the lesions appear in yellow or gold. Topical antifungals are currently the first line of treatment and systemic/oral antifungals are recommended for severe cases. Currently the most effective topical antifungal medications in treating pityriasis versicolor are selenium sulfide, zinc pyrithione, topical ketoconazole, and terbinafine. Ketoconazole is recommended once or twice daily for 14 days as topical ketoconazole cream or foam, and once weekly use of ketoconazole shampoo. Topical terbinafine cream recommended twice daily for 7 days. Treatment efficacy of topical formulations might be lower in more tropical climates. In oral treatment itraconazole 200 mg daily for 5 or 7 days, fluconazole 300 mg weekly for 2 weeks, and pramiconazole daily for 2 days are used.
    Ref:
    1. *Gupta AK, Foley KA. Antifungal treatment for pityriasis versicolor. J Fungi (Basel). 2015;1(1):13-29.*

15. **Ans. C**

    The skin eruption associated with secondary syphilis characteristically has a palmoplantar distribution, is pink or dark red and not pruritic. The appearance is typical of secondary syphilis. Treatment with single IM dose of penicillin G benzathine 2.4 million units is given.
    Ref:
    1. *Lamb CA, Mary Lamb EI, Mansfield JC, Sankar KN. Sexually transmitted infections manifesting as proctitis. Frontline Gastroenterol. 2013;4:32-40.*

16. Ans. B

Pityriasis rosea is a self-limiting, generally benign disorder for which the prognosis is excellent and the recurrence rate is low (approximately 2%). PR usually lasts for 6–8 weeks, but can last as long as 3–6 months.

Ref:
1. Schwartz RA, Janniger CK, Lichenstein R (2019). Pityriasis Rosea. [online] Available from https://emedicine.medscape.com/article/1107532-overview [Last accessed February, 2020].

17. Ans. D

This image suggests longitudinal melanonychia or longitudinal dark pigmentation of the nails which is characteristically associated with the use of zidovudine, hydroxyurea, minocycline, doxorubicin, and cyclophosphamide.

Ref:
1. Duan N, Zhang YH, Wang WM, Wang X. Mystery behind labial and oral melanotic macules: Clinical, dermoscopic and pathological aspects of Laugier-Hunziker syndrome. World J Clin Cases. 2018;6(10):322-34.

18. Ans. B

It is likely a voriconazole-induced periostitis. Hand radiographs show multifocal and asymmetrical periosteal reaction in the metacarpal shafts and phalanges. MRI demonstrates marked periosteal thickening of the phalangeal diaphysis, with preserved medullary cavities and congruent joints.

Ref:
1. Ladak K, Rubin L. Voriconazole-induced periostitis deformans: a mimicker of hypertrophic pulmonary osteoarthropathy. Clin Med Res. 2017;15:19-20.

19. Ans. D

These are vesiculopustular waxy lesions seen in keratoderma blenorrhagicum. These are often associated with sexually transmitted diseases.

Ref:
1. Dimitrova V, Valtchev V, Yordanova I, Haidudova H, Gospodinov D, Tisheva S. Keratoderma blenorrhagicum in a patient with Reiter syndrome. J of IMAB. 2008;14(1):68-71.

20. Ans. B

Orf virus is a *Parapoxvirus*. It is self-limiting, zoonotic viral disease that involving hands of people handling infected sheep and goats.

Ref:
1. Mola Selemon Review on Orf Virus on Shoat its Public and Economic Importance. SF J Flu Sci. 2019;2:1

21. Ans. D

Extrapulmonary TB can be conformed on biopsy, which reveals acid-fast bacilli, and tissue cultures for *M. tuberculosis* are positive. TB involving this region usually spares the tip of the finger.

Ref:
1. Mandal J, Margaretten M. Tuberculosis of the finger. N Engl J Med. 2018;379:1161.

22. Ans. D

The patient has developed pressure bed sore. The treatment involves aminoglycoside and clindamycin in combination.

Ref:
1. Trilla A. Skin and Soft Tissue Infections. International Society for Infectious Diseases; 2018

Pathogen	Empiric antibiotic	Active against MRSA?	Duration of initial therapy	Renal dose adjustment?
Mild infection			1–2 weeks	
Gram-positive cocci with or without MRSA	Amoxicillin/clavulanate (Augmentin)	No		Yes
	Cefdinir (Omnicef)	No		Yes
	Cephalexin (Keflex)	No		Yes
	Clindamycin*	Yes		No
	Dicloxacillin (Dynapen)	No		No
	Doxycycline	Yes		No
	Levofloxacin (Levaquin)	No		Yes
	Linezolid (Zyvox)	Yes (use if high risk of MRSA)		No
	Minocycline (Minocin)	Yes		Yes
	Trimethoprim/sulfamethoxazole	Yes		Yes
Moderate-to-severe infection			2–3 weeks	
Gram-positive cocci; gram-negative rods; anaerobes with or without multidrug-resistant organisms (e.g., MRSA, extended-spectrum beta-lactamase-producing strains, vancomycin-resistant *Enterococcus*)	Ampicillin/sulbactam (Unasyn)	No		Yes
	Cefoxitin	No		Yes
	Ceftriaxone (Rocephin)	No		No
	Clindamycin/fluoroquinolones	Somewhat		No/Yes
	Daptomycin (Cubicin)	Yes		Yes
	Ertapenem (Invanz)	No		Yes
	Imipenem/cilastin (Primaxin)	No		Yes
	Linezolid	Yes		No
	Moxifloxacin (Avelox)	No		No
	Piperacillin/tazobactam (Zosyn)	No		Yes
	Ticarcillin/clavulanate (Timentin)	No		Yes
	Tigecycline (Tygacil)	Yes		No
	Vancomycin	Yes		Yes

*Consider a double disk diffusion test before using for MRSA.
(MRSA: methicillin-resistant *Staphylococcus aureus*).
Source: Gemechu FW, Seemant F, Curley CA. Diabetic foot infections. Am Fam Physician. 2013;88(3):177-84.

23. Ans. D

For the supportive care in pressure bed sore, recommended management is removal of devitalized tissue, wound care in the form of cleansing with normal saline, keeping the surface free of moisture with appropriate positioning of the patient (image).

Ref:
1. ResearchGate (2016). Posture Recognition to Prevent Bedsores for Multiple Patients Using Leaking Coaxial Cable. [online] Available from https://www.researchgate.net/publication/309965747_Posture_Recognition_to_Prevent_Bedsores_for_Multiple_Patients_Using_Leaking_Coaxial_Cable [Last accessed February, 2020].

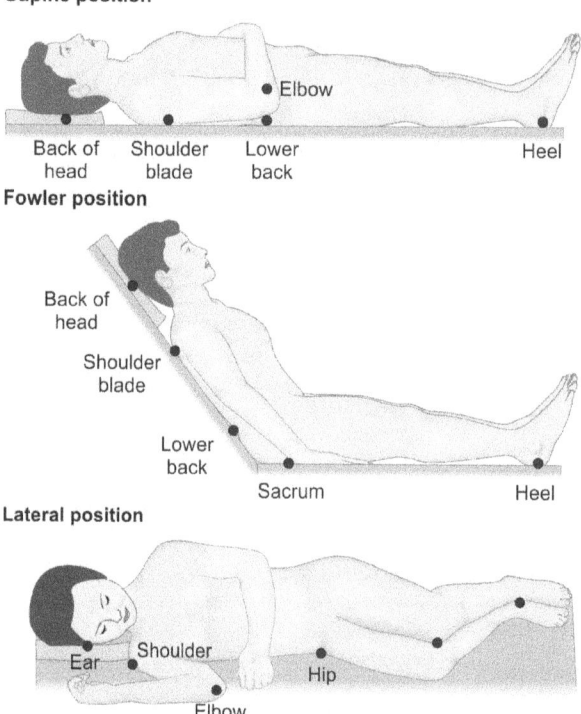

Source: ResearchGate (2016). Posture Recognition to Prevent Bedsores for Multiple Patients Using Leaking Coaxial Cable. [online] Available from https://www.researchgate.net/publication/309965747_Posture_Recognition_to_Prevent_Bedsores_for_Multiple_Patients_Using_Leaking_Coaxial_Cable [Last accessed February, 2020].

24. Ans. D

Amoxicillin-clavulanic acid 875 mg orally twice a day for 10 days is the appropriate antibiotic therapy. The management of diabetic ulcer is categorized according to the involvement of the structures. For a superficial ulcer with limited soft tissue, i.e., mild infection, the ulcer is cleansed and necrotic tissue and surrounding callus is debrided; an empiric oral antibiotic therapy is initiated which usually are targeted against *Staphylococcus aureus* and streptococci.

For deep or extensive infection, i.e., moderate or severe infection, the need for surgical intervention to remove necrotic tissue (debridement), compartment pressure is released or abscesses drained; also assessed for peripheral artery disease. Antibiotic therapy is aimed at common gram-positive and gram-negative bacteria, including obligate anaerobes.

Ref:
1. Lipsky BA, Berendt AR, Cornia PB, Pile JC, Peters EJG, Armstrong DG, et al. 2012 Infectious Diseases Society of America clinical practice guideline for the diagnosis and treatment of diabetic foot infections. Clin Infect Dis. 2012;54(12):e132-73.
2. Lipsky BA, Peters EJ, Senneville E, Berendt AR, Embil JM, Laveryet LA, et al. Expert opinion on the management of infections in the diabetic foot. Diabetes Metab Res Rev. 2012;28(Suppl 1):163-78.
3. Kosinski MA, Lipsky BA. Current medical management of diabetic foot infections. Expert Rev Anti Infect Ther. 2010;8(11):1293-305.
4. Schaper NC, van Netten JJ, Apelqvist J, Bus SA, Hinchliffe RJ, Lipsky BA (2019). IWGDF practical guidelines on the prevention and management of diabetic foot disease. International Working Group on the Diabetic Foot. [online] Available from https://iwgdfguidelines.org/wp-content/uploads/2019/05/01-IWGDF-practical-guidelines-2019.pdf [Last accessed February, 2020].

25. Ans. D

Most diabetic foot infections are polymicrobial. The most common pathogens are aerobic gram-positive cocci, mainly *Staphylococcus* species along with streptococci and *Bacteroides fragilis*. Methicillin-resistant *S. aureus* (MRSA) is present in 10–32% of diabetic infections and is associated with a higher rate of treatment failure in patients with diabetic foot infection.

Ref:
1. Gemechu FW, Seemant F, Curley CA. Diabetic Foot Infections. Am Fam Physician. 2013;88(3):177-84.
2. Vardakas KZ, Horianopoulou M, Falagas ME. Factors associated with treatment failure in patients with diabetic foot infections: an analysis of data from randomized controlled trials. Diabetes Res Clin Pract. 2008;80(3):344-51.
3. Kasper DL, Fauci AS, Hauser SL, Longo DL, Fauci A, Loscalzo J. Harrison's Principles and Practice of Medicine, 19th edition. New York, United States: McGraw Hill Education; 2015.

26. Ans. D

Erysipelas bacterial skin infection involving the upper dermis that characteristically extends into the superficial cutaneous lymphatics. It is a tender, intensely erythematous, and indurated plaque with a sharply demarcated border. Its well-defined margin can help differentiate it from other skin infections (e.g., cellulitis). Erysipelas is mainly caused by group A beta-hemolytic *Streptococcus, Streptococcus pyogenes*, rarely by another group of *Streptococcus*. The infection may enter the skin through abrasions or wounds such as

abrasions, sharp cuts, sheep scars, insect bites, surgical wounds, fissures of skin caused by injuries or by fungal infections, areas with necrosis such as foot ulcers in people with diabetes, chronic swollen areas such as hands, feet, arms, and legs.
Ref:
1. *Bonnetblanc JM, Bedane C. Erysipelas: recognition and management. Am J Clin Dermatol. 2003;4(3):157-63.*

27. **Ans. D**
US Food and Drug Administration (FDA) has approved ozenoxacin cream 1% for impetigo in patients aged 2 months and older. Ozenoxacin cream is a quinolone antimicrobial drug applied to the skin twice daily for 5 days.
Ref:
1. *Brown T (2017). FDA Approves Ozenoxacin Cream for Impetigo. [online] Available from https://www.medscape.com/viewarticle/890180 [Last accessed February, 2020].*

28. **Ans. E**
Cellulitis is commonly used to indicate a nonnecrotizing inflammation of the skin and subcutaneous tissues, usually from acute infection. Cellulitis caused by *S. aureus, S. pyogenes,* group A *Streptococcus,* and *S. epidermiditis.*
Ref:
1. *Kasper DL, Fauci AS, Hauser SL, Longo DL, Fauci A, Loscalzo J. Harrison's Principles and Practice of Medicine, 19th edition. New York, United States: McGraw Hill Education; 2015.*

29. **Ans. D**
Furuncle (Boil) and carbuncles are skin infections which are caused by *S. aureus.* These infections often form pockets in the skin filled with pus. A furuncle or a carbuncle is differentiated depending on its location and size. A furuncle is a painful infection of a single hair follicle. They occur on the buttocks, face, neck, armpits, and groin. Whereas a carbuncle is a deeper skin infection involving a group of infected hair follicles at a particular location. Carbuncles occur on the back of the neck, shoulders, hips and thighs, and are common in middle-aged or elderly men. People with diabetes are more likely to develop carbuncles.

Small furuncles are treated with moist heat; usually a warm or wet cloth is applied for 20–30 minutes, three or four times a day. This helps it to drain. Frequent washing of the affected area daily with antibacterial soap is advised to prevent the infection from spreading. Large furuncles and carbuncles are treated with antibiotics in combination with incision and drainage. Antibiotics are usually recommended for carbuncles, associated with fever, secondary infection (cellulitis).
Ref:
1. *www.health.harvard.edu/a_to_z/boils-and-carbuncles-a-to-z.*
2. *Ibler KS, Kromann CB. Recurrent furunculosis— challenges and management: a review. Clin Cosmet Investig Dermatol. 2014;7:59-64.*

30. **Ans. D**
Ecthyma gangrenosum (EG) is a well-recognized but uncommon cutaneous infection classically associated with *Pseudomonas aeruginosa* bacteremia. EG usually occurs in patients who are critically ill and immunocompromised; it is almost always a sign of pseudomonal sepsis. Rarely, other bacteria, including *Proteus* species, *Escherichia coli*, and methicillin-resistant *S. epidermidis* have been implicated in similar lesions. The characteristic lesions of EG are hemorrhagic vesicles or pustules that evolve into necrotic ulcers with a tender erythematous border.
Ref:
1. *Korte AKM, Vos JM. Ecthyma gangrenosum. N Engl J Med. 2017;377(23):e32.*
2. *Mouna K, Akkari H, Faten H, Yosra K, Hichem B, Maha M, et al. Ecthyma gangrenosum caused by Escherichia coli in a previously healthy girl. Pediatr Dermatol. 2015;32(4):e179-80.*
3. *Miyake S, Nobeyama Y, Baba-Honda H, Nakagawa H. Case of ecthyma gangrenosum in which only methicillin-resistant Staphylococcus epidermidis was detected. J Dermatol. 2016;43(4):460-2.*
4. *Firoz M, Jamal A, Ur Rehman SI. Non-pseudomonal ecthyma gangrenosum and idiopathic myelofibrosis in a two-year-old girl. Cureus. 2018;10(4):e2441.*

CHAPTER 9

Sexually Transmitted Infections

Surabhi Madan, Sneha Gohil

1. A 25-year-old unmarried male patient presented with complaints of penile ulceration with burning sensation for 10 days. There was no history of fever or any other comorbidities. He gave history of unprotected sexual intercourse about a week before the appearance of symptoms. On examination, there were multiple well-defined tender ulcers with polycyclic border on a background of diffuse erythema, with grouped vesicular lesions over the preputial skin. Bilateral firm, nonfluctuant, tender enlarged lymph nodes were present.

   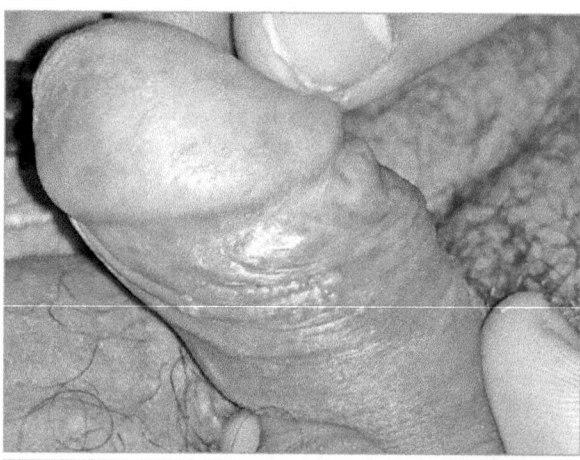
   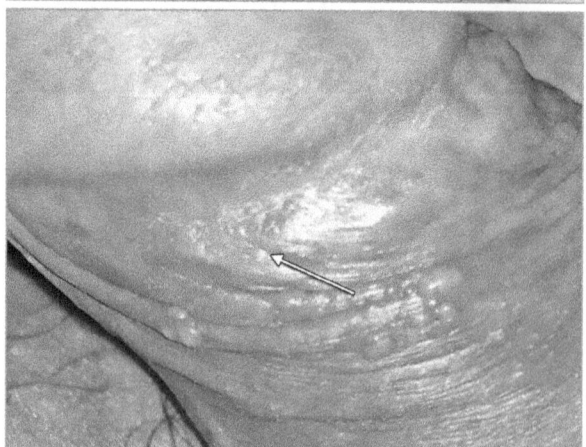

   Source: Dr Avanita Solanki, Associate Professor, Department of Dermatology, LG Hospital, Ahmedabad, Gujarat, India.

   What is the most likely diagnosis?
   A. Chancroid
   B. Herpes progenitalis
   C. Chancre
   D. Donovanosis

2. Which of the following is not true about herpetic genital infections?
   A. HSV DNA polymerase chain reaction (PCR) is the most sensitive test to diagnose HSV mucosal infections
   B. Sensitivity of all detection methods is higher in the recurrent episodes of infection
   C. Recurrence rates of genital herpes are more with HSV-2 than HSV-1
   D. Risk of mother-to-child transmission (MTCT) is highest when the infection is acquired near the time of labor

3. What is not true regarding treatment of herpetic infections?
   A. Acyclovir is the most frequently used agent used for treatment, in dose of 200 mg 5 times a day or 400 mg TDS, for 7–12 days
   B. Valacyclovir and famciclovir offer greater bioavailability than acyclovir and can be administered less frequently
   C. Treating the first episode of genital HSV eradicates the latent virus
   D. All patients are at risk of recurrent infections and may require additional antiviral therapy

4. A 30-year-old unmarried male patient presented with complaint of skin lesions over the penile shaft for almost a month. There were no burning, itching or other constitutional symptoms. History of unprotected sexual intercourse was present. On examination, there were pearly white papular lesions with central umbilication present over the penile shaft and pubic region. Lymph nodes appeared normal in size.

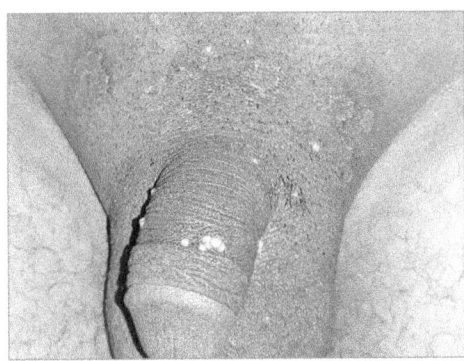

Source: Dr Avanita Solanki, Associate Professor, Department of Dermatology, LG Hospital, Ahmedabad, Gujarat, India.

What is the likely diagnosis?

A. Molluscum contagiosum
B. Genital warts
C. Herpes progenitalis
D. Lichen planus

5. **All of the following are the features of molluscum contagiosum, *except*:**

   A. The lesions may appear anywhere on the body except palms and soles
   B. It can affect both immunocompetent and immunosuppressed patients
   C. Cytoplasmic inclusion bodies (molluscum or Henderson–Paterson bodies) are seen by hematoxylin and eosin staining of the lesion
   D. Lesions resolve within few days in immunocompetent patients

6. **A 40-year-old diabetic male patient presented with history of skin lesions over the glans penis and preputial skin for last 4 months. Skin lesions had gradually increased over period of time. There was history of occasional bleeding from the skin lesions. However, there was no history of discharge, and burning or itching sensations. On examination, there were soft, pink, papilliferous masses, few of them with finger-like peduncles present over glans penis and preputial skin. What is the likely disease he is suffering from?**

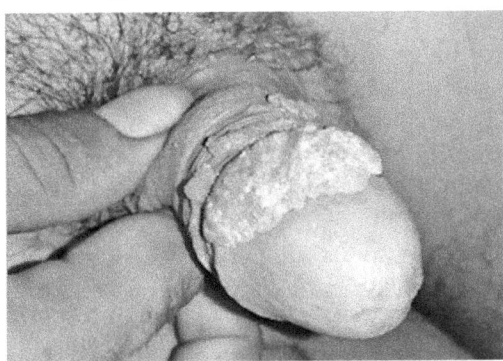

Source: Dr Avanita Solanki, Associate Professor, Department of Dermatology, LG Hospital, Ahmedabad, Gujarat, India.

A. Chancre
B. Chancroid
C. Condyloma acuminata
D. Herpes progenitalis

7. **A 50-year-old male patient presented with complaints of skin lesions over both palms and soles for last 1 month. He had history of skin lesions over penis 4–5 months back, which had healed after taking some oral and topical antibiotics. There was no history of pain over the genital lesions; however, mild burning sensation was present. There was no history of prior urogenital or enteric infection. On examination, there were dull, red papular eruptions of variable size on both palms and soles. Rounded, discrete lesions with characteristic collarette scaling were present over both palms, soles, and genitalia. He was diagnosed simultaneously with human immunodeficiency virus type 1 (HIV-1) infection.**

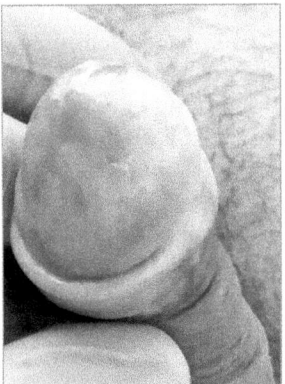

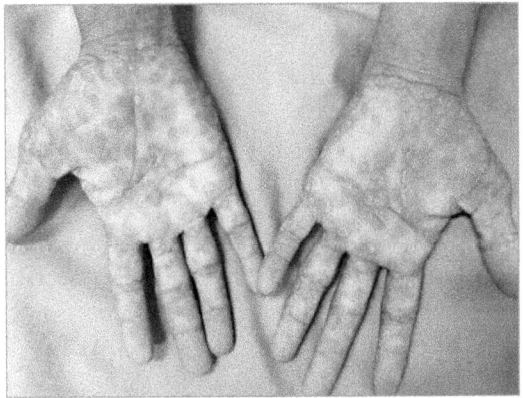

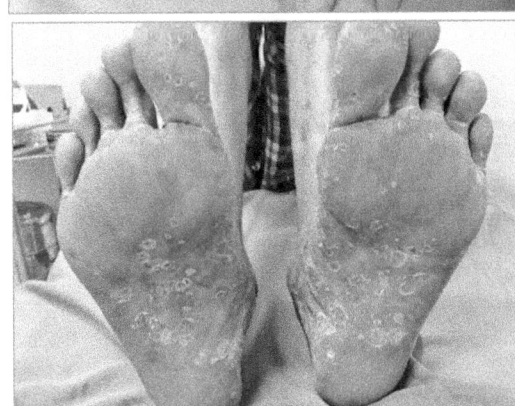

Source: Dr Avanita Solanki, Associate Professor, Department of Dermatology, LG Hospital, Ahmedabad, Gujarat, India.

What is the likely diagnosis?
A. Secondary syphilis
B. Reiter's disease
C. Disseminated gonococcal infection (DGI)
D. Chancroid

8. A 40-year-old male patient, diagnosed to have HIV-1 infection, with a CD4 count of 540 cells/mm^3, was found to be Venereal Disease Research Laboratory (VDRL) positive with a titer of 1 : 32. He was asymptomatic for syphilis and is presumed to have late latent syphilis. What should be the next step?
A. Cerebrospinal fluid (CSF) examination
B. Treat with penicillin G benzathine
C. Treat with aqueous crystalline penicillin G
D. No treatment

9. A 25-year-old unmarried male patient presented with complaint of urethral discharge for 7 days, along with burning micturition. He had history of unprotected sexual intercourse 10 days ago. There were no constitutional symptoms or itching. On examination, thick yellow urethral discharge was present at the urethral meatus. Rest of the glans penis and preputial skin was not affected. What is the likely organism to cause this syndrome?

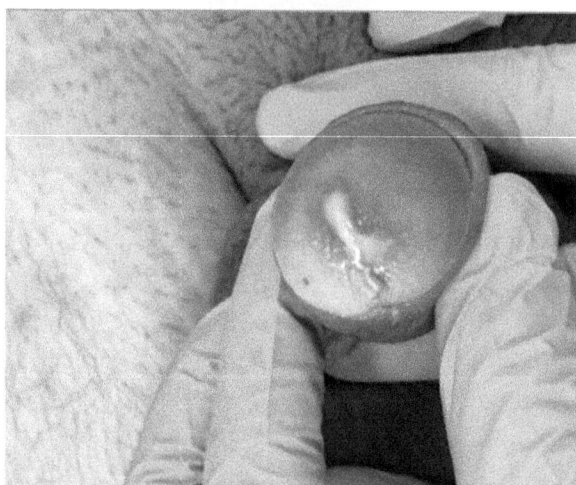

Source: Dr Avanita Solanki, Associate Professor, Department of Dermatology, LG Hospital, Ahmedabad, Gujarat, India.

A. *Chlamydia trachomatis*
B. *Neisseria gonorrhoeae*
C. *Trichomonas vaginalis*
D. *Mycoplasma genitalium*

10. What should be the first test to establish the diagnosis and cause of urethritis in men?
A. Gram stain
B. Culture
C. Multiplex nucleic acid amplification tests (NAATs)
D. Serology

11. What is the best treatment regimen for a patient with proven GU?
A. Ceftriaxone
B. Azithromycin
C. Ceftriaxone with azithromycin
D. Metronidazole

12. A 42-year-old married female patient presented with vaginal discharge for 10 days, with burning micturition and increased frequency of micturition. She complained of severe itching over the vulva at night with dyspareunia. Patient's husband also had skin lesions over glans penis, with itching and erosions over preputial skin. Examination revealed thick curdy white discharge around the introitus with surrounding mucosal erythema.

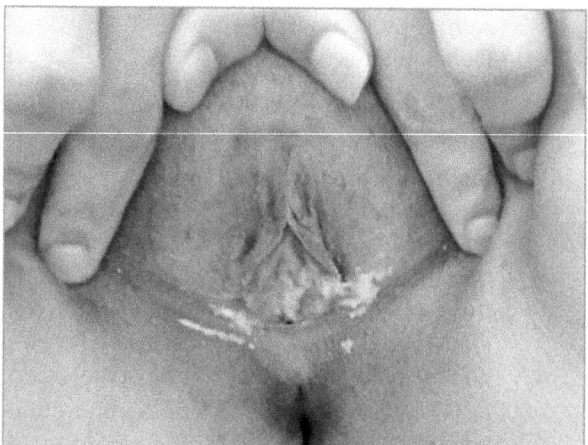

Source: Dr Avanita Solanki, Associate Professor, Department of Dermatology, LG Hospital, Ahmedabad, Gujarat, India.

What is the possible diagnosis?
A. *Trichomonas vaginalis*
B. Bacterial vaginosis
C. Vulvovaginal candidiasis
D. *Chlamydia trachomatis*

13. A 35-year-old diabetic female patient, presented with complaints of on and off per vaginal whitish discharge for 2–3 months, with increase in discharge and itching for 4–5 days. She also complained of severe dysuria and burning with difficulty in micturition for 5–6 days and appearance of vaginal ulcers for 6 days. On examination, there were multiple erosions and ulcers with polycyclic border with surrounding erythema over labia and in the gluteal fold, whitish discharge was present with edema of labia minora. Foley catheterization was done. Investigations revealed pyuria, with culture positive for *Escherichia coli* (colony count >10^5), extended-spectrum beta-lactamase (ESBL) pattern. Vaginal swab culture grew *Candida nonalbicans*.

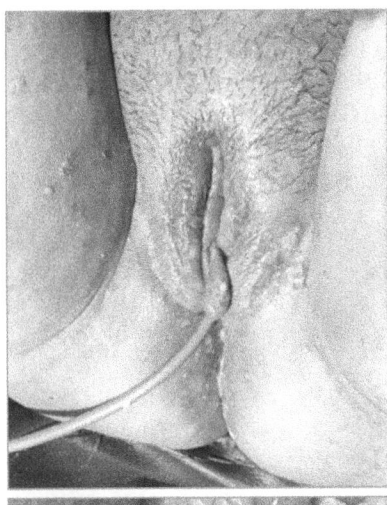

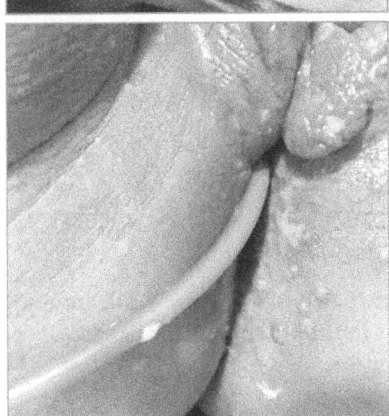

What other investigations should be done in this patient?

A. HSV-1 and HSV-2 PCR
B. Species identification and drug sensitivity testing for *Candida*
C. VDRL
D. Both A and B

14. Matrix-assisted laser desorption ionization time-of-flight (MALDI-TOF) identification of *Candida* was *Candida glabrata* (score 1.7). Which antifungal is least likely to act?

   A. Fluconazole   B. Voriconazole
   C. Posaconazole   D. Caspofungin

15. A 45-year-old female patient presented with history of 4–6 episodes of vaginal itching with scanty discharge P/V in last year, suggestive of recurrent candidiasis. Fungal culture of the vaginal swab was positive for fluconazole-sensitive *Candida albicans*. What is the best Rx option for her?

   A. Itraconazole
   B. Prolonged therapy with fluconazole
   C. Caspofungin
   D. Amphotericin B

16. A 40-year-old married male patient presented with history of genital ulceration since 5 days, complaint of pain at the site of ulceration with occasional blood staining of the undergarments. History of unprotected sexual intercourse 1 week ago was present. He also complained of painful swelling in the groin region since 5 days. There were no constitutional symptoms. On examination, two ulcers were present. One 2 × 2 cm ulcer was present over the frenulum, with sharp, rugged and undermined edges. The base of ulcer was nonindurated and was covered by yellowish necrotic exudate, covering the granulation tissue that bled readily on manipulation. The other ulcer was 0.5 × 0.5 cm with similar findings and was present over right side of frenulum.

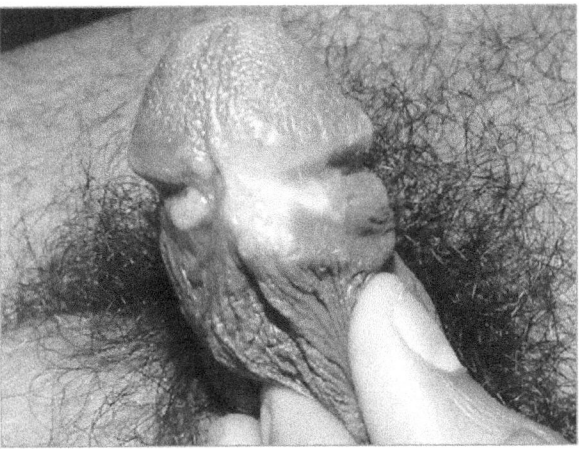

Source: Dr Avanita Solanki, Associate Professor, Department of Dermatology, LG Hospital, Ahmedabad, Gujarat, India.

What is the likely diagnosis?

A. Herpes progenitalis   B. Chancroid
C. Donovanosis   D. Chancre

17. A 30-year-old female patient, diagnosed with HIV for last 10 years and on tablets tenofovir disoproxil fumarate (TDF)/lamivudine (3TC)/efavirenz (EFV) for the same duration of time with excellent compliance, presented with progressive weight loss of about 15–17 kg over last 1 year, low-grade fever for 3 months. She was started on empirical anti-Koch's therapy (AKT) about 2 months ago elsewhere, as ultrasound examination revealed cervical lymphadenopathy, necrotic lymph nodes in the abdomen and splenic microabscesses. Fine-needle aspiration cytology (FNAC) of the cervical lymph node had shown presence of granulomas.

However, after 15 days of AKT, she developed severe vomiting and altered liver function tests (LFTs) [bilirubin—3.2 mg/dL, serum glutamic pyruvic transaminase (SGPT)—659 U/L, serum glutamic-oxaloacetic transaminase (SGOT)—2,040 U/L]. Also, there was no clinical improvement. On examination, she was cachexic, almost bed written. LFT were: bilirubin—8.04 mg/dL, direct—7.54 mg/dL, SGPT—508 U/L, SGOT—433 U/L, alkaline phosphatase—158 U/L, albumin—2.36 g/dL, globulin—2.2 g/dL. AKT was stopped. Computed tomography (CT) chest and abdomen with contrast was done which was suggestive of multiple enlarged inhomogeneously enhancing is to hypodense lymph nodes in neck, mediastinum and abdomen (largest 36 × 22 mm), without any calcification, multiple infiltrative lesions in the spleen. CD4 count was 113 cells/mm³ (49%), with CD4/CD8 ratio—2.3. HIV viral load was not detectable. Biopsy of cervical lymph node was done. What is the likely possibility?

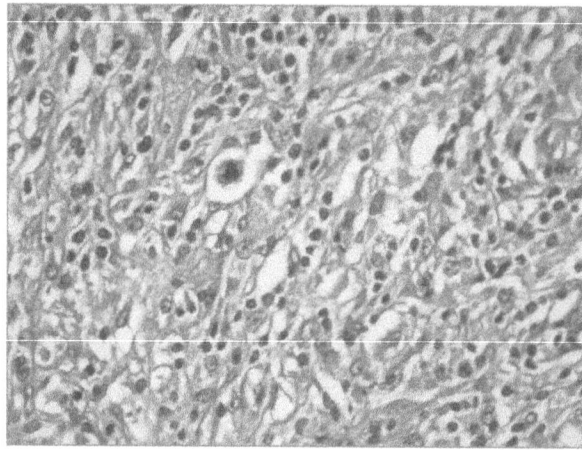

A. Tuberculosis (TB)   B. Lymphoma
C. Toxoplasmosis   D. Histoplasmosis

18. A 36-year-old male patient was brought by the relatives with history of altered conscious state (E3V1M4) for 7 days. Also, he had been suffering from fever for almost 6–8 months and had lost about 20 kg of weight. Recent workup done elsewhere revealed his positive retroviral status. Magnetic resonance imaging (MRI) brain was suggestive of multiple ring-enhancing lesions with possibility of abscesses with hemorrhagic areas. CT chest and abdomen revealed right-sided collapse consolidation (aspiration pneumonia). CSF examination showed 20 cells (90% lymphocytes), glucose—93.6 mg/dL [random blood sugar (RBS)—179], proteins—82; Gram stain, acid-fast bacillus (AFB) stain, India Ink and CSF cryptococcal antigen (CRAG) were all negative. His CD4 count was 11 cells/mm³ (3%), HIV RNA 440,300 IU/mL. *Toxoplasma* immunoglobulin G (IgG) was positive (154.8 IU/mL). What is the most likely diagnosis?

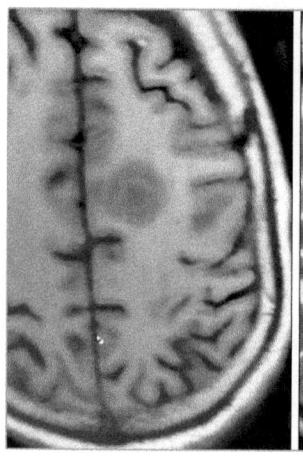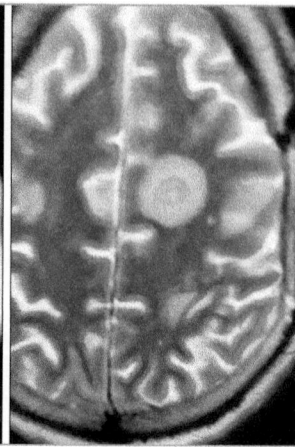

A. Cryptococcosis
B. Tuberculosis
C. Toxoplasmosis
D. Bacterial infection

19. What is the best immediate investigation which helps in the diagnosis of CNS toxoplasmosis in HIV patients?

A. Positive anti-toxoplasma IgG
B. Positive anti-toxoplasma IgM
C. Culture
D. Brain biopsy

20. A 57-year-old male patient presented elsewhere with fever and progressive weight loss for 1 year and headache with cough for a month. He was diagnosed as HIV reactive, CD4—78 cells/mm³ (7%) and was started on antiretroviral therapy (ART) [tenofovir + lamivudine + efavirenz (TLE)]. 15

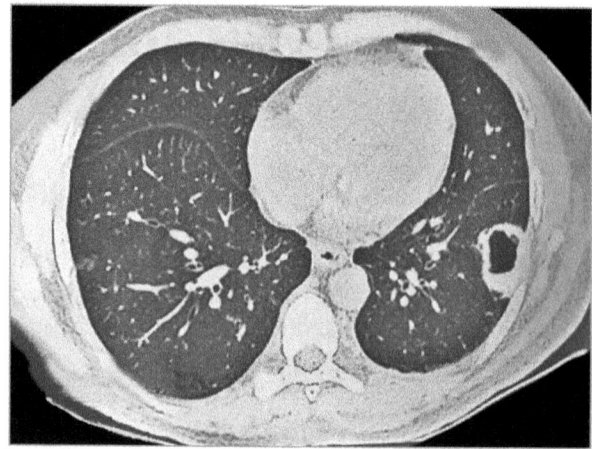

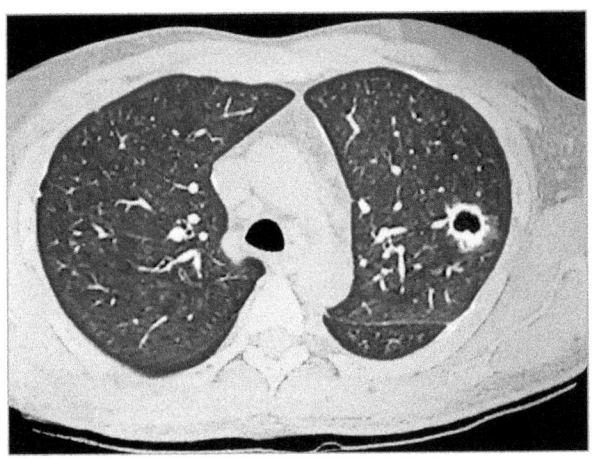

days later, AKT was started under directly observed treatment short-course (DOTS) based on his sputum positive for AFB. Almost a month after starting ART, he presented with progressively increasing headache. He looked poorly nourished; however, there were no focal deficits or neck rigidity.

MRI brain with contrast was normal. CT chest revealed cavitary lesions in left lung with multiple enhancing non-necrotic lymph nodes in the mediastinum without any consolidation or bronchiectasis.

Sputum was positive for AFB +2, repeated twice, with a negative GeneXpert test. CSF revealed 15 cells/mL, protein—43 mg/dL, glucose—59.8 mg/dL (RBS—120) with negative GeneXpert. CSF CRAG was positive by lateral flow assay. He was diagnosed to have cryptococcal meningitis [unmasking immune reconstitution inflammatory syndrome (IRIS)] with mycobacterial lung infection.

What is the next best intervention?

A. Bronchoscopy and investigations in bronchoalveolar lavage (BAL)
B. Line probe assay (LPA) from sputum
C. Continue ART, AKT and start Rx for cryptococcal meningitis
D. None of the above

ANSWERS WITH EXPLANATIONS

1. **Ans. B**

    A. *Chancroid*: It is an acute localized autoinoculable sexually transmitted genital ulcerative disease caused by gram-negative bacillus *Haemophilus ducreyi*. It is characterized by soft painful ulcer at the site of inoculation and is often associated with suppurative regional lymphadenitis. The edges of the ulcer are sharp, rugged and undermined, in contrast to the polycyclic border of ulcers seen in this patient. The base of ulcer is nonindurated and usually covered with a yellowish gray necrotic exudate covering granulation tissue that bleeds readily on manipulation.

    B. *Herpes progenitalis*: Genital herpes is acute, sexually transmitted genital ulcerative disease caused by herpes simplex virus (HSV). HSV-2 is more likely to cause genital recurrences as compared to HSV-1. The lesions start as grouped vesicles, but rapidly become pustular and ulcerate, coalescing to form an ulcer, with polycyclic margins. Lymph nodes are generally firm, nonfluctuant and extremely tender. It is a recurrent disease, and the first episode is usually associated with the systemic symptoms, involving multiple genital and extragenital sites.

    C. *Chancre*: It is the first lesion of primary syphilis, caused by *Treponema pallidum*, which usually goes unnoticed. The classical ulcer is painless, rounded, well-defined, indurated with dull red clean looking granular surface. It produces more serum than blood on manipulation, unlike chancroid. The lymph nodes are discrete, painless, small to moderate in size, of a firm rubbery consistency, and nonsuppurative.

    D. *Donovanosis*: It is also called granuloma inguinale, it is a chronic, indolent, sexually transmitted granulomatous ulceration of genitoinguinal region, caused by a bacillus known as *Calymmatobacterium granulomatis*. The primary lesion appears usually over genitals (90%) and inguinal (10%) regions, and very rarely at extragenital sites. It begins as a papule or a nodule that breaks down to form an ulcer, with a granulomatous base and beefy red margins. It characteristically bleeds on touch.

    Ref:
    1. Lawrence C. Herpes simplex virus infections. In: Kasper D, Fauci A, Hauser S, Longo D, Jameson J, Loscalzo J (Eds). Harrison's Principles of Internal Medicine, 19th edition. USA: McGraw Hill Companies; 2015. pp. 1175-82.

2. **Ans. B**

    A. Diagnosis of HSV genital infection can be made clinically when the lesions are characteristic. However, ulcerations may resemble other infections. Staining of the scrapings to detect giant cells or intranuclear inclusions of herpes virus infection can be done, the sensitivity of staining is 30%, and may resemble varicella-zoster virus (VZV) infections. Serological assays have limitations, and cannot differentiate between acute and old infections many a times. PCR is the most sensitive test to diagnose HSV mucosal infections.

B. Sensitivity of all detection methods is higher in the first rather than recurrent episodes. Similarly, vesicular lesions are associated with higher sensitivity as compared to ulcerative lesions. Also, sensitivity is more in immunosuppressed patients.

C. Though both HSV-1 and HSV-2 can cause genital and orofacial infections, and the infections caused by both are clinically indistinguishable, genital HSV-2 infection is twice as likely to reactivate and recur 8–10 times more frequently than genital HSV-1 infection.

D. When the infection is acquired in previously seronegative females, the risk of MTCT is highest when the infection is acquired near the time of labor. Also, first episode infections in pregnancy have more severe consequences for mother and infant. When women are seropositive for HSV-2 at the outset of pregnancy, no effects on neonatal outcomes are seen.

Ref:
1. Lawrence C. Herpes simplex virus infections. In: Kasper D, Fauci A, Hauser S, Longo D, Jameson J, Loscalzo J (Eds). Harrison's Principles of Internal Medicine, 19th edition. USA: McGraw Hill Companies; 2015. pp. 1175-82.

3. **Ans. C**

There is high risk of recurrences in patients with herpetic infections due to latent phase of virus in the body. Chronic suppressive therapy is a strategy for six or more recurrences per year.

Ref:
1. Lawrence C. Herpes simplex virus infections. In: Kasper D, Fauci A, Hauser S, Longo D, Jameson J, Loscalzo J (Eds). Harrison's Principles of Internal Medicine, 19th edition. USA: McGraw Hill Companies; 2015. pp. 1175-82.

4. **Ans. A**

A. *Molluscum contagiosum*: It is a benign papular condition that is often sexually transmitted, caused by a pox virus. The lesions begin as tiny white-colored papule that grows over several months, occasionally enlarging to produce giant molluscum. The skin-colored papules are smooth, firm and dome shaped, with a characteristic central umbilication from which caseous material can be expressed that contains molluscum body.

B. *Genital warts*: These are pedunculated, papular or macular lesions of genital mucosa and the adjoining area caused by human papillomavirus infection. These lesions are soft, pink, pedunculated papilliferous masses (cauliflower like) with finger-like peduncle and irregular surface.

C. *Herpes*: The lesions of herpes are grouped vesicular lesions, which often rupture to form ulcers with polycyclic margin.

D. *Lichen planus*: It is an inflammatory, papulosquamous disorder affecting either or all of the skin, mucous membranes, hair and nail. The typical lesion is a pruritic, purplish, plain top, polygonal papule.

Ref:
1. Marrazzo JM, Holmes KK. Sexually transmitted infections: overview and clinical approach. In: Kasper D, Fauci A, Hauser S, Longo D, Jameson J, Loscalzo J (Eds). Harrison's Principles of Internal Medicine, 19th edition. USA: McGraw Hill Companies; 2015. pp. 869-83.

5. **Ans. D**

Individual lesions usually spontaneously resolve within 2 months and the infection often clears completely in 6–12 months, disease may persist for 3–5 years in a minority of patients.

Ref:
1. Marrazzo JM, Holmes KK. Sexually transmitted infections: overview and clinical approach. In: Kasper D, Fauci A, Hauser S, Longo D, Jameson J, Loscalzo J (Eds). Harrison's Principles of Internal Medicine, 19th edition. USA: McGraw Hill Companies; 2015. pp. 869-83

6. **Ans. C**

Condyloma acuminata are pedunculated, papular or macular lesions of genital mucosa and its adjoining area caused by human papillomavirus infection. These lesions are soft, pink, pedunculated papilliferous masses (cauliflower like) with finger-like peduncle and irregular surface. They are usually seen on moist partially keratinized epithelium like preputial cavity, urinary meatus, labia minora, introitus, vagina, cervix, anus, and anal cavity.

The clinical features of chancre, chancroid and genital herpetic lesions have already been described above.

Ref:
1. Marrazzo JM, Holmes KK. Sexually transmitted infections: overview and clinical approach. In: Kasper D, Fauci A, Hauser S, Longo D, Jameson J, Loscalzo J (Eds). Harrison's Principles of Internal Medicine, 19th edition. USA: McGraw Hill Companies; 2015. pp. 869-83.

7. **Ans. A**

A. *Secondary syphilis*: Signs and symptoms of secondary syphilis usually develop 6–8 weeks after the development of primary chancre. Common signs are rash (75–100%), lymphadenopathy, and mucosal lesions. The papular syphilide is the most common and most characteristic lesion of secondary syphilis. Papules are dull red in color, variable in size, rounded, discrete, symmetrically distributed and usually polymorphic, with collarette scaling, and have a predilection for palms and soles as seen in our patient.

B. *Reiter's disease*: It is also known as oculo-urethro-synovial syndrome, manifests as nonsuppurative polyarthritis lasting for more than 1 month. It follows closely after lower urogenital or enteric infection with certain microorganisms. Common clinical manifestations includes arthritis, urethritis, cystitis, mucocutaneous eruptions like circinate balanitis, ulceration over tongue, keratoderma blenorragicum, conjunctivitis, uveitis, cardiac involvement in form of aortitis, aortic insufficiency, heart block.

C. *Disseminated gonococcal infection*: It most commonly follows asymptomatic mucosal infection and is more common in women. The clinical manifestations of DGI include vasculitis-like skin lesions, endocarditis, myocarditis, pericarditis, meningitis, and arthritis.

D. *Chancroid*: Chancroid is characterized by soft painful ulcer and is often associated with suppurative regional lymphadenitis. Mild constitutional symptoms such as malaise and low-grade fever may accompany the illness. However, *H. ducreyi* has not been shown to cause systemic infection.

Ref:
1. *Radolf JD, Tramont EC, Salazar JC. Syphilis (Treponema pallidum). In: Mandell GL, Douglas RG, Bennett JE (Eds). Principles and Practice of Infectious Diseases, 8th edition. Philadelphia: Elsevier Churchill Livingstone; 2015. pp. 2684-709.*

8. **Ans. B**

Cerebrospinal fluid examination is not routinely recommended in late latent syphilis to diagnose asymptomatic neurosyphilis. Several studies have suggested that a VDRL titer of ≥1:32 or CD4 <350 cells/mm^3 in HIV patients indicate higher risk of neurosyphilis, and CSF examination in this subgroup is advisable.

Treatment with 3 weekly injections of benzathine penicillin 2.4 million units (MU) for treatment of all non-neurological forms of late syphilis is recommended. 10- to 14-day course of aqueous penicillin G is recommended for neurosyphilis (3–4 MU IV every 4 hours).

Ref:
1. *Radolf JD, Tramont EC, Salazar JC. Syphilis (Treponema pallidum). In: Mandell GL, Douglas RG, Bennett JE (Eds). Principles and Practice of Infectious Diseases, 8th edition. Philadelphia: Elsevier Churchill Livingstone; 2015. pp. 2684-709.*

9. **Ans. B**

This is the syndrome of urethritis in men, which produces urethral discharge, dysuria or both, usually without frequency of urination. Common causes include *N. gonorrhoeae, C. trachomatis, M. genitalium, Ureaplasma urealyticum, T. vaginalis,* HSV, and adenovirus.

- *Chlamydia trachomatis* infection: *C. trachomatis* is gram-negative bacterium that causes infection of lower genital tract in both men and women. In men, it causes urethritis, and occasionally, epididymitis. It usually causes mucoid or mucopurulent discharge, less purulent than the typical discharge in gonorrhea. In women, it causes an odorless, mucoid vaginal discharge not associated with pruritus. Some women may develop urethritis manifesting with dysuria without frequency or urgency.
- *Gonorrhea*: Acute urethritis is the most common manifestation of gonorrhea in males. It manifests typically as acute anterior urethritis, characterized by a thick, yellow urethral discharge associated with symptoms of dysuria, meatal itching and burning. The incubation period is usually 2–7 days. The discharge becomes profuse and purulent within a day or two of onset of symptoms. In women, it causes odorless vaginal discharge, vaginal bleeding, dyspareunia and increased urinary frequency.
- *Trichomonas vaginalis* infection: *T. vaginalis* is an important cause of persistent or recurrent urethritis. In men, it manifests as subpreputial discharge with associated balanoposthitis in the uncircumcised men. Meatal moisture and mild irritation is the only finding in chronic cases. In women, it manifests as foul smelling, greenish-yellowish or lime green vaginal discharge, vaginal soreness with dyspareunia, lower abdominal pain and dysuria. The mucosa of vagina and cervix is edematous, inflamed and covered with punctate hemorrhages giving it a characteristic strawberry appearance. The surrounding skin of vulva is inflamed and red.

Ref:
1. *Marrazzo JM, Holmes KK. Sexually transmitted infections: overview and clinical approach. In: Kasper D, Fauci A, Hauser S, Longo D, Jameson J, Loscalzo J (Eds). Harrison's Principles of Internal Medicine, 19th edition. USA: McGraw Hill Companies; 2015. pp. 869-83.*

10. **Ans. A**

A. Gram stain of the urethral discharge/urethrogenital swab usually reveals ≥ 5 neutrophils per 1,000 × field in areas containing cells. Gram-negative intracellular bacilli suggestive of gonococci are typical of gonococcal urethritis (GU). This test is 98% sensitive for the diagnosis of gonococcal infection.

Microscopic examination of wet mounts of prostatic secretions and direct immunofluorescent antibody staining are used for diagnosis of *T. vaginalis*.

B. Culture may be positive when Gram stain is negative. Certain strains of *N. gonorrhoeae* can result in negative Gram stains in up to 30% of cases.
C. *NAATs*: Multiplex NAATs of first-voided urine may be yielding in gonococcal urethritis (GU) as well as nongonococcal urethritis (NGU), mainly caused by *C. trachomatis*.
D. *Serology*: It has no role in the diagnosis of these infections.

Ref:
1. Marrazzo JM, Holmes KK. Sexually transmitted infections: overview and clinical approach. In: Kasper D, Fauci A, Hauser S, Longo D, Jameson J, Loscalzo J (Eds). Harrison's Principles of Internal Medicine, 19th edition. USA: McGraw Hill Companies; 2015. pp. 869-83.

11. Ans. C

If gonococci are demonstrated by Gram stain or if urethritis is treated empirically, then single dose injection ceftriaxone 250 mg single dose/oral cefixime 400 mg along with oral azithromycin 1 g single dose/doxycycline 100 mg BD for 7 days to cover for *C. trachomatis* should be given, as the latter frequently causes coinfection in men with GU.

Metronidazole 2 g stat or 500 mg BD for 7 days should be considered in men with recurrent urethritis after treatment for NGU.

Ref:
1. Marrazzo JM, Holmes KK. Sexually transmitted infections: overview and clinical approach. In: Kasper D, Fauci A, Hauser S, Longo D, Jameson J, Loscalzo J (Eds). Harrison's Principles of Internal Medicine, 19th edition. USA: McGraw Hill Companies; 2015. pp. 869-83.

12. Ans. C

A. *Trichomonas vaginalis*: It is one of the common causes of vaginal discharge. It manifests as profuse, foul smelling, greenish-yellow, purulent vaginal discharge, vaginal soreness with dyspareunia, lower abdominal pain and dysuria. The mucosa of vagina and cervix is edematous, inflamed and covered with punctate hemorrhages giving it a characteristic strawberry appearance. The surrounding skin of vulva is inflamed and red.
B. *Bacterial vaginosis*: It is a syndrome that occurs due to disturbance in the vaginal microbial ecosystem, rather than a true tissue infection. The normal vaginal flora, especially the hydrogen peroxide producing lactobacilli, is replaced by organisms such as *Gardnerella vaginalis, Mycoplasma hominis* and several anaerobic bacteria. It is characterized clinically by a foul smelling grayish-white nonviscous homogeneous and uniformly adherent vaginal discharge.
C. *Vulvovaginal candidiasis*: It presents with intense vulval and vaginal pruritus, vaginal discharge, dysuria, dyspareunia, and postcoital irritation. A thick curdy white or cottage cheese-like vaginal discharge is pathognomonic. Satellite pustules may be seen on the labia, perineum and inner side of the thigh.
D. *Chlamydia trachomatis*: Chlamydia infection of the lower genital tract occurs in the endocervix, and causes mucopurulent cervicitis. It causes an odorless discharge from the cervical os, endocervical bleeding upon gentle swabbing; generally not associated with pruritus.

Ref:
1. Pappas PG, Kauffman CA, Andes DR, Clancy CJ, Marr KA, Ostrosky-Zeichner L, et al. Clinical practice guideline for the management of candidiasis: 2016 update by the Infectious Diseases Society of America. Clin Infect Dis. 2016:62:e1-50.

13. Ans. D

Vaginal ulcers appear to be herpetic ulcers, the diagnosis of which can be made best with the help of PCR. Per vaginal discharge and other symptoms can be attributed to vulvovaginal candidiasis, which mandates treatment. Hence, workup for *Candida* [ID and diploid sequence type (DST)] is needed.

Ref:
1. Pappas PG, Kauffman CA, Andes DR, Clancy CJ, Marr KA, Ostrosky-Zeichner L, et al. Clinical practice guideline for the management of candidiasis: 2016 update by the Infectious Diseases Society of America. Clin Infect Dis. 2016:62:e1-50.

14. Ans. A

Candida glabrata has dose-dependent susceptibility (DDS) to fluconazole, mostly due to changes in drug efflux. Fluconazole may be resistant in many cases. Hence it is not the antifungal of choice for this species, or may need very high doses. Isolates that are resistant to fluconazole may be resistant to voriconazole as well.

Ref:
1. Pappas PG, Kauffman CA, Andes DR, Clancy CJ, Marr KA, Ostrosky-Zeichner L, et al. Clinical practice guideline for the management of candidiasis: 2016 update by the Infectious Diseases Society of America. Clin Infect Dis. 2016:62:e1-50.

15. Ans. B

Complicated vulvovaginal candidiasis includes cases that occur ≥4 times per year, are unusually severe, are caused by nonalbicans species, or occur in women with uncontrolled diabetes mellitus (DM), immunosuppression or pregnancy. Sensitivity of *Candida* needs to be checked in all these cases. If the

Candida is fluconazole sensitive, then 10–14 days of fluconazole followed by a maintenance therapy with 200 mg every week for 6 months is advisable.
Ref:
1. *Pappas PG, Kauffman CA, Andes DR, Clancy CJ, Marr KA, Ostrosky-Zeichner L, et al. Clinical practice guideline for the management of candidiasis: 2016 update by the Infectious Diseases Society of America. Clin Infect Dis. 2016:62:e1-50.*

16. Ans. B

Chancroid: Chancroid is an acute localized autoinoculable sexually transmitted genital ulcerative disease caused by Gram negative bacteria (GNB) *H. ducreyi*. It is characterized by soft painful ulcer at the site of inoculation and is often associated with suppurative regional lymphadenitis. The edges of the ulcer are sharp, rugged and undermined. The base of ulcer is nonindurated and usually covered with a yellowish gray necrotic exudate covering granulation tissue that bleeds readily on manipulation. In males, most common sites of ulcer in order of frequency are the prepuce, frenulum and coronal sulcus. In females, the lesions are usually localized on the vulva, especially on the fourchette, vestibule and clitoris.
Ref:
1. *Marrazzo JM, Holmes KK. Sexually transmitted infections: overview and clinical approach. In: Kasper D, Fauci A, Hauser S, Longo D, Jameson J, Loscalzo J (Eds). Harrison's Principles of Internal Medicine, 19th edition. USA: McGraw Hill Companies; 2015. pp. 869-83.*

17. Ans. B

Tuberculosis is a strong differential. However, worsening of the clinical condition despite undetectable viral load, nature of the lymph nodes on CT scan and no response to AKT are points against the diagnosis of TB. With the use of highly active antiretroviral therapy (HAART), incidence of major acquired immunodeficiency syndrome (AIDS)-associated malignancies—Kaposi's sarcoma and high-grade non-Hodgkin lymphoma (HL) has gone down. However, among non-AIDS-defining cancers, an increased risk of HL has been observed. The aggressive histological subtypes of classical HL, i.e., mixed cellularity and lymphocyte depletion, predominate among HIV-HL. *This patient was found to have Hodgkin Lymphoma—mixed cellularity type.*

Toxoplasmosis is associated with very low CD4 counts (<100/mm³), and this is not the presentation of the disease.
Ref:
1. *National AIDS Control Organisation (NACO). National guidelines on prevention, management and control of reproductive tract infections including sexually transmitted infections. Ministry of Health and Family Welfare, Government of India, New Delhi; 2007*

18. Ans. C

Cryptococcal meningitis in HIV patients does not present radiologically with mass lesions usually, unlike TB and toxoplasmosis. The typical features are meningovascular enhancement, prominence of Virchow–Robin spaces (CT scan may be normal in 50% of patients and MRI is preferred). Also, CSF and serum CRAG > 90% sensitive and specific for diagnosis of cryptococcal meningitis in HIV patients.

Tuberculosis and toxoplasma are very close differential diagnoses due to similar radiological features. However, there are some differences on brain imaging which help to differentiate between them. CD4 count <100 cells/mm^3 is the major risk factor to develop central nervous system (CNS) toxoplasmosis.

CNS tuberculosis	CNS toxoplasmosis
Multiple stages may be seen—noncaseating granulomas, solid caseating granulomas, caseating granulomas with central necrosis, abscess	Classical lesion has hemorrhage presenting as blooming on susceptibility-weighted imaging (SWI), T1 hyperintensity
Nonrestricting solid caseating granulomas on diffusion-weighted imaging (DWI), restricting central necrosis	Restriction of peripheral rim
Areas of brain involved—sulci, basal cisterns, subcortical white matter. Infratentorial involvement is common	Along the vessels—grayish white matter junction, deep brain. Basal ganglia, thalami, periventricular regions are commonly involved
Usually thick and well-defined ring; conglomeration may be present	Usually ill-defined ring with edema out of proportion, presence of hemorrhage

Ref:
1. *National AIDS Control Organisation (NACO). National guidelines on prevention, management and control of reproductive tract infections including sexually transmitted infections. Ministry of Health and Family Welfare, Government of India, New Delhi; 2007.*

19. Ans. A

A presumptive diagnosis of CNS toxoplasmosis in patients with AIDS can be made by clinical presentation, radiology and positive IgG which suggests history of past exposure. When these criteria are used, the predictive value is as high as 80%. More than 90% of patients with AIDS and toxoplasmosis have IgG antibody to *Toxoplasma gondii* in serum.

Immunoglobulin M serum antibody is usually not detectable.

Brain biopsy is indicated in the above-mentioned category of patients, when they do not respond to therapeutic trial for toxoplasmosis, which should result in quantifiable clinical improvement by days 3–7.

Ref:
1. *National AIDS Control Organisation (NACO). National guidelines on prevention, management and control of reproductive tract infections including sexually transmitted infections. Ministry of Health and Family Welfare, Government of India, New Delhi; 2007.*

20. Ans. D

Any additional information from bronchoscopy is unlikely in this case as sputum is already positive for AFB. LPA is unlikely to be positive if GeneXpert is negative despite high bacterial load in sputum as in this case.

Probability of lung infection with nontuberculous mycobacteria (NTM) is high in this patient as compared to TB.

- Though clinical features of both NTM infection and TB may be similar, presence of following radiological features are more in favor of NTM infection: *Thin-walled cavities with less surrounding parenchymal opacities, less bronchogenic but more contiguous spread of disease, more marked involvement of pleura over the involved areas of the lungs, pleural effusion being rare and lesser of adenopathy.* Molecular tests like GeneXpert are negative in NTM infection. The gold old standard is culture for diagnosis.

- This patient was started on treatment for cryptococcal meningitis and NTM infection, along with ongoing ART.

AFB culture turned out to be positive for positive for *Mycobacterium kansasii.*

Registration Date and Time: 18 Jul, 2017; 00:37	Sample Type:
Sample Date and Time: 18 Jul, 2017; 00:36	Sample collected by: Non STMPL #
Report Date and Time: 31 Jul, 2017; 19:10	Accessioning Remarks: Normal
Test	Results
AFB culture (Bactec MGIT 960)	
Specimen	SPUTUM
ZN stain by petroffs method	AFB DETECTED (+)
AFB primary report	AFB culture is positive for NTMIMOTT on 10th day of incubation (Final report)
AFB intermediate report	
AFB culture final report	
Organism	*Mycobacterium* other than tuberculosis complex (MOTTINTM) confirmed by TB Ag MPT64 card

Ref:
1. *Griffith DE, Aksamit T, Brown-Elliott BA, Catanzaro A, Daley C, Gordin F, et al. An official ATS/IDSA statement: diagnosis, treatment, and prevention of nontuberculous mycobacterial diseases. Am J Respir Crit Care Med. 2007;175:367-416.*

CHAPTER 10

Tuberculosis and Its Variants

Amita Athavale, Rahul Bahot

PART I

1. Which of the following antibiotic regimens is suggested for adults with severe *Mycobacterium avium* complex (MAC) pulmonary disease?
   A. Rifampicin 600 mg daily + Ethambutol 25 mg/kg daily + Azithromycin 250 mg daily/Clarithromycin 500 mg twice daily + consider IV/nebulized amikacin
   B. Rifampicin 600 mg alternate day + Ethambutol 25 mg/kg alternate day + Azithromycin 250 mg daily/Clarithromycin 500 mg twice daily + consider IV/nebulized amikacin
   C. Rifampicin 600 mg daily + Ethambutol 25 mg/kg daily + Azithromycin twice a week/Clarithromycin 500 mg twice a week
   D. Rifampicin 600 mg thrice a week + Ethambutol 25 mg/kg thrice a week + Azithromycin 500 mg thrice a week/Clarithromycin 1 g in two divided doses thrice a week + consider IV/nebulized amikacin

2. Which of the following antibiotic regimens are suggested for adults with clarithromycin-resistant MAC pulmonary disease?
   A. Rifampicin 600 mg daily + Ethambutol 15 mg/kg daily + consider IV/nebulized amikacin
   B. Rifampicin 600 mg alternate day + Ethambutol 15 mg/kg daily + Isoniazid 300 mg (+ Pyridoxine 10 mg OD)/Moxifloxacin 400 mg OD + consider IV/nebulized amikacin
   C. Rifampicin 600 mg daily + Isoniazid 300 mg (+ Pyridoxine 10 mg OD)/Moxifloxacin 400 mg OD + consider IV/nebulized amikacin
   D. Rifampicin 600 mg daily + Ethambutol 15 mg/kg daily + Isoniazid 300 mg (+ Pyridoxine 10 mg OD)/Moxifloxacin 400 mg OD + consider IV/nebulized amikacin

3. What is the duration of treatment for MAC pulmonary disease?
   A. 6 months
   B. 9 months
   C. 18–24 months
   D. Minimum 12 months after culture conversion

4. Definition of culture conversion in nontuberculous mycobacteria (NTM) pulmonary disease:
   i. Three consecutive negative mycobacterial sputum cultures collected over a minimum of 3 months, with the time of conversion being the date of the first of the three negative mycobacterial cultures.
   ii. In patients unable to expectorate sputum, a single negative mycobacterial culture of a CT-directed bronchial wash is indicative of culture conversion.
   iii. Three consecutive negative mycobacterial sputum cultures collected over a minimum of 3 weeks, with the time of conversion being the date of the first of the three negative mycobacterial cultures.

   Which one of the following is correct answer?
   A. Statements i, ii, and iii all are correct
   B. Statements i and iii are correct
   C. Statements i and ii are correct
   D. Statements ii and iii are correct

5. Recurrence in NTM pulmonary disease is defined as:
   A. A positive mycobacterial culture 1 month after starting treatment
   B. A positive mycobacterial culture any time after completion of treatment
   C. Two positive mycobacterial cultures following culture conversion
   D. A positive mycobacterial culture following culture conversion

6. Refractory disease is defined as:
   A. Failure to culture—convert after 12 months of nontuberculous mycobacterial treatment
   B. Failure to culture—convert after 2 months of nontuberculous mycobacterial treatment
   C. Failure to culture—convert after 6 months of nontuberculous mycobacterial treatment
   D. Failure to culture—convert after 3 months of nontuberculous mycobacterial treatment

7. What is false about *Mycobacterium abscessus* (*M. abscessus*)?
   A. Pulmonary infection is the most common form of disease
   B. Approximately 80% of isolates of *M. abscessus* subsp. abscessus carry a functional *erm* gene with subsequent in vivo macrolide resistance
   C. Untreated isolates of *M. abscessus* subsp. massiliense are all macrolide susceptible
   D. Dual infection with MAC never occurs due to competitive colonization

8. Select the false statement:
   A. *Mycobacterium chelonae (M. chelonae)* is a rapid grower mycobacteria that causes skin and soft tissue disease
   B. *Mycobacterium fortuitum (M. fortuitum)* is a rare cause of lung disease, usually associated in patients with achalasia
   C. Most *M. fortuitum* isolates are macrolide resistant
   D. *M. fortuitum* commonly causes cavitary lung disease in patients with chronic obstructive pulmonary disease (COPD)

9. "Hot tub lung" refers to:
   A. Pulmonary infection by NTM in setting of acute inhalational burns
   B. Hypersensitivity lung disease
   C. Lung abscess caused by NTM in immunocompromised hosts
   D. Pulmonary NTM disease with cuts on skin being the point of entry of NTM

10. What is false about immunological response to NTM?
    A. Defects in IL-12 and interferon gamma production may make individuals with congenital immune deficiencies susceptible to NTM disease
    B. Defects in IL-3, IL-4 and IL-6 pathways may make individuals with chronic granulomatous diseases susceptible to NTM disease
    C. Tumor necrosis factor is also essential in the prevention of NTM disease activation
    D. NTM has not been shown to lead to latent infection in the immunologically normal host

PART II

11. The term "tuberculosis" was coined by:
    A. Johann Lukas Schönlein
    B. Sir Robert Koch
    C. Benjamin Marten
    D. None of the above

12. The organism responsible for causing tuberculosis was discovered by:
    A. Alexander Graham Bell
    B. Sir Robert Koch
    C. Hutchinson
    D. Thomas Edison

13. The environmental hygienic measures to promote prevention of tuberculosis include the following:
    A. Reduce overcrowding
    B. Houses to improve ventilation
    C. Discourage smoking in public places
    D. All of the above

14. The necrotizing granuloma is a feature of:
    A. *Mycobacterium tuberculosis*
    B. *Nocardia* spp.
    C. *Pneumocystis jirovecii*
    D. All of the above

15. Which of the following test used for the diagnosis of tuberculosis is key test in RNTCP?
    A. Sputum microscopy
    B. Sputum culture for tuberculosis
    C. Cartridge-based nucleic acid amplification test
    D. Chest X-ray

16. The WHO recommendations for the use GeneXpert for TB are not applicable to:
    A. Stool   B. Urine
    C. Blood   D. All of the above

17. A 32-year-old male was admitted with fever and neck stiffness along with altered sensorium in the emergency. He was suffering from pulmonary tuberculosis and the X-ray chest had worsened while on treatment. There was a clinical suspicion of tuberculous meningitis. Hence, cerebrospinal fluid was tapped and sent for GeneXpert for TB. Which of the following statements is correct?
    A. The volume of cerebral spinal fluid required for the GeneXpert is >0.1 mL
    B. The processing of cerebral spinal fluid depends upon the volume of CSF tapped
    C. Bloodstained or xanthochromic samples may give false-negative result in general support for the process
    D. All of the above

18. In case of nontreatment of tuberculosis the 5-year mortality rate for tuberculosis is:
    A. 30–40%   B. 40–50%
    C. 50–60%   D. 60–70%

19. The principles guiding the treatment of tuberculosis are all, *except*:
    A. Sputum examination can be overlooked in view of the presenting symptoms
    B. A single drug treatment of tuberculosis is not advocated
    C. Adding a single drop to the filling regiment strongly discouraged
    D. All the use of fluoroquinolones community-acquired pneumonia

20. The following measures are used for prevention of spread of tuberculosis to household contacts:
    A. Using sodium hypochlorite to disinfect the sputum
    B. Paper handkerchiefs active discarded by burning
    C. Use of 3 μm mask on patients' face
    D. All of the above

21. The differential diagnosis of pulmonary tuberculosis includes the following:
    A. Pulmonary echinococcosis
    B. Teratoma
    C. Wegner's granulomatosis
    D. Interstitial lung disease

22. The time taken for lymphadenopathy disappears after initiation of treatment is usually:
    A. 1 month
    B. 2 months
    C. 3 months
    D. 5 months

23. The differential diagnosis of tuberculosis lymphadenopathy includes the following, *except*:
    A. Lymphoma
    B. Leukemia
    C. Filariasis
    D. None of the above

24. The following statement is false about line probe assay:
    A. It can be done on smear positive and negative cases
    B. It yields results within 2 days
    C. This can detect rifampicin and isoniazid resistance
    D. It has less value in HIV and extrapulmonary TB

25. The 20-year-old gentleman was suffering from decrease appetite, evening rise in temperature followed by weight loss of 7 kg. The microbiological report of his sputum sample was *Mycobacterium tuberculosis* complex. The *Mycobacterium tuberculosis* complex includes the following:
    A. *Mycobacterium tuberculosis*
    B. *Mycobacterium africanum*
    C. *Mycobacterium bovis*
    D. All of the above

26. A 22-year-old male had been suffering from chronic cough for the past 6 months and weight loss of 10 kg in the same period. His uncle suffered from pulmonary tuberculosis died. His sputum smear was positive for acid fast bacilli. The DST report revealed resistance to streptomycin, ethambutol, and pyrazinamide. This patient has:
    A. Monodrug-resistant TB
    B. Multidrug-resistant TB
    C. Extensively drug-resistant TB
    D. Polydrug-resistant TB

27. A relative pays visit to sputum positive MDR-TB patient in the USA. Two weeks later he seeks medical attention. Which one of the following management options would be most appropriate?
    A. Immediate chest radiograph
    B. Tuberculin test or interferon-γ release assay (IGRA) in 6 weeks
    C. Prophylactic chemotherapy similar to that prescribed to the patient in the USA
    D. Treatment only if the tuberculin test or IGRA is positive
    E. Chest radiograph in 6 weeks

28. A 32-year-old woman who abuses intravenous drugs has a cough, blood-streaked sputum and a temperature of 38.8°C. She has lost 13 kg over the past 3 months. Chest radiography shows a right upper lobe infiltrate with cavitation. Three sputum smears are positive for acid-fast bacilli and culture results are pending. Gram staining of her sputum shows numerous leukocytes and scant gram-positive cocci in clusters. The tuberculin skin test shows 0 mm induration at 48 hours. The CD4+ T-cell count is 4.9×10^9/L. Her serum is positive for antibodies to HIV. The most likely diagnosis is pulmonary infection due to which one of the following?
    A. *Mycobacterium avium-intracellulare*
    B. *Mycobacterium kansasii*
    C. *Mycobacterium tuberculosis*
    D. *Staphylococcus aureus*
    E. Mixed anaerobic bacteria

ANSWERS WITH EXPLANATIONS

PART I

1. Ans. A

For severe MAC pulmonary disease (i.e., AFB smear-positive respiratory tract samples, radiological evidence of lung cavitation/severe infection, or severe symptoms/signs of systemic illness) the British Thoracic Society (BTS) 2017 guidelines recommends: Rifampicin 600 mg daily and ethambutol 15 mg/kg daily and azithromycin 250 mg daily or clarithromycin 500 mg twice daily and consider intravenous amikacin for up to 3 months or nebulized amikacin. Antibiotic treatment should continue for a minimum of 12 months after culture conversion.

2. Ans. D

Clarithromycin-resistant MAC pulmonary disease has to be treated with rifampicin 600 mg daily and ethambutol 15 mg/kg daily and isoniazid 300 mg (+pyridoxine 10 mg) daily or moxifloxacin 400 mg daily and consider intravenous amikacin for up to 3 months or nebulized amikacin. Antibiotic treatment should continue for a minimum of 12 months after culture conversion.

3. Ans. D

Antibiotic treatment should continue for a minimum of 12 months after culture conversion as per BTS guidelines 2017 for NTM

4. Ans. C

Culture conversion: Three consecutive negative mycobacterial sputum cultures collected over a minimum of 3 months, with the time of conversion being the date of the first of the three negative mycobacterial cultures. In patients unable to expectorate sputum, a single negative mycobacterial culture of a CT-directed bronchial wash is indicative of culture conversion.

5. Ans. C

Recurrence: Two positive mycobacterial cultures following culture conversion. If available, genotyping may help distinguish relapse from reinfection.

6. Ans. A

Refractory disease: Failure to culture—convert after 12 months of nontuberculous mycobacterial treatment.
Ref:
1. British Thoracic Society Guidelines, 2017.

7. Ans. D

Mixed infection with MAC and *Mycobacterium massiliense* (66%) was more common than mixed infection with MAC and *M. abscessus* (34%).

Ref:
1. Shin SH, Jhun BW, Kim SY, Choe J, Jeon K, Huh HJ, et al. Nontuberculous mycobacterial lung diseases caused by mixed infection with Mycobacterium avium complex and Mycobacterium abscessus complex. Antimicrob Agents and Chemother. 2018;62:e01105-18. doi. https://doi.org/10.1128/AAC.01105-18.

8. Ans. D

Mycobacterium fortuitum primarily associated with reflux esophagitis in achalsia cardia. It is a colonizer in lung damaged due to previous infections such as tuberculosis.
Ref:
1. Taiwo B, Glassroth J. Nontuberculous mycobacterial lung Diseases.b Infectious Disease Clinics of North America. 2010;24(3):769-89.
2. Park S, Suh GY, Chung MP, Kim H, Kwon OJ, Lee KS, et al. Clinical significance of Mycobacterium fortuitum isolated from respiratory specimens. Respir Med. 2008;102(3):437-42.

9. Ans. B

Hot tub lung is a hypersensitivity pneumonitis caused by *Mycobacterium avium* complex. The symptoms include cough, breathlessness, fever, chest tightness, and weight loss. The patients usually have an exposure to hot tub. The median time of diagnosis from symptom appearance ranges from 1 to 54 months. The chest X-ray shows diffuse nodular or interstitial infiltrates. HRCT chest shows diffuse ground-glass opacities with centrilobular micronodules. Specific anti-mycobacterial therapy is usually not required to manage most of this patients. Corticosteroid therapy seems to be helpful in severe cases. Complete recovery is achieved by further avoiding exposure to hot tub.
Ref:
1. Hanak V, Kalra S, Aksamit TR, Hartman TE, Tazelaar HD, Ryu JH. Hot tub lung: presenting features and clinical course of 21 patients. Respir Med. 2006;100(4): 610-5. doi: 10.1016/j.rmed.2005.08.005. Epub 2005, Sep 27.

10. Ans. B

A number of immunodeficiencies have been associated with NTM infection, including inherited disorders of IFNγ-IL12 pathway (e.g., IFNγR1 mutations), other cytokine signaling (e.g., STAT mutations), and macrophage and dendritic cell function (e.g., GATA2,83 NRAMP184), as well as acquired immunodeficiencies including HIV-AIDS85 and functional anti-interferon gamma antibodies.

The primary source of reference to all answers in Part I is British Thoracic Society guidelines for the management of non-tuberculous mycobacterial pulmonary disease (NTM-PD). The additional references as mentioned with the respective explanations.

PART II

11. Ans. A
Ref:
1. Barberis I, Bragazzi NL, Galluzzo L, Martini M. The history of tuberculosis: from the first historical records to the isolation of Koch's bacillus. J Prev Med Hyg. 2017;58(1):E9-E12.

12. Ans. B
Ref:
1. Barberis I, Bragazzi NL, Galluzzo L, Martini M. The history of tuberculosis: from the first historical records to the isolation of Koch's bacillus. J Prev Med Hyg. 2017;58(1):E9-E12.

13. Ans. D
Tuberculosis spreads via droplet infection. The reduction of overcrowding and improvement of the house of ventilation helps to reduce the transmission of droplet nuclei. Similarly smoking impairs the host defences against microorganisms. Thereby adapting these measures can reduce the risk of transmission of tuberculosis.
Ref:
1. Rieder HL, Chen-Yuan C, Gie RP, Enarson DA. Crofton's Clinical Tuberculosis, 3rd edition. New York City, United States: Macmillan Publishers Ltd; 2009.

14. Ans. D
Causes of necrotizing granulomas are:

Bacterial	Fungal	Parasites
Mycobacterium tuberculosis	Coccidioides immitis	Echinococcus granulosus
Nontuberculous mycobacteria	Coccidioides. posadasii	
Brucella	Cryptococcus neoformans	
Nocardia	Cryptococcus gattii	
	Histoplasma capsulatum	
	Blastomyces dermatitidis	
	Aspergillus spp.	
	Mucorales	
	Pneumocystis jirovecii	

Ref:
1. Shah KK, Pritt BS, Alexander MP. Histopathologic review of granulomatous inflammation. J Clin Tuberculos. Other Mycobacter Dis. 2017;7:1-12.

15. Ans. C
Cartridge-based nucleic acid amplification test is also known as TB GeneXpert test.
The turnaround time for this test is 1-2 days. The sensitivity and specificity of 95% and 98%, respectively in respiratory specimens whereas a nonrespiratory specimens the specificity is 95% while the sensitivity drops to 75-80%.

A positive test provides confirmation of the diagnosis of tuberculosis but however, a negative test does not exclude the disease.
Ref:
1. http://apiindia.org/wp-content/uploads/pdf/medicine_update_2017/ mu_022.pdf.

16. Ans. D
There is very little data on the clinical utility of GeneXpert for TB in the specimens like stool, urine, and blood. Hence, WHO does not recommend the use of GeneXpert for the above specimens.
Ref:
1. http://www.tbcindia.nic.in/showfile.php?lid=3255.

17. Ans. D
The volume of cerebrospinal fluid (CSF) < 0.1 mL is insufficient to run GeneXpert test for tuberculosis.
The volume of CSF tapped determines the processing method for GeneXpert, for example, if the volume of CSF is 5 mL or more the full sample has to be centrifuged and then it is mixed with 2 mL of reagent and if the volume of CSF tapped is 1-5 mL equal volume of the CSF to the sample reagent is added.
Blood stained and xanthochromic CSF samples may cause false negative Xpert MTB/RIF results.
Ref:
1. http://www.tbcindia.nic.in/showfile.php?lid=325.

18. Ans. C
The 5-year mortality rate of untreated tuberculosis is 50-60% and 20-25% experience spontaneous cure while chronic smear-positive TB develops in 20-25% immunocompetent individuals with smear-positive pulmonary tuberculosis.
Ref:
1. Varaine F, Rich ML (Eds). Rich ML. Chapter 2: Clinical presentation. In: Tuberculosis: Practical Guide for Clinicians, Nurses, Laboratory Technician and Medical Auxiliaries, 2014 edition. Geneva, Switzerland: Médecins Sans Frontieres; 2014.

19. Ans. A
It is mandatory to examine the sputum of the patient with probable diagnosis of pulmonary tuberculosis.
A single drug treatment for tuberculosis causes rapid development of resistance and hence is generally avoided.
If the patient is becoming worse get out culture sensitivity done for the tuberculosis bacilli. It is futile to add a single drug the failing regimen as resistance is likely to develop to this newly introduced single drug.
Ref:
1. Reider H, Chen-Yuan C, Gie RP, Enarson DA (Eds). General guidelines on the treatment of tuberculosis. In: Crofton's Clinical Tuberculosis, 3rd edition. New York City, United States: Macmillan Publishers Ltd; 2009.

20. Ans. D
Ref:
1. Rieder HL, Chen-Yuan C, Gie RP, Enarson DA. Crofton's Clinical Tuberculosis, 3rd edition. New York City, United States: Macmillan Publishers Ltd; 2009.

21. Ans. A
Cysts can mimic tuberculous cavities.
Ref:
1. Varaine F, Rich ML (Eds). Chapter 2: Clinical presentation. In: Tuberculosis: Practical Guide for Clinicians, Nurses, Laboratory Technician and Medical Auxiliaries, 2014 edition. Geneva, Switzerland: Médecins Sans Frontières; 2014.

22. Ans. C
Lymphadenopathy usually disappears within 3 months of starting antitubercular treatment. However, initially par may be observed in the form of increase in size of the lymph node, abscess formation, and fistula formation.
Ref:
1. Varaine F, Rich ML (Eds). Chapter 2: Clinical presentation. In: Tuberculosis: Practical Guide for Clinicians, Nurses, Laboratory Technicians and Medical Auxiliaries, 2014 edition. Geneva, Switzerland: Médecins Sans Frontières; 2014.

23. Ans. C
Ref:
1. Varaine F, Rich ML (Eds). Chapter 2: Clinical presentation. In: Tuberculosis: Practical Guide for Clinicians, Nurses, Laboratory Technicians and Medical Auxiliaries, 2014 edition. Geneva, Switzerland: Médecins Sans Frontières; 2014.

24. Ans. A

Line probe assay	GeneXpert
Can be done only in smear positive cases	Can be done in both smear positive and negative cases
Difficult to be done in crude clinical specimens	Can be done on crude clinical specimens
Results obtained in 2 days	Results obtained within 2 hours
Can detect both rifampicin and isoniazid resistance	Can detect only rifampicin resistance
Has less value in HIV and extrapulmonary TB	Has more value in HIV and extrapulmonary TB
Can only be used in national and regional level	Can be used in district and sub-district level
Technically less robust	Technically more robust
Less automated	More automated

Ref:
1. Varaine F, Rich ML (Eds). Chapter 3: Diagnostic investigation. In: Tuberculosis: Practical Guide for Clinicians, Nurses, Laboratory Technicians and Medical Auxiliaries, 2014 edition. Geneva, Switzerland: Médecins Sans Frontières; 2014.

25. Ans. D
The *Mycobacterium tuberculosis* complex consists of various species of *Mycobacterium* which can cause tuberculosis in humans. These are *M. tuberculosis*, *M. bovis*, *M. africanum*, *M. microti*, and *M. canetti*.
Ref:
1. Varaine F, Rich ML (Eds). Chapter 1: Introduction and epidemiology. In: Tuberculosis: Practical Guide for Clinicians, Nurses, Laboratory Technicians and Medical Auxiliaries, 2014 edition. Geneva, Switzerland: Médecins Sans Frontières; 2014.

26. Ans. D
Polydrug-resistant TB (PDR-TB): Resistance to more than one firstline antiTB drug, other than isoniazid and rifampicin.
Ref:
1. Varaine F, Rich ML (Eds). Chapter 2: Clinical presentation. In: Tuberculosis: Practical Guide for Clinicians, Nurses, Laboratory Technicians and Medical Auxiliaries, 2014 edition. Geneva, Switzerland: Médecins Sans Frontières; 2014.

27. Ans. B
Two weeks after contact, a chest radiograph would be unhelpful as the infection at contact would not have manifested yet. A positive tuberculin test or IGRA may indicate latent tuberculosis (TB) infection and a chest radiograph should only be performed after a positive result is obtained. Preventive anti-TB chemotherapy is not indicated for infection with MDR-TB because there is no evidence that it will be effective and because only a small proportion of infected contacts will develop TB. Contacts who test positively should be actively followed up for >2 years. Whether patients at elevated risk for developing active TB (such as HIV-infected patients) should receive preventive treatment for latent MDR-TB infection is currently unknown.
Ref:
1. National Institute for Health and Clinical Excellence. Tuberculosis: Clinical diagnosis and management of tuberculosis, and measures for its prevention and control. [online] Available from www.nice.org.uk/nicemedia/live/13422/53642/53642.pdf [Last accessed February, 2020].
2. Erkens CG, Kamphorst M, Abubakar I, Bothamley GH, Chemtob D, Haas W, et al. Tuberculosis contact investigation in low prevalence countries: a European consensus. Eur Respir J. 2010;36:925-49.

28. Ans. C
Immunocompromised patients especially early stages of HIV infection and intravenous drug abusers are highly susceptible for tuberculosis infection. The presence of acid fast bacilli in three consecutive samples clinched the diagnosis of mycobacterial infection. The sensitivity for tuberculin skin test is reduced in immunocompromised individuals. In HIV individuals *Mycobacterium avium* complex (MAC) and *Mycobacterium Kansasii* are the predominant nontuberculous mycobacteria causing infections. The constitutional symptoms of fever, night sweats,

weight loss, fatigue, diarrhea and pain in abdomen are typically present with MAC infections. They also have organomegaly (hepatomegaly and/or splenomegaly) with the lymphadenopathy. The diagnosis of disseminated MAC is made via demonstration of organism from bone marrow, blood or lymph node.

Ref:
1. Cobelens FG, Egwaga SM, Ginkel T, et al. Tuberculin skin testing in patients with HIV infection: limited benefit of reduced cutoff values. Clin Infect Dis. 2006;43(5):634-9.
2. Mandell LA, Wunderink RG, Anzueto A, et al. Infectious Diseases Society of America/American Thoracic Society consensus guidelines on the management of community-acquired pneumonia in adults. Clin Infect Dis. 2007;(Suppl 2):S27-S72.
3. Morris A, Crothers K, Beck JM, et al. An official ATS workshop report: Emerging issues and current controversies in HIV-associated pulmonary diseases. Proc Am Thorac Soc. 2011;8(1):17-26.
4. Perlman D, Salomon N, Perkins MP, Yancovitz S. Tuberculosis in drug users. Clin Infect Dis. 1995;21:1253-64.

CHAPTER 11

Central Nervous System Infections

Joy Desai, Azad Irani

CASE 1

A 30-year-old male presented with fever, headache, vomiting, and altered behavior since 5–7 days.
- On examination (O/E)—neck rigidity ++
- Cerebrospinal fluid (CSF): Proteins—80, sugar—normal, cells—100 with lymphocytic pleocytosis
- Tuberculosis (TB) polymerase chain reaction (PCR)—negative
- Herpes simplex virus (HSV) PCR—negative.

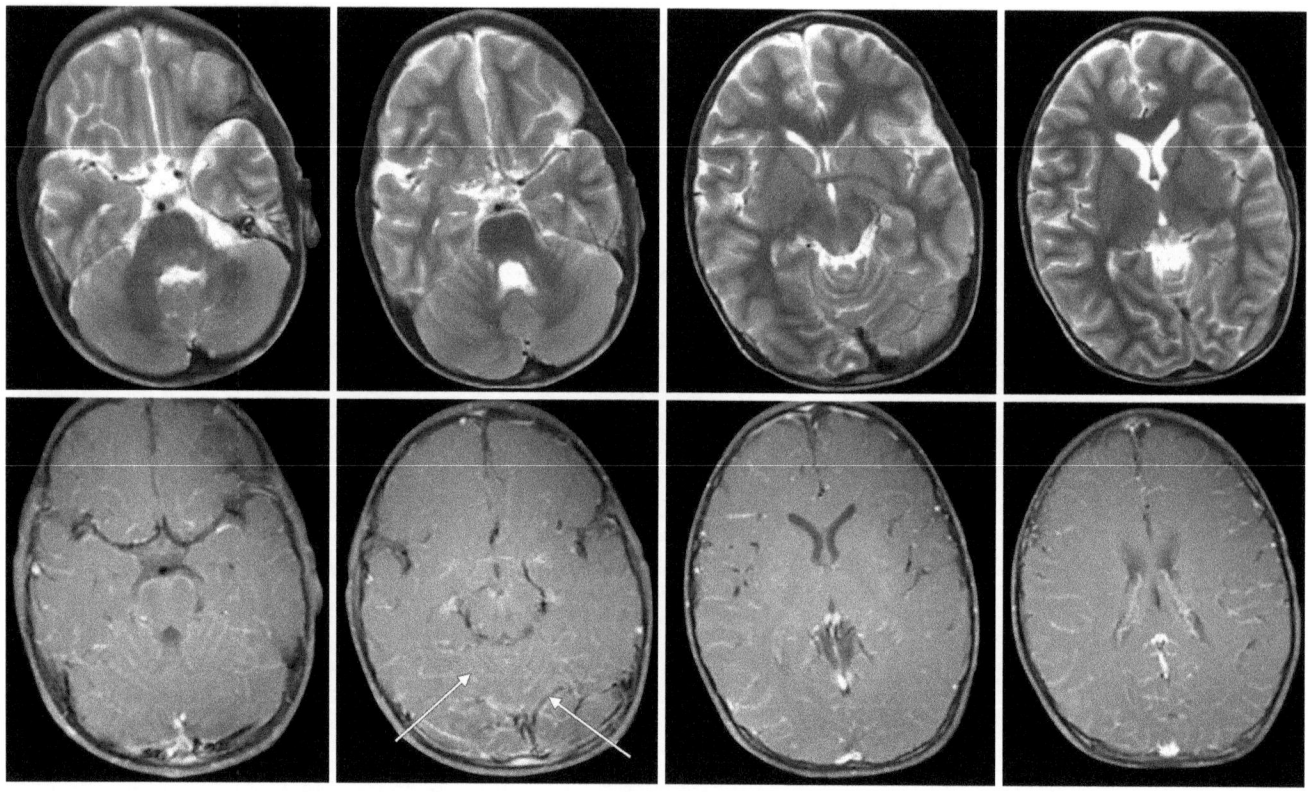

Postcontrast images showing enhancement along the meninges (arrows). No focal parenchymal lesion seen.

1. **The diagnosis that requires evaluation is:**
   A. Meningitis
   B. Encephalitis
   C. Tuberculosis
   D. Cryptococcosis

CASE 2

A 40-year-old seropositive male presented with right-sided weakness, fever, headache, vomiting, and altered sensorium.
- O/E—papilledema
- CSF—proteins—200, sugar—10/100, cells—500, 90% polymorphs, culture—negative.

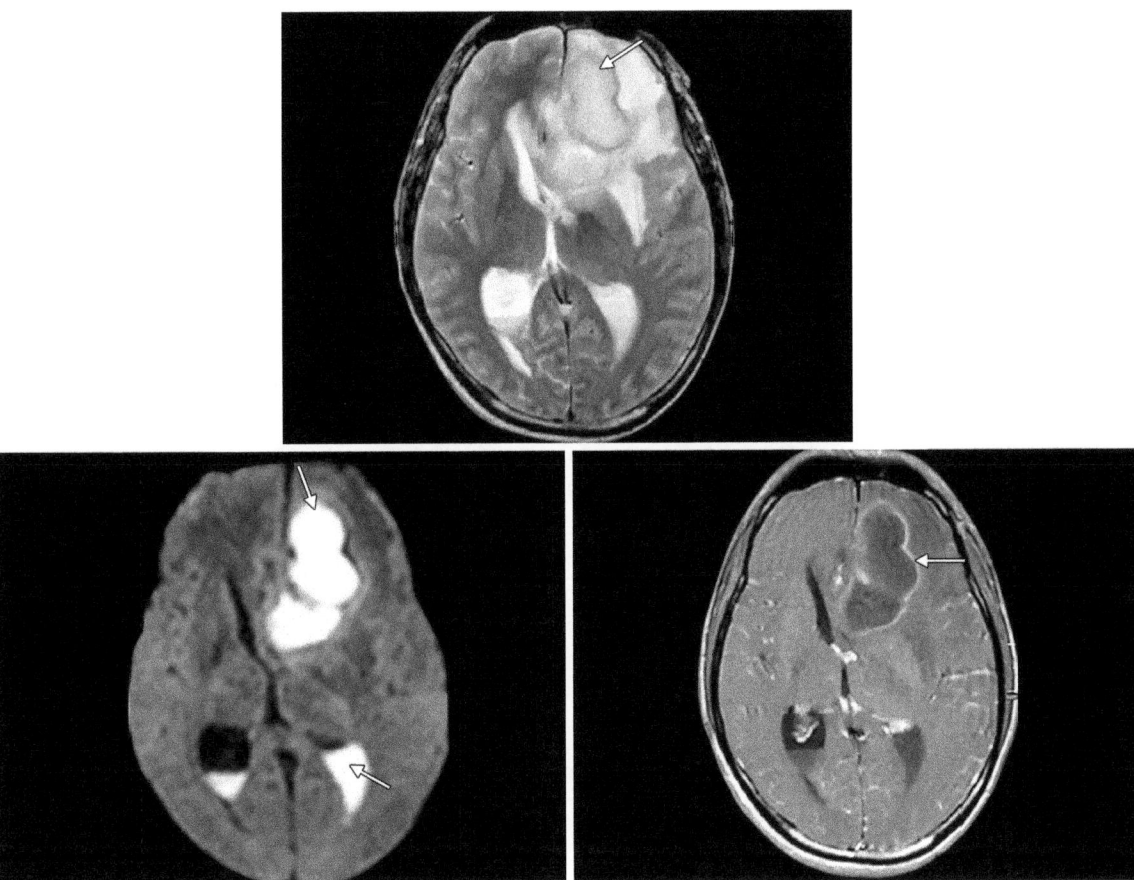

Well-defined T2 hyperintense ring-like enhancing conglomerate lesions showing intense diffusion restriction with perilesional edema with fluid level in ventricles.

2. **What is the most likely diagnosis?**
   A. Giant tuberculoma
   B. Tuberculous abscess
   C. Bacterial abscess
   D. Fungal abscess

CASE 3

A 43-year-old male presented with fever, headache, and left-sided weakness.
- O/E—power on left side grade 3
- CSF: Proteins—150, sugar—30/100, cells—200, 80% lymphocytes.

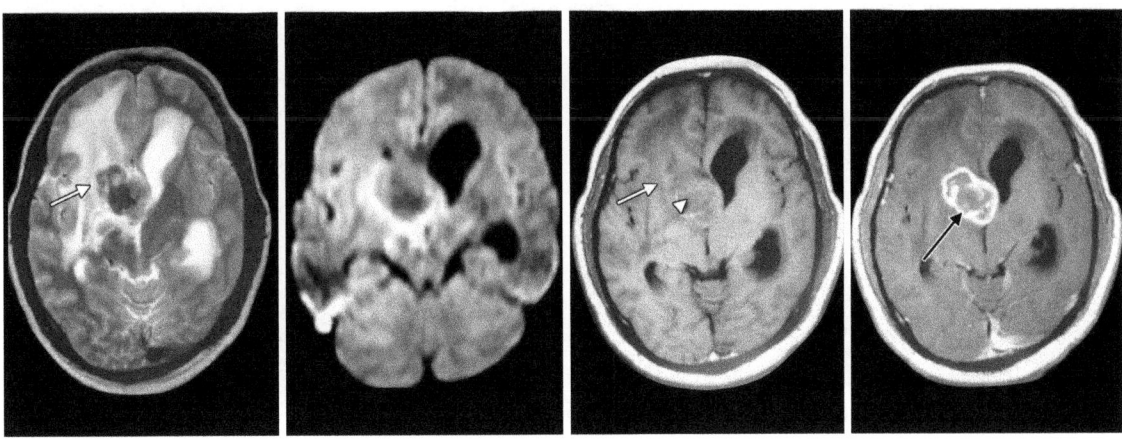

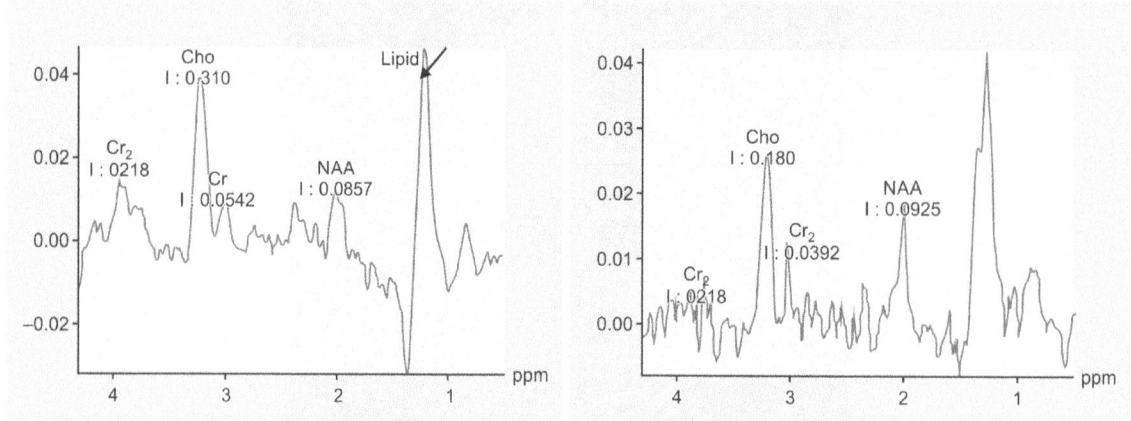

T2-hypointense (white arrow), T1-hyperintense (arrowhead) lesion in right caudate nucleus showing ring-like enhancement (black arrow) and high lipid peak on magnetic resonance spectroscopy.

3. What is the most likely diagnosis?
    A. Toxoplasmosis
    B. Aspergilloma
    C. Tuberculoma
    D. Blastomycosis

CASE 4

A 40-year-old seropositive male with CD4 count 50 presented with dull aching headache since 2 months, fever, and vomiting.
- CSF: Proteins—160 mg%, sugar—55/120, cells—80, 75% lymphocytes.

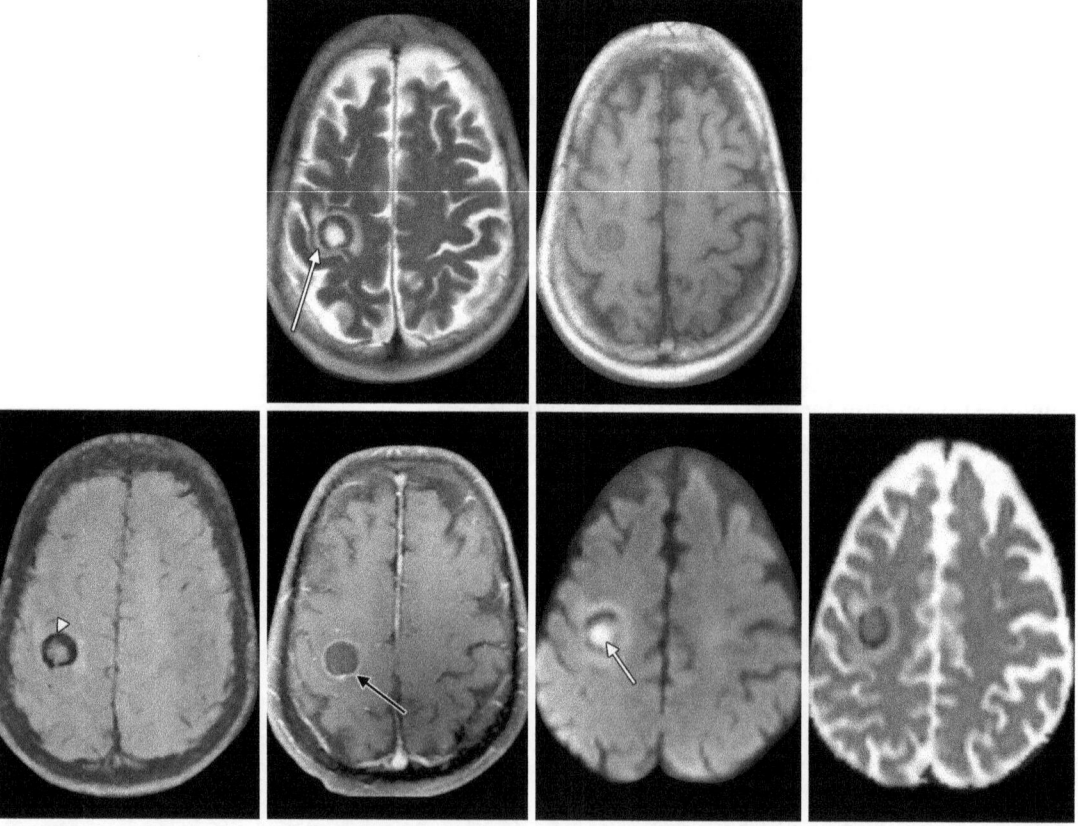

Thick-walled T2-hyperintense lesion showing susceptibility-weighted imaging (SWI) hypointensity in walls (arrowhead) and peripheral enhancement (black arrow).

4. What is the most likely diagnosis?
    A. Bacterial abscess
    B. Tubercular abscess
    C. Fungal abscess
    D. Toxoplasmosis

Central Nervous System Infections

CASE 5

A 6-year-old patient presented with focal convulsions.
- No history of (H/o) fever
- No neck stiffness
- No significant past history

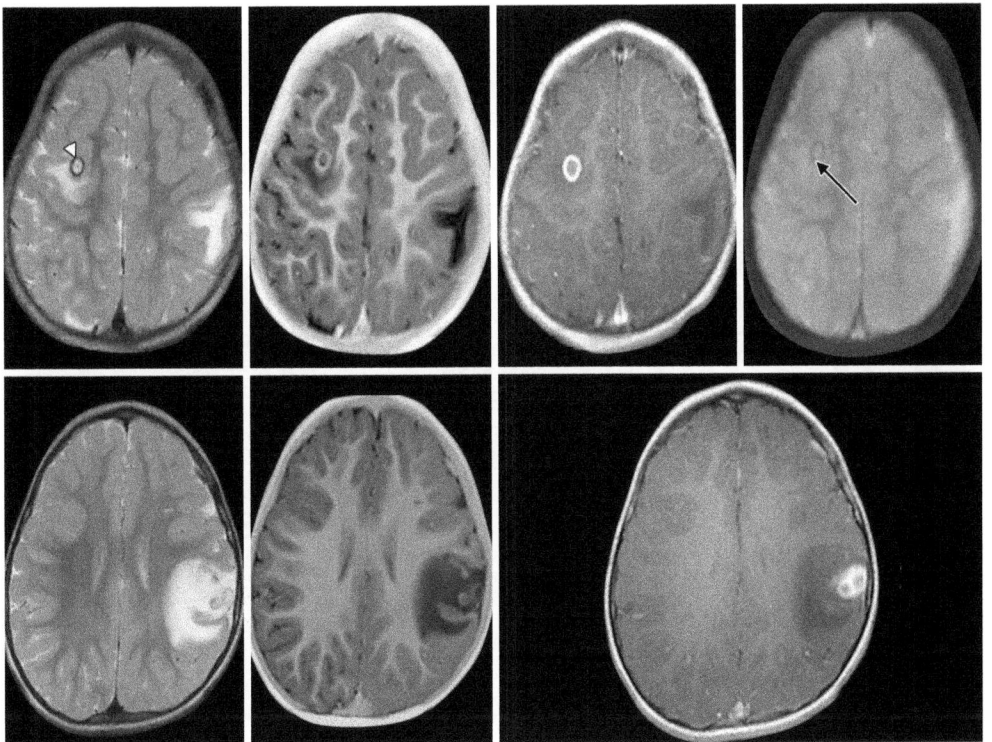

Multiple well-defined cystic lesions in both hemispheres with perilesional edema (arrowhead). Scolex seen in right-sided lesion (arrowhead). Susceptibility-weighted imaging (SWI) hypointensity also seen (black arrow).

5. What is the most likely diagnosis?
   A. Neurocysticercosis   B. Tuberculoma   C. Bacterial abscess   D. Fungal abscess

CASE 6

A 38-year-old HIV positive man being treated for cerebral tuberculomas with AKT and highly active antiretroviral therapy (HAART) undergoes MRI scanning for clinical worsening.
- *History*: Pyrexia of unknown origin (PUO) with bifrontal headache, vision and diplopia
- *Investigations*: Erythrocyte sedimentation rate (ESR)—59 mm, human immunodeficiency virus (HIV)—positive
- CD4 66, 15.2% and CD8 164, 37.8%
- CSF—200 cells, 80% lymphocytes, proteins—200.

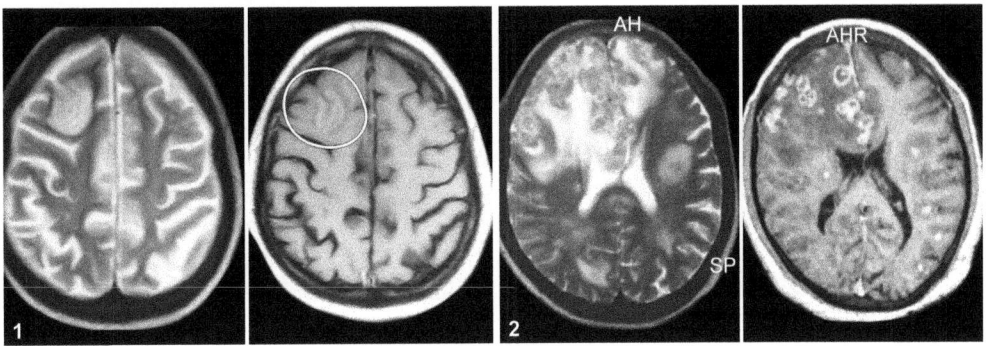

Scan 1: AKT plus HAART started;
Scan 2: Worsening of symptoms with flaring of lesions post-HAART.

104 Central Nervous System Infections

6. **What is the most likely diagnosis?**
    A. MDR-TB
    B. XDR-TB
    C. Immune reconstitution syndrome
    D. TB–Toxoplasma coinfection

CASE 7

A 27-year-old female presented with headache and convulsions.
- No H/o fever
- No comorbidities
- H/o drinking unpasteurized milk
- CSF: No organism grown, cytospin—negative, mildly elevated proteins and cells (lymphocyte).

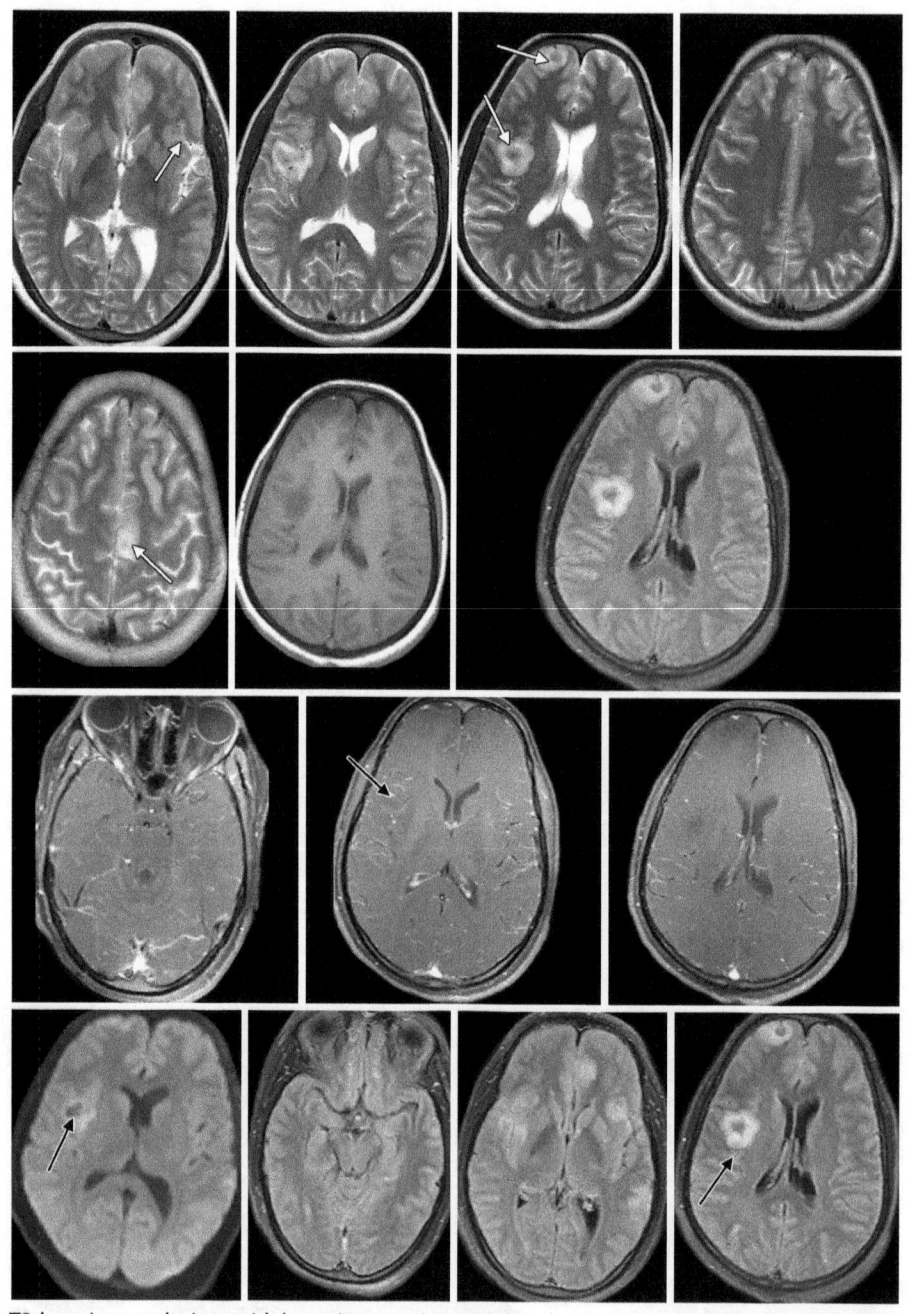

Ring-like enhancing T2-hypointense lesions with hyperintense rim, peripheral enhancement and associated meningeal enhancement.

7. **What is the most likely diagnosis?**
    A. Brucellosis
    B. Tuberculoma
    C. Toxoplasmosis
    D. Fungal infection

CASE 8

A 45-year-old seropositive male presented with fever, convulsion, and altered sensorium.
- CD4+ count—50
- CSF: 50 cells, 80% lymphocytes, sugar and protein—normal.

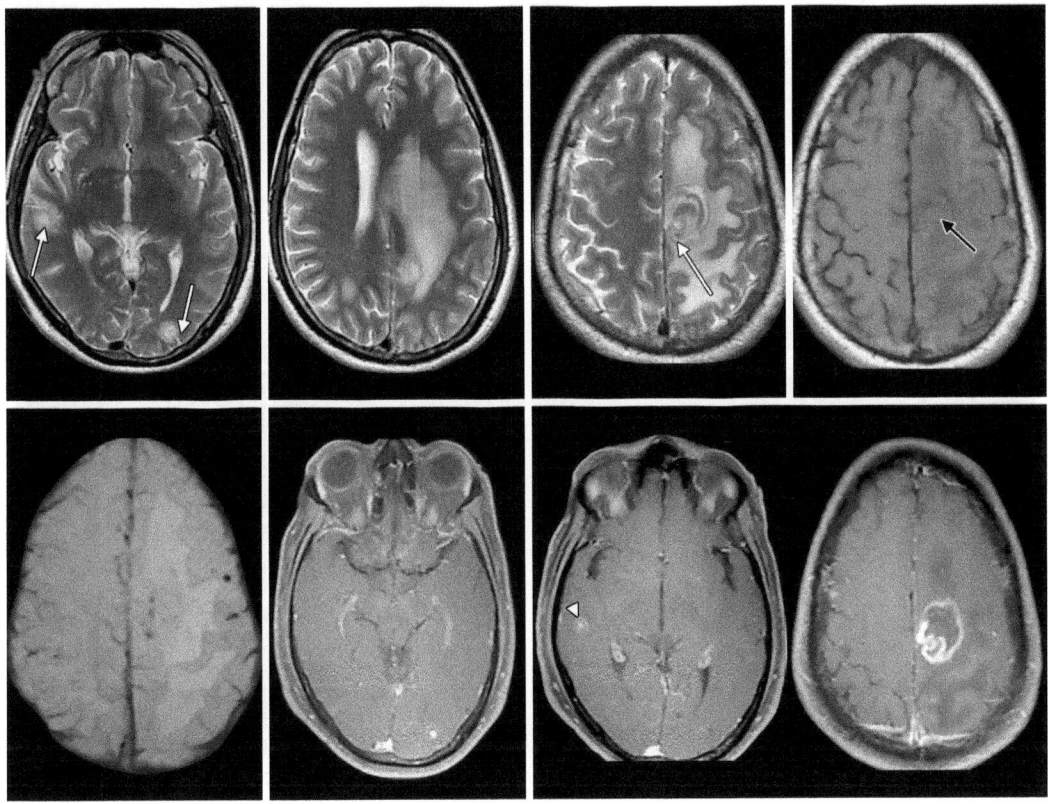

T2 mixed signal intensity lesions (white arrow) with mild central hemorrhage (black arrow) and target type of enhancement (arrowhead) at grey white matter interface.

8. **What is the most likely diagnosis?**
   A. Tuberculoma   B. Toxoplasmosis   C. Lymphoma   D. Fungal abscess

CASE 9

A 40-year-old seropositive male with CD4 count 50 presented with dull aching headache since 2 months, fever, and vomiting.
- O/E—left-sided weakness with bilateral extensor planters.

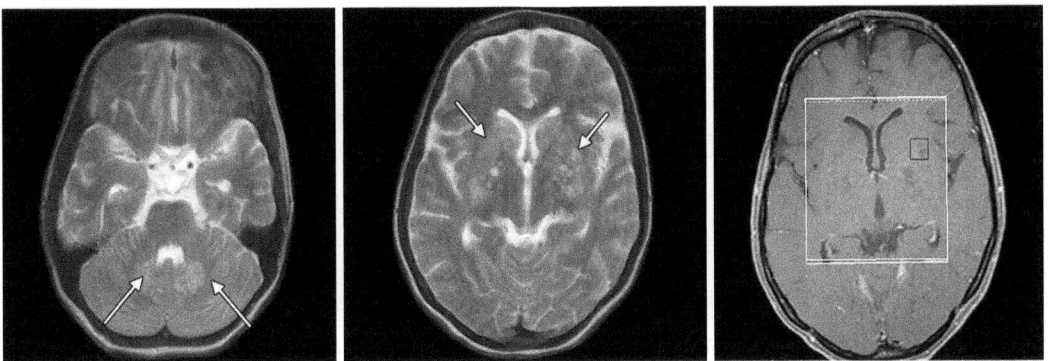

Nonenhancing T2-hyperintense lesions representing dilated Virchow-Robin spaces in basal ganglia and dentate nuclei.

9. **What is the most likely diagnosis?**
   A. Toxoplasmosis   B. Tuberculomas   C. Cryptococcosis   D. Neurocysticercosis

CASE 10

A 40-year-old male with H/o high fever, presented with drowsiness and signs of meningitis.
- Peripheral blood smear—positive for malarial parasite.

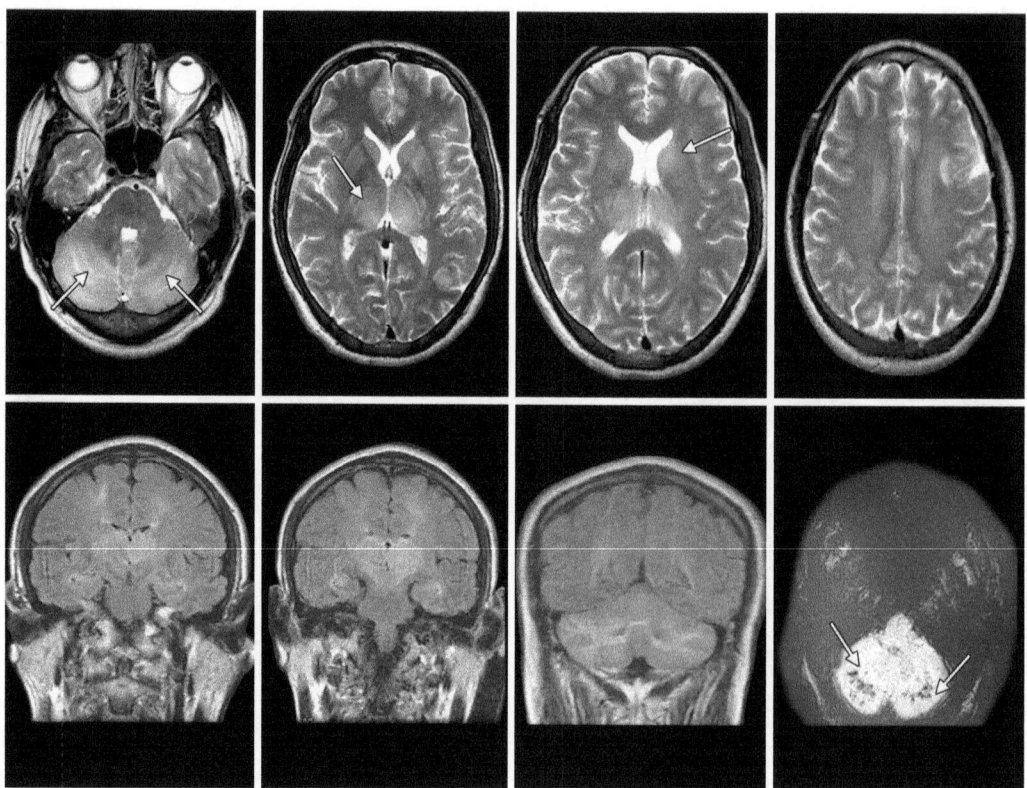

Symmetrical hyperintensities in thalami and cerebellum with hemorrhagic foci.

10. What is the most likely diagnosis?
    A. Cerebral malaria   B. Japanese B encephalitis   C. Toxoplasmosis   D. Cryptococcosis

CASE 11

A 15-year-old patient presented with fever, headache, and convulsions.
- CSF: Proteins—80, sugar—60, cells—40 (lymphocytes).

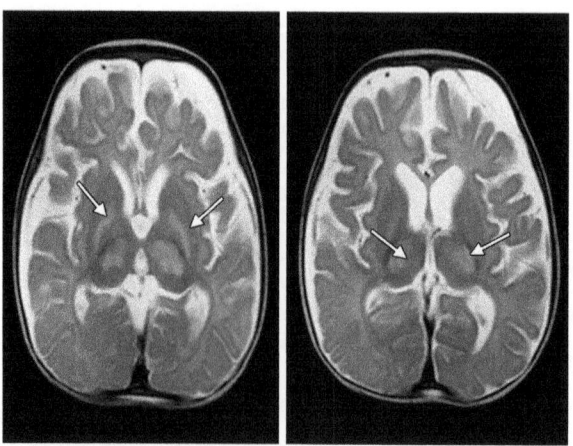

Symmetric hyperintensity in basal ganglia and thalami (arrows).

11. What is the most likely diagnosis?
    A. Cerebral malaria   B. Japanese B encephalitis   C. Toxoplasmosis   D. Cryptococcosis

CASE 12

A 54-year-old seropositive female complains of abnormal behavior since 2 months, associated with weakness in both upper limb and lower limb since 2 months.
- No H/o fever and vomiting
- CD4+—50
- CSF is normal.

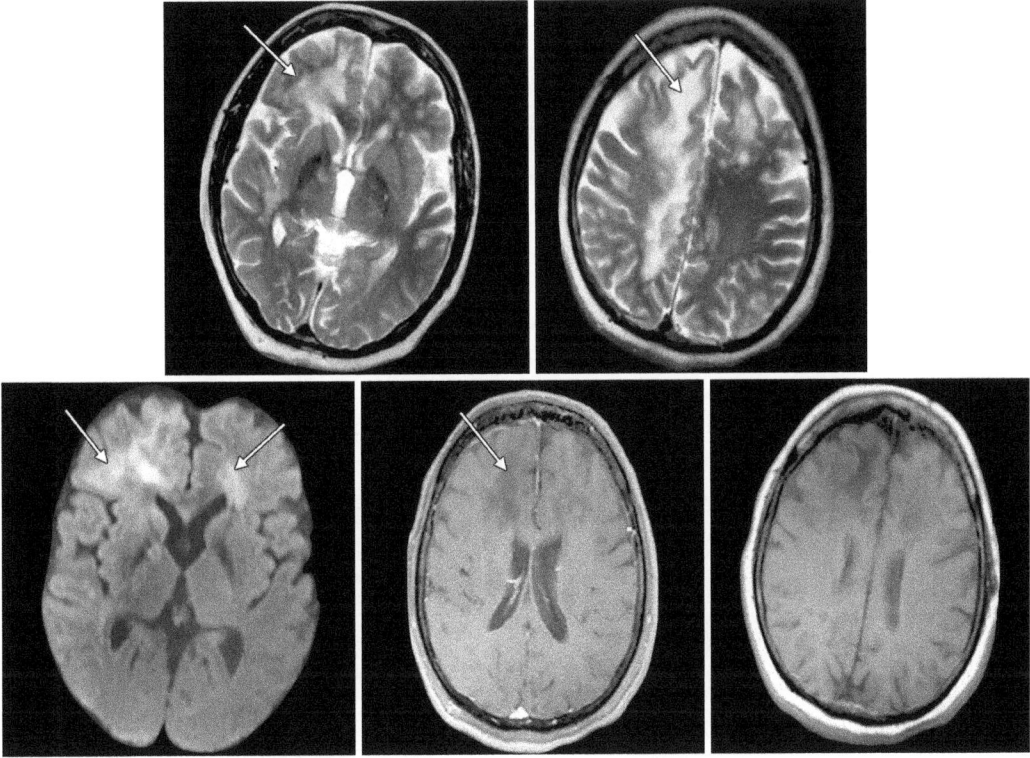

Asymmetric T2-hyperintense and T1-hypointense lesion in bilateral frontal white matter (right>>left) showing mild diffusion restriction with no significant enhancement.

12. **What is the most likely diagnosis?**
    A. Progressive multifocal leukoencephalopathy (PML)
    B. HIV encephalopathy
    C. HSV encephalitis
    D. CNS lymphoma

CASE 13

A 20-year-old male, who is a known seropositive, presented with decreased concentration, forgetfulness, slowing of thought, slowing of activities of daily living, and apathetic.

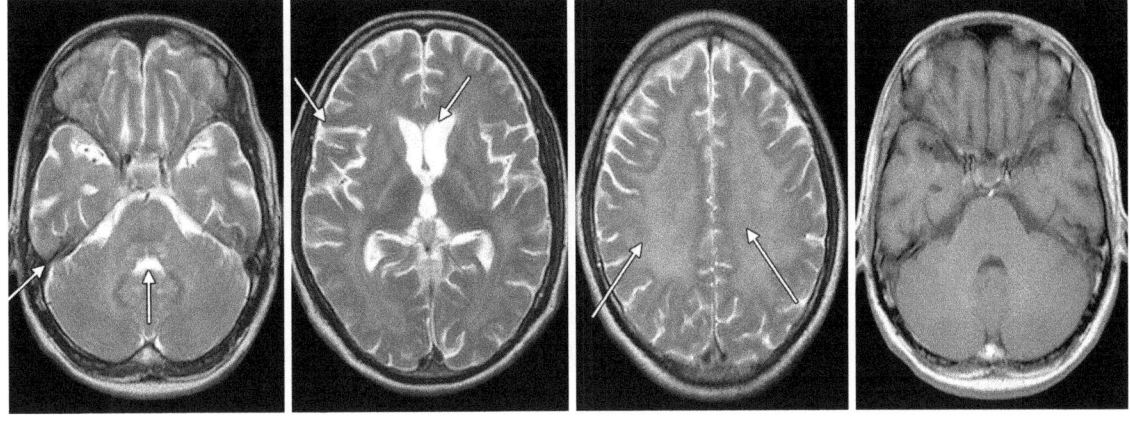

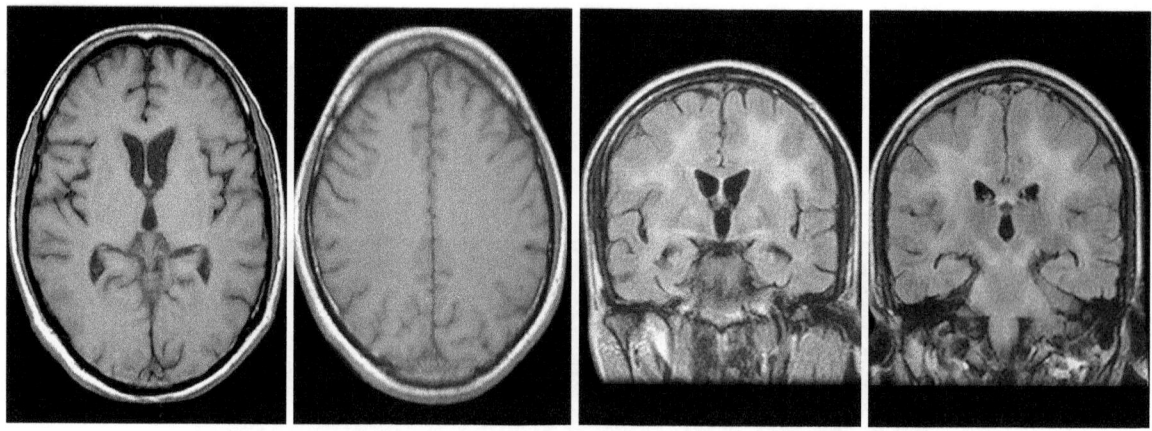

Bilaterally symmetric hyperintensity involving cerebral white matter and basal ganglia.

13. **What is the most likely diagnosis?**
    A. PML
    B. HIV encephalopathy
    C. HSV encephalitis
    D. CNS lymphoma

CASE 14

A 45-year-old seropositive male presented with fever, confusion and very minimal right-sided weakness.
- CSF: Proteins—high, sugar—normal, cells—60 cells, 80% lymphocytes

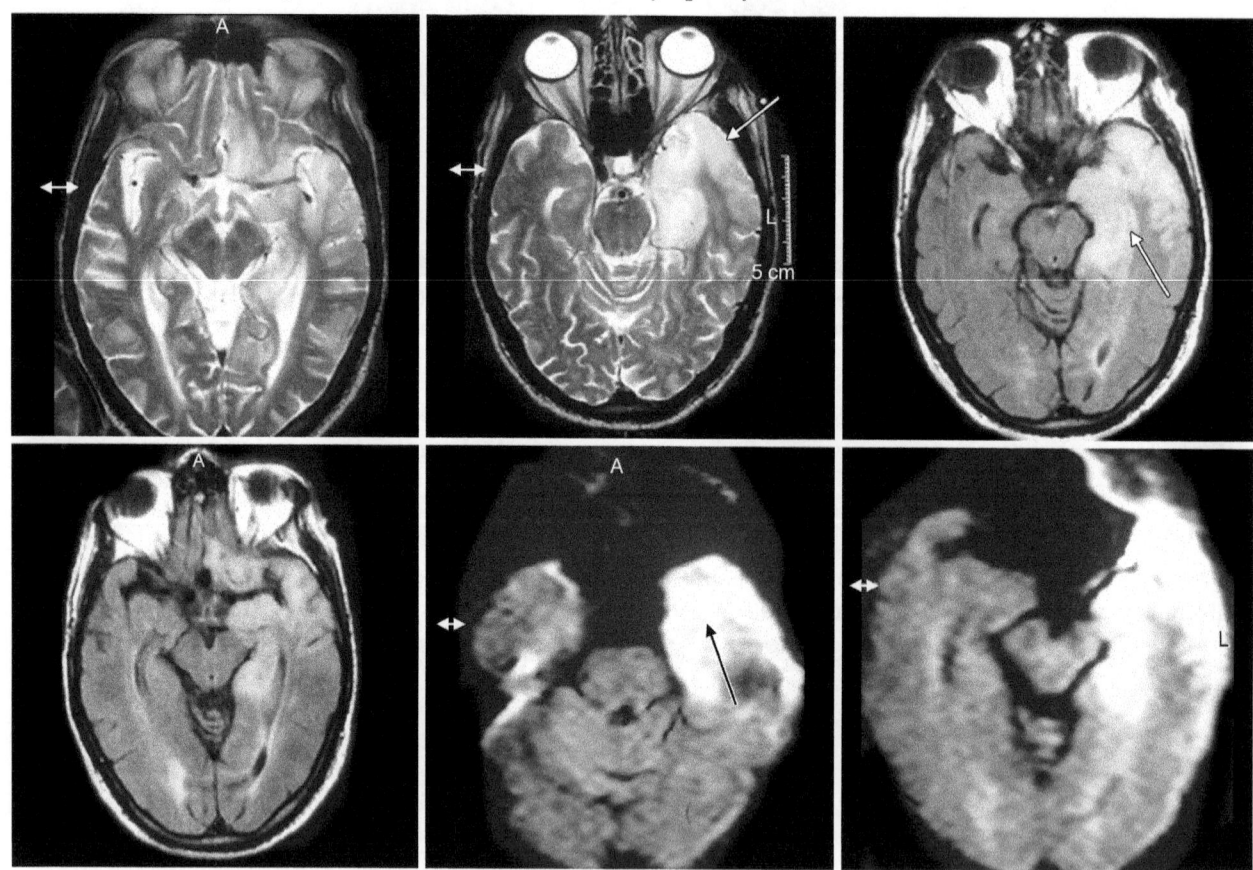

Asymmetric hyperintensity showing diffusion restriction (black arrow) in left temporal neocortex with involvement of medial temporal lobe.

14. **What is the most likely diagnosis?**
    A. PML
    B. Herpes simplex encephalitis
    C. HIV encephalitis
    D. Japanese B encephalitis

CASE 15

A 60-year-old female presented with rapidly progressive dementia, myoclonic jerks, and akinetic mutism.

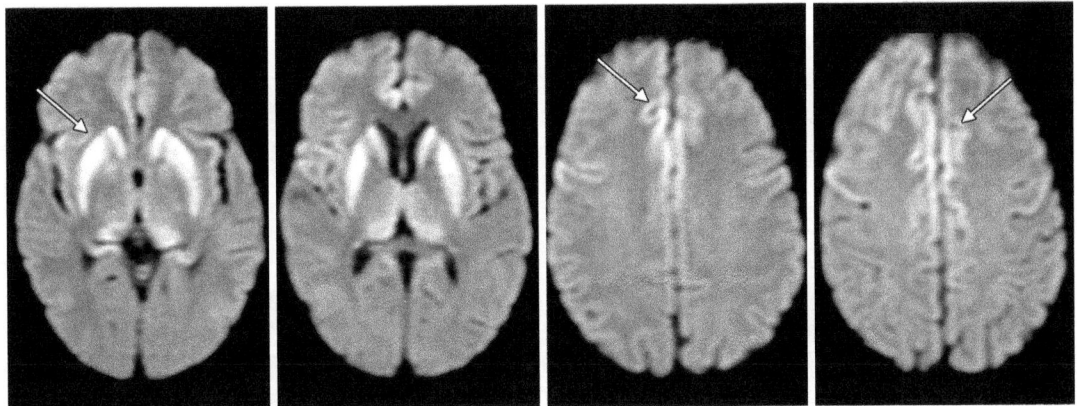

Symmetric hyperintensities in the basal ganglia and posteromedial thalami showing diffusion restriction along cortex.

15. What is the most likely diagnosis?
- A. Japanese B encephalitis
- B. Cryptococcosis
- C. Creutzfeldt–Jakob disease (CJD)
- D. Cerebral malaria

CASE 16

A 45-year-old seropositive male presented with fever, headache, and altered sensorium.
- CSF: 100 cells, lymphocyte predominant

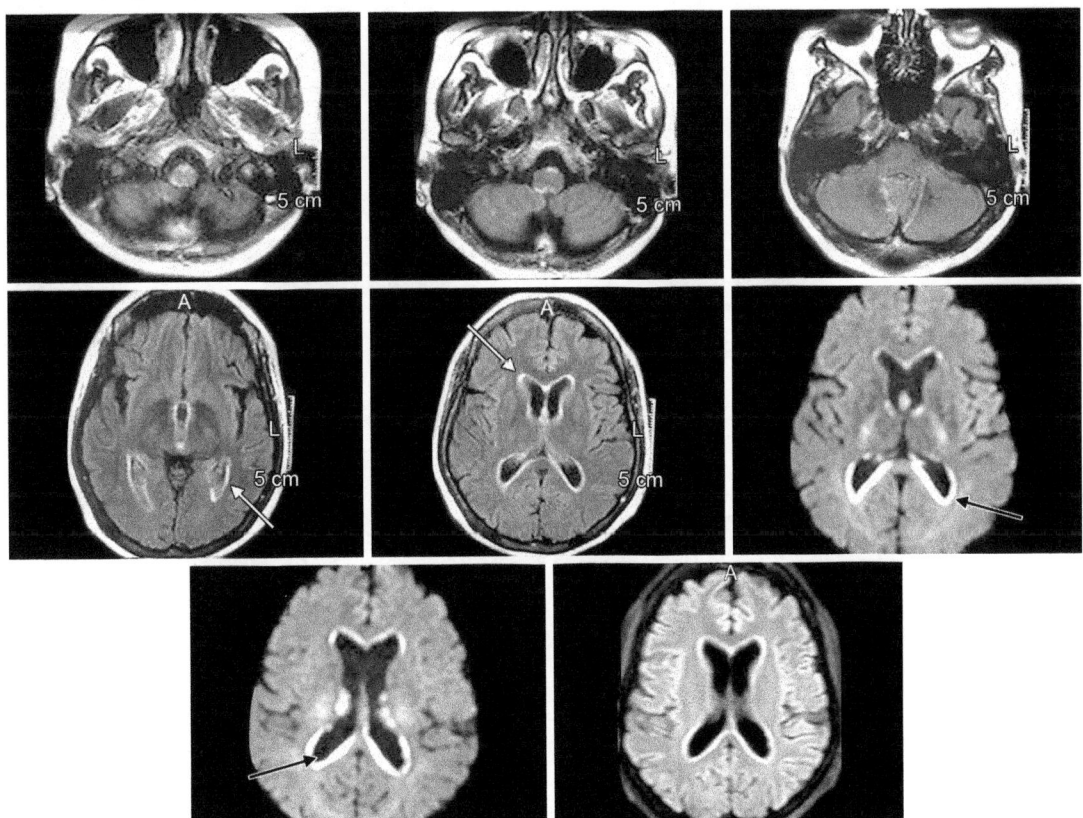

FLAIR hyperintensity along ependymal lining of lateral ventricles (white arrows) showing diffusion restriction (black arrows).

16. What is the most likely diagnosis?
- A. Infiltrative glioma
- B. CNS lymphoma
- C. PML
- D. CMV encephalitis

Central Nervous System Infections

CASE 17

- A 39-year-old male patient with alcoholic liver cirrhosis came with sudden loss of vision in right eye for 10 days.
- Went to local ophthalmologist—right-sided papilledema on fundoscopy.
- Patient was advised MRI brain with orbits.

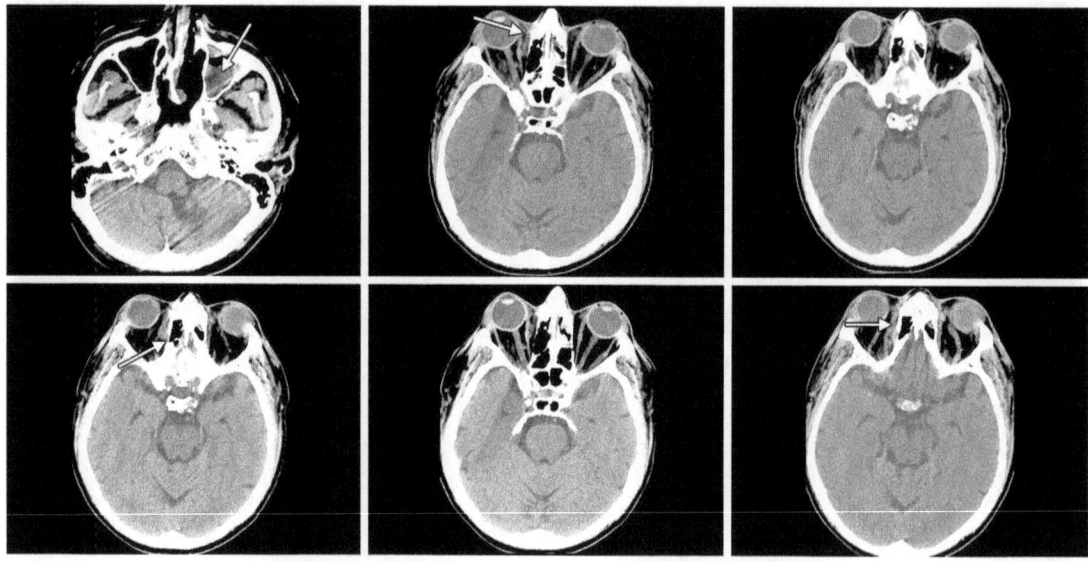

Left maxillary sinusitis with soft tissue in medial extraconal compartment of right orbit.

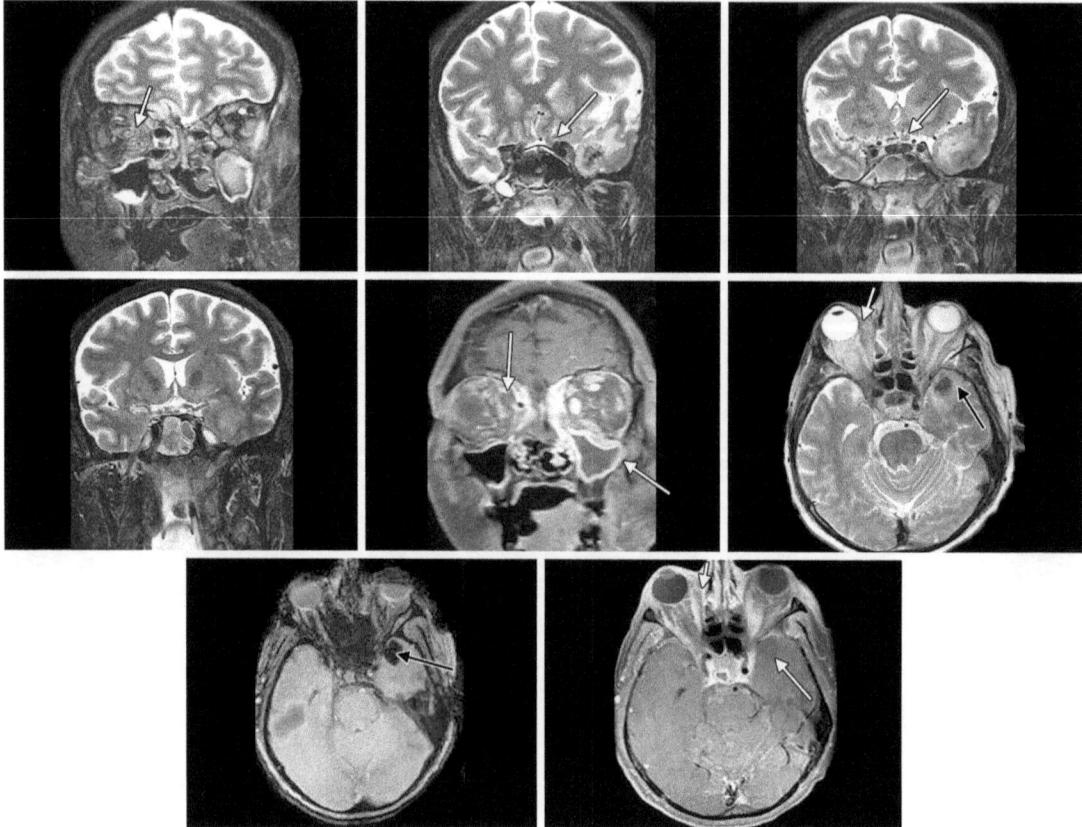

MRI with contrast showing intense enhancement of walls of left maxillary sinus and soft tissue in extraconal fat of right orbit with stranding in the retrobulbar fat. Associated SWI hypointense lesion in left anterior temporal lobe (black arrows).

17. **What is the most likely diagnosis?**
    A. Invasive fungal sinusitis with intracranial extension
    B. Pyogenic sinusitis
    C. Tuberculosis
    D. Base of skull osteomyelitis

CASE 18

A 65-year-old male with poorly controlled diabetes presented with persistent foul smelling discharge from left ear, earache, and headache.

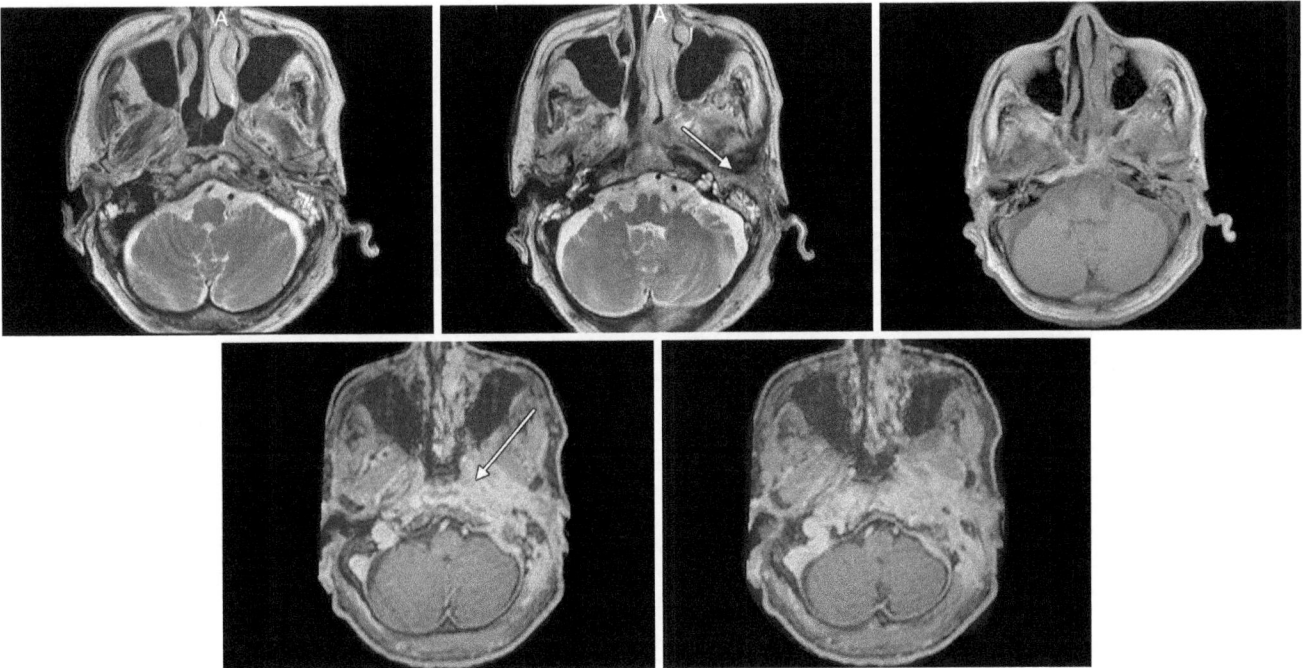

T2-hyperintense enhancing soft tissue in the left external, middle ear with involvement of mastoid, petrous bone and spreading into adjacent soft-tissues.

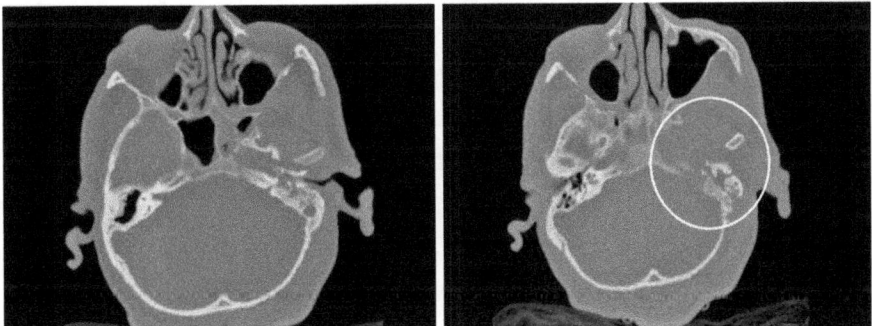

CT scan showing massive bone destruction of mastoid, petrous and squamous temporal bone.

18. **What is the most likely diagnosis?**
    A. Malignant otitis externa with skull base osteomyelitis
    B. Tuberculosis
    C. Otitis media with cholesteatoma
    D. Base of skull neoplasm

CASE 19

A 60-year-old male, a known case of chronic kidney disease (CKD), presented with 7th nerve palsy on the left.

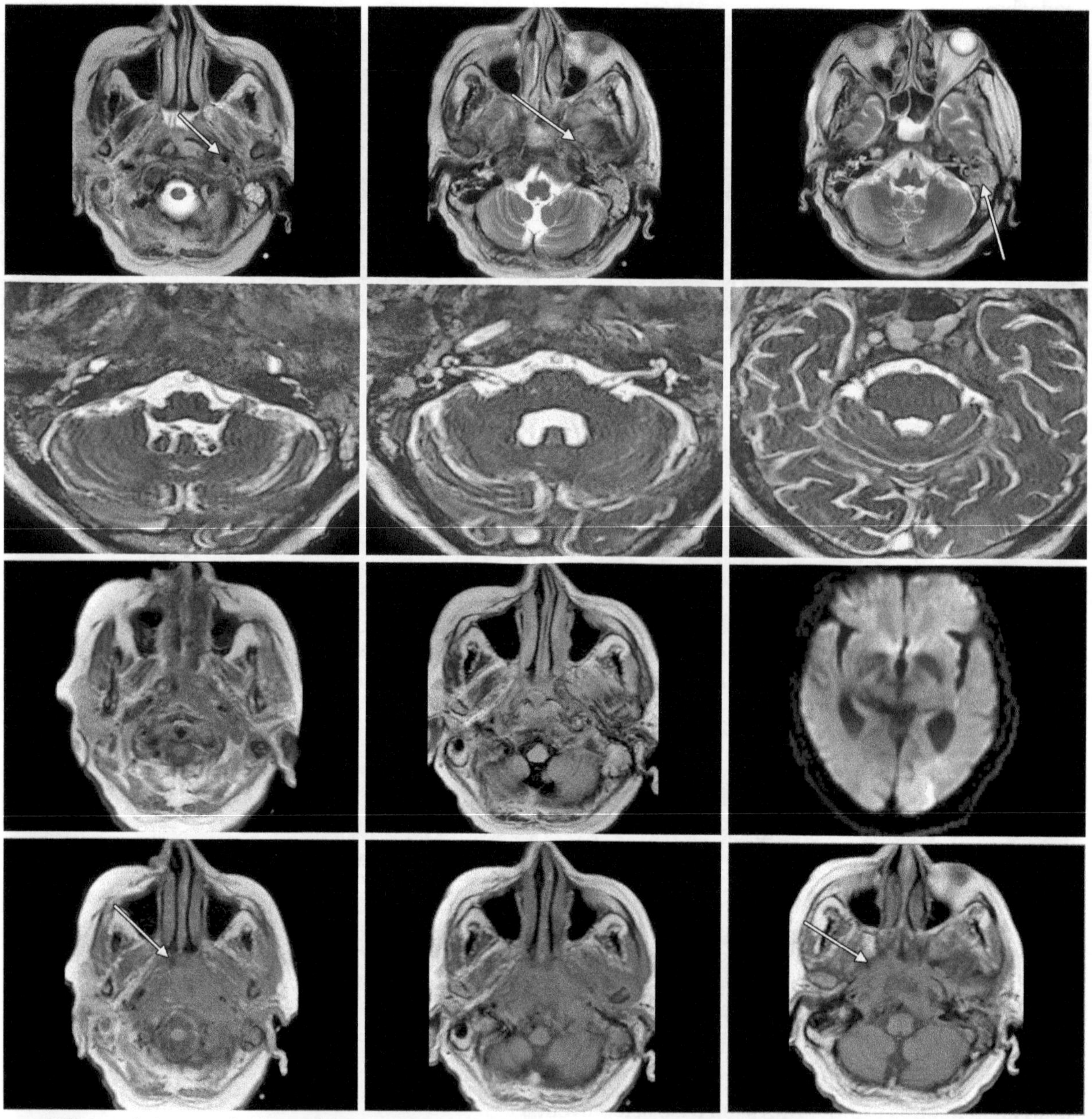

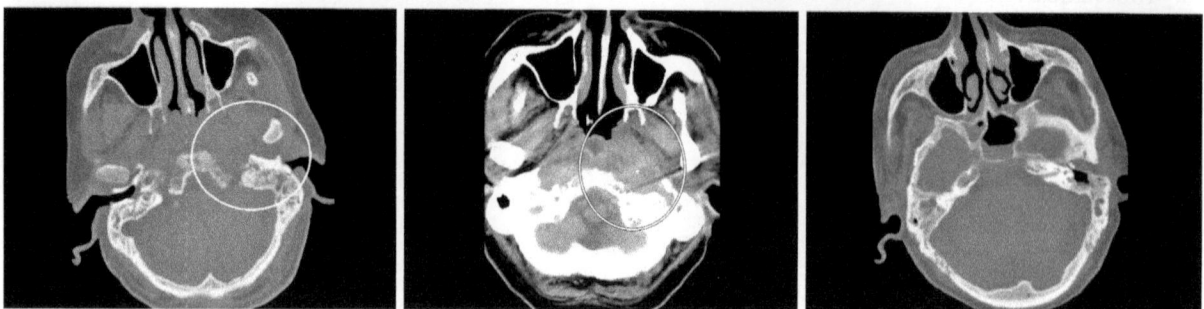

Diffuse soft tissue at the base of skull on left side extending into cisternal spaces with involvement of petrous bone.

Bone destruction seen on CT.

19. **What is the most likely pathological process leading to the patient's symptoms?**
    A. Fungal B. Granulomatous C. Neoplastic D. Bacterial

ANSWERS WITH EXPLANATIONS

1. **Ans. A**
   - *Leptomeningitis*, which is more commonly referred to as *meningitis*, represents inflammation of the subarachnoid space.
   - CT may be normal or show subtle hydrocephalus, leptomeningeal enhancement.
   - Hyperdensity around basal cisterns (especially in tuberculosis).
   - MRI better in detection of leptomeningeal enhancement.
   - Fluid-attenuated inversion recovery (FLAIR) hyperintensity in sulcal spaces.

   Ref:
   1. Vaswani AK, Nizamani WM, Ali M, Aneel G, Shahani BK, Hussain S, et al. Diagnostic Accuracy of contrast-enhanced FLAIR magnetic resonance imaging in diagnosis of meningitis correlated with CSF analysis. ISRN Radiol. 2014;2014:578986.
   2. Gupta RK, Lufkin RB. MR Imaging and Spectroscopy of Central Nervous System Infections. New York: Kluwer Academic Publishers; 2001.

2. **Ans. C**
   - Cerebral abscesses result from pathogens growing within the brain parenchyma. *Streptococcus* is the most common organism.
   - MRI has a greater ability to distinguish a cerebral abscess from other ring-enhancing lesions.
   - Stages of abscess include:
     - Early cerebritis
     - Late cerebritis
     - *Early encapsulation*:
       - Discrete lesion with thin, enhancing rim
       - Rim may be less well-defined along peripheral aspect of lesion (away from ventricles)
       - ± additional "daughter" collections
       - ± ventricular extension, with accompanying ventriculitis.
     - *Late encapsulation*: Progressive central necrosis, cavity shrinks, decreasing surrounding edema.

   MRI
   - Hyperintense on T2 and show central diffusion restriction
   - Diffusion helps in distinguishing from other ring-enhancing lesions
   - Magnetic resonance spectroscopy (MRS)—abscesses show peaks of various amino acids on MRS.

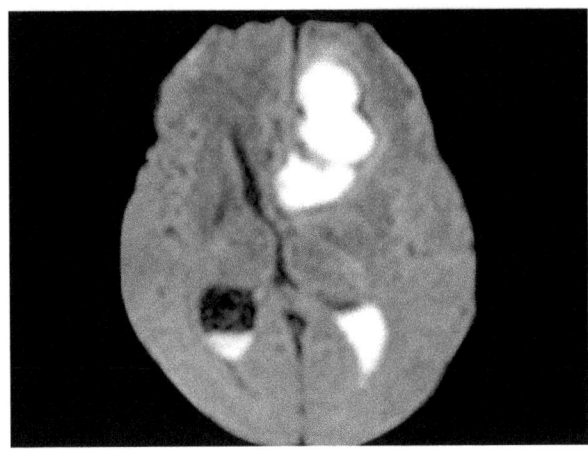

MR Spectroscopy

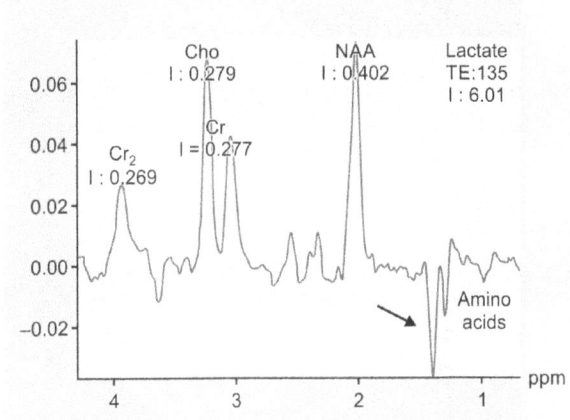

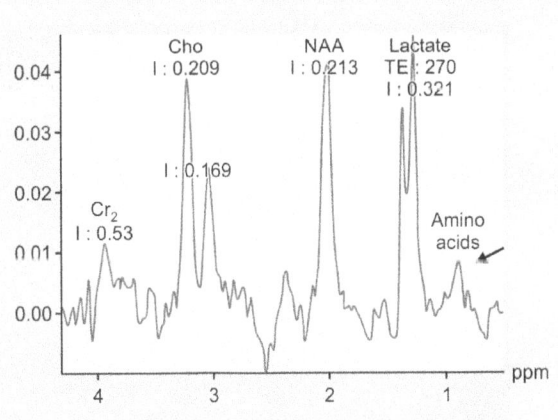

Valine, leucine, and isoleucine at 0.90 ppm to at 1.33 ppm—nonspecific marker; Lipid peaks at 0.90, 1.30, and 2.02 ppm; Succinate at 2.40 ppm and/or of acetoacetate at 1.92 ppm; Alanine at 1.47 ppm; Glycine at 3.56 ppm.

Ref:
1. Haimes AB, Zimmerman RD, Morgello S, Weingarten K, Becker RD, Jennis R, et al. MR imaging of brain abscesses. Am J Roentgenol. 1989;152(5):1073-85.
2. Holmes TM, Petrella JR, Provenzale JM. Distinction between cerebral abscesses and high-grade neoplasms by dynamic susceptibility contrast perfusion MRI. Am J Roentgenol. 2004;183(5):1247-52.

3. Ans. C

- Infection caused by *Mycobacterium tuberculosis*.
- Granulomatous reaction and caseous necrosis within lesion
- Solid on CT and shows ring-like or solid enhancement
- Calcification may be seen on treatment
- Imaging appearance on MRI depends on the degree of caseous necrosis and liquefaction
- Shows ring-like enhancement and no diffusion restriction in the center unlike abscesses

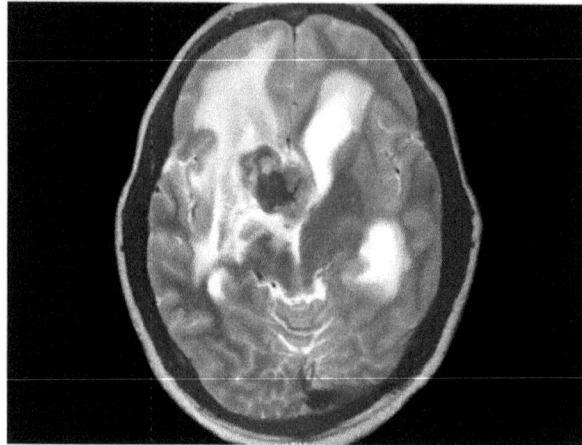

Caseating with solid center—predominantly T2 hypointense.

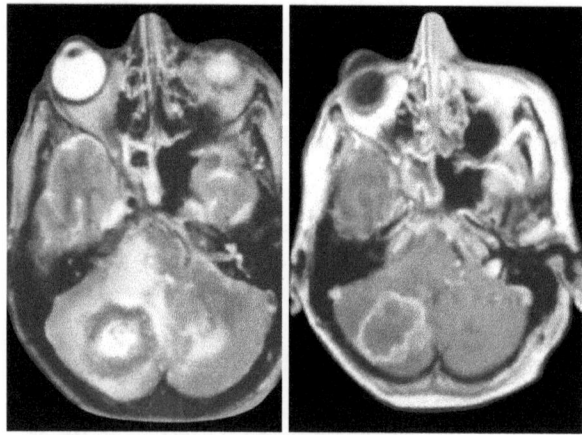

Caseation with liquefaction—hyperintense on T2.

- Tuberculomas show lipid peak on MRS unlike the amino acid peak in abscesses

- This is due to the presence of mycolic acid in the walls.

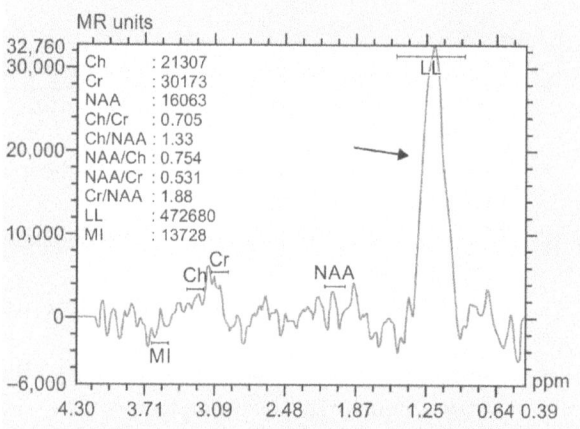

Ref:
1. Kim TK, Chang KH, Kim CJ, Goo JM, Kook MC, Han MH. Intracranial tuberculoma: comparison of MR with pathologic findings. Am J Neuroradiol. 1995;16(9):1903-8.
2. Khanna PC, Godinho S, Patkar DP, Pungavkar SA, Lawande MA. MR spectroscopy-aided differentiation: "giant" extra-axial tuberculoma masquerading as meningioma. Am J Neuroradiol. 2006;27(7):1438-40.

4. Ans. C

- *Aspergillus* is the most common pathogen
- Hyperintense with hypointense rim on T2-weighted images
- Hypointensity on susceptibility-weighted images in wall
- Rim enhancement on contrast.

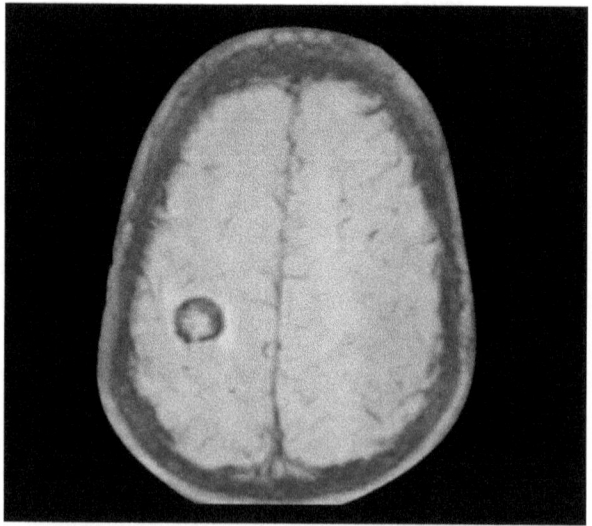

Susceptibility-weighted imaging hypointensity helps to distinguish from other ring-like enhancing lesions.

Central Nervous System Infections

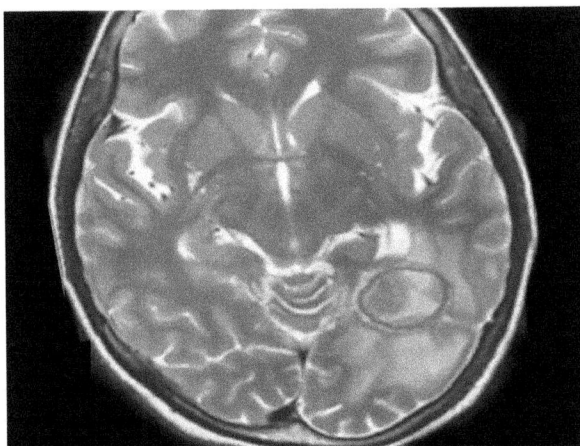

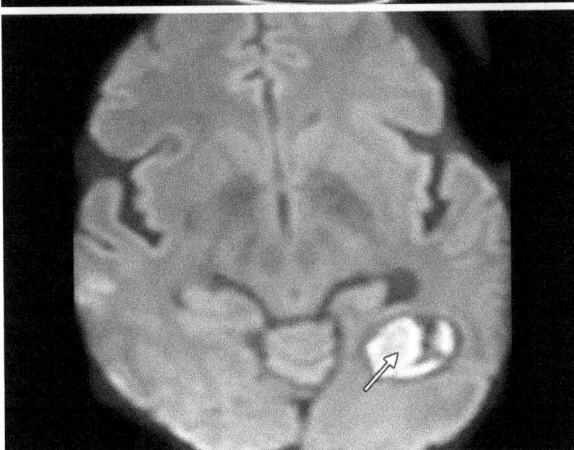

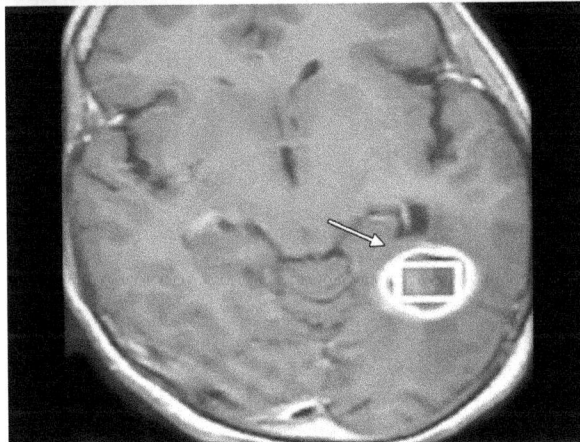

Intracavitary projections showing diffusion restriction also help in differentiating from other infections.

Ref:
1. Gaviani P, Schwartz RB, Hedley-Whyte ET, Ligon KL, Robicsek A, Schaefer P, et al. Diffusion-weighted imaging of fungal cerebral infection. Am J Neuroradiol. 2005;26:1115-21.

2. Luthra G, Parihar A, Nath K, Jaiswal S, Prasad KN, Husain N, et al. Comparative evaluation of fungal, tubercular, and pyogenic brain abscesses with conventional and diffusion MR imaging and proton MR spectroscopy. Am J Neuroradiol. 2007;28(7): 1332-8.

5. **Ans. A**
   - *Neurocysticercosis* is caused by the central nervous system (CNS) infection with the pork tapeworm *Taenia solium*.
   - There are four main stages (also known as Escobar's pathological stages):
     - *Vesicular:* Viable parasite with intact membrane and therefore no host reaction
     - *Colloidal vesicular:* Parasite dies within 4–5 years untreated or earlier with treatment and the cyst fluid becomes turbid. As the membrane becomes leaky, edema surrounds the cyst. This is the most symptomatic stage
     - *Granular nodular:* Edema decreases as the cyst retract further; enhancement persists.
     - *Nodular calcified:* End-stage quiescent calcified cyst remnant; no edema.
   - Parenchymal lesion is the most common.
   - Subarachnoid and cisternal lesions are common in South America.
   - Typically, the parenchymal cysts are small (1 cm) whereas the subarachnoid cysts can be much bigger.
   - Ring-like enhancement seen on CT and MRI, once the organism dies. Calcification may be seen in nodular stage.
   - Appearance on imaging depends on stage.

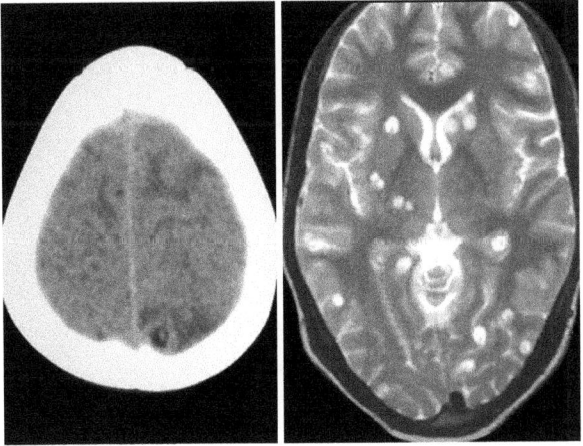

Vesicular—no enhancement, edema.

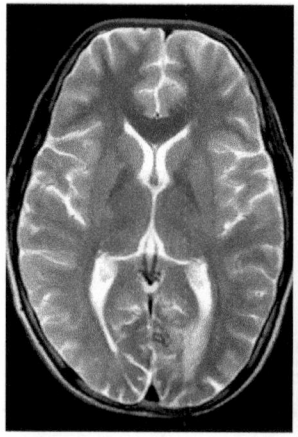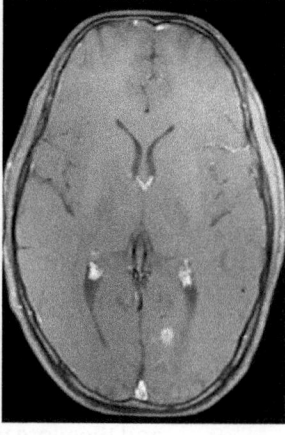

Granular nodular—edema and enhancement decrease.

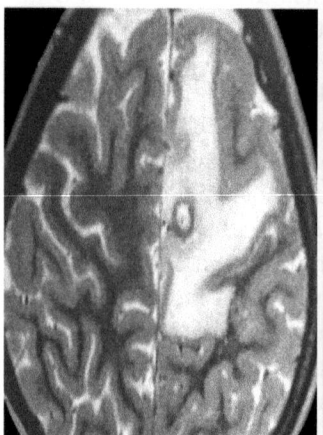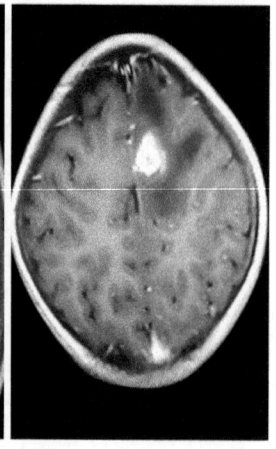

Colloidal vesicular—thick peripheral enhancement, edema.

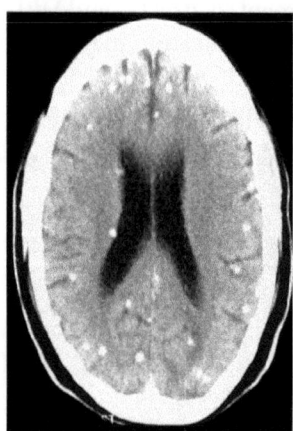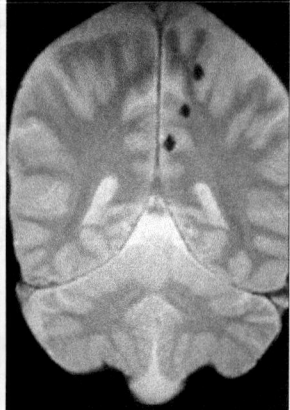

Nodular calcified—calcification.

Neurocysticercosis	Tuberculomas
Cysticerci are usually round in shape	Tuberculomas are usually irregular, solid, and larger than 20 mm in size
Cysticerci are usually 20 mm or less in size with ring enhancement or visible scolex	They are often associated with severe perifocal edema and focal neurologic deficit
The cerebral edema is not severe enough to produce midline shift or focal neurologic deficit	Associated meningitis

Ref:
1. Sheth TN, Pillon L, Keystone J, Kucharczyk W. Persistent MR contrast enhancement of calcified neurocysticercosis lesions. Am J Neuroradiol. 1998;19(1):79-82.
2. Teitelbaum GP, Otto RJ, Lin M, Watanabe AT, Stull MA, Manz HJ, et al. MR imaging of neurocysticercosis. Am J Roentgenol. 1989;153(4):857-66.
3. Kimura-Hayama ET, Higuera JA, Corona-Cedillo R, Chávez-Macías L, Perochena A, Quiroz-Rojas LY, et al. Neurocysticercosis: radiologic-pathologic correlation. Radiographics. 2010;30(6):1705-19.

6. **Ans. C**

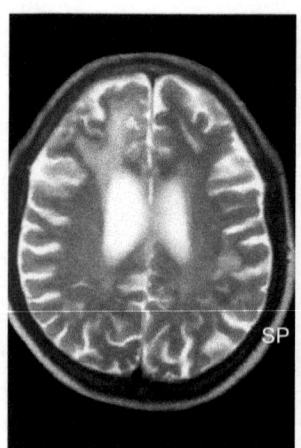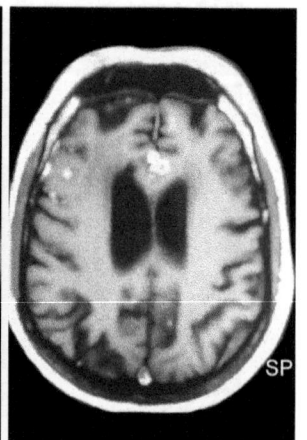

Scan 3 months later, post-steroid, AKT.

- Recently recognized disorder that arises from rapid restoration of immune system which targets infectious pathogens or their antigens to the detriment of the patient.
- Immune reconstitution inflammatory syndrome (IRIS) plays a role in several acquired immunodeficiency syndrome (AIDS)-related CNS disorders such as tuberculosis, cryptococcal disease, *Cytomegalovirus* (CMV) retinitis and progressive multifocal leukoencephalopathy (PML).

Proposed criteria for IRIS
- Patient had HIV or AIDS.
- Treatment with HAART has led to a decrease in HIV-1 RNA viral load.
- Symptoms are consistent with an infectious or inflammatory condition that appeared while the patient was on HAART.
- Symptom cannot be explained by a newly acquired infection, the expected course of a newly diagnosed opportunistic infection, or drug toxicity.

Ref:
1. Chen KC, Chen JY, Tung GA. Case 149: Immune reconstitution inflammatory syndrome. Radiology. 2009; 252(3):924-8.
2. Smith AB, Smirniotopoulos JG, Rushing EJ. From the archives of the AFIP: central nervous system infections associated with human immunodeficiency virus infection: radiologic-pathologic correlation. Radiographics. 2008;28(7):2033-58.

7. **Ans. A**
   - Patient gave history of drinking unpasteurized milk
   - Serum *Brucella* immunoglobulin M—positive.

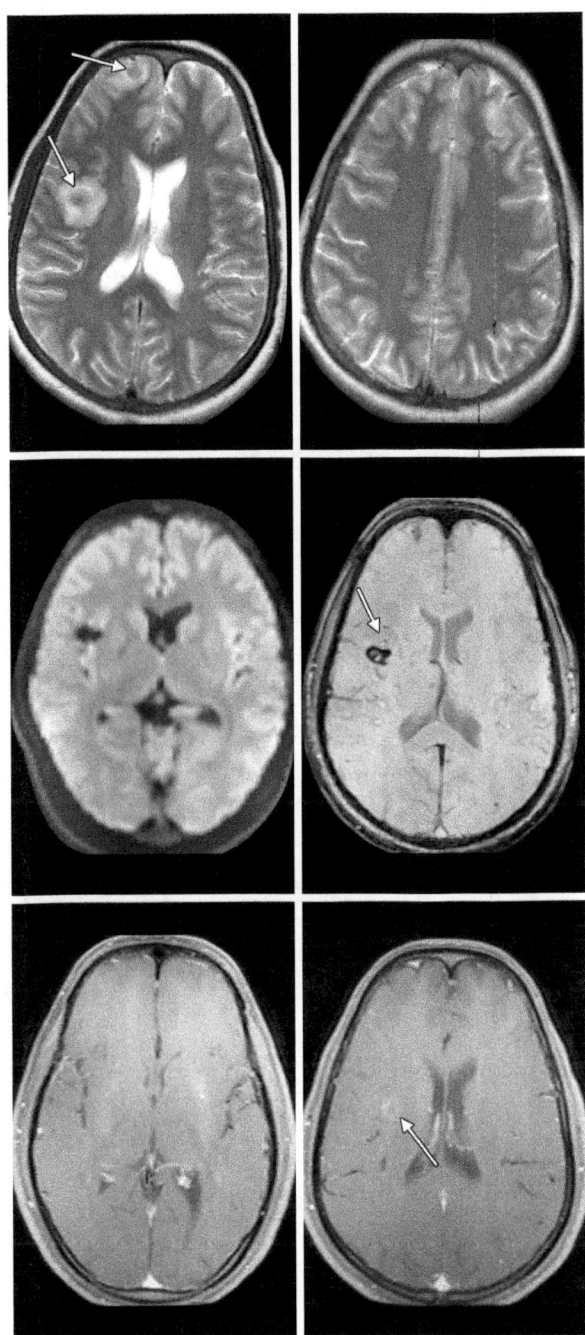

Follow-up after doxycycline shows resolution of the lesions.

Neurobrucellosis
- There are three types of CNS involvement—inflammation, white matter changes, and vascular insult:
  - Inflammation may cause granulomatous formation or enhancement of the meninges, perivascular space, or lumbar nerve roots
  - White matter changes—periventricular, and the third one is a focal demyelinating appearance
  - Vascular insult—inflammatory process of the small vessels or venous system causes lacunar infarcts, small hemorrhages, or venous thrombosis.

Ref:
1. Al-Sous MW, Bohlega S, Al-Kawi MZ, Alwatban J, McLean DR. Neurobrucellosis: clinical and neuroimaging correlation. Am J Neuroradiol. 2004; 25(3)395-401.

8. **Ans. B**
   - Caused by *Toxoplasma gondii*
   - Common locations include gray white matter interface and basal ganglia
   - T2-hyperintense to isointense
   - Concentric alternating zone of hypo/hyper/isointense signal
   - Target type of ring-like enhancement
   - Blood products in lesion

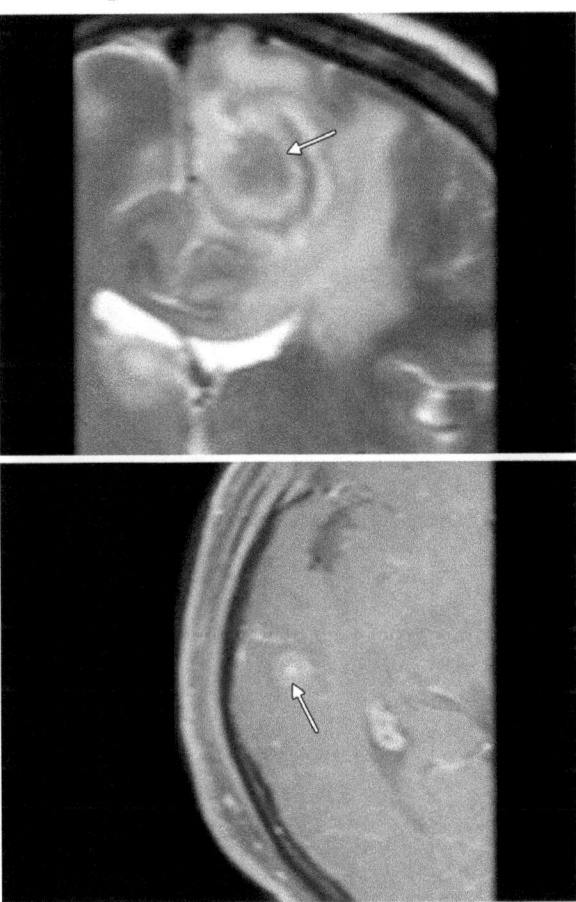

Toxoplasmosis should be differentiated from lymphoma, which also occurs in the same clinical setting and can show ring-like enhancement.

Toxoplasmosis	Lymphoma
Presence of blood products within lesion before treatment	Bleed only on treatment, ependymal enhancement
No elevated perfusion	Elevated perfusion
Low metabolic activity on single-photon emission computed tomography	Choline on magnetic resonance spectroscopy

Ref:
1. Chang L, Cornford ME, Chiang FL, Ernst TM, Sun NC, Miller BL. Radiologic-pathologic correlation. Cerebral toxoplasmosis and lymphoma in AIDS. Am J Neuroradiol. 1995;16(8):1653-63.
2. Ramsey RG, Gean AD. Neuroimaging of AIDS. I. Central nervous system toxoplasmosis. Neuroimaging Clin N Am. 1997;7(2):171-86.

9. **Ans. C**
   - CNS cryptococcosis results from infection of the CNS with the yeast-like fungus *Cryptococcus neoformans*.
   - Most common fungal infection and second most common opportunistic infection of the CNS.
   - In HIV/AIDS patients, cryptococcal infection of the CNS usually occurs when the CD4+ count drops below 100 cells/μL.
   - Meningitis causing hydrocephalus, the most common presentation.
   - Gelatinous pseudocysts appearing as dilated perivascular spaces, one of the most frequently described feature on MRI, are seen most commonly in basal ganglia.
   - Cryptococcomas can be seen as ring-like enhancing lesions.

   Ref:
   1. Lanzieri CF, Bangert BA, Tarr RW, Shah RS, Lewin JS, Gilkeson RC. Neuroradiology case of the day. CNS cryptococcal infection. Am J Roentgenol. 1997;169(1):295, 299.
   2. Andreula CF, Burdi N, Carella A. CNS cryptococcosis in AIDS: spectrum of MR findings. J Comput Assist Tomogr. 1993;17(3):438-41.

10. **Ans. A**

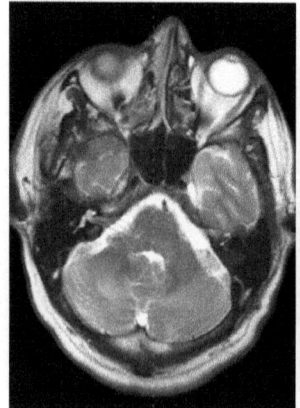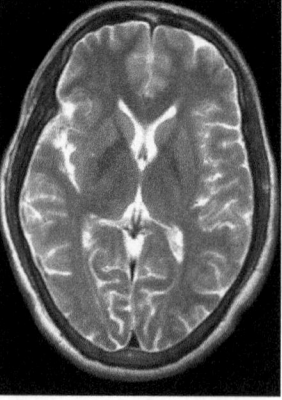

Follow-up MRI—symmetric hyperintensities in thalami and cerebellum with hemorrhage are seen which resolve on treatment.

Imaging patterns
- Normal scan
- Diffuse cerebral edema—both cytotoxic and vasogenic
- Bilateral thalamic hyperintensities/hemorrhages
- Bilateral thalamic and cerebellar hyperintensities
- Brain stem cerebrum and hippocampus rarely

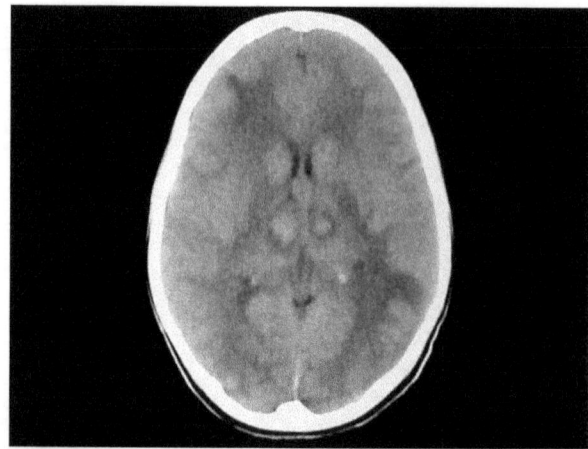
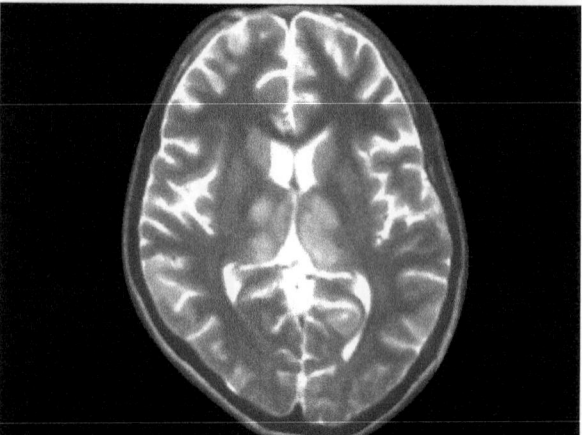
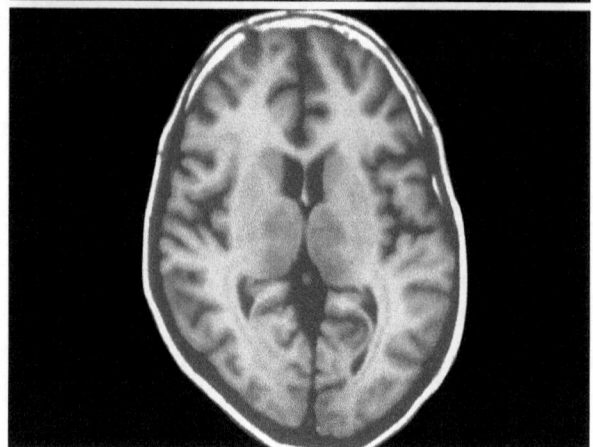

Ref:
1. Patankar TF, Karnad DR, Shetty PG, Desai AP, Prasad SR. Adult cerebral malaria: prognostic importance of imaging findings and correlation with postmortem findings. Radiology. 2002;224(3):811-6.
2. Nickerson JP, Tong KA, Raghavan R. Imaging cerebral malaria with a susceptibility-weighted MR sequence. Am J Neuroradiol. 2009;30(6):e85-6.

11. Ans. B

- Caused by the Japanese encephalitis virus, a single-stranded RNA *Flavivirus*
- Bilateral thalamic, substantia nigra, basal ganglia, brain stem, cerebellum, cerebral cortical, and white matter lesions
- Lesions are usually symmetric
- Coinfection with neurocysticercosis is known, as pigs are the intermediate host in both.

Ref:
1. Singh P, Kalra N, Ratho RK, Shankar S, Khandelwal N, Suri S. Coexistent neurocysticercosis and Japanese B encephalitis: MR imaging correlation. Am J Neuroradiol. 2001;22(6):1131-6.
2. Kumar S, Misra UK, Kalita J, Salwani V, Gupta RK, Gujral R. MRI in Japanese encephalitis. Neuroradiology. 1997;39(3):180-4.
3. Prakash M, Kumar S, Gupta RK. Diffusion-weighted MR imaging in Japanese encephalitis. J Comput Assist Tomogr. 2004;28(6):756-61.

12. Ans. A

- Infection caused by JC virus (John Cunningham virus)
- T2-hyperintense demyelinating lesions involving subcortical and deep white matter
- Hypointense on T1-weighted images
- Solitary, multifocal or widespread confluent
- Typically bilateral but asymmetric, no mass effect, may or may not enhance
- Propensity for parieto-occipital region, thalamus and basal ganglia
- May cavitate in later stages.

Ref:
1. Smith AB, Smirniotopoulos JG, Rushing EJ. From the archives of the AFIP: central nervous system infections associated with human immunodeficiency virus infection: radiologic-pathologic correlation. Radiographics. 2008;28(7):2033-58.
2. Mark AS, Atlas SW. Progressive multifocal leukoencephalopathy in patients with AIDS: appearance on MR images. Radiology. 1989;173(2):517-20.

13. Ans. B

- *HIV associated dementia (HAD),* previously referred to as *AIDS dementia complex (ADC),* corresponds to a neurological clinical syndrome seen in patients with HIV infection
- Brain atrophy
- Symmetric periventricular and deep white matter T2-hyperintensity with relative sparing of the subcortical white matter and posterior fossa structures
- Frontal predominance that may include involvement of the genu of the corpus callosum
- No mass effect or enhancement
- Increased signal in basal ganglia, thalami, and pons may be seen.

AIDS dementia complex	Progressive multifocal leukoencephalopathy
• Diffuse bilaterally symmetrical white matter hyperintensities	• Usually focal T2-hyperintense lesions
• No hypointensity on T1W1 images	• Hypointense on T1W1 images
• Basal ganglia involvement more common	• Basal ganglia involvement less common
• Magnetization transfer ratio (MTR) > 40	• MTR > 20
	• Callosal involvement

Ref:
1. Smith A, Smirniotopoulos J, Rushing E. From the archives of the AFIP: central nervous system infections associated with human immunodeficiency virus infection: radiologic-pathologic correlation. Radiographics. 2008;28(7):2033-58.
2. Clifford DB, Ances BM. HIV-associated neurocognitive disorder. Lancet Infect Dis. 2013;13(11):976-86.

14. Ans. B

- Herpes simplex encephalitis is the most common cause of fatal sporadic fulminant necrotizing viral encephalitis and has characteristic imaging findings.
- Childhood and adult herpes encephalitis are usually due to HSV-1 (90%).
- Pattern is quite typical and manifests as a bilateral asymmetrical involvement with T2-hyperintensities in the limbic system, medial temporal lobes, insular cortices and inferolateral frontal lobes.
- In immunocompromised patients, involvement can be more diffuse, and more likely to involve the brainstem.

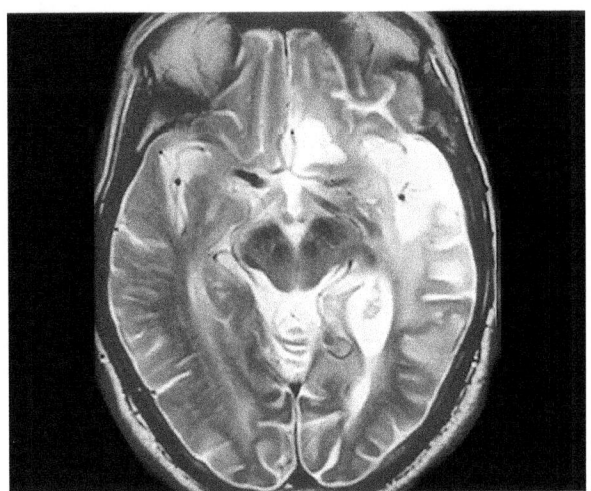

Central Nervous System Infections

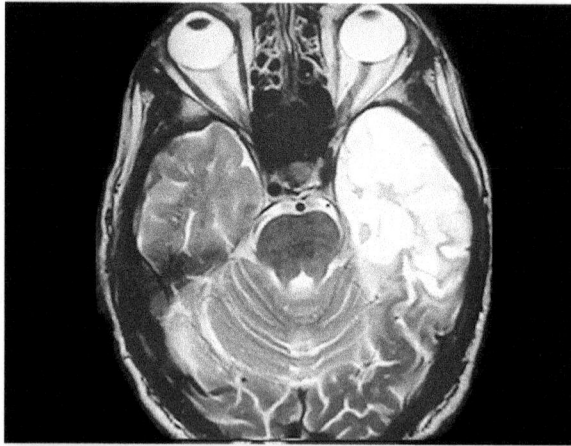
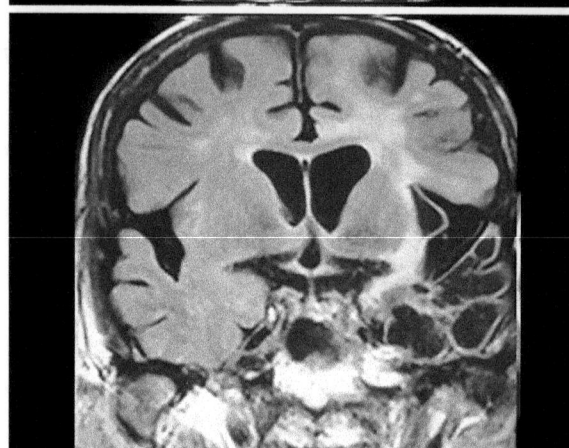
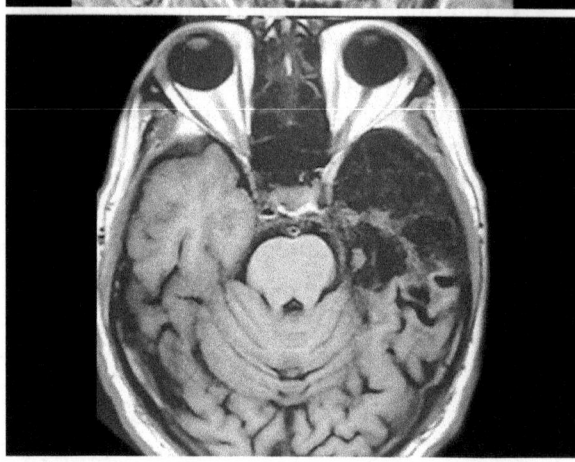

Scan after 21 days of acyclovir.

Ref:
1. Leonard JR, Moran CJ, Cross DT 3rd, Wippold FJ 2nd, Schlesinger Y, Storch GA. MR imaging of herpes simplex type 1 encephalitis in infants and young children: a separate pattern of findings. Am J Roentgenol. 2000;174(6):1651-5.
2. Zimmerman RD, Russell EJ, Leeds NE, Kaufman D. CT in the early diagnosis of herpes simplex encephalitis. Am J Roentgenol. 1980;134(1):61-6.

15. Ans. C

- Creutzfeldt-Jakob disease is a spongiform encephalopathy that results in a rapidly progressive dementia
- Four types have been described:
  - Sporadic Creutzfeldt-Jakob disease (sCJD):
    - Accounts for 85–90% of cases
    - Further divided into numerous subtypes according to molecular markers
  - Variant Creutzfeldt-Jakob disease (vCJD):
    - Bovine-to-human transmission of bovine spongiform encephalopathy
  - Familial Creutzfeldt-Jakob disease (fCJD):
    - 10% of cases
    - These individuals carry a PrPC mutation
  - Iatrogenic Creutzfeldt-Jakob disease (iCJD):
    - Following administration of cadaveric human pituitary hormones
    - Various transplants.

Imaging
- T2-hyperintensity in basal ganglia (putamen and caudate), thalamus, cortex, and white matter.
- Diffusion-weighted imaging (DWI) or apparent diffusion coefficient—persistent restricted diffusion.

Ref:
1. Lee H, Hoffman C, Kingsley PB, Degnan A, Cohen O, Prohovnik I. Enhanced detection of diffusion reductions in Creutzfeldt-Jakob disease at a higher B factor. Am J Neuroradiol. 2010;31(1):49-54.
2. Kallenberg K, Schulz-Schaeffer WJ, Jastrow U, Poser S, Meissner B, Tschampa HJ, et al. Creutzfeldt-Jakob disease: comparative analysis of MR imaging sequences. Am J Neuroradiol. 2006;27(7):1459-62.
3. Tschampa HJ, Kallenberg K, Kretzschmar HA, Meissner B, Knauth M, Urbach H, et al. Pattern of cortical changes in sporadic Creutzfeldt-Jakob disease. Am J Neuroradiol. 2007;28(6):1114-8.

16. Ans. D

Acquired Cytomegalovirus
- Common in immunocompromised patient
- Can cause meningitis, encephalitis, ventriculitis, transverse myelitis, radiculomyelitis and chorioretinitis
- Ventriculitis with fluid debris level with ependymal enhancement
- Cytomegalovirus encephalitis can present as a T2-hyperintense mass with variable enhancement.

Ref:
1. Smith A, Smirniotopoulos J, Rushing E. From the archives of the AFIP: central nervous system infections associated with human immunodeficiency virus infection: radiologic-pathologic correlation. Radiographics. 2008;28(7):2033-58.
2. Holland NR, Power C, Mathews VP, Glass JD, Forman M, McArthur JC. Cytomegalovirus encephalitis in acquired immunodeficiency syndrome (AIDS). Neurology. 1994;44(3):507-14.

17. Ans. A

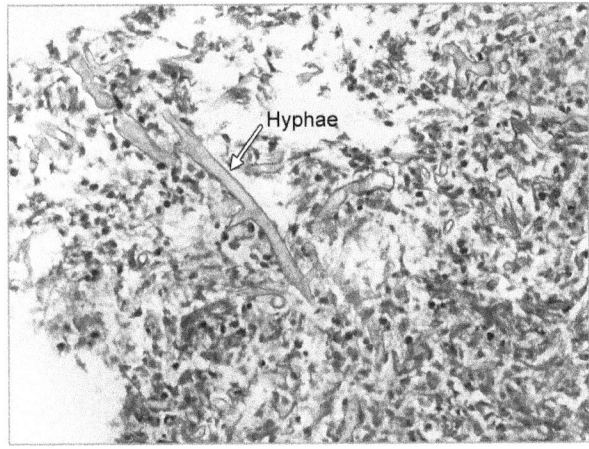

Pathophysiology
- Mucormycosis is an angioinvasive infection leads to infarction with or without hemorrhage.
- Occlusion of small perforating arteries leads to involvement of basal ganglia, thalamus, brain stem and corpus callosum.

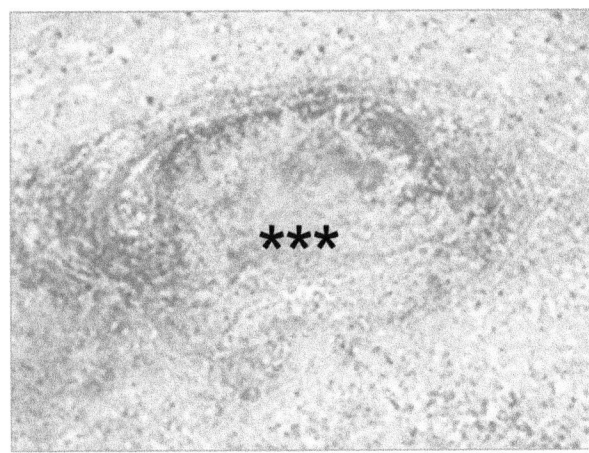

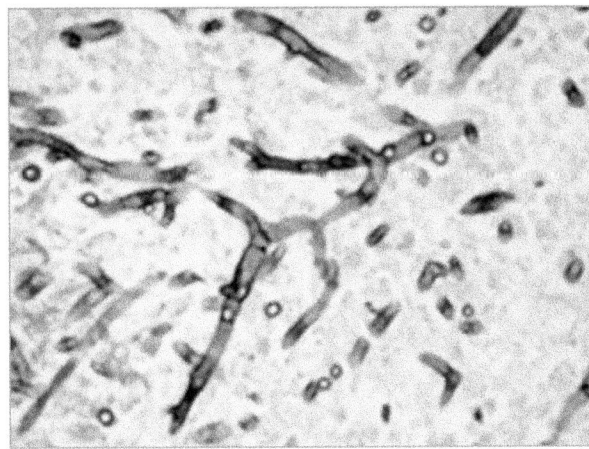

Imaging
- Sinusitis with collections showing high signal on T1W images

- Associated intense enhancement of sinus walls
- Associated bone erosion and destruction
- Extension into orbit, cavernous with resultant proptosis and visual complaints, ophthalmoplegia
- Intracranial extension with angioinvasion causing infarction and encephalitis.

Ref:
1. Gamba JL, Woodruff WW, Djang WT, Yeates AE. Craniofacial mucormycosis: assessment with CT. Radiology. 1986;160(1):207-12.
2. Ferguson BJ. Mucormycosis of the nose and paranasal sinuses. Otolaryngol Clin North Am. 2000;33(2): 349-65.

18. Ans. A

Malignant otitis externa with skull base osteomyelitis (Pseudomonas isolated)
- Necrotizing otitis externa (NOE), also known as malignant otitis externa, is a severe invasive infection of the external auditory canal (EAC) which can spread rapidly to involve the surrounding soft tissue, adjacent neck spaces, and skull base.
- *Pseudomonas aeruginosa* is the pathogen in 98% of cases.
- Thickening and enhancing soft-tissue in the region of the external auditory canal with or without formation of abscess.
- Soft-tissue can extend into adjacent structures.
- Base of skull osteomyelitis is a feared complication and associated with poor prognosis.

Ref:
1. Rubin Grandis J, Branstetter BF 4th, Yu VL. The changing face of malignant (necrotising) external otitis: clinical, radiological, and anatomic correlations. Lancet Infect Dis. 2004;4(1):34-9.
2. Grandis JR, Curtin HD, Yu VL. Necrotizing (malignant) external otitis: prospective comparison of CT and MR imaging in diagnosis and follow-up. Radiology. 1995;196(2):499-504.

19. Ans. A

Diagnosis: ?Fungal; ?Bacterial
Biopsy: Actinomycosis.

Cervicofacial actinomycosis
- Suppurative and granulomatous chronic infectious disease.
- Spreads into adjacent soft-tissues without regard for tissue planes or lymphatic drainage.
- May also be associated with a draining sinus tract.
- Cope classified actinomycosis infection into three distinct clinical forms—Cervicofacial (50%), pulmonothoracic (30%), and abdominopelvic (20%).
- Poor dental hygiene, caries, oral trauma, dental extraction, and an immunocompromised status.

Imaging
- CT-enhancing soft-tissue mass with a low-attenuating center associated with inflammatory change in the adjacent soft-tissue
- Invasion of the adjacent soft-tissue, including the muscles, can occur
- The lesions of the nasal, oral, and pharyngeal cavities contiguously extended to the adjacent neck space, crossing fascial planes
- T1- and T2-intermediate signal intensity associated with moderate contrast enhancement
- Regional lymphadenopathy is uncommon.

Osseous lesions in actinomycosis
- Slow process of absorption and a simultaneous formation of new bone
- Erode cortical and trabecular and even subchondral bone
- May resemble fungal, although incidence is lesser with actinomycosis.

Ref:
1. Park JK, Lee HK, Ha HK, Choi HY, Choi CG. Cervicofacial actinomycosis: CT and MR imaging findings in seven patients. Am J Neuroradiol. 2003;24(3):331-5.
2. Heo SH, Shin SS, Kim JW, Lim HS, Seon HJ, Jung SI, et al. Imaging of actinomycosis in various organs: a comprehensive review. Radiographics. 2014;34(1):19-33.

CHAPTER 12

Respiratory Infections

Rahul Bahot

1. A 28-year-old immunocompetent male patient was admitted to the hospital with prolonged recurrent fever, cough, anorexia, and weight loss. Admission investigations revealed anemia, while renal and liver functions were within normal limits. A chest radiograph showed patchy infiltrates and cavitation in the right upper lobe. Microbiological and molecular tests in sputum were positive for *Mycobacterium tuberculosis* and treatment with isoniazid, rifampicin, ethambutol, and pyrazinamide has been started. A few days later, the antituberculosis (anti-TB) drug susceptibility test shows isoniazid resistance. Which is the right treatment option for this patient?

    A. Category I treatment for 6 months
    B. Substitution of isoniazid with levofloxacin in category I treatment for 6 months
    C. Direct and supportive observation (DOTS)-plus regimen for multidrug-resistant TB assuming rifampicin resistance coexisting with isoniazid resistance
    D. Category II anti-TB treatment

2. A 55-year-old man presented with fever and mild dyspnea. He had a history of chronic renal failure secondary to membranoproliferative glomerulonephritis (MPGN) diagnosed 6 months prior to admission. He had been treated with 60 mg of prednisone daily for 6 months and mycophenolate mofetil for 4 months without improvement of his renal function. He had poor follow-up and was never placed on prophylaxis for pneumocystis pneumonia (PCP). His corticosteroids were tapered off 1 week prior to admission with the plan to initiate hemodialysis in the near future, but he became ill in the interim.

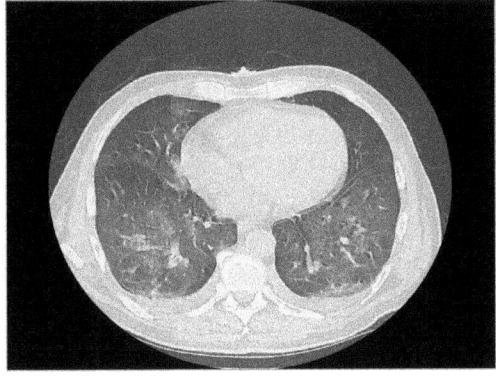

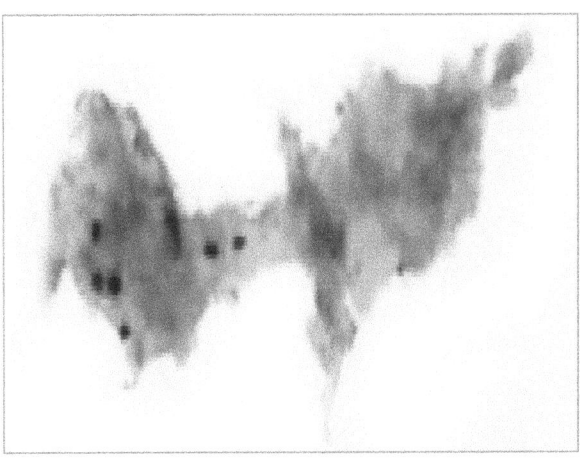

A high-resolution computed tomography (CT) scan of the thorax on day 4 of the admission demonstrated small bilateral pleural effusions with passive atelectasis and diffuse ground-glass opacification. Bronchoalveolar lavage (BAL) washings sent for culture showed cyst forms of *Pneumocystis jirovecii* stained with Grocott-Gomori's Methenamine Silver (GMS) nitrate.

Regarding *P. jirovecii* pneumonia in immunocompromised patients, which of the following statement(s) is false?

A. Most patients have CD4 counts <200 cells/μL at the time of diagnosis of their first episode of *P. jirovecii* pneumonia
B. Most patients with *P. jirovecii* pneumonia will have an elevated serum lactate dehydrogenase (LDH) level
C. Arterial blood gases (ABGs) in patients with *P. jirovecii* pneumonia frequently reveal respiratory alkalosis and a widened alveolar–arterial oxygen tension difference
D. A normal chest radiograph rules out the diagnosis

3. A 32-year-old, HIV-positive man presents with dyspnea, nonproductive cough, and fever. Physical examination reveals a temperature of 39.4°C; the chest examination is normal. His medical records show that he was hospitalized to an acquired immunodeficiency syndrome (AIDS) ward 6 weeks ago during an unrecognized outbreak of drug-resistant TB.

Which of the following tests would be helpful in the evaluation of this patient?

A. A chest radiograph and sputum culture for mycobacteria
B. GeneXpert
C. A tuberculin skin test (TST)
D. An interferon-γ release assay

4. A 46-year-old male presents to your outpatient clinic. He suffers from increasing shortness of breath, increasing amounts of sputum, and recurrent bronchopulmonary infections. He has infertility and had two operations for nasal polyposis and recurrent sinusitis. His lung function shows a combined obstructive–restrictive pattern. The CT scan of the thorax shows abnormalities in both lower lobes (below). Liver function tests and blood glucose concentration are within normal limits. Which of the following is the most likely diagnosis in this patient?

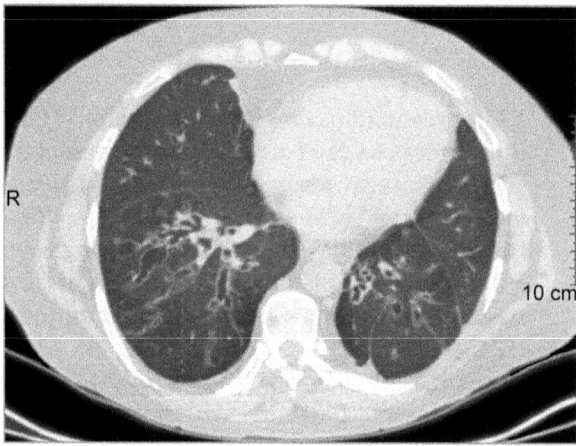

A. Allergic bronchopulmonary aspergillosis (ABPA)
B. Cystic fibrosis
C. Idiopathic bronchiectasis
D. Primary ciliary dyskinesia (PCD) (Young's syndrome)
E. Mounier-Kuhn syndrome

5. Which of the following statements about cystic fibrosis is false?

A. The most common mutation is Phe508del on chromosome 7
B. Pathogens such as *Pseudomonas aeruginosa*, *Burkholderia cepacia*, *Staphylococcus aureus*, and *Escherichia coli* are found in early stages of the disease
C. Congenital bilateral absence of the vas deferens leads to infertility in men with cystic fibrosis
D. Long-term, low-dose macrolide therapy (azithromycin) should be considered for patients who are chronically infected with *P. aeruginosa*

6. A 33-year-old male with cystic fibrosis presents to your clinic with a 4-week history of increasing dyspnea and decreased exercise tolerance. His chronic cough production of 90 mL greenish sputum per day has increased. He was hospitalized 2 years ago for a right pneumothorax. Current medications include pancreatic enzyme replacement, a multiple-vitamin supplement, and bronchodilators as needed. He admits to some noncompliance with his daily chest physiotherapy regimen. The patient weighs 60 kg and is 170 cm tall. His pulse rate is 86 beats/min, blood pressure 106/78 mm Hg, respiration rate 24 breaths/min, temperature 36.8°C, and SpO_2 93%. Chest examination reveals diffuse, coarse crackles, and expiratory rhonchi. His laboratory and spirometry results are as follows:

Hematocrit %	41
Leukocytes/μL	11,400
Neutrophils %	78
Lymphocytes %	16
Eosinophils %	2

	6 months ago	Current
FVC % predicted	74	62
FEV1 % predicted	48	40
FEV1/FVC %	70	62

His chest radiograph is shown below.

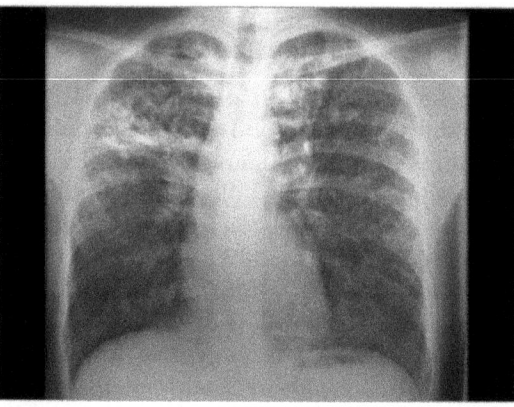

Which of the following is the most efficacious management option?

A. Initiate intensive inhaled bronchodilator therapy with ipratropium and β-agonists
B. Initiate intravenous antibiotic therapy with ticarcillin and tobramycin-pending sputum culture and sensitivity results
C. Initiate long-term continuous inhaled antibiotic therapy with high-dose tobramycin
D. Initiate regular therapy with inhaled recombinant human deoxyribonuclease (DNAse)
E. Reinstitute twice-daily chest physiotherapy with postural drainage and use of an airway oscillator

7. A 68-year-old male is admitted to the emergency room complaining about shortness of breath, fever, chills, and cough with purulent sputum production for the last 2 days. He is a nonsmoker without any previous medical history. The patient looks tired but other than that he is in good condition without any confusion. Vital signs are blood pressure 105/70 mm Hg, heart rate 110 beats/min, breathing rate 32 breaths/min, and temperature 38.9°C. Bronchial breath sounds are heard on auscultation of the right chest. Blood tests reveal a white blood cell count of $9,000 \times 10^9$/L with a left shift, hematocrit 46%, urea 22 mmol/L, creatinine 160 µmol/L, sodium 142 mmol/L, and oxygen saturation (room air) 92%. A chest radiograph demonstrates moderate cardiomegaly and a right lower lobe infiltrate with air bronchograms.
   Which of the following is the appropriate management decision for this patient?
   A. Treat as an outpatient, start empirical antibiotic therapy without further examinations
   B. Treat as an outpatient, take blood and sputum cultures, and start empirical antibiotic therapy
   C. Admit to hospital, start empirical antibiotic therapy within 4 hours of admission
   D. Admit to hospital, take blood and sputum cultures and Gram stains, and start antibiotic therapy according to results
   E. Treat in the intensive care unit and start empirical antibiotic therapy

8. A 48-year-old female with a 25 pack-year history of smoking presents with fever, cough, and purulent sputum production and her chest radiograph shows consolidation of the right middle lobe. She has a history compatible with chronic bronchitis but normal spirometry and she had a bronchitis exacerbation 2 months ago for which she received treatment with moxifloxacin. Her blood pressure is 115/75 mm Hg and her breathing rate is 18 breaths/min. She does not look severely ill but she is depressed and tired because her mother who was in the hospital died a week ago, 2 weeks after acquiring an influenza infection. The patient is anxious to get well soon and return to work because she has already taken a long time off.
   Which of the following is the appropriate treatment for this patient?
   A. Amoxicillin–clavulanate and macrolide
   B. Oseltamivir
   C. Moxifloxacin
   D. Piperacillin–tazobactam and ciprofloxacin
   E. Acyclovir and amoxicillin–clavulanate

9. A 60-year-old, previously fit and well man, presented with increased shortness of breath and a history of feeling generally unwell for 5 days. He had recently visited Dubai for a 10-day holiday and felt unwell on his return. He became acutely short of breath 24 hours before his admission, with an associated dry cough, malaise, and lethargy. He presented to his local Accident and Emergency Department and required admission to intensive care for mechanical ventilation. He continued to deteriorate from a respiratory perspective and was referred for extracorporeal membrane oxygenation (ECMO). The more sensitive diagnostic test for *Legionella* species is:
   A. Culture
   B. Urinary antigen
   C. Serology
   D. Direct fluorescence assay

10. The clinical case is same as Question 9. *Legionella* infection is commonly acquired through contamination of:
    A. Air
    B. Water
    C. Air conditioner
    D. None of the above

11. A 46-year-old nonsmoking patient suffers from recurrent purulent bronchitis. He complains of increased sputum production but is otherwise well. A CT scan shows bilateral, mainly lower lobe tubular bronchiectasis.
    Which of the following investigation(s) is for treatment decisions?
    A. Search for nontuberculous mycobacteria (NTM) in sputum
    B. α_1-antitrypsin (AAT) serum level
    C. Immunoglobulin G (IgG) and subclasses levels in serum
    D. Bacterial sputum cultures

12. A 66-year-old woman presents with 3 weeks of cough and sputum production, with hemoptysis and 2.3 kg weight loss in 1 month. She has a history of multiple episodes of childhood pneumonia. She does not smoke but says that she has had a chronic cough for 5 years, present throughout the day, with daily sputum production. Several times a year, she receives antibiotic therapy for purulent sputum. Her TST was positive 20 years ago. Chest radiography shows increased markings at the lung bases with "tramlines" and dilated bronchial shadows. Furthermore, an infiltrate with a 1-cm thin-walled cavity in the right upper lobe is seen. A sputum smear for acid-fast bacilli is positive.

Which of the following should be the next step in the management of this patient?

A. Start therapy with isoniazid, rifampicin, and ethambutol
B. Collect two additional sputum samples, and start therapy with isoniazid, rifampicin, ethambutol, and pyrazinamide
C. Collect two additional sputum samples for mycobacterial smears and culture, then start therapy with rifampicin, ethambutol, and clarithromycin
D. Collect three additional sputum samples for mycobacterial smears and culture, then await results before starting therapy
E. Perform bronchoscopy with transbronchial biopsy before starting therapy

13. A 65-year-old male is admitted to the hospital because of high fever and dyspnea associated with purulent sputum. Physical examination reveals dullness on percussion on the right lower chest and rales on auscultation. Chest radiography shows a pneumonic infiltrate in the right upper lobe and a small pleural effusion. Thoracentesis is performed. Which of the following results of the pleural fluid analysis indicates the need for chest-tube drainage?

A. Serosanguineous appearance
B. pH < 7.2
C. Glucose < 60 mmol/L
D. Negative Gram stain
E. LDH > 200 U/L

14. A 35-year-old male is admitted to hospital because of acute onset of fever (38°C), dry cough, severe dyspnea, and mental confusion. Arterial blood pressure is 140/80 mm Hg, heart rate is regular at 120 beats/min, and respiratory rate is 36 breaths/min. ABG analysis reveals a PaO_2 of 8 kPa (65 mm Hg), $PaCO_2$ of 5 kPa (42 mm Hg), bicarbonate concentration of 24.2 mmol/L, and a pH of 7.42. Chest radiography and CT show diffuse, bilateral pulmonary infiltrates. BAL reveals 920×10^9 cells/L with 35% eosinophils, 8% neutrophils, and 57% macrophages. A broad search for parasitic infestation is negative.
Which of the following statements about this case is correct?

A. Blood eosinophilia is required to support the diagnosis
B. The recommended treatment consists of broad-spectrum antibiotics
C. Thoracoscopic lung biopsy is required to support the diagnosis
D. Corticosteroids result in rapid resolution
E. The prevalence of this condition is reduced in smokers

15. A 40-year-old, HIV-positive male consults his physician because of a 2-week history of right chest pain, night sweats, and cough. His body temperature is 37.6°C and vital signs are normal, and there is dullness on percussion, reduced lung sounds, and some rales on the right lower chest. The chest radiograph is as shown below.
His C-reactive protein level is 119 mg/mL (normal <5 mg/mL) and white blood cell count is 6,570 cells/mm³. His CD4 cell count was 437 cells/μL 5 months ago.
Which further examination should be recommended first?

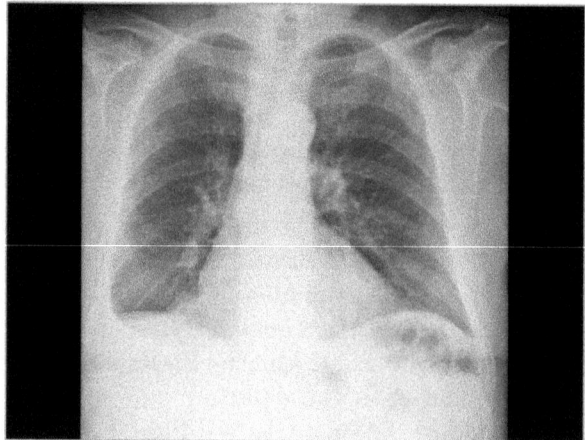

A. TST
B. Thoracentesis
C. Interferon-γ release assay
D. CT of the chest
E. Bronchoscopy

16. A 63-year-old healthy woman, who has never smoked, has been visiting her family, including three grandchildren. The children have been suffering from a febrile illness, passing it between one another, and two of them have had severe earaches. After being at their home for 2 weeks, the patient experiences a nonproductive cough, fever, and weakness. Her chest radiograph shows a right mid-lung infiltrate and a small pleural effusion. The white blood cell count of her pleural fluid is 560 cells/mm³. The cold agglutinin titer of her acute serum is 1:16. She responds to treatment with erythromycin. What could be done to confirm or rule out a diagnosis of *Mycoplasma pneumoniae*?

A. Obtain a second cold agglutinin titer 3–6 weeks later; if the titer fails to show at least a fourfold rise, this has to be considered strong evidence against the diagnosis
B. Obtain acute and convalescent titers of complement-fixing antibody against *M. pneumoniae*; if there is at least a fourfold increase in titer, this is a strong evidence confirming the diagnosis

C. Wait for results of throat washings cultured for *M. pneumoniae*; if the cultures are negative, this is a strong evidence against the diagnosis
D. Study the serum complement-fixing antibody against *Chlamydophila pneumoniae* (TWAR) because a titer of 1:16 or greater would strongly favor a diagnosis of chlamydial pneumonia
E. Avoid ordering additional tests because effusions are rare in *M. pneumoniae* and this makes the diagnosis most unlikely

17. A 52-year-old patient with severe late-onset intrinsic asthma and a history of sinusitis stopped taking systemic corticosteroids 4 weeks ago. Now, he is suffering from fever, malaise, and moderate weight loss. Due to severe chest pain that does not allow the patient to lie on his left side, he is referred to the intensive care unit. On auscultation, a pericardial friction rub is audible. On his skin, several new-onset hemorrhagic lesions are visible. His creatine kinase (CK) and CK-MB are elevated.
Which laboratory test could best help to support the suspected diagnosis?

A. Blood eosinophil count
B. Skin prick test for *Aspergillus spp.*
C. Antibasement membrane antibodies
D. Antisynthetase antibodies (Jo-1)
E. Troponin T

18. A 35-year-old male presents to the emergency room with productive cough and low-grade fever of approximately 6 weeks' duration. 6 months ago, he had received treatment with isoniazid, rifampicin, pyrazinamide, and ethambutol for smear-positive pulmonary TB. The treatment had led to rapid clinical improvement and he therefore stopped it upon return to London, after a duration of 8 weeks. Clinical examination at admission reveals a body mass index (BMI) of 18 kg/m² and a temperature of 37.8°C but no other abnormal findings. Chest radiography shows bilateral upper lobe infiltrates with a cavitary lesion in the right upper lobe. The sputum contains acid-fast bacilli. A HIV test is negative. Results of rapid molecular-based drug susceptibility tests are pending.
Which of the following should be recommended for this patient?

A. Initiate regimen with 2HRZES/1HRZE/5HRE
B. Await results of molecular susceptibility testing
C. Complete treatment with 4HR
D. Start prolonged treatment with 2HRZE/6HE
E. Restart standard regimen with 2HRZE/4HR

H: isoniazid; R: rifampicin; Z: pyrazinamide; E: ethambutol; S: streptomycin. Numbers before the letters denote the duration of treatment in months.

19. A 28-year-old female complains of a 1-week history of severe hacking dry cough, slight dyspnea, and weakness. On examination, she is mildly unwell but fully orientated and not cyanosed. However, she is pyrexial, pale, and slightly jaundiced. A full blood cell count shows normochromic anemia with Hb of 9 g/dL and neutrophil leukocytosis. Liver function tests show mild elevation of unconjugated bilirubin and raised LDH. Blood urea and electrolytes are normal. There is no proteinuria. Results of blood cultures are pending. The chest radiograph is shown below.

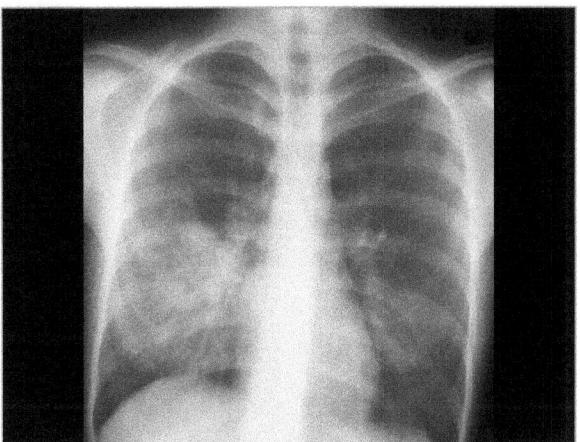

Which of the following additional investigations would be most likely to provide a diagnosis?

A. Chlamydia serology
B. Antineutrophil cytoplasmic antibody
C. Urine test for *Legionella*
D. *Mycoplasma* serology
E. Antibasement membrane antibody

20. A 45-year-old female is referred to you by her general practitioner because she has recurrent episodes (three to six per year) of bronchitis with fever for which she uses courses of antibiotics with good results. Between these episodes, she coughs up phlegm in considerable amounts (several spoonfuls a day). The color of the phlegm varies from white to yellow; she has never seen blood in her phlegm. She smoked approximately 20 cigarettes per day from the age of 18 years until the age of 30 years. Since then, she has stopped smoking. She has no complaints of shortness of breath, wheezing, or tightness of the chest. Her family history is uneventful. Her flow-volume curve was normal. Her chest radiograph and CT scan are shown on next page.

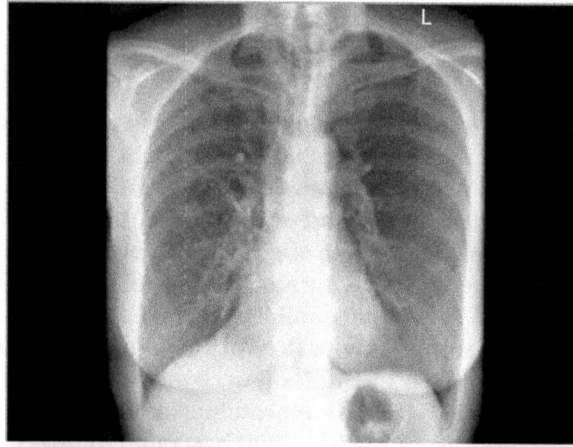
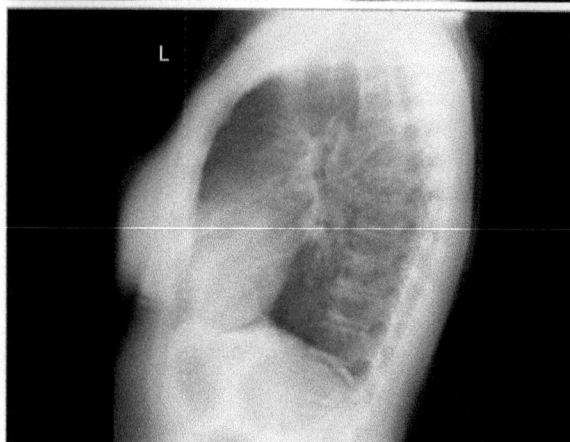
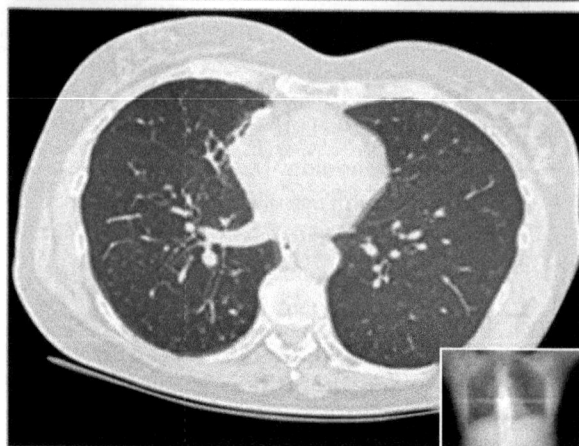

Which of the following is the most appropriate next action?

A. Lung resection surgery
B. Inhaled bronchodilators
C. Bronchoscopy
D. Maintenance antibiotic therapy with quinolones
E. Sputum culture

21. A 36-year-old immunocompetent male is admitted to the hospital with symptoms of recurrent fever, cough, anorexia, and weight loss. Admission baseline investigations show normal renal and liver function tests. A chest radiograph shows patchy infiltrates and cavitations in the right and left upper lobe. Microbiological and molecular tests in sputum are positive for *M. tuberculosis*. Initial molecular drug resistance testing of mutations associated with rifampicin and isoniazid resistance were negative. Which of the following is the recommended treatment for this patient?

A. Isoniazid, rifampicin, ethambutol, and pyrazinamide for 2 months, followed by isoniazid and rifampicin for 4 months
B. Isoniazid, rifampicin, ethambutol, and pyrazinamide for 6 months
C. Isoniazid, rifampicin, ethambutol, streptomycin, and pyrazinamide for 2 months, followed by rifampicin and isoniazid for 7 months
D. Isoniazid, rifampicin, and ethambutol for 6 months
E. Isoniazid, rifampicin, ethambutol, and pyrazinamide for 2 months, followed by rifampicin, isoniazid, and ethambutol for 4 months

22. A 34-year-old man has pulmonary TB with the lung lesion confined to the left upper lobe, where there is a 3-cm cavity with extensive interstitial infiltration. He has had hematuria and pyuria for 4 weeks, and an intravenous pyelogram shows deformed collecting structures in the upper pole of the left kidney. Sputum and urine cultures are positive for *M. tuberculosis*. A serum test for HIV infection is negative.
Which of the following is the treatment regimen of choice for this patient?

A. Isoniazid and rifampicin daily for 9 months
B. Isoniazid and rifampicin daily for 12 months
C. Isoniazid, rifampicin, and ethambutol daily for 9 months
D. Isoniazid, rifampicin, pyrazinamide, and ethambutol daily for 2 months, followed by rifampicin and isoniazid daily for 4 months
E. Isoniazid and rifampicin daily, together with streptomycin five times weekly for 2 months, followed by isoniazid and rifampicin daily for 10 more months

23. A 43-year-old male complains of sudden bilateral chest pain, aggravated by inspiration, and accompanied by malaise and slight fever. Physical examination shows some tenderness on both sides of the chest but normal breath sounds. His chest radiograph appears normal but ultrasound reveals small bilateral pleural effusions. The patient reports that 1 week ago, one of his children was admitted to the hospital with acute meningitis.
Which of the following is the most likely microorganism causing his illness?

A. Varicella zoster virus
B. Coxsackievirus B
C. Influenza virus
D. Epstein–Barr virus
E. Adenovirus

24. Which of the following organisms is least likely to be a part of the upper respiratory flora?
    A. *S. pneumoniae*
    B. *H. influenzae*
    C. *E. coli*
    D. *Legionella pneumophila*
    E. *Bacteroides fragilis*

25. A 55-year-old, HIV-positive male is admitted to the hospital because of fever and severe dyspnea. Physical examination shows tachypnea and tachycardia. Chest auscultation reveals bilateral fine crackles. Radiography shows extensive, bilateral, and patchy lung infiltrates. ABG analysis on room air reveals a PaO_2 of 45 mm Hg, $PaCO_2$ of 11 mm Hg, and pH of 7.56. He is intubated, and positive-pressure ventilation is initiated with an inspiratory oxygen fraction (FiO_2) of 0.5 and a positive end-expiratory pressure of 6 cmH_2O. ABG analysis after half an hour demonstrates a PaO_2 of 50 mm Hg, $PaCO_2$ of 22 mm Hg, and pH of 7.52. Brain natriuretic peptide concentration is normal, and echocardiography shows normal systolic and diastolic function as well as normal respiratory variation of the inferior vena cava size.
    Which of the following statements regarding this patient is false?
    A. A diagnosis of acute respiratory distress syndrome (ARDS) can be made
    B. The alveolar–arterial oxygen tension difference is corrected by oxygen administration
    C. The intrapulmonary shunt increases with increasing FiO_2
    D. Prone position during positive-pressure ventilation improves survival

26. Which of the following statements about anti-TB drugs is false correct?
    A. Anti-TB drugs have three major principles of action: bactericidal action, sterilization, and prevention of emergence of bacterial resistance
    B. Streptomycin is included in the standard recommended regimen for the treatment of TB as it has a lower resistance rate than ethambutol
    C. If pyrazinamide cannot be used, the standard recommended regimen for the treatment of TB has to be given for 12 months
    D. Initial cavitation and positive sputum culture after 2 months of correct treatment justify the prolongation of the continuation phase of anti-TB therapy to give a total duration of 6 months

27. A 58-year-old male smoker with a history of COPD (postbronchodilator FEV_1 57% predicted) presents to the emergency department with a cough of >24 hours duration accompanied by increased purulent sputum production. The patient has no history of lower respiratory tract infections and has received no antibiotics in the past 12 months. Physical examination: temperature 38.6°C, heart rate 112 beats/min, respiratory rate 34 breaths/min, and blood pressure 132/84 mm Hg. Examination of the chest reveals crackles in the right lower lung field. The chest radiograph shows consolidation of the right lower lobe. Laboratory tests show a leukocyte count of 22,000 cells/μL with 90% neutrophils; sputum Gram stain shows mixed flora and many squamous epithelial cells. The patient is hospitalized.
    Which empiric antibiotic therapy should be started in this patient?
    A. Erythromycin
    B. Azithromycin plus ceftriaxone
    C. Ceftazidime plus amikacin
    D. Cotrimoxazole
    E. Ciprofloxacin

28. A 75-year-old ex-smoker with COPD (Global Initiative for Chronic Obstructive Lung Disease grade 2) using long-acting bronchodilators has had shortness of breath, increased sputum expectoration, and fever for 5 days. His heart rate is 115 beats/min, respiratory rate is 36 breaths/min, blood pressure is 100/65 mm Hg, and body temperature is 38.6°C, and he seems slightly confused. On lung auscultation, you hear crackles, mainly in the right lung, and diffuse wheezes.
    Which of the following is the best choice for the further management of this patient?
    A. Hospitalization, intravenous antibiotics, and corticosteroids
    B. Amoxicillin/clavulanic acid and a short-acting bronchodilator
    C. Levofloxacin and corticosteroids
    D. Ciprofloxacin and inhaled corticosteroids
    E. Increased bronchodilator and clarithromycin

29. A 22-year-old woman presented with an 8-day history of fever associated with coughing, chills, and rigors. Although her coughing was initially dry, she had begun producing yellow-green sputum on day 5 and developed shortness of breath on day 7. The patient reported having recently undertaken a trip 1 week prior with her classmates, some of whom had also developed coughs. Upon initial examination, the patient appeared ill, dehydrated, febrile, and tachycardic. Her temperature was 40.3°C, her heart rate was 134 beats/min and her respiratory rate was 18 breaths/min. Pulse oximetry indicated an oxygen saturation of 97% on room air. Auscultation of the chest revealed reduced breath sounds in the right base. A chest X-ray showed consolidation of the right

middle and lower lobes, with right-sided pleural effusion and partial lower lobe collapse.

Two days after admission, a chest examination revealed absent breath sounds and stony dullness involving the middle and lower chest. A repeat chest X-ray confirmed that the right-sided pleural effusion had worsened.

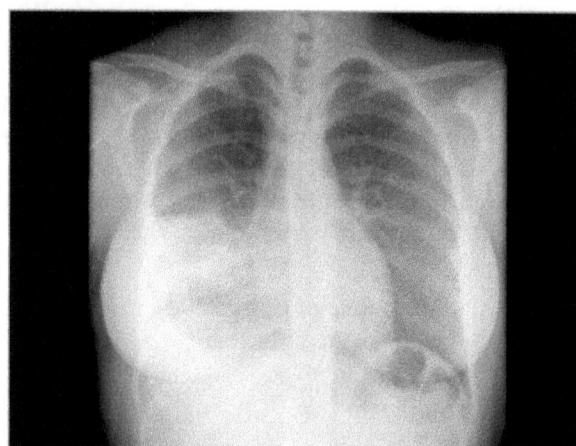

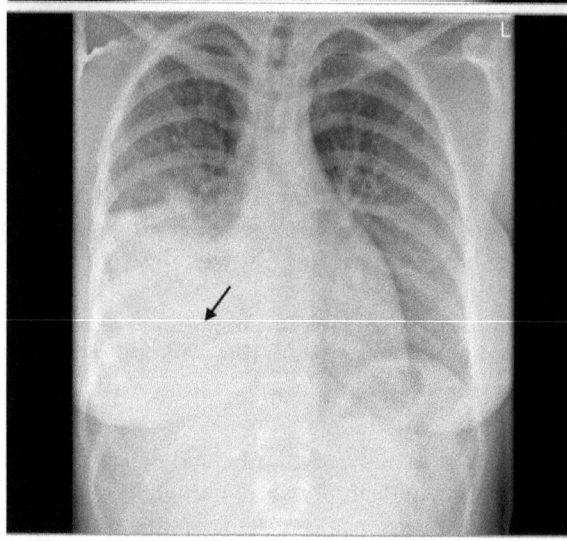

Accordingly, a drainage procedure was performed, during which 2 L of exudative fluid consisting predominantly of lymphocytes (80%) was drained via a pigtail catheter over a 24-hour period. In view of her worsening condition, a nasopharyngeal aspirate sample was sent for serological and polymerase chain reaction (PCR) testing.

The PCR test results were positive for *M. pneumoniae*, while the serology was positive for IgA, IgM, and IgG. As the serology test was qualitative, exact titers were not available.

The gold standard investigation for the diagnosis of *M. pneumoniae* is:

A. Sputum culture
B. Serological investigations
C. Molecular methods
D. None of the above exercise

30. The extrapulmonary manifestations of *M. pneumoniae* are all, *except*:

    A. Stevens–Johnson syndrome
    B. Cardiac thrombus
    C. Aseptic meningitis
    D. Acute conjunctivitis

31. You see an otherwise healthy 32-year-old female who has been treated by her general practitioner for 10 days with oral amoxicillin presents with fever up to 39°C and cough. 7 days after finishing the antibiotic therapy, she still feels weak. Her temperature is 37.2°C (oral). On examination, her respiratory rate is 20 breaths/min; there is dullness to percussion and breath sounds in the left base are absent.
The chest radiograph is shown below.
Which of the following statements is false?

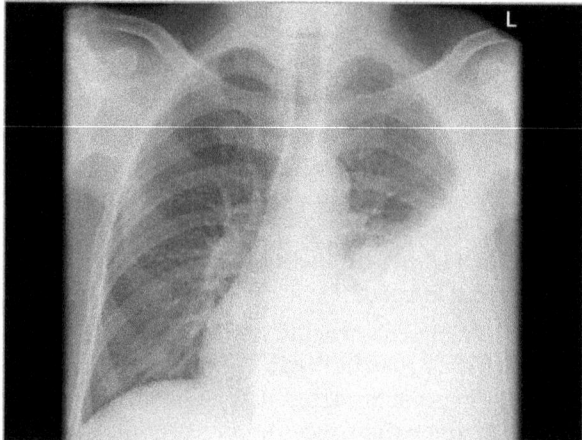

A. A diagnostic thoracentesis should be performed
B. A course of diuretics will reduce dyspnea
C. A pleural fluid pH > 7.4 suggests a simple parapneumonic effusion
D. A pleural fluid pH < 7.2 indicates the need for chest tube drainage

32. A 68-year-old male presents with cough, sputum production, and fever up to 39.5°C in the past 48 hours. He has COPD (Global Initiative for Chronic Obstructive Lung Disease grade 4), and uses daily tiotropium and albuterol as needed. His diabetes mellitus is well controlled with metformin. He has a confirmed allergy to amoxicillin. On physical examination, he is tachypneic (30 breaths/min) and tachycardic (110 beats/min), with a blood pressure of 130/90 mm Hg. He is alert and fully oriented. On auscultation, he has bilateral wheezing and crepitation on the right lung base. His laboratory tests reveal white blood cell count 14,000 cells/μL, C-reactive protein 30 mg/L, blood urea concentration 10 mmol/L, and SpO_2 82%, on inhaled oxygen fraction 0.21. Chest radiography shows consolidation in the right upper and lower lung fields.

Which of the following is the most appropriate antibiotic regimen for this patient?

A. Oral azithromycin
B. Oral ciprofloxacin
C. Intravenous ceftriaxone and azithromycin
D. Intravenous moxifloxacin and azithromycin
E. Intravenous aztreonam and moxifloxacin

33. A 47-year-old woman comes to your clinic with 3 days of fever, shortness of breath, and cough with mucoid sputum. On physical examination, she is alert but slightly confused; her temperature is 40°C, respiratory rate is 34 breaths/min, and blood pressure is 110/50 mm Hg. Examination of the chest shows bibasal crackles; the chest radiograph shows bilateral lower lobe infiltrates. ABGs with the patient breathing room air are PaO_2 46 mm Hg and $PaCO_2$ 28 mm Hg. She is admitted to the hospital, and therapy with ceftriaxone and clarithromycin is started. *Legionella* pneumonia is suspected.
Which of the following is/are clinically useful tests for guiding the treatment of this patient?

A. Urinary antigen test for *Legionella*
B. Sputum culture for *Legionella* on selective medium
C. Acute serum titers for *Legionella* antibodies
D. DNA probe study of bronchoscopically obtained lower respiratory tract secretions

34. A 65-year-old man was hospitalized for an exacerbation of newly diagnosed COPD. He was discharged 4 weeks ago and now presents to your clinic for a regular check-up in late spring. You perform a spirometry test with the following results: FVC, 2.52 L (77% predicted); FEV_1, 1.53 L (54% predicted); and FEV_1/FVC, 61%. He has now recovered and feels well. He has never received any vaccinations since childhood.
Which preventive approach against pneumonia is appropriate at this time?

A. Pneumococcal vaccine
B. Pseudomonas vaccine
C. *H. influenzae* type b vaccine
D. Influenza vaccine
E. None of the above

35. An 83-year-old male patient is referred to you because of a cough that started 6 months ago. He brings up some yellow phlegm and he recently noticed a little blood staining within his phlegm. Furthermore, he felt extremely tired. He had consulted his family physician who had prescribed antibiotics for 10 days which did not change the cough but the color of the phlegm turned white. The chest radiograph revealed an enlarged right hilum.

On further evaluation, the patient complains about painful ankles and wrists, a diminished appetite and a weight loss of 5 kg in the last month. In the last month, he lost a lot of energy, most of the day he is lying in his bed or sitting in a chair. He also needs some help with his personal hygiene. Further investigations revealed a squamous cell carcinoma of his right upper lobe and liver metastases.
Which of the following would be your most appropriate next therapeutic option?

A. Best supportive care
B. Gemcitabine
C. Platinum-containing doublet chemotherapy
D. Erlotinib
E. Bevacizumab

36. A 32-year-old man, known to be HIV-positive for 4 years, is referred to you for evaluation of pulmonary complaints and possible sputum induction. Approximately 2 years ago, the patient developed a chronic, productive cough that has persisted. The sputum color varies, ranging from white to yellow and green. Several courses of antibiotic therapy have cleared the sputum color to white each time, but sputum purulence recurs. He has had intermittent fever but does not have night sweats. He is dyspneic only on extreme exertion. He has not received anti-HIV medication or trimethoprim and sulfamethoxazole. He does not smoke cigarettes. He smoked marijuana in the past but quit 7 months ago. Physical examination reveals a thin, tired-looking man. The remainder of the physical examination is normal. A chest radiograph shows increased markings, primarily in the lung bases, but is unchanged compared with 3, 6, and 9 months ago. The CD4 count is 253 cells/mm^3, and serum LDH is 120 U/L. ABGs while breathing room air are PaO_2 88 mm Hg, $PaCO_2$ 36 mm Hg, and pH 7.44.
What should be recommended?

A. Induced sputum sample to test for *P. jirovecii*
B. CT scan of the chest
C. Sweat chloride test
D. Empiric therapy with trimethoprim and sulfamethoxazole
E. Biopsy of the nasal mucosa

37. A 75-year-old man with COPD has been treated with low-dose oral corticosteroids. He has had multiple acute exacerbations, which were treated with amoxicillin; the most recent one was 3 weeks ago. He now presents with pleuritic chest pain of acute onset, cough with purulent sputum, fever up to 38.5°C, and right lower lobe consolidation on

chest radiography. A sputum sample shows sheets of neutrophils with intra- and extracellular gram-positive *Diplococci*. The patient is admitted to the hospital.

Which of the following is the best initial empiric therapy for this patient?

A. Erythromycin, 250 mg intravenously every 6 hours
B. Ceftriaxone, 2 g intravenously every 24 hours
C. Doxycycline, 100 mg intravenously every 24 hours
D. Penicillin G, 500 mg intravenously every 4 hours
E. Trimethoprim–sulfamethoxazole, 160 mg trimethoprim plus 800 mg sulfamethoxazole, intravenously every 8 hours

38. A 55-year-old healthy, nonsmoking, HIV-negative woman with no known exposure to persons with TB has a TST as part of a routine check-up examination. Induration of 18 mm is noted. Her chest radiograph is normal.

What is the appropriate medication regimen for this person?

A. Isoniazid daily for 12 months
B. Isoniazid and rifampicin daily for 4 months
C. Rifampicin, pyrazinamide, and ethambutol daily for 4 months
D. Pyrazinamide and ciprofloxacin daily for 6 months
E. No antituberculous medications

ANSWERS WITH EXPLANATIONS

1. **Ans. B**

    The new guidelines recommend that patients with confirmed isoniazid-resistant and rifampicin-susceptible TB (abbreviated to Hr-TB) are treated for 6 months with a regimen composed of rifampicin (R), ethambutol (E), pyrazinamide (Z), and levofloxacin (Lfx). The exclusion of rifampicin resistance ahead of start of this regimen is critical. It is further recommended not to add streptomycin (S) or other injectable agents to the treatment regimen. The recommendations apply both to isoniazid resistance detected ahead of start and during TB treatment.

    Ref:
    1. World Health Organization (2018). [online] Available from: https://www.who.int/tb/publications/2018/FAQ_TB_policy_recommendations_guidelines.pdf?ua=1 [Last accessed on February, 2020].

2. **Ans. D**
    - Most patients have CD4 counts <200 cells/µL at the time of diagnosis of their first episode of *P. jirovecii* pneumonia.
    - Most patients with *P. jirovecii* pneumonia will have an elevated serum LDH level.
    - ABGs in patients with *P. jirovecii* pneumonia frequently reveal respiratory alkalosis and a widened alveolar–arterial oxygen tension difference.

    Two studies performed in the 1990s showed that a CD4 count of <200 cells/µL in patients with human immunodeficiency virus (HIV) infection carries an increased risk of *P. jirovecii* pneumonia. In one of these studies, over 95% of *P. jirovecii* pneumonia patients had a CD4 count of <200 cells/µL. Increased serum LDH is present in >90% of patients; a normal LDH has a high negative predictive value. A widened alveolar–arterial oxygen tension difference with hypoxemia is frequently seen in patients with *P. jirovecii* pneumonia. The resulting hyperventilation induces hypocapnia with (compensated) respiratory alkalosis. About 25% of patients with *P. jirovecii* pneumonia present with a normal chest radiograph.

    Ref:
    1. Miller RF, Huang L, Walzer PD. Pneumocystis pneumonia associated with human immunodeficiency virus. Clin Chest Med. 2013;34(2):229-41.
    2. Phair J, Muñoz A, Detels R, Kaslow R, Rinaldo C, Saah A. The risk of Pneumocystis carinii pneumonia among men infected with human immunodeficiency virus type 1. N Engl J Med. 1990;322(3):161-5.
    3. Stansell JD, Osmond DH, Charlebois E, LaVange L, Wallace JM, Alexander BV, et al. Predictors of Pneumocystis carinii pneumonia in HIV-infected persons. Am J Respir Crit Care Med. 1997;155(1):60-6.
    4. Zaman MK, White DA. Serum lactate dehydrogenase levels and Pneumocystis carinii pneumonia. Diagnostic and prognostic significance. Am Rev Respir Dis. 1988;137(4):796-800.

3. **Ans. A**

    After close contact with a person with active TB, as in this case, active TB has to be vigorously sought by microscopic sputum examination and culture, chest radiography, and other clinical examinations as appropriate. The TST has no role in the diagnosis of active TB because it cannot differentiate between latent and active disease; additionally, the TST is often falsely negative in HIV-infected patients due to their impaired immune response. The same holds true for the interferon-γ release assay, although its specificity for *M. tuberculosis* is greater than that of the skin test.

    Ref:
    1. Sester M. Tuberculosis in the immunocompromised host. In: Palange P, Simonds AK (Eds). ERS Handbook of Respiratory Medicine, 2nd edition. Sheffield: European Respiratory Society; 2013. pp. 245-57.

2. Sotgiu G, Migliori GB. Pulmonary tuberculosis. In: Palange P, Simonds AK, (Eds). ERS Handbook of Respiratory Medicine, 2nd edition. Sheffield: European Respiratory Society; 2013. pp. 229-40.
3. World Health Organization. WHO Guidelines on Tuberculosis. [online] Available from: www.who.int/ publications/ guidelines/tuberculosis/en/ [Last accessed on February, 2020].

4. **Ans. D**

The complex symptoms described here fit a diagnosis of PCD, a genetic disorder of cilia structure and function. Cells lining the nasopharynx, the middle ear, the paranasal sinuses, the lower respiratory tract, and the reproductive tract contain cilia and are generally affected in PCD when the disease is fully expressed. PCD leads to chronic infections of the upper and lower respiratory tract, impaired fertility, and disorders of organ laterality.

In contrast to cystic fibrosis, pancreatic function is preserved and hepatobiliary disease is usually absent. The clinical course is milder than in cystic fibrosis, without nutritional problems and diabetes. In ABPA, the localization of bronchiectasis would be central or in the upper lobes. Nasal polyposis and infertility are not associated with ABPA. Idiopathic bronchiectasis is equally not associated with nasal polyps and infertility. Mounier-Kühn's disease refers to tracheobronchomegaly. The disease may be associated with collagen tissue diseases such as Ehlers–Danlos syndrome. Symptoms are chronic unproductive cough, recurrent bronchopneumonia and irritative respiratory symptoms. On CT scan, the trachea would show enlargement.

Ref:
1. Bilton D, Jones AL. Bronchiectasis: epidemiology and causes. In: Floto RA, Haworth CS (Eds). Bronchiectasis (ERS Monograph). Sheffield: European Respiratory Society; 2011. pp. 1-10.
2. Flight WG, Jones AM. Cystic fibrosis, primary ciliary dyskinesia and non-cystic fibrosis bronchiectasis: update 2008-11. Thorax. 2012;67(7):645-9.

5. **Ans. B**

Cystic fibrosis is a genetic disease. It is caused by mutations in the cystic fibrosis transmembrane conductance regulator (CFTR), the most frequent of which is the Phe508del on chromosome 7. Deranged chloride transport leads to thick, viscous secretions in the lungs, pancreas, liver, intestine, and reproductive tract. The symptoms include persistent pulmonary infection and pancreatic insufficiency. A positive sweat chloride test and/or genetic analysis confirms the diagnosis. The viscous mucus also disturbs the embryological development of the vas deferens, which leads to male infertility. As the disease progresses, but not in the early stages of cystic fibrosis, bacteria such as *P. aeruginosa* and *S. aureus*, which are not seen in healthy lungs, colonize the airways of cystic fibrosis patients. *E. coli* has only recently been recognized as a critical pathogen in cystic fibrosis. Recent studies have shown that long-term, lose-dose macrolide therapy can reduce the frequency of exacerbations in cystic fibrosis patients colonized with *P. aeruginosa*.

Ref:
1. Yankaskas JR, Marshall BC, Sufian B, Simon RH, Rodman D. Cystic fibrosis adult care: consensus conference report. Chest. 2004;125(Suppl 1):1S-39S.
2. British Thoracic Society. Cystic fibrosis guideline 2013. [online] Available from: https://www.brit-thoracic.org.uk/clinical-information/cystic-fibrosis/ [Last accessed on February, 2020].

6. **Ans. B**

This patient's symptoms are indicative of a pulmonary exacerbation, which is usually due to *Pseudomonas* infection. Moreover, the patient has a history of pneumothorax, which is prognostically unfavorable. Therefore, the patient will need antipseudomonal antibiotic treatment. More intensive physiotherapy would help, but it would not be the most efficacious measure for the patient. Guidelines state that there is insufficient evidence for the concurrent use of inhaled and systemic antibiotic treatment, so the patient will need IV treatment for the exacerbation. Inhaled treatment may be used in the long term in patients with chronic *Pseudomonas* infection.

Ref:
1. lume PA, Mogayzel PJ Jr, Robinson KA, Goss CH, Rosenblatt RL, Kuhn RJ, et al. Cystic fibrosis pulmonary guidelines: treatment of pulmonary exacerbations. Am J Respir Crit Care Med. 2009;180(9):802-8.

7. **Ans. C**

Pneumonia is a condition caused by microbial infection within the lung parenchyma. Pneumonia is classified according to the origin as community-acquired pneumonia (CAP) or hospital-acquired pneumonia (HAP; nosocomial pneumonia). According to the definition, CAP occurs in the absence of immune compromise or prior hospital admission within the previous 7 days. The decision regarding the most appropriate site of care, including whether hospitalization of a patient with CAP is warranted, is the first and single most important decision in the overall management of CAP. This decision is best performed by an accurate assessment of the severity of illness at presentation and the likely prognosis. Clinical assessment of disease severity is dependent on the experience of the attending clinician, but such clinical judgment has been shown to result in apparent underestimation of severity. Therefore, various severity scoring systems and predictive models have been developed in an attempt to help the clinician identify patients with pneumonia and a poor prognosis at an early stage. The six-point CURB-65 score, one point for each of confusion, urea >7 mmol/L, respiratory rate >30 breaths/min, low systolic (<90 mm Hg) or diastolic (≤60 mm Hg) blood pressure, and age >65 years, is based on information available at initial hospital assessment and enables patients to be stratified according to increasing risk of mortality (score 0: 0.7%; score 1: 2.1%; score 2: 9.2%; and scores 3–5: 15–40%). Patients who have a CURB-65 score of 3 or more (as the patient in this question, with a CURB-65 score of 3) are at high risk of death. These patients require urgent hospital admission. Patients with CURB-65 scores of 4 and 5 should be assessed with specific consideration to the need for transfer to a critical care unit (high dependency unit or intensive care unit). Microbiological tests (blood and sputum cultures) are recommended in patients with moderate and high severity CAP admitted to the hospital. All patients should receive antibiotics as soon as the diagnosis of CAP is confirmed. The objective for any service should be to confirm a diagnosis of pneumonia with chest radiography and initiate empirical antibiotic therapy within 4 hours of presentation to the hospital.

Ref:
1. Lim WS, Baudouin SV, George RC, Hill AT, Jamieson C, Le Jeune I, et al. BTS guidelines for the management of community acquired pneumonia in adults: update 2009. Thorax. 2009;64 (Suppl 3):iii1-iii55.
2. Mandell LA, Wunderink RG, Anzueto A, Bartlett JG, Campbell GD, Dean NC, et al. Infectious Diseases Society of America/American Thoracic Society consensus guidelines on the management of community-acquired pneumonia in adults. Clin Infect Dis. 2007;44 (Suppl 2): S27-72.
3. Woodhead M, Rohde G. Pneumonia. In: Palange P, Simonds AK (Eds). ERS Handbook of Respiratory Medicine, 2nd edition. Sheffield: European Respiratory Society; 2013. pp. 199-202.

8. **Ans. A**

The patient has been exposed to a hospice environment and therefore this is healthcare-related pneumonia. Her pneumonia involves one lobe only, the patient is not severely ill and has no increased risk; so, according to the guidelines, she can be treated with aminopenicillin plus β-lactamase inhibitor, a second-generation cephalosporin or a respiratory quinolone. This patient has had treatment with a quinolone <3 months ago and she should not be treated with moxifloxacin. She has been exposed to influenza but that was >2 weeks ago and, therefore, this is too long for her to develop influenza. Aciclovir is used for the treatment of herpes infections and therefore is not indicated here. Piperacillin–tazobactam and ciprofloxacin are indicated for healthcare-related pneumonia but when risk factors for multidrug resistance (MDR) are suspected or after a long hospitalization. Amoxicillin–clavulanate and macrolide are appropriate as this treatment covers streptococcal infection which is still very probable.

Ref:
1. Blasi F, Gramegna A, Di Pasquale M. Hospital-acquired pneumonia. In: Palange P, Simonds AK, (Eds). ERS Handbook of Respiratory Medicine, 2nd edition. Sheffield: European Respiratory Society; 2013. pp. 203-6.
2. Torres A, Ewig S, Lode H, Carlet J; European HAP working group. Defining, treating and preventing hospital acquired pneumonia: European perspective. Intensive Care Med. 2009;35(1):9-29.
3. Woodhead M, Blasi F, Ewig S, Garau J, Huchon G, Ieven M, et al. Guidelines for the management of adult lower respiratory tract infections—summary. Clin Microbiol Infect. 2011;17 (Suppl 6):1-24.

9. **Ans. B**

All the above tests are used for diagnosis of *Legionella* species.

The sensitivity pattern of the tests is as follows:
- *Culture*: 20–80%
- *Urinary antigen*: 70–100%
- *Serology*: 80–90%
- *Direct fluorescence assay*: 25–75%

Ref:
1. Sharma L, Losier A, Tolbert T, Dela Cruz CS, Marion CR. Atypical pneumonia: updates on Legionella, Chlamydophila, and Mycoplasma Pneumonia. Clin Chest Med. 2017;38(1):45-58.

10. **Ans. B**

Contaminated water or soil are responsible for majority of the infections caused by *Legionella*. Using compost manure in garden, rainfall, and high humidity are the risk factors for *Legionella* infection.

Ref:
1. Sharma L, Losier A, Tolbert T, Dela Cruz CS, Marion CR. Atypical pneumonia: updates on Legionella, Chlamydophila, and Mycoplasma Pneumonia. Clin Chest Med. 2017;38(1):45-58.

11. **Ans. B**

Risk factors for NTM infections include chronic lung diseases, such as bronchiectasis and chronic obstructive pulmonary disease (COPD), and various forms of immunodeficiency. When NTM are inhaled by susceptible individuals, infection can lead to a chronic progressive and sometimes fatal lung disease. α_1-antitrypsin deficiency is classically associated with predominantly lower lobe emphysema. Bronchiectasis has also been associated with the enzyme deficiency. Whether this is a direct consequence of the deficiency or secondary to the emphysema-associated airway obstruction is not clear. In a study of patients with severe AAT-deficiency, the vast majority of subjects had some evidence of bronchiectasis on a high-resolution CT scan (70 out of 74 subjects). However, AAT augmentation therapy is not indicated in the described patient. Although it has been demonstrated to slow the progression of emphysema in CT studies, AAT augmentation has no role in the therapy of bronchiectasis.

Immunodeficiencies may predispose to bronchiectasis. The immune defects most strongly associated with bronchiectasis are those resulting in hypogammaglobulinemia. These include the primary immunodeficiencies, common variable immunodeficiency and X-linked agammaglobulinemia and the secondary immunodeficiencies caused by lymphoproliferative malignancy, allogeneic bone marrow transplantation, and chemoimmunotherapy. Conditions resulting in T-cell dysfunction, e.g., HIV infection or immunosuppression, reduced bacterial opsonization, complement deficiencies, failure of phagocyte migration (leukocyte adhesion deficiency), and impaired intracellular killing of bacteria (chronic granulomatous disease) may also predispose to bronchiectasis.

Sputum microbiology is a key investigation tool in the diagnosis of patients with bronchiectasis. *Haemophilus influenzae* is the most frequently isolated pathogen and found in up to 35% of patients. *Staphylococcus aureus*, *Streptococcus pneumoniae*, *Moraxella catarrhalis*, and *Pseudomonas aeruginosa* are also commonly identified. *Aspergillus spp.* may also be found and may be associated with ABPA. The presence of *P. aeruginosa* in sputum from patients with bronchiectasis is associated with more severe lung disease and may also indicate a worse prognosis.

Ref:
1. Bilton D, Jones AL. Bronchiectasis: epidemiology and causes. Eur Respir Monogr. 2011;52:1-10.
2. Daley C. Nontuberculous mycobacterial infections. Eur Respir Monogr. 2011;52:115-29.
3. Pasteur MC, Bilton D, Hill AT; British Thoracic Society Bronchiectasis non-CF Guideline Group. British Thoracic Society guideline for non-CF bronchiectasis. Thorax. 2010;65(Suppl 1):i1-58.

12. **Ans. B**

The patient's history and chest radiography suggest that she has bronchiectasis, probably due to recurrent bacterial bronchial infections during childhood. Furthermore, she had latent TB in the past, as evidenced by her positive TST 20 years ago. She also has a thin-walled cavity in her right upper lobe, a sputum smear showing acid-fast bacilli, and a recent history of coughing with sputum production and considerable weight loss. These findings are suggestive of TB.

A differential diagnostic consideration should be a nontuberculous mycobacterial infection. In light of this, additional sputum cultures should be collected (in total, at least three sputum samples should be collected, one of which is a morning sample) and then treatment against TB should be initiated. This treatment should be adjusted if the results of the definitive sputum cultures and resistance patterns warrant this.

A rapid diagnostic test for resistance patterns might be performed if available, particularly in a setting with a high likelihood of resistance. This is not the case for this patient.

If TB is suspected, therapy with isoniazid, rifampicin, pyrazinamide, and ethambutol should be initiated. Furthermore, at least two additional sputum samples should be collected. In the case of possible active TB, one should not wait until the results of the definitive cultures are available, as this may take several weeks. A transbronchial biopsy is not necessary to diagnose an active TB or NTM infection in this case.

Ref:
1. Griffith DE, Aksamit T, Brown-Elliott BA, Catanzaro A, Daley C, Gordin F, et al. An official ATS/IDSA statement: diagnosis, treatment, and prevention of non-tuberculous mycobacterial diseases. Am J Respir Crit Care Med. 2007;175(4):367-416.
2. National Institute for Health and Care Excellence (2011). Tuberculosis: clinical diagnosis and management of tuberculosis, and measures for its prevention and control. [online] Available from: www.nice.org.uk/guidance/cg117 [Last accessed on February, 2020].

13. **Ans. B**

Infection of the pleural space accompanying pneumonia leads to the invasion of inflammatory cells (neutrophils) associated with acidosis, low glucose levels, and high LDH levels. Parapneumonic effusions that require tube drainage are termed complicated parapneumonic effusions. The most accurate predictor of the need for chest tube drainage is a pH <7.2. A low glucose (<3.4 mmol/L) and high LDH level (>1,000 U/L) do not improve diagnostic accuracy but may be used to assess the need for chest tube drainage, if the pH cannot be measured. The glucose concentration is usually <3.4 mmol/L if the pH is <7.2. Identification of microorganisms in the Gram stain indicates empyema requiring tube drainage. A serosanguineous appearance, a negative Gram stain, normal glucose, and an only slightly elevated LDH are nonspecific and not helpful in assessing the need for tube drainage.

Ref:
1. Davies HE, Davies RJ, Davies CW; BTS Pleural Disease Guideline Group. Management of pleural infection in adults: British Thoracic Society pleural disease guideline 2010. Thorax. 2010;65 (Suppl 2):ii41-53.
2. Clive A, Falconer W, Hooper C, Maskell N. Pleural infection and lung abscess. In: Palange P, Simonds AK (Eds). ERS Handbook of Respiratory Medicine, 2nd edition. Sheffield: European Respiratory Society; 2013. pp. 215-21.

14. Ans. D

The high eosinophil count in the BAL fluid suggests the presence of a form of eosinophilic lung disease. Acute eosinophilic pneumonia (AEP) is usually accompanied by dyspnea, fever, and hypoxia and develops within <1 week. It responds well to corticosteroids. The described case is consistent with this diagnosis and lung biopsy is not required. Chronic eosinophilic pneumonia is subacute with progressive symptoms of breathlessness, night sweats, weight loss, cough, fever, and wheezing. The etiology of AEP is unknown. It has been shown that in the initial phase of AEP, blood eosinophilia is not present, in contrast to marked eosinophilia (>25%) in the BAL fluid. Several drugs, including antibiotics, and chemical and physical agents may induce AEP. A few studies have suggested a relationship between smoking and AEP, particularly new-onset smoking. Other reasons for pulmonary eosinophilia include helminth infections, coccidioidal infections, drugs (e.g., inhaled cocaine), several toxins (particulate metals, aluminum silicate, solvents, etc.), medication (nonsteroidal anti-inflammatory drugs, ampicillin, sulfonamides, etc.), eosinophilic granulomatosis with polyangiitis, ABPA, and hypereosinophilic syndrome.

Ref:
1. Badesch DB, King TE Jr, Schwarz MI. Acute eosinophilic pneumonia: a hypersensitivity phenomenon? Am Rev Respir Dis. 1989;139(1):249-52.
2. Menzies-Gow A, McBrien C. Eosinophilic disease. In: Palange P, Simonds AK (Eds). ERS Handbook of Respiratory Medicine, 2nd edition. Sheffield: European Respiratory Society; 2013. pp. 395-8.
3. Philit F, Etienne-Mastroïanni B, Parrot A, Guérin C, Robert D, Cordier JF. Idiopathic acute eosinophilic pneumonia: a study of 22 patients. Am J Respir Crit Care Med. 2002;166(9):1235-9.
4. Solomon J, Schwarz M. Drug, toxin, and radiation therapy-induced eosinophilic pneumonia. Semin Respir Crit Care Med. 2006;27(2):192-7.

15. Ans. B

The clinical and radiological pattern is highly suggestive of pleurisy, which in an HIV-positive patient, is likely to be tuberculous, depending also on the local epidemiology of TB and on the TB prevention measures that are in place. With a 2-week history, bacterial pneumonia is less likely. The TST is frequently negative in active TB in HIV-infected patients, including in pleural TB. However, a positive TST does not contribute to the differential diagnosis as it will only confirm TB infection, which is frequently latent. The same considerations are relevant for the interferon-γ release assay. Although chest CT and bronchoscopy might bring some useful information (including lung lesions not visible on chest radiography and bacteriological confirmation of *M. tuberculosis*, respectively), thoracentesis is the first investigation to be recommended. Pleural fluid analysis may suggest a parapneumonic effusion by a predominance of neutrophils, low pH, and/or isolation of bacteria. Conversely, it may show a lymphocytic-predominant effusion and cultural growth of mycobacteria, which would prove TB.

Ref:
1. Light RW. The undiagnosed pleural effusion. Clin Chest Med. 2006;27(2):309-19.

16. Ans. B

Mycoplasma pneumoniae can present with cough and chest pain, and be accompanied by wheezing. Nonrespiratory symptoms, such as arthralgia and headache, might also suggest *Mycoplasma* infection. The complement fixation test (CFT) is still regarded as the gold standard for diagnosis of *M. pneumoniae* pneumonia. Elevated CFT titers are detected no earlier than 10–14 days after the onset of *Mycoplasma* infection. Titration of antibodies in acute- and convalescent-phase serum specimens is usually performed. A fourfold increase in titer can confirm the diagnosis. If cold agglutinins are present in a patient with CAP, the higher the cold agglutinin titer (>1:64), the more likely the cold agglutinins are due to *M. pneumoniae*. *M. pneumoniae* infections may also be diagnosed by cultivation of the organism on complex agar medium. Because of the slow growth of the organism, partly reflecting fastidious nutrient requirements, culture techniques are expensive and slow.

Ref:
1. Lim WS, Baudouin SV, George RC, Hill AT, Jamieson C, Le Jeune I, et al. BTS guidelines for the management of community acquired pneumonia in adults: update 2009. Thorax. 2009;64 (Suppl 3):iii1-55.
2. Harris M, Clark J, Coote N, Fletcher P, Harnden A, McKean M, et al. British Thoracic Society guidelines for the management of community acquired pneumonia in children: update 2011. Thorax. 2011;66(Suppl 2):ii1-23.

17. Ans. A

Peripheral blood eosinophils >10% are a hallmark of eosinophilic granulomatosis with polyangiitis. This multisystem disorder is characterized by asthma, blood eosinophilia, sinusitis and, in some cases, mononeuritis multiplex, pericarditis, and cardiac arrhythmia.

Skin prick test for *Aspergillus spp.* would help in the diagnosis of allergic pulmonary aspergillosis, another disease associated with asthma. Antibasement membrane antibodies are elevated in Goodpasture syndrome, which is associated with renal glomerular disease and pulmonary alveolar hemorrhage. Antisynthetase antibodies (Jo-1; antiaminoacyl transfer RNA antibodies) are elevated in idiopathic anti-inflammatory diseases with arthritis, myopathy, and Raynaud's syndrome, which can be associated with interstitial lung disease. Cardiac troponin T is expected to be elevated in this patient with probable perimyocarditis, as suggested by an elevated CK-MB; however, elevated troponin would not help to secure the diagnosis, as the suspected cardiac involvement is just one manifestation of the vasculitic disease.

Ref:
1. Frankel SK, Schwarz MI. The pulmonary vasculitides. Am J Respir Crit Care Med. 2012;186(3):216-24.
2. Mouthon L, Dunogue B, Guillevin L. Diagnosis and classification of eosinophilic granulomatosis with polyangiitis (formerly named Churg-Strauss syndrome). J Autoimmun. 2014;48-49:99-103.

18. Ans. B

This patient presents with active TB after default interruption of treatment. Previous treatment is a strong determinant of drug resistance and MDR. A global survey has revealed that 15% of previously treated patients had MDR, compared with 3% of new cases. Therefore, particular precautions should be taken to avoid inappropriate treatment and thereby promote and spread MDR. Prompt MDR identification enables the physician to specifically select an appropriate combination of drugs. This enhances the chance of cure and contributes to the prevention of spread of resistant strains. Using rapid molecular-based tests, MDR can be confirmed or excluded within 1-2 days. Such tests are available in many European countries (as in the described case) and the results should be used to guide treatment.

If rapid drug susceptibility tests are not available, empirical treatment should be started based on the likelihood of MDR-TB. This likelihood is considered high in patients with treatment failure, who should receive empirical treatment for MDR-TB. Conversely, in patients returning with a relapse or after defaulting, the likelihood of MDR is lower (in countries with a low MDR prevalence) and a retreatment regimen containing first-line drugs is acceptable, i.e., 2HRZES/1HRZE/5HRE is the recommended empirical retreatment in this setting. If the results of susceptibility testing become available, treatment should be adapted accordingly. A treatment failure, a second or subsequent relapse or default of a previous treatment, a high local rate of MDR, and coexistent HIV infection are important criteria for selection of the retreatment regimen.

Ref:
1. Sotgiu G, Migliori GB. Pulmonary tuberculosis. In: Palange P, Simonds AK (Eds). ERS Handbook of Respiratory Medicine, 2nd edition. Sheffield: European Respiratory Society; 2013. pp. 229-40.
2. World Health Organization. Treatment of Tuberculosis: Guidelines for National Programmes, 4th edition. Geneva: World Health Organization; 2010.

19. Ans. D

From the patient's history, pneumonia is likely but the radiology does not suggest pneumococcal or other bacterial etiology, although blood cultures have been performed to evaluate this possibility as recommended in severe pneumonia. Atypical infection is, therefore, probable but the degree of anemia is unusual. The associated jaundice indicates that she may be hemolyzing. In the context of atypical pneumonia, this suggests *M. pneumoniae* pneumonia with hemolytic anemia due to cold agglutinins. Severe hemolysis in *M. pneumoniae* pneumonia is uncommon but well recognized. It can usually be controlled by keeping the patient warm. Serology would confirm the diagnosis, and tests for cold agglutinins and Coombs test would be positive. Hemolytic anemia does not fit the typical presentation of legionnaires' disease or Chlamydia infection. The association of pulmonary infiltrates and anemia suggest pulmonary hemorrhage due to vasculitic disease or Goodpasture's disease, but the absence of hemoptysis or significant proteinuria or renal failure does not support these possibilities.

Ref:
1. Cunha BA. The atypical pneumonias: clinical diagnosis and importance. Clin Microbiol Infect. 2006;12(Suppl. 3):12-24.
2. Lim WS, Baudouin SV, George RC, Hill AT, Jamieson C, Le Jeune I, et al. BTS guidelines for the management of community acquired pneumonia in adults: update 2009. Thorax. 2009;64(Suppl. 3):iii1-55.

20. Ans. E

The history and the CT are consistent with bronchiectasis. Surgery is not an option because conservative treatment options have to be optimized first. As the spirometry result is normal, bronchodilators are not indicated. In patients with airflow obstruction, reversibility to β-adrenergic and anticholinergic bronchodilators should be tested, and therapy initiated if lung function or symptoms improve on therapy. Bronchoscopy might be useful if there is hemoptysis to localize the source of bleeding, but this examination is not currently necessary in this patient. Three recently published randomized, double-blind, placebo-controlled studies showed that low-dose macrolides (azithromycin or erythromycin) taken for 6-12 months led to significant reductions in exacerbation rate and reduced the decline in lung function. In all studies, macrolides were generally well tolerated. The advantages of macrolide maintenance therapy need to be balanced against the risks, which include emergence of bacterial resistance, cardiotoxicity, and ototoxicity. Long-term quinolones should not be used until further studies are available. Apart from infection, bronchiectasis may be due to several specific causes, such as cystic fibrosis, antibody deficiency syndromes, and immotile cilia. Therefore, these diagnoses should be evaluated by performing a sweat test and measuring Ig levels. Furthermore, sputum samples should be investigated for particular microorganisms including mycobacteria and resistant bacteria.

Ref:
1. Haworth CS, Bilton D, Elborn JS. Long-term macrolide maintenance therapy in non-CF bronchiectasis: evidence and questions. Respir Med. 2014;108:1397-408.
2. Pasteur MC, Bilton D, Hill AT; British Thoracic Society Bronchiectasis non-CF Guideline Group. British Thoracic Society guideline for non-CF bronchiectasis. Thorax. 2010;65:(Suppl 1):i1-58.
3. Chalmers JD. Bronchiectasis. Palange P, Rohde G (Eds). ERS Handbook of Respiratory Medicine. Sheffield: European Respiratory Society; 2019.

21. Ans. A

Tuberculosis is an infectious disease caused by *M. tuberculosis*. World Health Organization (WHO) estimates that 9.27 million new cases of TB occurred in 2007 and of them 44% were infectious (new pulmonary sputum smear-positive cases). Sputum smear microscopy is still the most widely used technique for the diagnosis of pulmonary TB. Drug susceptibility testing using molecular techniques can enhance TB diagnosis and help physicians to choose the appropriate treatment. Due to their higher bacillary burden, individuals with active, smear-positive TB are the main source of TB transmission in the community. The highest priority in TB control programs is the rapid identification of these cases and effective treatment. The WHO and Centers for Disease Control and Prevention (CDC) recommends that for patients in whom TB is proved or strongly suspected, treatment should be initiated with isoniazid, rifampicin, pyrazinamide, and ethambutol for the initial 2 months. A repeat smear and culture should be performed after 2 months of treatment have been completed. If cavities were seen on the initial chest radiograph or the acid-fast smear is negative at completion of 2 months of treatment, the continuation phase of treatment should consist of isoniazid and rifampicin daily or twice weekly for 4 months to complete a total of 6 months of treatment. If cavitation was present on the initial chest radiograph and the culture at the time of completion of 2 months of therapy is positive, the continuation phase should be lengthened to 7 months (total of 9 months of treatment). Although clinical trials have shown that the efficacy of streptomycin is approximately equal to that of ethambutol in the initial phase of treatment, the increasing frequency of resistance to streptomycin globally has made the drug less useful. Thus, streptomycin is not recommended as being interchangeable with ethambutol.

Ref:
1. Blumberg HM, Burman WJ, Chaisson RE, Daley CL, Etkind SC, Friedman LN, et al. American Thoracic Society/Centers for Disease Control and Prevention/Infectious Diseases Society of America: treatment of tuberculosis. Am J Respir Crit Care Med. 2003;167:603-62.
2. Sotgiu G, Migliori GB. Pulmonary tuberculosis. In: Palange P, Simonds AK (Eds). ERS Handbook of Respiratory Medicine, 2nd edition. Sheffield: European Respiratory Society; 2013. pp. 229-40.

22. Ans. D

The British Thoracic Society guideline on TB recommends a 6-month, four-drug initial regimen (6 months of isoniazid and rifampicin, supplemented in the first 2 months with pyrazinamide and ethambutol) to treat active respiratory TB in adults not known to be HIV positive, adults who are HIV positive, and children. The reason for using four drugs in the initial phase is that, in most cases, the resistance pattern will not be known.

The addition of pyrazinamide in the initial phase (2 months) results in quicker sputum conversion and allows the reduction of the total treatment period from 9 to 6 months. The recommended regimen for renal TB is the same as for pulmonary TB.

Ref:
1. National Institute for Health and Care Excellence (2011). Tuberculosis: clinical diagnosis and management of tuberculosis, and measures for its prevention and control. [online] Available from: www.nice.org.uk/guidance/cg117 [Last accessed on February, 2020].

23. Ans. B

This patient's history and the simultaneous diagnosis of meningitis in his child point to an infectious disease. Bilateral chest pain aggravated by breathing movements is typical of epidemic pleurodynia (also known as Bornholm disease or epidemic myalgia), which is often caused by Coxsackievirus B infection. The pain is usually caused by involvement of the intercostal muscles. The disease can be accompanied by headache, pleuritis, meningitis, and myocarditis. Analgesics, narcotics, and heating pads are the mainstays of therapy. Patients generally recover completely within 1 week.

Ref:
1. Hind M. Chest pain. In: Palange P, Simonds AK (Eds). ERS Handbook of Respiratory Medicine, 2nd edition. Sheffield: European Respiratory Society; 2013. pp. 59-60.
2. Ikeda RM, Kondracki SF, Drabkin PD, Birkhead GS, Morse DL. Pleurodynia among football players at a high school. An outbreak associated with coxsackievirus B1. JAMA. 1993;270(18): 2205-6.

24. Ans. D

Pneumonia due to *S. pneumoniae*, *H. influenzae*, or *E. coli* is due to microaspiration from the oropharynx; thus, these bacteria may colonize the upper airways. *B. fragilis* is an anaerobic bacterium that can be found in the upper airways and can result in lung infection in cases of macroscopic aspiration. *Legionella* infection usually occurs through inhalation of contaminated aerosols produced by water systems such as cooling towers, showers, hot water distribution systems, and taps. Consequently, *Legionella* is the least likely to colonize the upper airways.

Ref:
1. Carratalà J, Garcia-Vidal C. An update on Legionella. Curr Op Infect Dis. 2010;23(2):152-7.

25. Ans. B

The diagnosis of ARDS is based on chest radiography (i.e., bilateral infiltrates not fully explained by effusions, lobar/lung collapse, or nodules), ABG findings (i.e., PaO_2/FiO_2 ratio ≤300 mm Hg) and the presence of respiratory failure not fully explained by cardiac failure or fluid overload, verified by objective assessment (echocardiography and brain natriuretic peptide). In the present case, arterial hypoxemia is only partially corrected by oxygen administration (PaO_2/FiO_2 100 mm Hg). It has been demonstrated that the degree of intrapulmonary shunting increases with increasing FiO_2; the clinician should be aware of this when assessing the severity of respiratory failure by using the PaO_2/FiO_2 ratio. A recent trial has shown that early application of prone-position ventilation in patients with severe ARDS decreases 28- and 90-day mortality.

The alveolar–arterial oxygen tension difference is not corrected by oxygen administration. In addition to increasing intrapulmonary shunting, oxygen administration does not correct underlying pathophysiological changes that occur due to capillary endothelial damage and alveolar epithelial damage, i.e., interstitial edema due to increased protein influx into the interstitial space and consecutive increase in oncotic pressure, and filling of the alveoli with edema fluid and cellular debris. Additional loss of surfactant leads to alveolar collapse.

Ref:
1. Guérin C, Reignier J, Richard JC, Beuret P, Gacouin A, Boulain T, et al. Prone positioning in severe acute respiratory distress syndrome. N Engl J Med. 2013;368(23):2159-68.
2. Karbing DS, Kjaergaard S, Smith BW, Espersen K, Allerød C, Andreassen S, et al. Variation in the PaO_2/FiO_2 ratio with FiO_2: mathematical and experimental description, and clinical relevance. Crit Care. 2007;11(6):R118.
3. Schönhofer B, Karagiannidis C. Lung injury. In: Palange P, Simonds AK (Eds). ERS Handbook of Respiratory Medicine, 2nd edition. Sheffield: European Respiratory Society; 2013. pp. 159-61.
4. Taccone P, Pesenti A, Latini R, Polli F, Vagginelli F, Mietto C, et al. Prone positioning in patients with moderate and severe acute respiratory distress syndrome. A randomized controlled trial. JAMA. 2009;302(18):1977-84.
5. West JB. Pulmonary Physiology and pathophysiology: an integrated, case-based approach, 2nd edition. Philadelphia: Lippincott Williams Wilkins and Wolters Kluwer; 2007.

26. Ans. A

Anti-TB drugs have the major actions listed above. The initial standard regimen includes the four drugs isoniazid, rifampicin, pyrazinamide, and ethambutol for 2 months followed by isoniazid and rifampicin for an additional 4 months, if *Mycobateriae* are sensitive to these drugs. Streptomycin is not included in the standard regimen because it has more undesirable effects, such as renal toxicity and ototoxicity, has a higher resistance rate than ethambutol, and is injectable and therefore difficult to administer. If the bactericidal drug pyrazinamide cannot be used, the treatment has to be given for 9 months instead of the standard 6 months. The CDC states that cavitation and positive culture after 2 months of treatment justify a prolongation of the continuation phase to 9 months, since the relapse rate in patients with these risk factors is 10 times as high as that in patients without cavitation or positive culture after 2 months (21% vs. 2%).

Ref:
1. World Health Organization (2010). Treatment of Tuberculosis: Guidelines for National Programmes, 4th edition. WHO/HTM/TB/2009.420. [online] Available from: http://whqlibdoc.who.int/publications/2010/9789241547833_eng.pdf [Last accessed on February, 2020].
2. Yew WW, Lange C, Leung CC. Treatment of tuberculosis: update 2010. Eur Respir J. 2011;37(2):441-62.
3. Blumberg HM, Burman WJ, Chaisson RE, Daley CL, Etkind SC, Friedman LN, Fujiwara P, Grzemska M, Hopewell PC, Iseman MD, Jasmer RM, Koppaka V, Menzies RI, O'Brien RJ, Reves RR, Reichman LB, Simone PM, Starke JR, Vernon AA. American Thoracic Society/Centers for Disease Control and Prevention/Infectious Diseases Society of America. Treatment of tuberculosis. Am J Respir Crit Care Med. 2003;52:1-77.

27. Ans. B

The most common cause for the CAP of this patient is *S. pneumoniae*. Due to high antibiotic resistance for erythromycin, and possibly cotrimoxazole in this case, these are not preferable options for empirical antibiotic treatment. Regimens including antipseudomonal β-lactams (such as ceftazidime) and aminoglycosides (such as amikacin) are indicated in cases with increased risk for *Pseudomonas* infections. However, this is not the case for the vignette case with moderate airflow obstruction and no history of antibiotic use in the past year. The preferred treatment option is a nonantipseudomonal β-lactam (such as ceftriaxone) plus a newer macrolide (such as azithromycin) or a respiratory fluoroquinolone (such as moxifloxacin or levofloxacin), but not ciprofloxacin.

Ref:
1. Woodhead M, Blasi F, Ewig S, Garau J, Huchon G, Ieven M, et al. Guidelines for the management of adult lower respiratory tract infections–full version. Clin Microbiol Infect. 2011;17(Suppl 6):E1-59.

28. Ans. A

This patient has suspected CAP, defined by acute illness with cough meeting at least one of the following criteria: new focal chest signs, fever for >4 days or dyspnea/tachypnea, and no other obvious cause. A definitive diagnosis of pneumonia would be supported by a chest radiograph showing consolidation. CAP is a common and potentially very serious disease, especially in the elderly and in the presence of comorbidities. This 75-year-old patient with COPD has an increased respiratory rate (>30 breaths/min) and is slightly confused. Although his blood pressure is not <90 mm Hg systolic or <60 mm Hg diastolic, several factors associated with an increased risk of mortality are present and he should thus be hospitalized. The CRB-65 score (confusion, respiratory rate >30 breaths/min, blood pressure <90 mm Hg systolic or <60 mm Hg diastolic, and age >65 years) is 3. A score ≥1 (other than age >65 years alone) should prompt hospitalization.

Ref:
1. Bauer TT, Ewig S, Marre R, Suttorp N, Welte T; CAPNETZ Study Group. CRB-65 predicts death from community-acquired pneumonia. J Intern Med. 2006;260:93-101.
2. Lim WS, van der Eerden MM, Laing R, Boersma WG, Karalus N, Town GI, et al. Defining community acquired pneumonia severity on presentation to hospital: an international derivation and validation study. Thorax. 2003;58(5):377-82.

29. Ans. A

Diagnosis of Mycoplasma pneumoniae

Diagnostic test	Sample type	Advantages/Disadvantages of test
Culture	Sputum	*Advantage:* If positive, 100% specific and considered the gold standard *Disadvantage:* Long growth period that provides limited clinical utility
Serology	Serum	*Advantage:* Test has ability to quantify expression amount *Disadvantages:* • Poor sensitivity and specificity • Requires paired sera (acute and convalescent phases) leading to retrospective results High false-positive rate likely due to carrier state
Molecular	Sputum, nasopharyngeal aspirate (NPA), nasopharyngeal swab (NPS), and oropharyngeal swab (OPS)	*Advantages:* Readily available with fast results; high specificity *Disadvantages:* • Expensive commercial kits • Improved standardization among kits required to determine optimal sample specimen

Ref:
1. Sharma L, Losier A, Tolbert T, Dela Cruz CS, Marion CR. Atypical pneumonia: updates on Legionella, Chlamydophila, and Mycoplasma Pneumonia. Clin Chest Med. 2017;38(1):45-58.

30. Ans. D

The extrapulmonary manifestations of *M. pneumoniae* are as follows:
- *Dermatologic*:
  - Erythema nodosum
  - Cutaneous leukocytoclastic vasculitis
  - Stevens–Johnson syndrome
- *Cardiovascular*:
  - Cardiac thrombi
  - Kawasaki's disease
- *Central nervous system*:
  - Encephalitis
  - Aseptic meningitis
- *Gastrointestinal*: Acute hepatitis

Ref:
1. Sharma L, Losier A, Tolbert T, Dela Cruz CS, Marion CR. Atypical pneumonia: updates on Legionella, Chlamydophila, and Mycoplasma Pneumonia. Clin Chest Med. 2017;38(1):45-58.

31. Ans. B

A complicated parapneumonic effusion must be considered in the context of persistent fever in patients with pneumonia. Since the infection may persist in the pleural space, C-reactive protein or procalcitonin are poor measures of disease severity and requirement for further measures. Therefore, a diagnostic thoracentesis should be performed. A pleural fluid pH < 7.2 indicates a complicated parapneumonic effusion. Spontaneous resolution is highly unlikely. Thus, intensified treatment is necessary. Although they are often negative, blood cultures and cultures from the pleural effusion should be taken. Therapy includes IV antibiotics and chest tube drainage guided by ultrasound. Small-bore (12–14 f) chest tubes are not inferior to large-bore tubes. If antibiotics and chest tube drainage do not lead to a clear improvement, thoracic surgery should be considered. A pH >7.4 indicates a simple parapneumonic effusion with a good prognosis.

Chest tube drainage is not necessary in this case.

Ref:
1. Clive A, Falconer W, Hooper C, Maskell N. Pleural infection and lung abscess. In: Palange P, Simonds AK (Eds). ERS Handbook of Respiratory Medicine. 2nd edition. Sheffield: European Respiratory Society; 2013. pp. 215-21.
2. Wrightson JM, Davies RJ. The approach to the patient with a parapneumonic effusion. Semin Respir Crit Care Med. 2010;31(6):706-15.

32. Ans. E

The patient has severe CAP (CURB-65 score 3) (**Table 1**) involving at least two lobes. Therefore, and because of his comorbidities (COPD and diabetes) and severe hypoxemia, he needs to be treated in the hospital, ideally in a high-dependency or intensive care unit. The risk of pseudomonal infection should be assessed to guide empirical antibiotic therapy. *P. aeruginosa* infection in COPD patients should be considered in the presence of at least two of the following: (1) Recent hospitalization, (2) frequent exacerbations (more than four courses of antibiotics per year), (3) severe COPD (FEV_1 <30% predicted), and (4) oral steroid use (>10 mg prednisolone daily in the past 2 weeks). Thus, there is no evidence of *P. aeruginosa* infection in this patient.

Table 1: The CURB-65 and CRB-65 indices.

	Sign/finding	CURB-65	CRB-65
C	Mental confusion	•	•
U	Blood urea concentration > 7 mmol/L	•	
R	Respiratory rate ≥30 breaths/min	•	•
B	Systolic blood pressure <90 mm Hg or diastolic blood pressure ≤60 mm Hg	•	•
65	Age ≥ 65 years	•	•

The preferred regimen in this setting would be a non-antipseudomonal third-generation cephalosporin and a respiratory fluoroquinolone (moxifloxacin or levofloxacin) or a macrolide (a new macrolide, such as azithromycin, would be preferred over erythromycin). However, the patient is allergic to penicillin. Therefore, the usual cephalosporin has to be substituted with aztreonam, a monobactam, which has been shown to be safe to use in patients with penicillin allergy. Oral antibiotics are not an option in severely ill patients. Several scores have been developed to assess severity of pneumonia and associated mortality. Two well-validated and simple scores are the CURB-65 and its derivative that does not require a laboratory study, the CRB-65. Lim et al. compared the two scores. Using the CURB-65 index, pneumonia is considered mild (score 0–1, mortality 1.5%), moderate (score 2, mortality 9.2%), or severe (score 3–5, mortality 22%). Using the CRB-65 index, pneumonia is considered mild (score 0, mortality 1.5%), moderate (score 1–2, mortality 8.2%), or severe (score 3–4, mortality 31%). In patients with a CRB-65 ≥ 1 (except age ≥ 65 years alone), hospitalization should be seriously considered.

Ref:
1. Lim WS, van der Eerden MM, Laing R, Boersma WG, Karalus N, Town GI, et al. Defining community acquired pneumonia severity on presentation to hospital: an international derivation and validation study. Thorax. 2003;58(5):377-82.
2. Mandel LA, Wunderink RG, Anzueto A, Bartlett JG, Campbell GD, Dean NC, et al. Infectious Diseases Society of America/American Thoracic Society consensus guidelines on the management of community-acquired pneumonia in adults. Clin Infect Dis. 2007;44(Suppl 2): S27-72.
3. Woodhead M, Blasi F, Ewig S, Garau J, Huchon G, Ieven M, et al. Guidelines for the management of adult lower respiratory tract infections-summary. Clin Microbiol Infect. 2011;17(Suppl 6):1-24.

33. Ans. C

The urinary antigen test is currently the most helpful rapid test. This enzyme immunoassay is highly specific (>95%), and its sensitivity ranges between 65 and 80%, but it only detects the most frequent type of *Legionella* (*L. pneumophila* serogroup 1; ~90% of all *Legionellaceae* infections). Nevertheless, its use has been shown to reduce both mortality and the need for intensive care. The results are available within hours.

Culture from respiratory samples (usually sputum) is important and should be specifically ordered on suspicion of *Legionella* pneumonia together with the urinary antigen test. The cultures serve for confirmation and detection of non-*L. pneumophila* serogroup 1 *Legionella* infections. Culture results are usually available within 3–4 days.

While antibody serology used to be the mainstay test, it has become less important with the availability of urinary antigen testing, direct immunofluorescence staining, and PCR. Because the definitive criterion for serological diagnosis requires a fourfold rise in antibody titer (IgG, or IgM and IgG) and/or the appearance of IgM titers, repeat serology is required up to 12 weeks after the onset of infection. A single elevated titer has been shown in up to 16% of healthy adults. Serology alone is, therefore, not very useful for clinical decision-making and treatment. DNA amplification testing for *Legionella* by real-time PCR offers results within hours with a high specificity and sensitivity. This test is particularly useful in patients with suspected legionellosis but a negative urine antigen test. *Legionella spp.* other than *L. pneumophila* are fastidious and difficult to grow in culture but can be detected with PCR assays where available.

Ref:
1. Ieven M, Matheeussen V. Microbiology testing and interpretation. In: Palange P, Simonds AK (Eds). ERS Handbook of Respiratory Medicine. 2nd edition. Sheffield: European Respiratory Society; 2013. pp. 183-9.
2. Lim WS, Baudouin SV, George RC, Hill AT, Jamieson C, Le Jeune I, et al. BTS guidelines for the management of community acquired pneumonia in adults: update 2009. Thorax. 2009;64(Suppl 3):iii1-55.
3. Murdoch DR, Podmore RG, Anderson TP, Barratt K, Maze MJ, French KE, et al. Impact of routine systematic polymerase chain reaction testing on case finding for Legionnaires' disease: a pre-post comparison study. Clin Infect Dis. 2013;57(9):1275-81.

34. Ans. A

Pneumococcal polysaccharide vaccine is recommended for COPD patients aged ≥65 years as well as in younger patients with significant comorbid conditions, such as cardiac disease. In addition, this vaccine has been shown to reduce the incidence of CAP in COPD patients aged <65 years with an FEV_1 <40% predicted. Pneumococcal conjugate vaccine protects against pneumonia even in patients aged >65 years.

Despite the recognition of *P. aeruginosa* as an opportunistic pathogen in severe COPD patients, to date, no vaccine against this bacterium has obtained market authorization. Persons considered at increased risk for invasive *H. influenzae* type b disease include those with functional or anatomic asplenia, HIV infection, Ig deficiency (including IgG2 subclass deficiency), or early component complement deficiency, recipients of a hematopoietic stem cell transplant, and those receiving chemotherapy or radiation therapy for malignant neoplasms. *H. influenzae* type b vaccination is not indicated for COPD patients.

Influenza vaccination can reduce serious illness (such as lower respiratory tract infections requiring hospitalization) and death in COPD patients. Vaccines containing killed or live, inactivated viruses are recommended as they are more effective in elderly patients with COPD. The strains are adjusted each year for appropriate effectiveness and should be given once each year. The CDC recommends that influenza vaccinations begin soon after the vaccine becomes available, ideally by October. However, as long as influenza viruses are circulating, it is not too late to vaccinate COPD patients, even in January or later. While seasonal influenza outbreaks can happen as early as October, most of the time influenza activity peaks between December and February. Since it takes about 2 weeks after vaccination for antibodies to develop, it is best that people are vaccinated in time to be protected before influenza viruses begin spreading in their community; so, influenza vaccination in the late spring is not recommended.

Ref:
1. *Global Strategy for the Diagnosis, Management and Prevention of COPD. Global Initiative for Chronic Obstructive Lung Disease (GOLD), 2015. [online] Available from: www.goldcopd.org [Last accessed on February, 2020].*
2. *Grohskopf LA, Olsen SJ, Sokolow LZ, Bresee JS, Cox NJ, Broder KR, et al. Prevention and control of seasonal influenza with vaccines: recommendations of the Advisory Committee on Immunization Practices (ACIP)—United States, 2014-15 Influenza Season. MMWR Morb Mortal Wkly Rep. 2014;63(32):691-7.*
3. *Miravitlles M. Exacerbations of COPD. In: Palange P, Simonds AK (Eds). ERS Handbook of Respiratory Medicine, 2nd edition. Sheffield: European Respiratory Society; 2013. pp. 293-9.*
4. *Briere EC, Rubin L, Moro PL, Cohn A, Clark T, Messonnier N, et al. Prevention and Control of Haemophilus influenzae type b disease: Recommendations of the Advisory Committee on Immunization Practices (ACIP). MMWR Recomm Rep. 2014;63(RR-01):1-14.*
5. *Bonten MJM, Huijts SM, Bolkenbaas M, Webber C, Patterson S, Gault S, et al. Polysaccharide conjugate vaccine against pneumococcal pneumonia in adults. N Engl J Med. 2015;372(12):1114-25.*

35. Ans. A

This patient has stage IV squamous cell carcinoma with a poor performance score [WHO/Eastern Cooperative Oncology Group (ECOG) stage 3-4] for which (palliative) chemotherapy is not indicated, except erlotinib for epidermal growth factor receptor (EGFR) mutation positive patients. Because of the low incidence (<3.6%) of EGFR mutations, routine testing for them should not be performed. Two-drug regimens are preferred. A third drug improves only response rate, not survival. Platinum-based therapy prolongs survival, improves symptom control, and quality of life in nonsmall cell lung cancer patients. In squamous cell carcinoma, the gemcitabine/cisplatin combination shows superior efficacy compared with pemetrexed/cisplatin. Gemcitabine would be an adequate maintenance therapy after a platinum/gemcitabine doublet therapy in the absence of disease progression. Bevacizumab blocks the vascular endothelial growth factor and is a recommended option for fit patients (WHO/ECOG stage 0-1) with nonsquamous cell carcinoma who are EGFR mutation negative. Bevacizumab is not a recommended treatment for squamous cell carcinoma.

Ref:
1. *National Comprehensive Cancer Network (NCCN). NCCN Clinical practice guidelines in oncology: non-small cell lung cancer, version 3.2011. National Comprehensive Cancer Network, 2011. [online] Available from: www.nccn.org [Last accessed on February, 2011].*
2. *Socinski MA, Evans T, Gettinger S, Hensing TA, VanDam Sequist L, Ireland B, et al. Treatment of stage I and II non-small cell lung cancer: treatment of stage IV non-small cell lung cancer: diagnosis and management of lung cancer, 3rd ed: American College of Chest Physicians evidence-based clinical practice guidelines. Chest. 2013;143(Suppl 5):e341S-68S.*
3. *Tufman A, Huber RM. Chemotherapy and molecular biological therapy. In: Palange P, Simonds AK (Eds). ERS Handbook of Respiratory Medicine, 2nd edition. Sheffield: European Respiratory Society; 2013. pp. 460-5.*

36. Ans. B

The patient's clinical history is suggestive for bronchiectasis, due to the recurrent bacterial lower respiratory tract infections in the past occurring because of an impaired immunological defense. Another differential diagnostic consideration would be lymphocytic interstitial pneumonitis in patients with HIV who have a long-standing infiltrate.

The patient's clinical history is not suggestive for a *Pneumocystis* infection. Furthermore, the patient is not hypoxemic and his LDH is normal findings that are commonly encountered in patients with a pneumocystis infection.

The sweat chloride test is used to screen for cystic fibrosis, which is not likely in this case; most cystic fibrosis patients will have health problems since early childhood.

Empiric therapy with trimethoprim and sulfamethoxazole might resolve this episode of a lower respiratory tract infection but will not give an answer for the recurrent episodes of lower respiratory tract infections. However, trimethoprim and sulfamethoxazole might be indicated as a prophylaxis for *Pneumocystis* infections as his CD4 count is low. Any WHO clinical stage of HIV infection with CD4 <350 cells/mm^3 or WHO clinical stage 3 or 4 irrespective of CD4 count should receive *P. jirovecii* pneumonia prophylaxis.

A nasal biopsy might be performed in a case where PCD is suspected. If this would be the diagnosis, one would expect the patient to have complaints of recurrent respiratory tract infections from childhood onward.

Ref:
1. *Pasteur MC, Bilton D, Hill AT; British Thoracic Society Bronchiectasis non-CF Guideline Group. British Thoracic Society guideline for non-CF bronchiectasis. Thorax. 2010;65(Suppl 1):i1-58.*
2. *World Health Organization. Consolidated Guidelines on HIV Prevention, Diagnosis, Treatment and Care for Key Populations. Geneva: WHO Press; 2014.*
3. *World Health Organization. Guidelines on Co-trimoxazole Prophylaxis for HIV-related Infections Among Children, Adolescents and Adults. Geneva: WHO Press; 2006.*

37. **Ans. B**

The diagnosis is CAP and the sputum sample is indicative of the presence of *S. pneumoniae*. As the patient has been treated with amoxicillin many times lately, the risk of resistance of *S. pneumoniae* is considered high not only to penicillins, but also to macrolides, tetracyclines, and trimethoprim-sulfamethoxazole; therefore, treatment with ceftriaxone is a reasonable choice.

Ref:
1. *Woodhead M, Blasi F, Ewig S, Garau J, Huchon G, Ieven M, et al. Guidelines for the management of adult lower respiratory tract infections–full version. Clin Microbiol Infect. 2011;17(Suppl 6):E1-59.*

38. **Ans. E**

The goal of testing for latent TB infection is to identify individuals who are at increased risk for developing active TB and would therefore benefit from preventive treatment. This healthy woman has no risk factors for reactivation of TB and therefore should not have been tested, and thus should not receive treatment regardless of the test result. Moreover, her age indicates that she may have received bacille Calmette–Guérin vaccination in early childhood, which can also explain her TST reaction. None of the proposed regimens is recommended for preventive therapy. Isoniazid prophylaxis is associated with increasing side effects with age above 35 years.

Ref:
1. *Horsburgh CR Jr, Rubin EJ. Clinical practice. Latent tuberculosis infection in the United States. N Engl J Med. 2011; 364(15):1441-8.*
2. *Targeted tuberculin testing and treatment of latent tuberculosis infection. This official statement of the American Thoracic Society was adopted by the ATS Board of Directors, July 1999. This is a Joint Statement of the American Thoracic Society (ATS) and the Centers for Disease Control and Prevention (CDC). This statement was endorsed by the Council of the Infectious Diseases Society of America. (IDSA), September 1999, and the sections of this statement. Am J Respir Crit Care Med. 2000;161(4 Pt 2):S221-47.*

CHAPTER 13

Genitourinary Tract Infections

MM Bahadur, Ashay Shingare

1. A 36-year-old lady had developed acute onset dysuria, frequency, and urgency 2 weeks ago. She had completed 5 days course of nitrofurantoin with relief of her symptoms. She has presented with reappearance of dysuria and frequency for past 3 days. Her urine routine examination shows presence of 20 pus cells/mm^3, however urine culture is negative. Which of the following best describes her urine examination findings?
   A. Asymptomatic bacteriuria (ASB)
   B. Clinically significant bacteriuria
   C. Sterile pyuria
   D. Colonization

2. A 66-year-old gentleman has presented with 1 month history of urinary frequency, weight loss, and intermittent hematuria. His urine examination shows presence of pyuria, however, urine culture is negative. Which of the following is least likely cause of sterile pyuria?
   A. Genitourinary tuberculosis (GUTB)
   B. *Klebsiella* cystitis
   C. Schistosomiasis
   D. Bladder tumor

3. A 32-year-old lady with history of pulmonary tuberculosis 2 years ago has now presented with low grade fever for past 1 month. She also has complaints of intermittent hematuria. Her urine examination has revealed sterile pyuria. Which of the following is most common mode of spread in renal tuberculosis?
   A. Hematogenous   B. Adjacent spread
   C. Retrograde   D. Droplets

4. A 60-year-old gentleman with poorly controlled type 2 diabetes mellitus has presented with 2 months history of right flank pain, intermittent dysuria, and gross hematuria. He has received three courses of oral antibiotics and urine culture is sterile. He has been advised urine culture for *Mycobacterium tuberculosis* and imaging studies. Which of the following is least likely imaging finding in renal tuberculosis?
   A. Renal calcification
   B. Calyceal distortion
   C. Ureteric stricture
   D. Emphysematous pyelonephritis

5. Which of the following statement is not true regarding treatment of GUTB?
   A. Rifampicin should be avoided in renal transplant recipients on tacrolimus
   B. Ethambutol does not require dose reduction in GUTB with chronic kidney disease (CKD)
   C. Streptomycin use can be associated with ototoxicity and nephrotoxicity
   D. Surgical stenting may be required for ureteric strictures secondary to GUTB

6. A 26-year-old male has presented with complaints of fever, myalgia, suprapubic pain, and cough for past 2 weeks. He had recently travelled to Africa 2 months ago and had visited Lake Malawi. His blood picture has revealed eosinophilia. Urine examination shows presence of eggs of *Schistosoma haematobium* with terminal spike. What is the most likely diagnosis?
   A. Katayama fever
   B. Urinary tuberculosis
   C. African trypanosomiasis
   D. Yellow fever

7. Which of the following is not associated with urinary schistosomiasis?
   A. Obstructive uropathy
   B. Vesicoureteric reflux
   C. Adenocarcinoma of the urinary bladder
   D. Small capacity bladder

8. A 40-year-old male was diagnosed with human immunodeficiency virus (HIV) infection 8 years ago and is not on antiretroviral therapy. He has presented with 3 months history of edema feet and frothing in urine. His serum creatinine is 2.3 mg/dL and 24 hours urine protein is 3,800 mg per day. Ultrasound examination has revealed normal sized kidneys. Which of the following is the most likely diagnosis?
   A. HIV-associated nephropathy (HIVAN)
   B. HIV-associated immune-complex kidney disease
   C. HIV-associated thrombotic microangiopathy
   D. Nephrotoxicity of antiretroviral therapy

9. A 40-year-old male with HIV infection was started on zidovudine-, tenofovir-, and efavirenz-based antiretroviral therapy 6 months ago. His serum creatinine at the time of antiretroviral therapy initiation was 1.2 mg/dL. He was prescribed a course of fluconazole 1 month ago for oral candidiasis. He has presented with complaints of easy fatigability for past few weeks and vomiting for the past 3 days. There is no history of edema or oliguria. However, his serum creatinine has risen to 4.6 mg/dL and urine examination shows presence of glycosuria with no active sediment and plasma blood glucose is 110 mg/dL. Which of the following drug is most likely cause of his renal dysfunction?
    A. Zidovudine B. Tenofovir
    C. Efavirenz   D. Fluconazole

10. A 50-year-old lady was diagnosed with HIV infection 10 years ago and is on antiretroviral therapy. She is also on conservative management for CKD for the past 3 years. Her kidney disease has progressed gradually to stage 5 CKD and she has been advised regarding future requirement of renal replacement therapy. Which of the following statement is true about CKD in HIV?
    A. HIV patients should not undergo hemodialysis due to risk of transmission of infection
    B. HIV patients should not undergo peritoneal dialysis due to risk of peritonitis
    C. HIV is a contraindication for undergoing kidney transplant
    D. Organs from HIV-infected donors can be transplanted into HIV positive recipients

11. A 60-year-old male had undergone deceased donor kidney transplant 3 months ago with antithymocyte globulin as the induction agent and had delayed graft function in immediate post-transplant period. He has presented with allograft dysfunction in the form of rise in serum creatinine from 1.2 mg/dL to 2.6 mg/dL over the past 4 weeks. His current immunosuppression includes tacrolimus, mycophenolate mofetil, and prednisolone and the tacrolimus trough level is high. Ultrasonography of the transplant kidney has revealed stenosis at the distal end of the transplant ureter with resultant hydroureteronephrosis. Which of the following virus can cause ureteric stenosis?
    A. BK virus
    B. *Cytomegalovirus* (CMV)
    C. Epstein–Barr virus (EBV)
    D. Parvovirus B19

12. A 21-year-old female had undergone live donor kidney transplant 6 months ago. She had developed antibody mediated rejection 3 months post-transplant due to poor medication adherence and had received antirejection treatment. She has presented with rising serum creatinine over the past 1 month. Her urine examination has revealed epithelial cells with large basophilic nuclear inclusions suggestive of decoy cells and transplant kidney biopsy is suggestive of BK virus-associated tubulointerstitial nephritis. Which of the following is not useful for treatment of BKVAN?
    A. Azathioprine
    B. Cidofovir
    C. Leflunomide
    D. Reduction in immunosuppression

13. A 23-year-old female medical intern had undergone health check tests 5 days ago. Her urine routine test had revealed 20 pus cells/hpf, whereas rest of her reports were unremarkable. Following this, she had herself submitted a urine sample for culture testing. Her urine culture shows growth of >10^5 CFU/mL of *Escherichia coli*. She has no history of fever, frequency, dysuria or suprapubic pain. Which of the following should be next step for management of her UTI?
    A. Repeat urine routine
    B. Reassurance and no treatment
    C. Send urine fungal culture
    D. Treat according to antibiotic sensitivity

14. Screening and treatment for ASB is not recommended in which of the following?
    A. Pregnancy
    B. Prior to lithotripsy for real calculi
    C. Diabetes mellitus
    D. Prior to transurethral resection of the prostate (TURP)

15. A 65-year-old male with diabetes mellitus and ischemic heart disease was admitted to intensive care unit (ICU) 8 days ago for congestive cardiac failure. He had undergone urinary catheterization on admission. After improvement in his condition, he was shifted out of the ICU and urinary catheter was removed on the sixth day. He has now developed fever and dysuria for past 2 days. His urine culture has revealed growth of 10^5 CFU/mL of *E. coli*. Which of the following is most likely diagnosis?
    A. ASB
    B. Colonization
    C. Catheter-associated urinary tract infection (CAUTI)
    D. Clinically insignificant bacteriuria

16. Which is of the following is not recommended for prevention of CAUTI?
    A. Early catheter removal when indwelling catheter is no longer indicated

B. Use of condom catheter when appropriate
C. Adherence to a closed collecting system
D. Prophylaxis with systemic antimicrobials

17. **Which of the following is not true about bacterial UTIs?**
    A. *Escherichia coli* is the predominant causative agent of uncomplicated cystitis
    B. Urinary tract obstruction is a risk factor for complicated UTI
    C. Urine culture should be performed in all suspected cases of uncomplicated cystitis
    D. Leukocyte esterase and nitrites on dipstick urine test are suggestive of UTI

18. **A 25-year-old lady has presented with dysuria and urinary frequency for 3 days. There is no history of fever or flank pain. She had similar episode 8 months ago and was treated with oral antimicrobials. Which of the following is not a first-line therapy drug for treatment of acute uncomplicated cystitis?**
    A. Ciprofloxacin
    B. Fosfomycin
    C. Trimethoprim–sulfamethoxazole (TMP-SMX)
    D. Nitrofurantoin

19. **Which of the following is not a recommended strategy for prevention of recurrent cystitis?**
    A. Abstinence from sexual intercourse
    B. Topical estrogen in postmenopausal women
    C. Using spermicides
    D. Voiding after intercourse

20. **A 70-year-old male has complaints of difficulty in initiating urination, poor urinary stream, nighttime urine frequency, and feeling of incomplete bladder emptying for the past 6 months. He has presented now with high grade fever, chills, dysuria, and urinary urgency for the past 3 days. Which of the following is not preferred for treatment of acute prostatitis?**
    A. Nitrofurantoin
    B. Piperacillin–tazobactam
    C. Ceftriaxone plus gentamicin
    D. Ciprofloxacin

21. **A 40-year-old lady with poorly controlled diabetes mellitus for past 7 years, has presented with high grade fever and right flank pain for past 3 days. On further evaluation she is found to be in septic shock with blood pressure 90/50 mm Hg. On urine routine examination, innumerable pus cells are seen and hemogram shows hemoglobin 9 g/dL and total leukocyte count 45,900/mm³ with 90% neutrophils. CT scan shows bulky right kidney with extensive diffuse gas in the cortex and collecting system.**

    Which of the following is the definitive treatment for this patient?
    A. Antimicrobial agents targeting gram-negative and gram-positive bacteria
    B. Broad-spectrum antibacterial and antifungal agents
    C. Antibiotics and CT-guided percutaneous nephrostomy
    D. Antibiotics and right side nephrectomy

22. **Which of the following is least likely cause of emphysematous pyelonephritis?**
    A. *Escherichia coli*
    B. *Pseudomonas aeruginosa*
    C. *Klebsiella pneumoniae*
    D. *Clostridium perfringens*

23. **A 35-year-old primigravida with 12 weeks gestation was detected to have ASB on screening. Her urine culture has revealed > 10^5 CFU/mL of *K. pneumoniae*. Which of the following is not true regarding UTI in pregnancy?**
    A. Screening for ASB is recommended during pregnancy
    B. Vesicoureteric reflux is a risk factor for UTI in pregnancy
    C. Perineal bacteria enter the urinary tract via retrograde route
    D. Treatment of ASB in pregnancy will not reduce further risk of pyelonephritis

24. **Which of the following is true regarding pyelonephritis in pregnancy?**
    A. Pyelonephritis in pregnancy is most common in the first trimester
    B. Enterococcus is the most common cause of UTI in pregnancy
    C. Pyelonephritis in pregnancy is more common on the left side
    D. Dilated ureters predispose to development of pyelonephritis in pregnancy

25. **Which of the following is not true about use of fosfomycin in UTIs?**
    A. Fosfomycin is contraindicated for treatment of ASB in pregnancy
    B. Oral fosfomycin single dose can be used for uncomplicated cystitis in nonpregnant state
    C. Fosfomycin is excreted in the urine
    D. Diarrhea is a common adverse effect

26. **A 60-year-old diabetic male was admitted to ICU 2 weeks ago with acute ischemic stroke. His hospital course was complicated by ventilator-associated pneumonia and he is presently on carbapenem therapy. He has now developed fever for past 3 days**

and urine routine shows pyuria in the absence of bacteriuria. Urine culture has revealed growth of *Candida albicans*. Which of the following is not a risk factor for candida UTI?
   A. Broad-spectrum antibiotics
   B. Admission to ICU
   C. Male gender
   D. Diabetes mellitus

27. Which of the following is not true about *Candida* UTI?
   A. *Candida* can appear in urine due to improper sample collection
   B. Candiduria in the presence long term urinary catheter is diagnostic of *Candida* UTI
   C. *Candida* pyelonephritis can present as fever, flank pain, and renal angle tenderness
   D. *Candida* UTI can present as fungus ball in the collecting system

28. Which of the following is the drug of choice for treatment of cystitis caused by *C. albicans*?
   A. Liposomal amphotericin B (AmB)
   B. Anidulafungin
   C. Fluconazole
   D. Posaconazole

29. Treatment with antifungal agents for asymptomatic candiduria is not recommended in which of the following?
   A. Neutropenic patients
   B. Very low-birth-weight infants
   C. Urological surgery
   D. HIV infection

30. Which of the following is preferred drug for treatment of lower UTI caused by *Candida auris*?
   A. AmB deoxycholate
   B. Anidulafungin
   C. Fluconazole
   D. Liposomal AmB

ANSWERS WITH EXPLANATIONS

1. **Ans. C**
Pyuria is presence of 10 or more pus cells/mm^3 in urine. Presence of 10^5 bacterial colony forming units (CFU)/mL in midstream urine culture is regarded as clinically significant. However, lower bacterial counts may be present in case of current antibiotic use or recent treatment for urinary tract infection (UTI). ASB is the presence of 10^5 bacterial CFU/mL in two separate midstream urine samples in the absence of symptoms of UTI. Absence of bacterial CFU in urine culture in the presence of pyuria is called sterile pyuria.
Ref:
  1. Wise GJ, Schlegel PN. Sterile pyuria. N Engl J Med. 2015;372(11):1048-54.

2. **Ans. B**
Sterile pyuria can be caused by infective as well as noninfective causes. For patients presenting with urinary or urethral symptoms, it is important to rule out sexually transmitted infections such as gonorrhea, chlamydia, and genital herpes. Prostatitis in males and pelvic inflammatory disease in females should also be considered. For patients with systemic symptoms, urine culture should be repeated. Recent use of antibiotics or ongoing antibiotic therapy can alter urine culture findings. GUTB is an important cause of sterile pyuria. Other infective causes include fungal infections and schistosomiasis.

Noninfective causes include urinary catheter, renal calculi, urinary tract tumors, pelvic irradiation, papillary necrosis, and recent urological procedure.

Imaging studies, cystoscopy, and biopsy procedure will help in evaluating for noninfective causes.
Ref:
  1. Wise GJ, Schlegel PN. Sterile pyuria. N Engl J Med. 2015;372(11):1048-54.

3. **Ans. A**
Genitourinary tuberculosis is the second most common site of extrapulmonary tuberculosis after lymph node tuberculosis. Kidney is most commonly involved organ in the genitourinary system and the most common mode of spread to kidney is hematogenous. Renal involvement can be in the form of cortical granulomas or medullary caseous foci which can rupture into the collecting system. Further fibrosis and scarring of the collecting system and ureters will lead to strictures and obstruction. Renal calcification and papillary necrosis can occur in renal tuberculosis.

Genital involvement can occur from hematogenous or retrograde spread and can present as scrotal or epididymal mass, epididymitis or chronic prostatitis in males. Penile and urethral involvement may present as penile ulcers, urethral strictures or fistulae, and papulonecrotic skin lesions. Involvement of the female genital tract can present as infertility secondary to salpingitis, pelvic pain, secondary amenorrhea, and tender adnexal masses.
Ref:
  1. Abbara A, Davidson RN. Etiology and management of genitourinary tuberculosis. Nat Rev Urol. 2011;8(12): 678-88.

4. Ans. D

For diagnosis of urinary tract TB, early morning urine samples for three consecutive days should be sent for TB culture. *Mycobacterium smegmatis* can appear as acid-fast bacillus on staining and give false positive results. Nucleic acid amplification tests help in rapid diagnosis, offer higher sensitivity and specificity, and can detect drug resistance.

Intravenous urography (IVU) may reveal erosion of the tip of the calyx, calyceal distortion, multiple ureteral strictures (beaded or corkscrew ureter), hydronephrosis, hydroureter, or nonvisualization of the kidney (autonephrectomy). Urinary bladder wall may appear irregular with distortion secondary to fibrosis and vesicoureteric reflux may occur. Computed tomography (CT) will identify renal calcification, cortical thinning, scarring, and cavitatory lesions. CT-IVU will identify calyceal and ureteric lesions. Distal ureter is the most common site for ureteric strictures.

Cystoscopic findings include mucosal ulceration, granulomas, scarring or a contracted bladder. Scarring at the vesicoureteric junction may give cystoscopic appearance of golf hole ureteric orifice. Biopsy can be taken for histopathological examination and TB culture.

Ref:
1. Abbara A, Davidson RN. Etiology and management of genitourinary tuberculosis. Nat Rev Urol. 2011;8(12): 678-88.

5. Ans. B

Treatment of GUTB involves use of rifampicin, isoniazid, pyrazinamide, and ethambutol in initial intensive phase for 2 months followed by rifampicin and isoniazid for 4 months in maintenance phase. Drug resistance is of concern and sensitivity testing will help in guiding further treatment. Ethambutol and streptomycin require dose reduction in patients with CKD. Allergic interstitial nephritis can occur in patients receiving rifampicin.

Surgical treatment may involve stenting for ureteric strictures and reconstructive surgeries for obstruction in the form of pyeloplasty and ureteroureterostomy. Ureteric reimplantation may be necessary for vesicoureteric reflux with repeated secondary infections. Augmentation cystoplasty may be required if bladder capacity has reduced to <100 mL. Excision surgery in the form of nephrectomy may be required in patients with secondary sepsis, bleeding, uncontrolled hypertension, or persistent positive urinary cultures. Abdominal hysterectomy may be indicated for women with recurrent endometrial TB or excessive uterine bleeding; however, there is risk of developing postoperative fistulae.

Ref:
1. Abbara A, Davidson RN. Etiology and management of genitourinary tuberculosis. Nat Rev Urol. 2011;8(12): 678-88.

6. Ans. A

Schistosomiasis (bilharziasis) is a parasitic disease caused by trematode of the genus *Schistosoma*. Three species—*S. haematobium*, *S. mansoni*, and *S. japonicum* cause human disease. Adult worms reside in the venules of the human host whereas fresh water snails act as intermediate hosts. Acute schistosomiasis (Katayama fever) is seen in travelers visiting endemic region. Presentation includes fever, headache, myalgia, dyspnea, and eosinophilia few weeks after visiting endemic region and is an allergic reaction to the schistosomal egg antigen.

Ref:
1. Colley DG, Bustinduy AL, Secor WE, King CH. Human schistosomiasis. Lancet. 2014;383(9936):2253-64.
2. Ross AG, Vickers D, Olds GR, Shah SM, McManus DP. Katayama syndrome. Lancet Infect Dis. 2007; 7(3):218-24.

7. Ans. C

Urinary schistosomiasis is caused by granulomatous response to eggs of *S. haematobium* in urinary bladder. Multiple granulomas coalesce to form pseudotubercles in the bladder wall followed by ulceration and hematuria. Healing by fibrosis leads to distorted, calcified, and small capacity bladder. Obstructive uropathy, ureteric strictures, and vesicoureteric reflux may be seen. Transitional cell carcinoma and squamous cell carcinoma of the urinary bladder are associated with urinary schistosomiasis. Genital tract involvement can cause sandy patches (neovascularization) on the cervix, stress incontinence, and infertility in females and hematospermia and oligospermia in males. *Schistosoma mansoni* can cause immune complex mediated glomerular disease due to circulating immune complexes containing schistosomal antigens.

Diagnosis involves detection of schistosomal eggs in urine, feces or tissue biopsies. Serological tests are useful for diagnosis of acute schistosomiasis in travelers, but cannot differentiate recent or past infection in people from endemic region.

Praziquantel is the drug of choice for schistosomiasis. Dose of 40 mg/kg is used for *S. haematobium* and *S. mansoni* whereas 60 mg/kg is used for *S. japonicum*. Repeat treatment with praziquantel may be required for suspected treatment failure. Artemisinin derivatives have activity against immature larval forms and can be used in common point-source outbreaks. Steroid therapy may be required for Katayama fever to reduce the severity of allergic reaction.

Ref:
1. Colley DG, Bustinduy AL, Secor WE, King CH. Human schistosomiasis. Lancet. 2014;383(9936):2253-64.
2. Ross AG, Vickers D, Olds GR, Shah SM, McManus DP. Katayama syndrome. Lancet Infect Dis. 2007;7(3): 218-24.

8. **Ans. A**

    Kidney diseases in patients with HIV infection include HIVAN, HIV immune-complex kidney disease (HIVIC), thrombotic microangiopathies, and nephrotoxicity of antiretroviral therapy. Also, coinfection with hepatitis B and hepatitis C virus can present with glomerular disease. HIVAN presents with nephrotic range proteinuria, edema, high viral load, low CD4 count, and preserved kidney sizes on ultrasonography. Classical glomerular lesion seen on kidney biopsy in HIVAN is collapsing variety of focal segmental glomerulosclerosis (FSGS). Patients of African descent have increased genetic susceptibility to HIVAN associated with *APOL1* gene variants, encoding for apolipoprotein L1. HIVIC presents as a nephritic illness with microscopic hematuria, proteinuria, and hypocomplementemia. Mainstay of treatment for HIVAN is antiretroviral therapy. Renin-angiotensin system blockers help in reduction of proteinuria.
    Ref:
    1. *Cohen SD, Kopp JB, Kimmel PL. Kidney diseases associated with human immunodeficiency virus infection. N Engl J Med. 2017;377(24):2363-74.*
    2. *Jotwani V, Atta MG, Estrella MM. Kidney disease in HIV: moving beyond HIV-associated nephropathy. J Am Soc Nephrol. 2017;28(11):3142-54.*

9. **Ans. B**

    Nucleoside reverse transcriptase inhibitors (NRTIs) and maraviroc require dose reduction in CKD. Indinavir and atazanavir can cause crystalluria and crystal nephropathy. Tenofovir disoproxil fumarate can get accumulated in proximal tubular cells and cause Fanconi's syndrome characterized by glycosuria, phosphaturia, aminoaciduria, and uricosuria. Acute tubular necrosis may also be observed as part of tenofovir toxicity. Tenofovir alafenamide (TAF) is a prodrug which does not get accumulated in proximal tubular cells and hence is associated with lesser nephrotoxicity.
    Ref:
    1. *Cohen SD, Kopp JB, Kimmel PL. Kidney diseases associated with human immunodeficiency virus infection. N Engl J Med. 2017;377(24):2363-74.*
    2. *Jotwani V, Atta MG, Estrella MM. Kidney disease in HIV: moving beyond HIV-associated nephropathy. J Am Soc Nephrol. 2017;28(11):3142-54.*

10. **Ans. D**

    Increased risk of CKD progression in HIV is seen with black race, hepatitis C virus coinfection, use of tenofovir disoproxil fumarate, and metabolic disorders (e.g., diabetes and hyperlipidemia) associated with antiretroviral therapy. Patients with HIV and end-stage renal disease can undergo hemodialysis or peritoneal dialysis. However, the best modality of treatment for such patients is kidney transplant. Effective HIV viral suppression for more than 6 months and absence of active opportunistic infection and malignancy are the criteria for including HIV patients into kidney transplant programs. Organs from HIV-infected donors can be transplanted into HIV positive recipients.
    Ref:
    1. *Cohen SD, Kopp JB, Kimmel PL. Kidney diseases associated with human immunodeficiency virus infection. N Engl J Med. 2017;377(24):2363-74.*
    2. *Jotwani V, Atta MG, Estrella MM. Kidney disease in HIV: moving beyond HIV-associated nephropathy. J Am Soc Nephrol. 2017;28(11):3142-54.*

11. **Ans. A**

    BK virus belongs to the family of polyomaviruses. Other polyomavirus which causes human disease is John Cunningham (JC) virus causing progressive multifocal leukoencephalopathy. BK virus resides in the renal tubular cells and transitional epithelium of the urinary tract and causes disease in immunocompromised individuals, especially transplant recipients. It causes BK virus-associated nephropathy (BKVAN) characterized by tubulointerstitial nephritis. It also causes obstructive uropathy due to multiple ureteral strictures. Risk factors for BKVAN include higher degree of immunosuppression use, antirejection treatment, use of lymphocyte depleting antibodies, ureteric stents, and deceased donor renal transplant. Most cases of BKVAN occur in first 2–6 months post-transplant and can present as graft dysfunction or obstructive uropathy on imaging study.
    Ref:
    1. *Elfadawy N, Yamada M, Sarabu N. Management of BK polyomavirus infection in kidney and kidney-pancreas transplant recipients: a review article. Infect Dis Clin North Am. 2018;32(3):599-613.*

12. **Ans. A**

    Diagnosis of BK virus infection is done by quantitative polymerase chain reaction (PCR) on urine and blood. Plasma BK virus PCR is the preferred method. Urine may reveal decoy cells which are shed urothelial cells in the urine with basophilic nuclear inclusions. Renal allograft biopsy staining with simian virus 40 (SV40) will also identify tubular cells with viral inclusions. Primary measure for treatment of BK virus infection is reduction in immunosuppression. Leflunomide which inhibits BK virus replication and cidofovir with some anti-BK virus activity may be tried. Intravenous immunoglobulin (IVIG) may be used in the setting of BK virus infection alongside allograft rejection.
    Ref:
    1. *Elfadawy N, Yamada M, Sarabu N. Management of BK polyomavirus infection in kidney and kidney-pancreas transplant recipients: a review article. Infect Dis Clin North Am. 2018;32(3):599-613.*

13. **Ans. B**

    Asymptomatic bacteriuria is the presence of 10^5 bacterial CFU/mL in midstream urine sample in the absence of symptoms of UTI. For female patients, urine culture should be repeated within 2 weeks to confirm presence of bacteriuria as 10–60% bacteriuria will have resolved on repeat testing. In men, single positive urine culture is sufficient for defining ASB. ASB is common in healthy women and persons with abnormalities of the genitourinary tract. Treatment for ASB is as an important contributor to inappropriate antimicrobial use and leads to emergence of antimicrobial resistance.

Ref:
1. Nicolle LE, Gupta K, Bradley SF, Colgan R, DeMuri GP, Drekonja D, et al. Clinical Practice Guideline for the Management of Asymptomatic Bacteriuria: 2019 Update by the Infectious Diseases Society of America. Clin Infect Dis. 2019;68:e83-110.

14. **Ans. C**

Screening and treatment for ASB is recommended in pregnant women. Urine culture testing should be done during early pregnancy. ASB is found in 2–7% women during pregnancy. Treatment of ASB during pregnancy decreases the risk of developing pyelonephritis as well as preterm delivery and low birth weight. Bacterial clearance rates achieved with single dose antimicrobials during pregnancy are less. Hence 4–7 days of nitrofurantoin or β-lactam antimicrobials are recommended for treatment of ASB during pregnancy. Screening and treatment for ASB is also recommended for patients who will be undergoing endoscopic urological procedures associated with mucosal trauma such as TURP or bladder tumor, ureteroscopy, lithotripsy, and percutaneous stone surgery. Short course (one or two doses) of antimicrobial therapy is recommended in these situations for reducing the risk of sepsis and symptomatic UTI.

Screening and treatment for ASB is not recommended in children, healthy nonpregnant women, diabetics, renal transplant recipients >1 month after surgery, any nonrenal solid organ transplant recipients, bladder dysfunction following spinal cord injury, and patients with indwelling urinary catheters.

Ref:
1. Nicolle LE, Gupta K, Bradley SF, Colgan R, DeMuri GP, Drekonja D, et al. Clinical Practice Guideline for the Management of Asymptomatic Bacteriuria: 2019 Update by the Infectious Diseases Society of America. Clin Infect Dis. 2019;68:e83-110.

15. **Ans. C**

A CAUTI is associated with urinary catheter use that has been in place for more than 2 days and presence of at least one sign or symptom (temperature > 38°C, urinary urgency, urinary frequency, dysuria, suprapubic tenderness, or costovertebral angle pain or tenderness) along with a positive urine culture. Urinary urgency, frequency, or dysuria may not be present if the catheter is still in place. CAUTI increases the hospital stay and healthcare cost. Incidence of bacteriuria is 3–10% per day of indwelling catheterization.

Host level risk factors for CAUTI include female gender, elderly, diabetes, and CKD. Duration of catheterization is the most important modifiable risk factor for developing CAUTI. Other modifiable risk factors include nonadherence to aseptic catheter care, opening a closed catheter system, catheter insertion outside operating room, and catheter insertion after sixth day of hospitalization. Bacteriuria is universal after long-term catheterization (≥30 days). Also, pyuria does not differentiate symptomatic from asymptomatic UTI, and hence diagnosis of CAUTI can be difficult. Urine culture may show significant growth if improperly collected.

Ref:
1. Shuman EK, Chenoweth CE. Urinary catheter-associated infections. Infect Dis Clin North Am. 2018;32(4):885-97.
2. Hooton TM, Bradley SF, Cardenas DD, Colgan R, Geerlings SE, Rice JC, et al. Diagnosis, prevention, and treatment of catheter-associated urinary tract infection in adults: 2009 International Clinical Practice Guidelines from the Infectious Diseases Society of America. Clin Infect Dis. 2010;50(5):625-63.

16. **Ans. D**

Routine screening or treatment is not recommended for catheter-associated ASB because it does not reduce the risk of complications and can lead to emergence of antimicrobial resistance. For symptomatic UTI, urine culture should be collected from a freshly placed catheter if indwelling catheter has been present for a few days. Also, response to antimicrobial therapy is improved if catheter is changed at the time of initiation of antibiotics. 7 days is the recommended duration of antimicrobial treatment for patients who have prompt resolution of symptoms and 10–14 days if response is delayed.

Complications of catheterization include bacteriuria, often with drug-resistant flora, cystitis, pyelonephritis, sepsis, catheter obstruction, stone formation, and rare complications in long-term like fistula formation and bladder cancer.

Preventive strategies for CAUTI include catheter insertion only for appropriate indications, sterile insertion, prompt removal, use of alternatives to indwelling catheterization (intermittent catheterization and condom catheter) when appropriate, strict adherence to a closed collecting system, and avoiding routine bladder irrigation. Catheters coated with silver alloy and antimicrobials such as nitrofurazone, minocycline, and rifampicin appear to be effective in reducing bacteriuria in patients catheterized for less than 7 days. However, their efficacy in reducing bacteriuria in patients with long-term indwelling catheter is unclear.

Ref:
1. *Shuman EK, Chenoweth CE. Urinary catheter-associated infections. Infect Dis Clin North Am. 2018;32(4):885-97.*
2. *Hooton TM, Bradley SF, Cardenas DD, Colgan R, Geerlings SE, Rice JC, et al. Diagnosis, prevention, and treatment of catheter-associated urinary tract infection in adults: 2009 International Clinical Practice Guidelines from the Infectious Diseases Society of America. Clin Infect Dis. 2010;50(5):625-63.*

17. Ans. C

Risk factors for uncomplicated cystitis and pyelonephritis include sexual intercourse, use of spermicidals, previous UTI, multiple sexual partners, and a history of UTI in a first-degree female relative. Genetic risk factors include lower expression of *CXCR1* (interleukin-8 receptor) and nonsecretors of ABO blood group antigens. Blood group P1 phenotype is a risk factor for recurrent pyelonephritis.

Escherichia coli is the predominant causative agent of uncomplicated cystitis and pyelonephritis. Other organisms include *Klebsiella pneumoniae*, *Staphylococcus saprophyticus*, and *Enterococcus faecalis*. Complicated UTI includes underlying functional, metabolic, or anatomical conditions that may increase the risk of treatment failure or serious outcomes (e.g., obstruction, stone, indwelling catheter, diabetes, neurogenic bladder, vesicoureteric reflux, and immunosuppression).

Cystitis presents as dysuria, frequency, suprapubic pain, and hematuria. Symptoms of pyelonephritis include fever, chills, and flank pain. Presence of renal-angle tenderness is suggestive of pyelonephritis. Assessment for pyuria and bacteriuria is often performed with the use of commercially available dipstick urine tests. Presence of leukocyte esterase (released by leukocytes) or nitrites (bacterial reduction of urinary nitrates to nitrites) in these tests is suggestive of UTI. Urine culture may not be performed in uncomplicated cystitis; however, should be done in suspected cases of pyelonephritis and complicated UTI.

Ref:
1. *Hooton TM. Clinical practice. Uncomplicated urinary tract infection. N Engl J Med. 2012;366(11):1028-37.*

18. Ans. A

Recommended first-line therapy drugs for empirical treatment of acute uncomplicated cystitis include nitrofurantoin (100 mg twice daily for 5 days), trimethoprim–sulfamethoxazole (160/800 mg twice daily for 3 days) and fosfomycin (3 g sachet in a single dose). In patients with history of allergy and areas with high prevalence of resistance to first-line agents, alternatives include fluoroquinolones (ciprofloxacin 250 mg twice daily for 3 days and levofloxacin 500 mg once daily for 3 days) and beta-lactams (amoxicillin-clavulanate for 3–7 days). Their use should be minimized to prevent the emergence of resistance.

Fluoroquinolones, oral beta-lactams, and trimethoprim–sulfamethoxazole can be used for empirical outpatient treatment of acute uncomplicated pyelonephritis. However, therapy should be guided by urine culture. Intravenous antibiotic therapy is required for patients with hemodynamic instability, urinary tract obstruction, renal calculi, diabetes, and pregnancy.

Ref:
1. *Hooton TM. Clinical practice. Uncomplicated urinary tract infection. N Engl J Med. 2012;366(11):1028-37.*
2. *Gupta K, Hooton TM, Naber KG, Wullt B, Colgan R, Miller LG, et al. International clinical practice guidelines for the treatment of acute uncomplicated cystitis and pyelonephritis in women: A 2010 update by the Infectious Diseases Society of America and the European Society for Microbiology and Infectious Diseases. Clin Infect Dis. 2011;52(5):e103-20.*

19. Ans. C

Recurrent cystitis despite treatment can occur due to antimicrobial-resistance or relapse. Treatment of recurrent cystitis should be guided by urine culture. Nonantimicrobial strategies for prevention of recurrent cystitis include abstinence or reduction in frequency of intercourse, voiding after intercourse, use of topical estrogen in postmenopausal women, avoiding spermicides, avoiding delay in urination, and wiping front to back after defecation. Cranberry juice and D-mannose powder have possible role in blocking adhesion of uropathogens to uroepithelial cells and can be tried as preventive strategies for recurrent cystitis.

Women with ≥ 3 UTI in 12 months or ≥ 2 UTI in 6 months despite nonantimicrobial preventive strategies can follow self-diagnosis and self-treatment at the onset of UTI symptoms. Alternatively, postcoital antimicrobial prophylaxis (single dose nitrofurantoin, TMP-SMX or cephalexin) or continuous antimicrobial prophylaxis with same agents can be tried.

Ref:
1. *Hooton TM. Clinical practice. Uncomplicated urinary tract infection. N Engl J Med. 2012;366(11):1028-37.*

20. Ans. A

Acute prostatitis presents as fever associated with frequency, urgency, and dysuria. Patients can complain of poor stream or straining at urination in the presence of benign prostatic hyperplasia causing obstruction. Chronic bacterial prostatitis can present as recurrent cystitis. In the absence of fever, symptoms may be attributed to lower urinary tract obstruction. If the bacterial CFU/mL on culture of expressed prostatic secretions and postprostatic massage urine is 10 times higher than preprostatic massage urine, then it is diagnostic of bacterial prostatitis. Identification of the same strain in repeat infections suggests bacterial persistence within the urinary tract. CT scan and USG are useful in evaluating for prostatic hyperplasia with obstruction, urethral stricture, bladder or renal stones, and bladder cancer.

Parenteral antibiotics such as piperacillin–tazobactam, ceftriaxone plus gentamicin, and fluoroquinolones are used for the treatment of acute bacterial prostatitis. Parenteral therapy should be followed by oral antibiotics for 2 weeks in clinically stable patients and 4 weeks in patients with severe illness or bacteremia. Nitrofurantoin is not effective due to poor penetration into prostatic tissue. Bacteremia may be observed in 25% patients with acute bacterial prostatitis. It can progress to septic shock and can be fatal. Other complications include development of prostatic abscess in 5–10% and progression to chronic prostatitis in 5%.

Alpha-blockers and catheterization may be considered in patients with difficulty in urination. Agents for treatment of chronic bacterial prostatitis include levofloxacin, ciprofloxacin or trimethoprim–sulfamethoxazole for 30 days. In patients with obstructive uropathy, transurethral resection of prostate may be considered to relieve obstruction, and prevent recurrences.

Ref:
1. Schaeffer AJ, Nicolle LE. Clinical practice. Urinary tract infections in older men. N Engl J Med. 2016;374(6): 562-71.
2. Lipsky BA, Byren I, Hoey CT. Treatment of bacterial prostatitis. Clin Infect Dis. 2010;50(12):1641-52.

21. Ans. D

Emphysematous pyelonephritis is a fulminant necrotizing infection of the renal parenchyma characterized by production of gas. Renal parenchymal collection of gas can be focal or diffuse, and can spread to the collecting system and perinephric space. Emphysematous pyelitis comprises gas collection only in the collecting system and has better prognosis than emphysematous pyelonephritis.

Treatment of emphysematous pyelonephritis involves achieving hemodynamic stability, blood glucose control, and broad spectrum antimicrobials targeting gram-negative bacteria. Ureteric obstruction if present must be relieved by percutaneous nephrostomy or ureteric stenting. CT-guided percutaneous drainage is the preferred method in patients who have focal gas collection with preserved surrounding renal tissue. Nephrectomy is indicated in patients with nonfunctioning kidney, fulminant renal damage, extension of gas into perinephric or pararenal space, and multiple underlying risk factors.

Ref:
1. Pontin AR, Barnes RD. Current management of emphysematous pyelonephritis. Nat Rev Urol. 2009;6(5):272-9.

22. Ans. D

The most common organisms isolated in urine and kidney tissue cultures in emphysematous pyelonephritis are E. coli and K. pneumoniae. Other organisms include Acinetobacter, Proteus, Streptococcus, and Pseudomonas. Histological examination of the infected kidney reveals vascular occlusion, intra-arterial infection and microabscesses. Hyperglycemia, impaired renal perfusion due to vascular occlusion, and infection with gas-forming organisms will together lead to accumulation of gas, which is commonly composed of carbon dioxide, nitrogen, and hydrogen.

Risk factors for developing emphysematous pyelonephritis include females with diabetes, urinary tract obstruction, renal transplant recipients, and underlying immune deficiency. Presentation includes fever, flank pain, renal angle tenderness, nausea, and vomiting. Rapid progression will lead to altered sensorium, renal failure, and septic shock. Pyuria is a common finding on urine routine examination.

X-ray imaging may reveal gas in the collecting system or perinephric space if extensive and renal calculi. CT scan is the investigation of choice for diagnosis of emphysematous pyelonephritis and shows the extent of renal involvement, spread to collecting system, and perinephric space. It is also useful for detection of renal calculi and ureteric obstruction.

Ref:
1. Pontin AR, Barnes RD. Current management of emphysematous pyelonephritis. Nat Rev Urol. 2009;6(5):272-9.

23. Ans. D

Risk factors for UTI in pregnancy include coexistent genital tract infection, diabetes, urinary tract abnormalities, vesicoureteric reflux, and previous UTIs. ASB is seen in 2–7% of pregnant women. Screening and treatment of ASB is recommended during pregnancy to prevent further development of pyelonephritis. Overall incidence of pyelonephritis in pregnancy is 1%; however, it is seen in 30–40% of women with ASB. Treatment of ASB will reduce the incidence of pyelonephritis by 80%. ASB and UTI in pregnancy can be associated with adverse maternal and fetal outcomes such as preterm delivery and low birth weight because of progression to pyelonephritis. Repeat screening of patients treated for ASB is recommended as they can have recurrent bacteriuria.

Ref:
1. Glaser AP, Schaeffer AJ. Urinary tract infection and bacteriuria in pregnancy. Urol clin North Am. 2015;42(4):547-60.

24. Ans. D

Perineal bacteria enter the urinary tract via retrograde route and cause UTI. Dilated ureters and relative urinary stasis contribute to further ascent and development of pyelonephritis. E. coli is the most common organism causing UTI in pregnancy. Other enterobacteriaceae and gram-positive organisms (group B streptococci) are also common.

Pyelonephritis in pregnancy most commonly occurs in the second or third trimester. It is more common on the right side, probably due to dilated ureter. Other risk factors include abnormalities of the urinary tract and gestational diabetes. Pyelonephritis in pregnancy presents with fever, flank pain, and dysuria.

Initial treatment of pyelonephritis in pregnancy includes resuscitation with intravenous fluids and parenteral antibiotics. Oral antibiotics can be started after fever subsides and total duration of therapy is 2 weeks. Urine culture should be repeated after the course. Ultrasound evaluation will help in identification of renal calculi, pyonephrosis, and renal abscess. Prophylactic antibiotics (nitrofurantoin or cephalexin) throughout pregnancy are recommended for women with recurrent UTI and persistent ASB despite treatment.

Ref:
1. Glaser AP, Schaeffer AJ. Urinary tract infection and bacteriuria in pregnancy. Urol Clin North Am. 2015;42(4):547-60.

25. **Ans. A**

Fosfomycin use for treatment for UTIs has regained popularity due to activity against resistant organisms. Fosfomycin was discovered in 1969 and is produced by *Streptomyces* species. It exhibits activity against gram-positive pathogens such as *Enterococcus*, *Staphylococcus aureus*, and *Staphylococcus epidermidis*. Fosfomycin also exhibits considerable activity against gram-negative pathogens, such as *Salmonella* spp., *Shigella* spp., *E. coli*, *Klebsiella*, and *Enterobacter* spp., *Serratia* spp., *Citrobacter* spp., and *Proteus mirabilis*.

Acinetobacter, *Stenotrophomonas*, and *Morganella morganii* demonstrate inherent resistance to fosfomycin. Activity against *Pseudomonas* is variable. However, combining fosfomycin with cefepime or meropenem for *Acinetobacter* and aminoglycoside for *P. aeruginosa* can have synergistic effect. Toxicity of aminoglycosides, glycopeptides, and polymyxin B can be reduced by combination with fosfomycin as lower drug doses can be used.

Fosfomycin is excreted into the urine and peak urine concentrations are reached within 4 hours of oral dose administration. Drug concentration remains high in urine and bladder tissue for next 1–2 days. Following intravenous fosfomycin administration, >90% drug is excreted unchanged in the urine.

Oral fosfomycin 3 g single dose is recommended for treatment of uncomplicated cystitis. For complicated UTI, 3 g oral fosfomycin every 2–3 days for three doses may be used. Intravenous fosfomycin is administered as 8 g of fosfomycin twice daily. However, 24 g total daily dose can be administered in patients with central nervous system (CNS) or other severe infections. Common side effects include diarrhea, nausea, and abdominal pain. Single dose fosfomycin can be used for treatment of ASB and cystitis in pregnancy.

Ref:
1. Falagas ME, Vouloumanou EK, Samonis G, Vardakas KZ. Fosfomycin. Clin Microbiol Rev. 2016;29(2):321-47.

26. **Ans. C**

Fungal UTI is most commonly caused by *C. albicans*. Spread to the kidneys can occur by hematogenous route or retrograde involvement. In the presence of candidemia, yeast forms will penetrate renal tubules followed by interstitium and form cortical and medullary fungal abscesses. Entry of the yeast forms into the collecting system can lead to formation of fungus balls in renal pelvis. *Candida* species show poor adherence to the urothelium. However, candidal invasion of the bladder and retrograde spread to kidney is possible with underlying urinary tract obstruction, concomitant bacteriuria or immunosuppression. Biofilm formation is more common with latex and silicone urinary catheters than polyvinylchloride or polyurethane catheters.

Predisposing factors for candiduria and *Candida* UTIs include extremes of age, female gender, diabetes, kidney transplant, urinary tract obstruction, renal calculi, indwelling urinary catheters, instrumentation of the urinary tract, broad-spectrum antibiotics, and admission to ICU.

Ref:
1. Fisher JF, Kavanagh K, Sobel JD, Kauffman CA, Newman CA. Candida urinary tract infection: pathogenesis. Clin Infect Dis. 2011;52 (Suppl 6):S437-51.
2. Achkar JM, Fries BC. Candida infections of the genitourinary tract. Clin Microbiol Rev. 2010;23(2):253-73.

27. **Ans. B**

Candiduria can commonly appear due to contamination during sample collection and most patients are asymptomatic. Most of them do not have a fungal UTI. Symptomatic patients with cystitis can present with frequency, urgency, dysuria, suprapubic pain, and fever. Fungal pyelonephritis can present as fever, flank pain, and renal angle tenderness. Oliguria, strangury (difficult and painful urination), passage of particulate matter or pneumaturia suggest a complication such as presence of a fungus ball. Neutropenic patients and critically ill patients may remain asymptomatic due weak inflammatory response and difficulty in communication.

Yeasts can appear in urine due to contamination during sample collection. Repeating a clean-voided, midstream sample is useful to confirm the presence of funguria. For patients with indwelling urinary catheter, change of catheter and fresh urine sample collection through this new catheter is suggested. In the presence of indwelling catheter, pyuria does not help in differentiating *Candida* UTI form colonization. Pyuria in the absence of indwelling catheter or bacteriuria is suggestive of *Candida* UTI.

Ultrasonography in *Candida* pyelonephritis may reveal hypoechoic renal abscess, fungus ball in the collecting system, and hydronephrosis. In males, prostatic abscess due to *Candida* infection may be present. CT urogram is useful for evaluation of pyelonephritis and renal abscess.

Ref:
1. Kauffman CA, Fisher JF, Sobel JD, Newman CA. Candida urinary tract infections—diagnosis. Clin Infect Dis. 2011;52 (Suppl 6):S452-6.

28. **Ans. C**

Elimination of predisposing factors is important step in management of fungal UTI. Fluconazole 200–400 mg orally once daily for 2 weeks is the drug of choice for candida cystitis. *Candida glabrata* and *Candida krusei* may demonstrate fluconazole resistance. Fluconazole is water soluble and excreted into the urine as active drug. However, other azoles have minimal excretion of the active compound into urine (itraconazole 1%, voriconazole 5%, and posaconazole 1%) and hence are not useful for treatment of cystitis. Alternatives include oral flucytosine and parenteral AmB. For patients with indwelling urinary catheters, continuous irrigation of the bladder with local AmB (50 mg AmB diluted in 1 L of sterile water) for 5–7 days may be used as an alternative. Although resolution of cystitis may be seen in 90%, relapse rates are high. Fluconazole is also the drug of choice for *Candida* pyelonephritis. AmB deoxycholate is an alternative for invasive renal parenchymal infection or systemic involvement. Lipid formulations of AmB have reduced nephrotoxicity, but urinary excretion is low. Hence they are not recommended for treatment of *Candida* pyelonephritis or cystitis.

Ref:
1. Pappas PG, Kauffman CA, Andes DR, Clancy CJ, Marr KA, Ostrosky-Zeichner L, et al. Clinical Practice Guideline for the Management of Candidiasis: 2016 Update by the Infectious Diseases Society of America. Clin Infect Dis. 2016;62(4):e1-50.
2. Achkar JM, Fries BC. Candida infections of the genitourinary tract. Clin Microbiol Rev. 2010;23(2): 253-73.

29. **Ans. D**

Elimination of predisposing factors, such as indwelling catheters, whenever feasible is recommended for treatment of asymptomatic candiduria. Treatment with antifungal agents is recommended for neutropenic patients, very low-birth-weight infants (<1,500 g), and patients who will undergo urologic manipulation to prevent disseminated candidiasis. Neutropenic patients and very low-birth-weight infants should be treated as for candidemia and disseminated candidiasis. Patients undergoing urologic procedures should be treated with 400 mg fluconazole once daily or AmB deoxycholate (0.3–0.6 mg/kg daily) for several days before and after the procedure.

Ref:
1. Pappas PG, Kauffman CA, Andes DR, Clancy CJ, Marr KA, Ostrosky-Zeichner L, et al. Clinical Practice Guideline for the Management of Candidiasis: 2016 Update by the Infectious Diseases Society of America. Clin Infect Dis. 2016;62(4):e1-50.

30. **Ans. A**

Candida auris is a nonalbicans *Candida* that is difficult to identify, often multidrug resistant is associated with outbreaks in ICUs. Even after treatment for invasive infection, patients may remain colonized with *C. auris* for long periods. It may persist in the environment and withstand many routinely used disinfectants. Transmission despite the implementation of enhanced infection prevention and control practices is a particular concern. Risk factors for colonization include contact with patients known to harbor *C. auris* or their environment. *C. auris* has been reported to cause candidemia, respiratory tract, urogenital system, abdominal, skin and soft tissue, surgical wound site infections, and central venous catheter-associated infections.

Candida auris is commonly misidentified as *Candida haemulonii* due to phylogenetic relationship. *C. auris* spectra included in the matrix-assisted laser desorption/ionization time-of-flight mass spectrometry (MALDI-TOF MS) database can identify it reliably. Other methods include molecular methods for deoxyribonucleic acid (DNA) sequencing of genetic loci and PCR assays.

Due to reported multidrug resistance, echinocandins (anidulafungin, caspofungin, micafungin) are recommended for initial therapy. Liposomal AmB is an alternative for patients with persistent fungemia for >5 days and no clinical improvement with echinocandins. However, echinocandins due to heavy molecular weight have minimal excretion of the active compound into urine as well as limited penetration into cerebrospinal fluid. Hence, AmB is suggested for the treatment of UTI caused by *C. auris*. 5-flucytosine may be added for improving outcomes.

Ref:
1. Jeffery-Smith A, Taori SK, Schelenz S, Jeffery K, Johnson EM, Borman A, et al. Candida auris: a Review of the Literature. Clin Microbiol Rev. 2017;31(1):e00029-17.
2. Centers for Disease Control and Prevention (2019). Candida auris. Information for Laboratorians and Health Professionals. [online] Available from: https://www.cdc.gov/fungal/candida-auris/health-professionals.html. [Last accessed on February, 2020].

CHAPTER 14

Bone and Joint Infections

Gautam Zaveri, Harshad Argekar

PART 1

1. *Staphylococcus aureus* is the normal flora in which part of the body?
   A. Nasal cavity
   B. Axillary folds
   C. Sebaceous glands
   D. Hair follicles

2. The most abundant bacterium on the human skin is:
   A. *Staphylococcus epidermidis*
   B. *Staphylococcus aureus*
   C. *Escherichia coli*
   D. *Streptococcus pyogenes*

3. Preoperative skin preparation with chlorhexidine:
   A. Eliminates all skin bacteria
   B. Prevents further growth of skin organisms
   C. Reduces resident microbial count
   D. Prevents skin sebum from being secreted

4. Removal of hair from operative site:
   A. To be done 24 hours before surgery
   B. Not necessary at all
   C. Use of hair clippers just before surgery, if hair interferes with surgery
   D. Use a razor just before incision

5. Currently recommended method for wound lavage in open wounds is:
   A. High-pressure pulse jet lavage
   B. Antibiotic solution wash
   C. Wash with povidone iodine
   D. Low-pressure wash with soap solution

6. Peak elution of vancomycin from impregnated cement beads is achieved in:
   A. 24 hours
   B. 4 days
   C. 3 weeks
   D. 6 weeks

7. Best method to obtain specimen for culture in a periprosthetic joint infection (PJI) is:
   A. From a discharging sinus
   B. Predebridement sample from open wounds
   C. Intraoperative wound swab
   D. Multiple deep tissue samples

8. *Streptococcus* is the most common cause of:
   A. Infantile osteomyelitis
   B. Juvenile osteomyelitis
   C. Adult osteomyelitis
   D. Chronic osteomyelitis

9. The epiphysis is crossed by blood vessels in:
   A. Infants (<1 year of age)
   B. Children up to 4 years of age
   C. Never at any age
   D. Crosses at all ages

10. In hematogenous osteomyelitis, earliest radiographic changes are seen at:
    A. In 24 hours
    B. At 3 weeks
    C. In 7–14 days
    D. Only after 6 weeks

11. What is *not* a common radiologic feature of acute osteomyelitis?
    A. Soft-tissue swelling
    B. Moth-eaten trabecular destruction
    C. Periosteal new bone formation
    D. Sequestrum

12. In children, the best investigation for detection of early changes of osteomyelitis is:
    A. MRI
    B. Ultrasonography
    C. Plain X-ray
    D. CT scan

13. Which statement related to helpfulness of MRI in osteomyelitis is *false*?
    A. Helps in detection of sequestra
    B. Better differentiation of osteomyelitis from tumors after contrast
    C. Differentiation between reactive edema and inflammation of osteomyelitis
    D. Visualization of fistulous tracts

PART 2

14. Patients with sickle cell disease are prone to osteomyelitis caused by:
    A. *Salmonella*
    B. *Staphylococcus aureus*
    C. *Klebsiella*
    D. *Staphylococcus epidermidis*

15. Which of the following antibiotic can be used as an effective alternative to intravenous (IV) vancomycin for the treatment of severe soft tissue infections caused by methicillin-resistant *Staphylococcus aureus* (MRSA)?
    A. Ciprofloxacin
    B. Linezolid
    C. Clindamycin
    D. Gentamicin

16. New bone formation surrounding a sequestrum as a result of osteomyelitis is known as:
    A. Osteophyte
    B. Osteosarcoma
    C. Sequestrum
    D. Involucrum

17. The X-ray below shows:

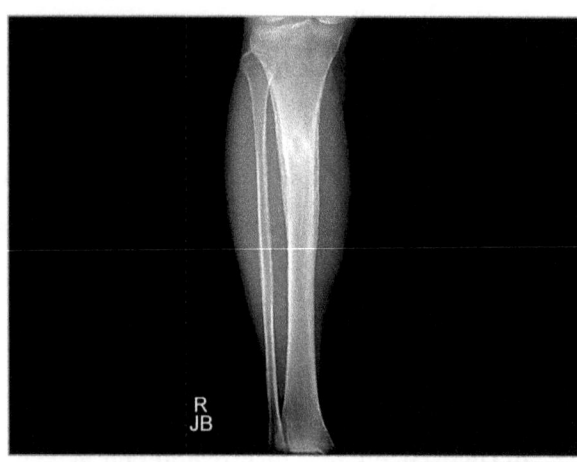

    A. Osteoid osteoma
    B. Acute osteomyelitis
    C. Brodie's abscess
    D. Enchondroma

18. Discharging sinus of chronic osteomyelitis is indicative of:
    A. Resistant organism
    B. Unresolved abscess
    C. Presence of sequestrum
    D. Acute on chronic osteomyelitis

19. End result of pyogenic arthritis is:
    A. Fibrous ankylosis
    B. Bony ankylosis
    C. Painful but mobile joint
    D. Painless mobile joint

20. Hematogenous osteomyelitis seeds in:
    A. Synovium
    B. Diaphysis
    C. Epiphysis
    D. Metaphysis

21. Madura foot is:
    A. Tuberculosis of the foot
    B. Chronic neuropathic foot infection
    C. Chronic bacterial osteomyelitis
    D. Fungal osteomyelitis of foot

22. End result of tuberculosis osteomyelitis is:
    A. Bony ankylosis
    B. Neuropathic joint
    C. Painful mobile joint
    D. Fibrous ankylosis

23. Osteomyelitis of short bones is mostly caused by:
    A. *Salmonella*
    B. *Mycobacterium tuberculosis*
    C. *Candida*
    D. *Escherichia coli*

24. Wandering acetabulum is a feature of:
    A. Developmental dysplasia of the hip
    B. Perthes disease
    C. Tuberculosis of hip
    D. Unreduced central dislocation of hip

25. Which of the following antibiotics cannot be used with poly methyl methacrylate (PMMA) as a carrier for local drug delivery?
    A. Gentamycin
    B. Piperacillin
    C. Tobramycin
    D. Ciprofloxacin

26. The release of antibiotics from PMMA bone cement occurs:
    A. In two phases
    B. As a continuous slow process
    C. Within first 24 hours
    D. Initial peak at 24 hours followed by another peak at 3 weeks

27. For an antibiotic to be used with PMMA as a drug carrier, all of the following features are required, except:
    A. Must remain stable at higher temperatures
    B. Should be hydrophilic
    C. Should react chemically with PMMA to form a compound enabling slow release
    D. Should be bactericidal

28. Which of the following is not true regarding tubercular osteomyelitis of long bones?
    A. It is a secondary tuberculosis (TB)
    B. Periosteal reaction is seen
    C. Sequestration is uncommon
    D. Inflammation is minimum

29. Pathological changes of tuberculous arthritis include:
    A. Synovial membrane is markedly thickened and transformed to tuberculous granulation tissue

B. No spasm or wasting of the surrounding muscles
C. Destruction of epiphyseal cartilage occurs first then erosion of the underlying bones
D. Dislocation of joint never occurs.

30. **Clinical presentation of tuberculous arthritis includes:**
    A. High-grade fever and malaise
    B. Constant and severe pain
    C. Sharp pain occurs at night
    D. Localized abscess with redness and warmth

31. **The common site of bone rarefaction of tuberculous arthritis of the hip joint is:**
    A. Upper part of the acetabulum
    B. Superior pubic ramus
    C. Lesser trochanter
    D. Lower part of the neck of femur close to epiphysis

PART 3

32. **Based on the classification developed by the National Academy of Sciences, an operative wound in which a viscus has entered under controlled circumstances and without unusual contamination is classified as:**
    A. Clean   B. Clean-contaminated
    C. Contaminated   D. Dirty

33. **The Centre for Disease Control and Prevention (CDC), USA and the Health Care Infection Control Practices Advisory Committee (HICPAC) have labeled infections of the incision, organ, or operative space as SSIs, if they occur:**
    A. Within 1 week of surgery and up to 1 month after surgery in patients receiving implants.
    B. Within 30 days of surgery and up to 1 year after surgery in patients receiving implants.
    C. Within 3 months of surgery and up to 1 year after surgery in patients receiving implants.
    D. At any time after surgery.

34. **Pyrexia within 24 hours of surgery is most unlikely due to:**
    A. Stress of surgery
    B. Pyrogenic reactions from IV infusions/blood transfusions
    C. Surgical site infection
    D. Adverse reaction to administered drugs

35. **Antibiotic prophylaxis for joint replacement surgery must be administered:**
    A. 24 hours before the surgery
    B. Between 3 and 24 hours prior to the incision
    C. Within ½ hour after making the incision
    D. Between ½ and 2 hours prior to the incision

36. **Repeating the antibiotic during orthopedic surgery is recommended in all of the following conditions, *except*:**
    A. Procedures > 4 hours duration
    B. Blood loss > 1,500 mL
    C. Patient also has extensive burns
    D. Patents with renal insufficiency

37. **The most specific and sensitive test to detect wound infection following spine surgery is:**
    A. Raised WBC count
    B. Raised C-reactive protein (CRP) and erythrocyte sedimentation rate (ESR)
    C. MRI scan
    D. Plain X-rays

38. **All of the following are common with brucellar spondylodiskitis, *except*:**
    A. History of contact with farm animals
    B. Undulant fever pattern with back pain
    C. Dorsal spine involvement
    D. MRI showing severe disk destruction with minimal adjacent bone destruction

39. **In a suspected case of tuberculous spondylodiskitis, the biopsy specimen must be sent for all of the following tests, *except*:**
    A. Tubercular smear, culture, and drug sensitivity
    B. Pyogenic smear, culture, and drug sensitivity
    C. GeneXpert
    D. Histopathological examination
    E. Tubercular IgG and IgM

40. **A 15-year-old girl presents with severe back pain, localized kyphotic deformity, fever, weight loss, and anorexia for 1 month. X-ray is as shown. Which among the following tests is the most sensitive test to confirm the diagnosis of tubercular spondylodiskitis?**

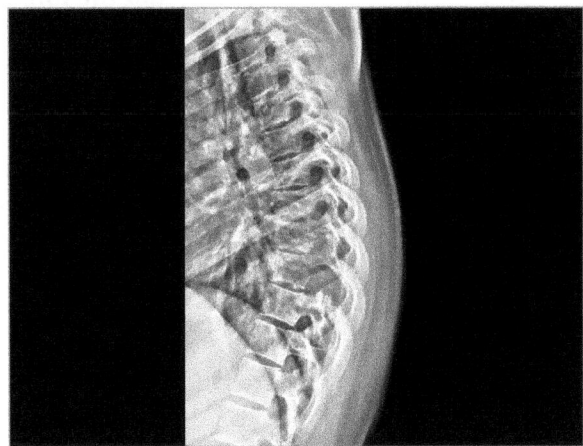

    A. Mantoux test
    B. Sputum for acid-fast bacilli (AFB)

C. Tubercular IgG and IgM
D. MRI

41. In 2011, which of the following Indian cities was reported to have the highest incidence of multidrug-resistant tuberculosis (MDR-TB)?
    A. Bengaluru
    B. New Delhi
    C. Ernakulam
    D. Mumbai

42. For osteoarticular tuberculosis, current recommendations from WHO suggest that antitubercular chemotherapy should be continued for:
    A. 6 months
    B. 9–12 months
    C. 18–24 months
    D. 36 months

43. A 36-year-old male presented with progressive mid back pain for the past 3 months, which was accompanied by constitutional symptoms of low-grade fever, weight loss, and anorexia. He had suffered from spinal and pulmonary tuberculosis 10 years ago for which a biopsy had been done, which showed that the organisms were sensitive to all antitubercular drugs. He had taken full course of treatment and stopped medications only after 1 year on the advice of a doctor. His current MRI picture is as shown:

What is the most appropriate next step?
    A. Start primary line of antitubercular drugs
    B. Start treatment for multidrug-resistant tuberculosis
    C. Perform a core biopsy
    D. Surgery

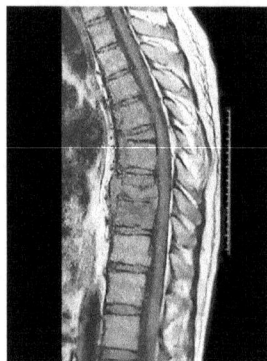
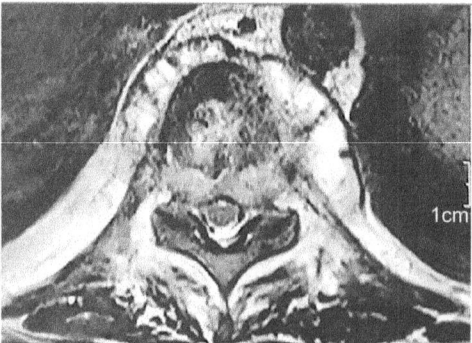
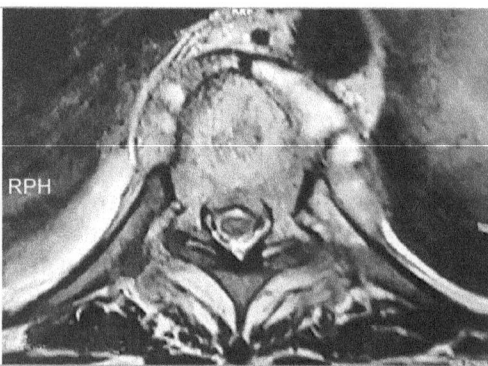

44. Indications for surgery in spinal tuberculosis include all of the following, *except*:
    A. Severe neurologic deficit
    B. Spinal instability
    C. Kyphosis > 40°
    D. Large disease load

45. A 34-year-old lady presented with fever, anorexia, weight loss, and severe back pain, power—MRC grade 4 in both lower limbs, and the following MRI picture. Her total WBC count was 6,000/mm^3, ESR was 110 mm/h, and CRP was 1:36. A vertebral biopsy revealed *Mycobacterium tuberculosis* that was sensitive to all drugs. She was started on four drug ATT including INH + R + Z + E. At the 6-week follow-up, improvement is most likely to be observed in which of the following?
    A. ESR
    B. Neurologic deficit
    C. Constitutional symptoms
    D. MRI

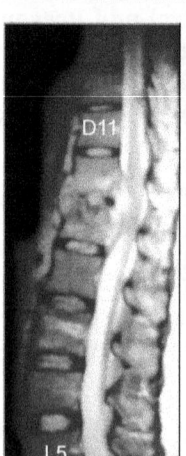
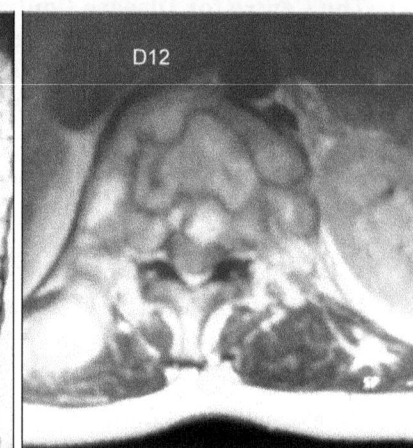

46. A 22-year-old lady presented with severe back pain, constitutional symptoms of fever, loss of appetite and weight loss, and early neurologic deficit—mild spasticity, brisk reflexes, and upgoing plantar reflex. She was biopsied and found to be rifampicin sensitive on GeneXpert. She was started on four drugs ATT (INH + R + Z + E). Her subsequent culture reports revealed that she had infection due

to *Mycobacterium tuberculosis* that was sensitive to all drugs. At the 3-month follow-up, the patient had significant reduction in back pain, neurologic deficit, and constitutional symptoms. However, a repeat MRI showed a slight increase in the size of the paraspinal abscess and of the vertebral collapse. What is the next most appropriate treatment?

A. Start second-line ATT for MDR tuberculosis
B. Add linezolid to the existing regime
C. Repeat a biopsy
D. Continue present line of management

47. A 45-year-old lady presented to a general surgeon with a swelling over the back as shown. Her total WBC count was 7,200/mm³, ESR was 74 mm Hg, and the CRP was 1:24. She was HIV negative. The next most appropriate step would be:

A. Aspiration of the abscess
B. Obtaining a X-ray/MRI
C. Starting IV antibiotics
D. Drainage of the abscess

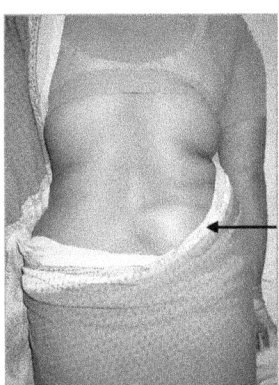

ANSWERS WITH EXPLANATIONS

PART 1

1. **Ans. A**

   The most common aerobic bacteria are *Staphylococcus epidermidis* (79%), diphtheroids (41%), and *Staphylococcus aureus* (34%).
   Ref:
   1. Savolainen S, Ylikoski J, Jousimies-Somer H. The bacterial flora of the nasal cavity in healthy young men. Rhinology. 1986;24(4):249-55.

2. **Ans. A**

   Historically, *Staphylococcus epidermidis* and other coagulase-negative *Staphylococci* (CONS) have been regarded as the primary bacterial colonizers of the skin. *S. epidermidis* is a major inhabitant of the skin, and in some areas, it makes up more than 90% of the resident aerobic flora.
   Ref:
   1. Baron S. Medical Microbiology, 4th edition. Galveston (TX): University of Texas Medical Branch at Galveston; 1996.

3. **Ans. C**

   As microorganisms tend to colonize the deeper layers of the stratum corneum, they are not shed with desquamation. There are two types of microorganisms on the skin—(1) commensals, which are normally resident, and (2) transients, which are not consistently present and are easily exchanged between individuals.

   The transient organisms are easily removed, whereas, it has been suggested that the commensals are difficult to remove completely.
   Ref:
   1. Dumville JC, McFarlane E, Edwards P, Lipp A, Holmes A. Preoperative skin antiseptics for preventing surgical wound infections after clean surgery. Cochrane Database Syst Rev. 2013;(3):CD003949.

4. **Ans. C**

   Do not remove hair at the operative site unless it will interfere with the operation; do not use razors—if necessary, remove by clipping or by use of a depilatory agent just before surgery.
   Ref:
   1. Centers for Disease Control and Prevention. Top CDC Recommendations to Prevent Healthcare-Associated Infections. [online] Available from: https://www.cdc.gov/HAI/pdfs/hai/top-cdc-recs-factsheet.pdf [Last accessed on February, 2020].

5. **Ans. D**

   Certain solutions may be more effective in removing bacteria from bone than mechanical irrigation with saline solution alone. Among the various solutions examined, the soap solution preserved the number and activity of osteoblasts the most. Low-pressure lavage with soap solution resulted in the greatest removal of adherent bacteria from bone. Use of povidone iodine or chlorhexidine as a solution for wash may decrease the number and activity of the osteoblasts resulting in alteration in bone activity.

Ref:
1. Bhandari M, Adili A, Schemitsch EH. The efficacy of low-pressure lavage with different irrigating solutions to remove adherent bacteria from bone. J Bone Joint Surg Am. 2001;83(3):412-9.

6. **Ans. A**

The release of vancomycin and gentamycin was measured in the drainage fluid on a daily basis. The drains were left in situ until less than 50 mL was produced per day. The elution of both antibiotics was determined by fluorescence polarization immunoassay. Systemic antibiotics were given postoperatively according to antibiogram. If possible, no gentamicin or vancomycin was given. Peak mean concentrations from beads and spacers were reached for gentamicin [1,160 (12–371) µg/mL and 21 (0.7–39) µg/mL, respectively] and for vancomycin [80 (21–198) µg/mL and 37 (3.3–72) µg/mL] on Day 1. The last concentrations to be determined were 3.7 µg/mL gentamicin and 23 µg/mL vancomycin in the beads group after 13 days, and 1.9 µg/mL gentamicin and 6.6 µg/mL vancomycin in the spacer group after 7 days.

Ref:
1. Anagnostakos K, Wilmes P, Schmitt E, Kelm J. Elution of gentamicin and vancomycin from polymethylmethacrylate beads and hip spacers in vivo. Acta Orthopaedica. 2009;80(2):193-7.

7. **Ans. D**

The greatest accuracy of PJI diagnosis is obtained when three periprosthetic tissue specimens are obtained and inoculated into blood culture bottles, or four periprosthetic tissue specimens are obtained and cultured using standard plate and broth cultures. Increasing the number of specimens to five or more, per current recommendations, does not improve accuracy of PJI diagnosis.

Ref:
1. Peel TN, Spelman T, Dylla BL, Hughes JG, Greenwood-Quaintance KE, Cheng AC, et al. Optimal periprosthetic tissue specimen number for diagnosis of prosthetic joint infection. J Clin Microbiol. 2016;55(1):234-43.
2. Schnettler R, Steinau HU. Septic Bone & Joint Surgery. New York: Thieme; 2011.

8. **Ans. A**

Infantile osteomyelitis (up to age of 12 months) is an acutely progressive disease that often shows multicentric and articular involvement. Sites of predilection are the femoral metaphyses, hips, and humerus. The diaphyseal, metaphyseal, and epiphyseal blood vessels create potential pathways for epiphyseal and subperiosteal spread. The main causative organisms are *Streptococci*.

9. **Ans. A**

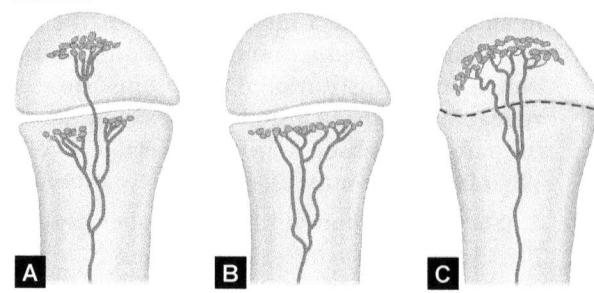

During the first year of life, the vessels cross the epiphyseal plate (A). From approximately 2–16 years of age, the vessels become obliterated and the epiphysis forms a barrier to hematogenous spread (B). By skeletal maturity, the blood vessels again establish a connection between the epiphysis and the metaphysis (C).

10. **Ans. C**

Hematogenous osteomyelitis produces radiographically detectable bone changes by 7–14 days at the earliest. Trabecular bone at that time may show ill-defined margins with a geographic, moth-eaten, or permeative pattern of bone destruction. The lesion margins are indistinct. The cortex is initially eroded from the inside before varying degrees of cortical destruction can be seen. Note that destructive changes are more difficult to detect in trabecular bone than in compact bone. The infection may spread outward through the cortical bone, elevating the periosteum and causing radiographically detectable periosteal new bone formation. If the spread of infection deprives bony areas of their blood supply, these areas will become necrotic and will eventually appear on radiographs as sequestra. Reactive new bone formation may completely isolate the sequestrum from surrounding bone (involucrum). Marked associated soft-tissue swelling, especially about joints, will often develop within 3–5 days in infants and small children.

11. **Ans. D**

Sequestrae are a feature of chronic osteomyelitis. In acute osteomyelitis, the soft tissue swelling is visible after 3–4 days and bone changes after 7–14 days. The bone changes in acute osteomyelitis include trabecular bone destruction (geographic, moth eaten and permeative) and subperiosteal new bone formation.

12. **Ans. A**

The value of ultrasound in acute osteomyelitis is inversely proportional to patient age. In infants, the early phase of osteomyelitis is initially marked by edematous swelling of the deeper soft tissues. This is followed later by the appearance of thin echo-free subperiosteal fluid collection that visibly elevates the periosteum; however, these changes are nonspecific and there is a substantial incidence of false-positive (40%) and false-negative findings.

Computed tomography has a minor role in pediatric cases due to its high radiation.

13. **Ans. C**

It is difficult for MRI to distinguish between inflammatory tissue and reactive edema, between active and inactive inflammation in chronic osteomyelitis and among periosteitis, osteomyelitis, and reactive bone edema associated with primary soft-tissue inflammation.

PART 2

14. **Ans. A**

Salmonellosis is one of the most frequent serious infections in sickle cell patients and remains a significant cause of morbidity and mortality in this population. Capillary occlusion secondary to intravascular sickling may devitalize and infarct the gut, permitting *Salmonella* invasion. Reduced function of the liver and spleen, together with interference with reticuloendothelial system function due to erythrophagocytosis, suppresses clearing of these organisms from the bloodstream.

15. **Ans. B**

Linezolid can be given orally, 600 mg every 12 hours, and it is well tolerated. No adverse effects were reported in various studies. It has the advantage of oral administration and being safer than vancomycin. Some studies have shown a higher clinical cure rate with linezolid (94%) as compared to (84%) with vancomycin.

16. **Ans. D**

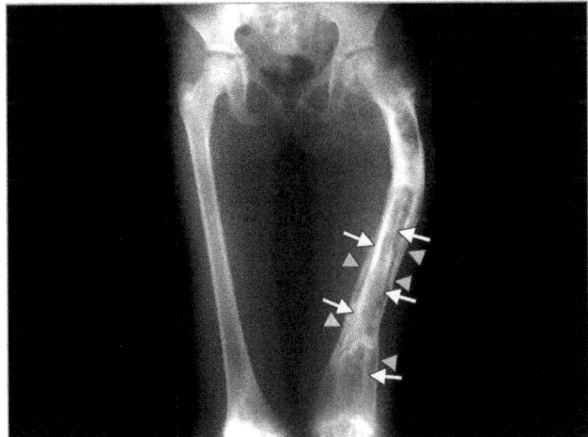

White arrows pointing at the sequestrum while the arrowheads pointing at the involucrum.

Infection causes the periosteum to be elevated from bone. This causes formation of new bone, which surrounds the infected bony tissue. The infected bone eventually forms the sequestrum, whereas the new bone produced is called the involucrum.

17. **Ans. C**

Subacute osteomyelitis is a distinct form of osteomyelitis, and Brodie abscess is one type of subacute osteomyelitis. Subacute osteomyelitis appears to depend on the interplay between the infecting bacteria and the immune mechanism of the host. True primary subacute osteomyelitis represents a favorable host-pathogen response. The pyogenic organisms' initial attack is presumed to be controlled by the host, and presumably no spread to large areas of cancellous tissue or to the subperiosteal region has occurred. A central area of suppurative necrosis in the metaphyseal region becomes enclosed by a wall of fibrous tissue and granulations, the offending organisms are destroyed, and the pus may be sterile.

18. **Ans. C**

A sequestrum is an avascular bone, which serves as a reservoir of bacteria. Chronic persistent discharge indicates presence of a sequestrum in an otherwise vascular area.

19. **Ans. B**

Septic arthritis in adults leads to complete destruction of cartilage and finally a fusion across the joint. Chronic tuberculosis arthritis is more likely to cause a fibrous ankylosis.

20. **Ans. D**

The majority of pediatric osteomyelitis cases are secondary to hematogenous spread. The infection seeds in the metaphysis where blood flow is rich but sluggish, as the capillaries approach the epiphyseal plate, they reverse direction by forming a loop and then merge into a network of sinusoidal venous blood lakes.

21. **Ans. D**

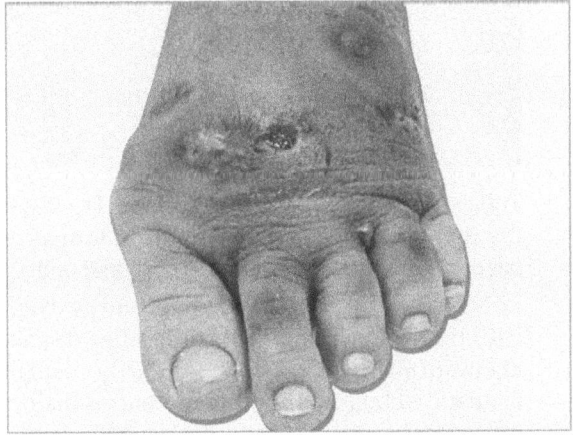

It is a chronic granulomatous fungal disease of humans, affecting mainly the limbs, and sometimes the abdominal and chest walls or the head. Mycetoma pedis (mycetoma of the foot), the most common form of mycetoma, is known widely as the Madura foot. The infection is endemic in Africa, India, and Central and South America.

22. **Ans. D**

Septic arthritis in adults leads to complete destruction of cartilage and finally a fusion across the joint. Chronic tuberculosis arthritis is more likely to cause a fibrous ankylosis.

23. **Ans. B**

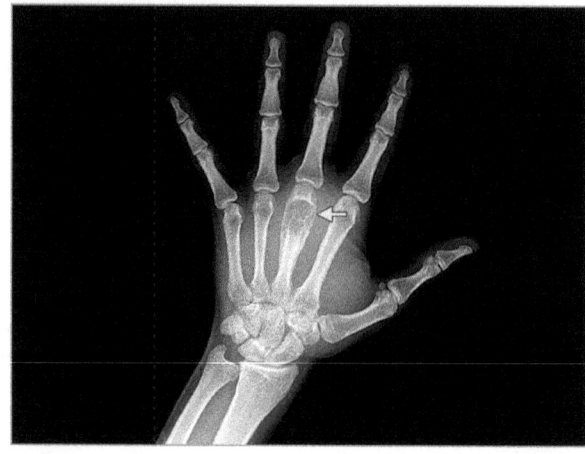

Whereas long bone infection is mostly caused by pyogenic organisms, osteomyelitis of small bones of the hands, feet is more likely to be caused by *Mycobacteria* (spina ventosa).

24. **Ans. C**

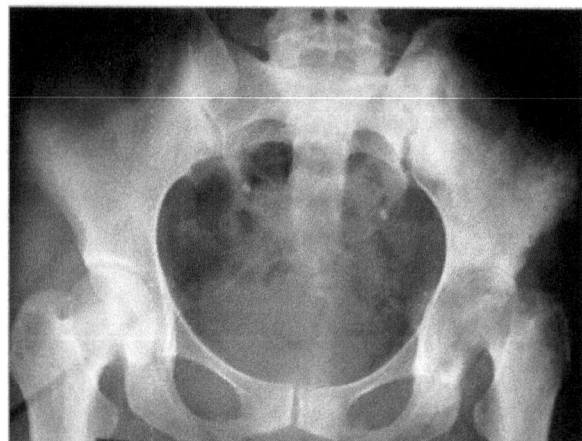

Tuberculous affection of the hip joint. Destruction of the roof of the acetabulum results in formation of a false acetabulum superior to the original one.

In a dislocated hip, the acetabulum is dysplastic with deficient sloping roof. In Perthes disease, the acetabulum is affected secondarily resulting in arthritic changes. Unreduced central dislocation causes protrusion. Tuberculosis involving the dome of acetabulum (most common site of origin) is the cause of a wandering acetabulum.

25. **Ans. D**

Ciprofloxacin is not heat stable and cannot be used as a locally acting drug with PMMA bone cement.

26. **Ans. A**

A rapid release of antibiotic takes place from the carrier cement in the first 24–48 hours. This is followed by a rapid decline in the next 48 hours and then a very gradual reduction over next 2–3 weeks.

27. **Ans. C**

The release of antibiotic from PMMA cannot occur, if it is chemically bound to the cement components.

28. **Ans. B**

Tubercular osteomyelitis more commonly affects the ends of the long bone, unlike pyogenic osteomyelitis, which affects the metaphysis.
- Bone and joint tuberculosis is always secondary to some primary focus in the lungs, lymph nodes, etc. The mode of spread from the primary focus may be either hematogenous or by direct extension from a neighboring focus.
- Tubercular osteomyelitis presents as a well-defined area of bone destruction, typically with minimal reactive new bone formation. This is unlike a pyogenic infection where reactive periosteal new bone formation is an important feature.
- As the condition proceeds, radiology shows bone destruction without the periosteal reaction so typical of pyogenic infection.
- Characteristic features of acute bacterial infection (osteomyelitis):
  - Periosteal reaction is characteristic.
  - Sequestrum is seen.
  - Involucrum is seen.
  - Abscess formation with signs of inflammation.

29. **Ans. A**

Tuberculous infection causes significant hypertrophy of the involved synovium and formation of a pannus, which spreads to destroy the cartilage and underlying bone.

Pain and effusion cause spasm and deformity of the affected joints. There is wasting of muscles of the joint involved.

Tuberculosis begins in the bone or synovium and epiphyseal cartilage is not involved primarily.

Long-standing TB affection results in destruction and dislocation of the joint.

30. **Ans. C**

"Night cries" occurs commonly in TB arthritis. This is because the spasmodic muscles relax when the patient sleeps. This causes the joint surfaces to move against each other, resulting in pain and sleep disturbance. TB being an insidious infection, the acute signs of inflammation are absent.

31. **Ans. A**

Upper part of the acetabulum is the most common site of affliction in tuberculosis, if hip is the supra-acetabular area.

Second most common site is the weight-bearing area of the femoral epiphysis.

The medial metaphyseal area and the greater trochanter are the least common sites of involvement.

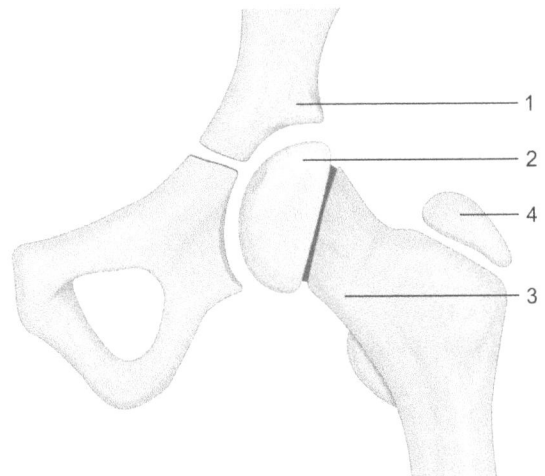

PART 3

32. Ans. B

A widely accepted wound classification system has been developed by the National Academy of Sciences and the National Research Council based upon the degree of expected microbial contamination during surgery. It stratifies wounds as clean, clean-contaminated, contaminated, or dirty using the following definitions:

- Clean wounds are uninfected operative wounds in which no inflammation is encountered and the wound is closed primarily. By definition, a viscus (respiratory, alimentary, genital, or urinary tract) is not entered during a clean procedure.
- Clean contaminated wounds are operative wounds in which a viscus is entered under controlled conditions and without unusual contamination.
- Contaminated wounds are open, fresh accidental wounds, operations with major breaks in sterile technique, or gross spillage from a viscus. Wounds in which acute, nonpurulent inflammation was encountered also were included in this category.
- Dirty wounds are old traumatic wounds with retained devitalized tissue, foreign bodies, or fecal contamination or wounds that involve existing clinical infection or perforated viscus.

Several studies have found a moderate correlation between the wound classification and the surgical site infection (SSI) rate. SSI rates were higher in dirty wound as compared to clean wounds.

Ref:
1. *Onyekwelu I, Yakkanti R, Protzer L, Pinkston CM, Tucker C, Seligson D. Surgical wound classification and surgical site infections in the orthopaedic patient. J Am Acad Orthop Surg Glob Res Rev. 2017;1(3):e022.*
2. *Anderson DJ, Sexton DJ. Antimicrobial prophylaxis for prevention of surgical site infection in adult. United States: UpToDate. 2015. pp. 1-31.*
3. *Olson M, O'Connor M, Schwartz ML. Surgical wound infections. A 5-year prospective study of 20,193 wounds at the Minneapolis VA Medical Center. Ann Surg. 1984;199(3):253-9.*
4. *Culver DH, Horan TC, Gaynes RP, Martone WJ, Jarvis WR, Emori TG, et al. Surgical wound infection rates by wound class, operative procedure, and patient risk index. National Nosocomial Infections Surveillance System. Am J Med. 1991;91(3B):152S-7S.*

33. Ans. B

Surgical site infections are infections of the incision, organ, or operative space that occur up to 30 days after surgery (or up to 1 year after surgery in patients receiving implants) and are a common type of health care-associated infection (HAI) as defined by the CDC and the Healthcare Infection Control Practices Advisory Committee (HICPAC).

Surgical site infections are placed into three categories depending on the extent or depth of infection:

- *Superficial incisional SSI*—skin or subcutaneous tissue is involved, occurs within 30 days postoperatively, and fulfilling one of the following additional criteria:
  - Purulent drainage from incision with or without diagnostic laboratory testing (culture)
  - Isolated organisms from aseptically obtained fluid or tissue culture in incision
  - At least one sign or symptom of clinical infection—localized pain, edema, erythema, warmth, and the superficial incision—is deliberately opened by a surgeon (unless culture of incision is negative)
  - Diagnosis of a superficial incisional SSI by a surgeon or attending physician.
- *Deep incisional SSI*—involves deep soft tissues such as fascia or muscle within the incision, occurs within 30 days postoperatively in wounds without an implant, occurs within 1 year if implant is in place and infection appears to be directly related to the surgical procedure, and must fulfill one of the following additional criteria:
  - Purulent drainage from incision but not from the organ/operative space
  - Dehiscence or deliberate opening by the surgeon from the deep incision when the patient has at least one of the following signs or symptoms of clinical infection (fever >100.4°F, localized pain or edema, unless culture is negative).
  - Abscess or other evidence of infection involving the deep incision is found during examination

of incision, reoperation, or pathological or radiological examination.
- Diagnosis of a deep incisional SSI by a surgeon or attending physician
- *Organ/space SSI*—involves any part of the anatomy other than the incision, occurs within 30 days postoperatively in cases without an implant, occurs within 1 year, if implant is in place and infection appears to be directly related to surgical procedure, and must fulfill one of the following:
  - Purulence from a drain that was placed via stab incision into the organ/space (infection of drain site is not an SSI)
  - Isolated organisms from aseptically obtained fluid or tissue from the organ/space
  - Abscess or other evidence of infection involving the deep incision is found during examination of incision, reoperation, or pathologic or radiological examination
  - Diagnosis of an organ/space SSI by a surgeon or attending physician

Ref:
1. *Anderson DJ, Sexton DJ. Antimicrobial prophylaxis for prevention of surgical site infection in adults. United States: UpToDate; 2015. pp. 1-31.*

34. Ans. C

Postoperative fever is not uncommon. The temperature elevation is usually <2° above the baseline of 98.6°F. Rise of temperature up to 103°F is not worrisome. The most common cause of postoperative fever is surgical stress. Adverse reactions to administered medications, pyrogenic reactions following intravenous infusions or blood transfusions, respiratory problems such as pneumonia or atelectasis, urinary tract infections, thrombophlebitis or deep vein thrombosis, and infected central lines are some of the other causes of postoperative pyrexia.

Unless there has been gross contamination of the surgical site at the time of surgery, as with unsterile instruments, it is rare for SSI to manifest within the first 48 hours after surgery.

35. Ans. D

It is critical to administer the prophylactic antibiotic at the correct time in order to provide maximum protection. The drug should ideally be administered within 30 minutes and certainly within 2 hours of the time of incision. Studies have shown that patients receiving antibiotic prophylaxis within the 2-hour window have lower SSI rates than those who receive it more than 3 hours before surgery. This ensures serum and tissue concentrations that exceed the minimum inhibitory concentration for the most probable organisms at the surgical site during the procedure. The first dose should always be given before the skin incision is performed. Antibiotics can also be used during an operation, if necessary, especially in procedures that last several hours. Administration of vancomycin or a fluoroquinolone should begin 120 minutes before surgical incision because of the prolonged infusion times required for these drugs.

Ref:
1. *Anderson DJ, Sexton DJ. Antimicrobial prophylaxis for prevention of surgical site infection in adults. United States: UpToDate; 2015. pp. 1-31.*
2. *Crader MF, Varacallo M (2020). Preoperative Antibiotic Prophylaxis. [online] Available from: https://www.ncbi.nlm.nih.gov/books/NBK442032/ [Last accessed on February, 2020].*

36. Ans. D

Repeat dosing is considered:
- For longer procedures (duration of surgery >3 hours), where it is readministered at intervals of one or two times the half-life of the drug (using the same dose).
- When there is excessive blood loss (>1,500 mL).
- In the setting of factors that shorten antimicrobial half-life, such as extensive burns.

Redosing may not be required for patients in whom the antimicrobial half-life is prolonged, such as renal insufficiency and for clean and clean-contaminated procedures, following closure of the surgical incision, even in the presence of a drain.

Ref:
1. *Anderson DJ, Sexton DJ. Antimicrobial prophylaxis for prevention of surgical site infection in adults. United States: UpToDate; 2015. pp. 1-31.*

37. Ans. C

Magnetic resonance imaging is the most sensitive (93%) and specific (96%) test for the evaluation of wound infections following spine surgery. The diagnostic features of SSI can be detected as early as 3–5 days postoperatively. Characteristic findings include decreased disk height, loss of end-plate definition, and high-intensity signal within the intervertebral disk and the vertebral endplates on T2-weighted images due to edema. Paravertebral or intradiskal fluid collection suggests the diagnosis of diskitis. STIR sequences on MRI are helpful in differentiating infection (higher signal intensity) from normal postoperative changes such as hematoma, reparative changes, and fibrosis. However, metal artifacts from spinal implants may render the MRI images unclear. In some cases, degenerative or inflammatory disease may mimic the MRI picture of infection.

Radiographs performed up to 4 weeks post the index procedure are usually normal. A decrease in intervertebral height may be observed between the 4th and 6th week postoperatively, while osteolysis, deformity, and endplate destruction are only expected to appear after 6 weeks.

The total white cell count, erythrocyte sedimentation rate (ESR), and C-reactive protein (CRP) are the most frequently used tests for both the diagnosis and follow-up of patients suspected to have SSI following spine surgery. The WBC count may be elevated in less than 50% cases of SSI, thus making it an unreliable marker of infection. Both CRP and ESR are routinely elevated in the postoperative period. The CRP levels peak on Day 3 postoperatively, and return to baseline by 10–14 days. ESR levels peak at around Day 14 after surgery, and take 6 weeks to return to baseline. CRP is more sensitive in the diagnosis of SSI than ESR (95% vs. 80%); however, it has a low positive predictive value (31%). A decreasing trend of these two parameters indicates that the initial rise was secondary to surgery. However, if the CRP is higher on Day 7 as compared to Day 3, then it may suggest the possibility of infection. A persistently elevated ESR and CRP value more than 15 days after surgery strongly suggests infection, but normal ESR and/or CRP values do not exclude this diagnosis.

Ref:
1. Hadjipavlou AG, Mader JT, Necessary JT, Muffoletto AJ. Hematogenous pyogenic spinal infections and their surgical management. Spine. 2000;25(13):1668-79.
2. Thelander U, Larsson S. Quantitation of C-reactive protein levels and erythrocyte sedimentation rate after spinal surgery. Spine (Phila Pa 1976). 1992;17(4):400-4.
3. Takahashi J, Ebara S, Kamimura M, Kinoshita T, Itoh H, Yuzawa Y, et al. Early-phase enhanced inflammatory reaction after spinal instrumentation surgery. Spine (Phila Pa 1976). 2001;26(15):1698-704.
4. Tyrrell PN, Cassar-Pullicino VN, McCall IW. Spinal infection. Eur Radiol. 1999;9:1066-77.

38. Ans. C

Brucella spondylitis is one of the most common differential diagnoses for tuberculous spondylitis. They share many common features including—(1) chronicity, (2) latency in clinical manifestation, (3) similar clinical features (back pain, fever, and elevated inflammatory markers), and (4) granulomatous lesions. In a history of direct contact (working) with domestic animals, undulant fever pattern may be suggestive of diagnosis. MRI findings to differentiate brucella from tuberculosis are enumerated in **Table 1**. The diagnosis, however, is best established by isolation of the causative organism on blood culture or biopsy and agglutination reaction with a brucella antibody.

Ref:
1. Gao M, Sun J, Jiang Z, Cui X, Liu X, Wang G, et al. Comparison of tuberculous and brucellar spondylitis on magnetic resonance images. Spine (Phila Pa 1976). 2017;42(2):113-21.

Table 1: MRI findings to differentiate brucella from tuberculosis.

Tuberculous spondylitis	Brucella spondylitis
Predominant dorsal involvement • Relative disk preservation • Mainly bone destruction • Significant destruction of vertebral architecture • Gibbous deformity common	Mainly affects the lumbar spine • Severe disk destruction • Mainly peridiskal bone destruction • Intact vertebral architecture • Minimal associated paraspinal soft tissue involvement • Absence of gibbous deformity
Diffuse, abnormal signals from the whole involved body	• Diffuse, abnormal signal mainly surrounding the peridiskal part of the vertebral body • Fan-shaped hyperintensity is a typical feature
• Typical psoas abscesses • More extensive subligamentous spread	Focal abscess with minimal subligamentous spread
Diffusion path → Body to body spread mode	Diffusion path → Body (disk) to disk (body) to body (disk) spread mode

39. Ans. E

The diagnosis of spinal tuberculosis is difficult. The yield rates are not very high. Hence, it is vital to send obtain adequate material for testing by performing a core biopsy with a wide-bore bone biopsy needle. The biopsy can be performed under CT guidance or fluoroscopy guidance. The material must be sent for routine microbiological examination for tubercular bacilli. However, this may take 6–12 weeks to obtain a positive result. GeneXpert is a PCR test that amplifies the nucleic acid of the tubercle bacilli. It can detect up to the limit of 130 colony-forming units (CFUs) per milliliter, compared with 10,000 CFU/mL in cultures. Another advantage is its rapid turnaround time, which is less than a day. It can also detect rifampicin resistance via the detection of mutations in the *rpoB* gene and thus aid in starting MDR treatment early in the course of therapy.

Ref:
1. Held M, Laubscher M, Zar H, Dunn R. GeneXpert polymerase chain reaction for spinal tuberculosis. Bone Joint J. 2014;96-B(10):1366-9.

40. Ans. D

Tubercular IgG and IgM have high specificity but lack sensitivity in endemic areas. WHO in 2011 issued an official statement that there is no evidence that these serological assays improve the management of patients. There is vast proportion of false-positive and false-negative results, which leads to adverse impact on patient safety. At present, there is no role of these investigations in management of tuberculosis.

Tuberculin skin testing (TST) or Mantoux test has limited role in diagnosing active TB disease in India. Asia and Africa are endemic zones for tuberculosis, where most of the population is either infected with bacilli in its life span or BCG vaccinated, so a positive TST does not always suggest an active disease. Similarly, several immunocompromised states as described above may have low or no TST reaction even in active disease state. TST still has an adjuvant diagnostic role in children less than 4 years, where sensitivity and specificity are more favorable.

Sputum AFB is usually negative in patients with spinal tuberculosis. Concomitant tubercular infection of the spine and lungs is not very common.

Although not very specific, MRI is extremely sensitive in diagnosing spinal infection. Hyperintensity signal within the paradiskal region appears early in the course of the disease.
Ref:
1. *Chatterjee K, Mandal P, Chaudhuri N, Mukherjee S, Chaudhuri N, Sen S. Status of enzyme-linked immunosorbent assay test for tuberculosis serology in low socio economic status and undernourished children with suspected pulmonary tuberculosis. Int J Contemp Pediatr. 2016;3(4):1348-54.*

41. Ans. D

Reported incidence of MDR-TB within India is 24% in Mumbai, 1.1% in Bengaluru and New Delhi, and 2% in Ernakulam.
Ref:
1. *Sharma SK, Kaushik G, Jha B, George N, Arora SK, Gupta D, et al. Prevalence of multidrug-resistant tuberculosis among newly diagnosed cases of sputum-positive pulmonary tuberculosis. Indian J Med Res. 2011;133:308-11.*

42. Ans. B

The WHO recommends 9–12 months of antitubercular chemotherapy for osteoarticular tuberculosis. The intensive phase where four drugs—isoniazid (INH), rifampicin (R), pyrazinamide (Z), and ethambutol (E)—are given lasts for 2 months while the maintenance phase requires administration of isoniazid and rifampicin for 7–10 months.
Ref:
1. *World Health Organization. Treatment of Tuberculosis: Guidelines for National Programmes, 4th edition. Geneva: World Health Organization; 2009.*

43. Ans. C

Although the patient had a previous infection with drug-sensitive *Mycobacterium*, it cannot be assumed that the same organism is the cause of the reinfection. Secondary resistance to antitubercular drugs is common among previously treated patients. Hence, a transpedicular biopsy of the lesion is recommended prior to starting antitubercular treatment (ATT). There are no indications for surgery in this patient presently.

44. Ans. D

Uncomplicated spinal tuberculosis is essentially a medical disease. Majority of patients can be treated successfully with antitubercular chemotherapy alone. Currently, indications for surgery include a severe neurologic deficit, so that the patient is unable to ambulate or the appearance of a fresh neurologic deficit while on ATT, presence of significant spinal instability or severe vertebral destruction leading to kyphosis. In the days before effective ATT was available, a large disease load was considered to be an indication for surgery. Drainage of large cold abscesses and debridement of dead and necrotic tissue reduced the amount of dead/necrotic tissue and promoted neovascularization of the diseased area, promoting healing.

45. Ans. C

Periodic follow-up is absolutely essential in all patients with tuberculosis in order to assess improvement/deterioration of the spinal infection as well as to look for side effects of ATT. The follow-up visit consists of clinical and radiological evaluation along with estimation of the ESR and CRP. The total WBC count, liver, and renal function tests are obtained to look for side effects of the ATT.

The first signs of infection control are an improvement in the constitutional symptoms with a feeling of well-being, improved appetite, and weight gain along with a reduction in the level of C-reactive proteins. The ESR takes a much longer time to normalize. Although the severe pain of acute infection starts reducing, it takes a longer time to become pain free. Neurologic deficits also take a longer time to normalize. Radiological signs of improvement typically lag behind the clinical improvement by about 3 months. Hence, an X-ray or MRI when obtained within the first 3 months of starting ATT may actually show worsening rather than improvement.

46. Ans. D

The patient has shown significant clinical improvement. A slight deterioration in the radiological presentation is not uncommon and must be expected within the first 2–3 months after starting ATT. Hence, the current treatment must be continued.

Even if this was MDR-TB, adding a single drug to a failing regime of ATT increases the risk of resistance and failure of treatment. Also, starting second-line ATT without appropriate cultures is not recommended. Hence, in case MDR-TB is strongly suspected, a repeat biopsy must be performed.

47. Ans. B

Whenever a patient presents with an abscess, especially in the extremities, the underlying bone/joint must be evaluated for evidence of infection. In case the bony infection is not diagnosed and adequately treated, the surgical wound may not heal and the infection may persist. The above patient had an underlying tubercular infection of the sacroiliac joint, which was undiagnosed. She landed up developing a nonhealing ulcer over the incision site.

CHAPTER 15

Human Immunodeficiency Virus

Om Shrivastav

1. **The biggest involvement in *Pneumocystis jirovecii* outside lungs is:**
   A. Gut
   B. Kidney
   C. Brain
   D. Adrenal gland

2. **The backbone of treatment in toxoplasma infection is:**
   A. Clindamycin and atovaquone
   B. Trimethoprim and dapsone
   C. Augmentin and albendazole
   D. Pyrimethamine and sulfadiazine

3. **A 36-year-old male presents with altered sensorium, fever, and weight loss of 22 kg in 10 weeks. His CD4 count is 15 cells/mm³, white cell count is 2,100/mm³, and Hb 3 g%. His chest X-ray is shown. He is transferred to an intensive care unit (ICU) because his blood gas shows PO_2 66, PCO_2 95, and HCO_3 17. A bone marrow was sent for examination from the ICU. The most likely diagnosis is:**

   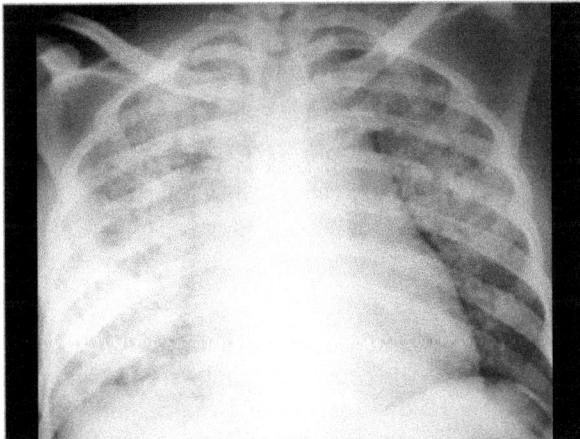

   Source: Kisembo HN, Den Boon S, Davis JL, Okello R, William W, Cattamanchi A, et al. Chest radiographic findings of pulmonary tuberculosis in severely immunocompromised patients with the human immunodeficiency virus. Br J Radiol. 2012;85(1014):e130-9.

   A. Histoplasmosis
   B. *Aspergillus* infection
   C. Coccidioidomycosis
   D. Disseminated tuberculosis

4. **In the patient mentioned in Question 3, what would be the approach in further management?**
   A. Cerebrospinal fluid (CSF) examination and culture with GeneXpert
   B. Blood culture with GeneXpert with CSF culture
   C. Commence empirical therapy with antifungal and antibiotic therapy
   D. Await results of bone marrow examination

5. **A 66-year-old male defaulter on his antiretroviral therapy (ART) presents to the emergency with fever, vomiting, and pain in the abdomen for 5 days. His last CD4 count 1 year ago was 170 cells/mm³ with a viral load of 230 copies/mL. His ultrasound and positron emission tomography-computed tomography (PET-CT) shows:**

   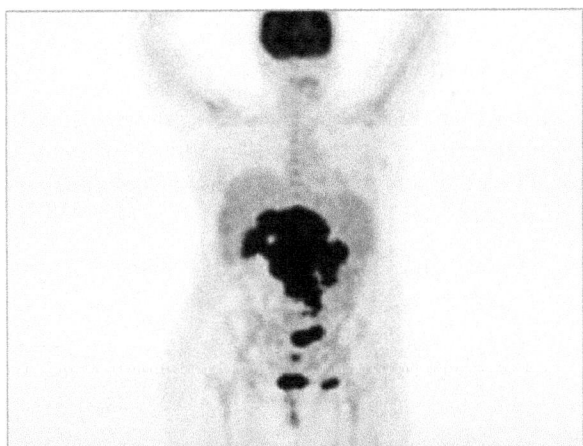

   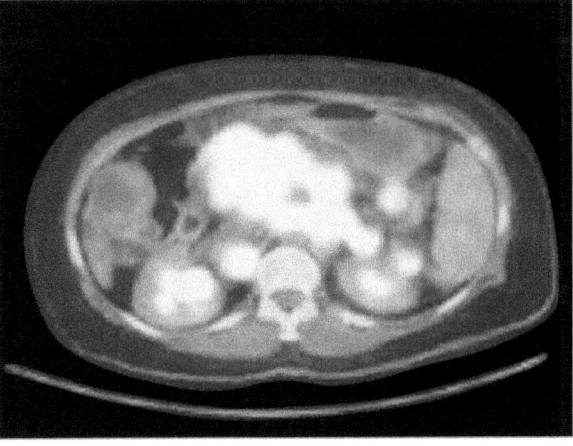

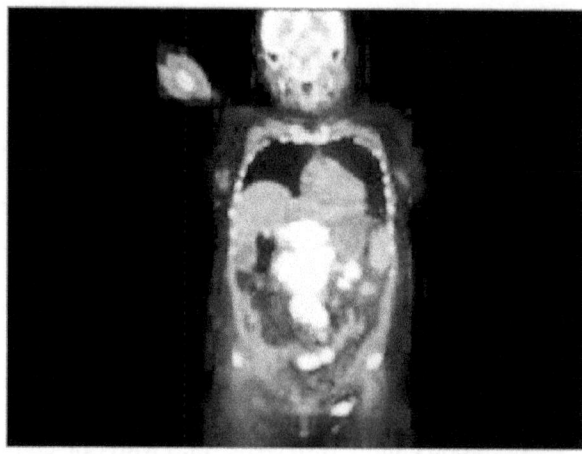

Source: Farghaly H, Nasr H, Qarni AA, Elhussein W. 18F-FDG PET/CT for first follow-up postchemotherapy in lymphoma: is it mandatory to do whole body scan? J Cancer Res Ther. 2015;3:20-5.

He is transferred to the ICU and stabilized with conservative treatment for an acute abdomen. He undergoes a CT-guided biopsy that shows non-necrotic tissue with large spindle cells. The sample test is positive for CD20. The most likely diagnosis is:

A. Hodgkin's lymphoma
B. Abdominal tuberculosis
C. Non-Hodgkin's lymphoma
D. Blastomycosis

6. A 21-year-old female presents with headache, blurring of vision, and swelling in her neck of 3 weeks duration. Her ultrasonography of neck shows:

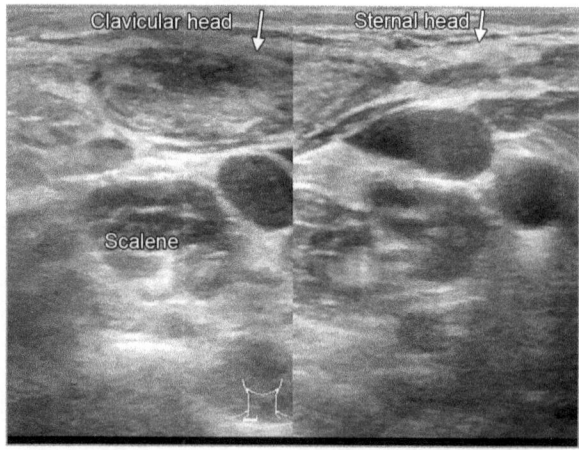

Source: Iqbal S, Gaillard F, et al. (2008). Tuberculous cervical lymphadenitis. [online] Available from https://radiopaedia.org/articles/tuberculous-cervical-lymphadenitis [Last accessed February, 2020].

She has recently been diagnosed with retroviral disease and is commenced on triple-drug therapy. 5 days after treatment, she has worsening headache and difficulty in swallowing. The most likely cause is:

A. Non-Hodgkin's lymphoma (of head and neck)
B. Rapidly growing *Mycobacteria*
C. Immune reconstitution inflammatory syndrome (IRIS)
D. Drug hypersensitivity

7. In the same patient, the best treatment option/approach would be:

A. Add a fourth drug to the existing ART
B. In dual infection with tuberculosis, treat tuberculosis first
C. Commence methylprednisolone for 5 days
D. Commence antitubercular therapy 2 weeks after ART

8. A 33-year-old asymptomatic female shows you her reports of the last 1 year.

	CD4 count (cells/mm^3)	Viral load (copies/mL)	CD4:CD8 ratio	CD4 (%)
June, 2018	290	670	0.3	8
September, 2018	310	110	0.1	11
January, 2019	276	<20	0.2	14
May, 2019	305	<20	0.2	16

What are the possibilities in her scenario?
A. Virological failure
B. Clinical failure
C. Immunological failure (IF)
D. None of the above

9. In the same person:
A. The treatment should be altered to increase CD4
B. A fourth drug should be added for better response
C. HIV genotype resistance testing as indicated
D. Observe the patient

10. A 44-year-old female with an 8-month history of nonresolving cough, weight loss, and fever presents with a 12-day history of streaky hemoptysis. Her CT chest reveals necrotic mediastinal lymph nodes and a right-sided cavitary lesion. She is failing antitubercular treatment (ATT) for the last 4 months. A bronchoscopy is done. Her CD4 count on ART is 112 cells/mm^3 with a viral load of 27,000 copies/mL. The most likely diagnosis is:

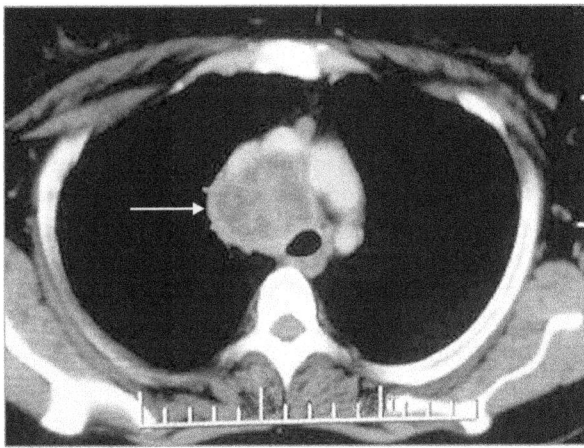

Source: Madan K, Ayub II, Jain D, Mohan A, Guleria R. Necrotic mediastinal lymph node enlargement in a middle-aged female. Lung India 2015;32(3):293-5.

A. Multidrug-resistant pulmonary tuberculosis
B. Atypical mycobacteria with dissemination
C. Histoplasmosis with aspergillus ball in the pulmonary cavity
D. Blastomycosis with pulmonary tuberculosis

11. Kitten litter exposure to immune-compromised patients, especially with CD4 count <100 cells/mm^3, are likely to reactivate which of the following conditions?
    A. *Bartonella henselae* and cat-scratch disease
    B. Toxoplasmosis
    C. Bacteroides fragilis
    D. Rabies

12. A 21-year-old female presents this year a fifth episode of salmonellosis in her blood culture. She has a history of 8 kg of weight loss in 1 year and a general feeling of growing lethargy and lack of appetite. In her workup, the tests that she needs are:
    A. CT abdomen with contrast
    B. Neutrophil myeloperoxidase deficiency evaluation
    C. Resistance testing for antityphoid treatment
    D. ELISA (enzyme-linked immunosorbent assay) for HIV, hepatitis B, and hepatitis C

13. A 71-year-old symptomatic male with a 100 pack-year history of smoking on ART presents with a history of weight loss. His reports are as follows:

	CD4 count	Viral load
January, 2019	260 cells	Undetectable
April, 2019	295 cells	Undetectable
August, 2019	220 cells	Undetectable

    The patient wants to change the treatment based on these reports. Your best advice is:
    A. Switch to second-line ART with protease inhibitor-based therapy
    B. Add a fourth drug to the existing regimen
    C. No change is required given the patient's history
    D. Evaluate for other opportunistic infections

14. A 38-week-old pregnant woman presents to emergency with labor pain. Her husband says that she was diagnosed with retroviral infection but she has discontinued the medication for the last 5 months and she does not remember her last CD4 count or viral load. Your advice is:
    A. No role for ART at this stage since it may not work
    B. Cesarean section with emergency ART for the neonate
    C. Single-dose nevirapine/raltegravir immediately and ART for the neonate
    D. Four-drug therapy for mother and child for the next 6 weeks

15. A 37-year-old sailor meets you with a history of unprotected sexual exposure 4 days ago. He is keen to start postexposure prophylaxis immediately. The regimen that you will advise is:
    A. Zidovudine + Lamivudine + Efavirenz
    B. Lopinavir + Ritonavir + Atazanavir
    C. No therapy at this stage
    D. Four-drug regimen with Darunavir + Cobicistat + Lamivudine + Raltegravir

16. In the same patient, the role of sulfamethoxazole-trimethoprim prophylaxis is indicated for:
    A. TB extrapulmonary
    B. Salmonellosis
    C. *Nocardia* and *Pneumocytis jirovecii* with toxoplasma prevention
    D. *Isospora belli* gut infection

17. A 38-year-old male was admitted to an ICU in a state of obtundation, severe dehydration, and fever of 3 days duration. He has just tested positive for retroviral infection with the CD4 count of 30 cells/mL and viral load of >35 black copies. A stool culture shows multiple oocytes on concentration smear.

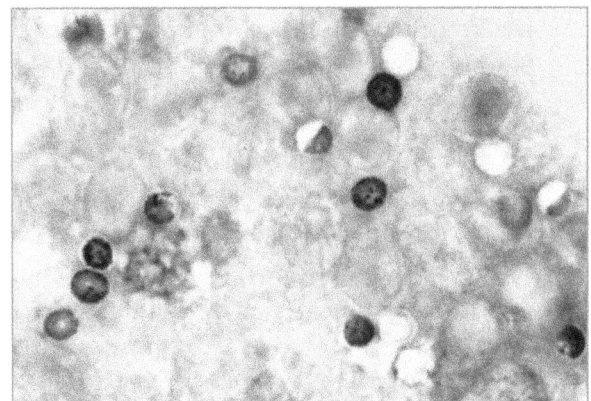

The most likely microorganism is:
A. Disseminated candida
B. *Salmonella* paratyphi
C. Cryptosporodia
D. *Isospora belli*

18. The treatment of choice for this infection is:
A. Doxycycline
B. 50% dextrose with electrolyte correction
C. Ceftriaxone + Metronidazole
D. Cotrimoxazole

19. A 36-year-old female presents with seizures and severe dysphagia. Her imaging of head and neck shows multiple intracranial lesions and masses impending on the nasopharyngeal space. She had a previous history of infectious mononucleosis 8 years ago. She also had three episodes of genital herpes and a varicella zoster infection 5 years ago. Her last CD4 count was 370 cells/mm^3 with a viral load of 185 copies/mL. A CSF study shows 900 white cells with 28% atypical lymphocytes, besides low glucose and high proteins. The most likely diagnosis is:
A. Viral encephalitis
B. Disseminated tuberculosis
C. Systemic lymphoma with nasopharyngeal carcinoma
D. Primary CNS Burkitt lymphoma

20. The most likely mechanism for cancer in HIV is:
A. Uncontrolled viral load
B. Inappropriate ART
C. Reduced immune surveillance and virus-driven oncogenesis
D. IRIS

21. A 23-year-old girl presents with Grade IV orthopnea. On evaluation, she has bilateral pleural effusion, ascites, and a liver span of 18 cm. Her bedside 2D-ECHO shows severely dilated right atrium, right ventricle, and severely elevated pulmonary artery pressure. Her ultrasound of abdomen shows early cirrhotic changes in the liver. She is noncompliant with her ART over the last 5 years and is a chronic smoker. She also has a history of injectable substance abuse and alcohol. Her most likely diagnosis is:
A. Hepatitis B-Hepatitis C infection
B. HIV-induced pulmonary arterial hypertension (PAH) and right-sided failure
C. Alcohol-induced liver cirrhosis
D. Substance-induced multiorgan damage

22. The incidence of acquiring active tuberculosis in patients who are carrying the immune-deficiency virus is:
A. 0 if the viral load is completely suppressed
B. 8–10% every year
C. 1–3% every year
D. 20–25% every year

23. A 37-year-old female is commenced on dolutegravir and lopinavir with ritonavir and abacavir. She breaks into mild rash. Her primary physician withholds the treatment for 2 weeks and then recommences on the same regimen. She now presents to the hospital with: fever and maculopapular rash accompanied by constitutional symptoms (fatigue, malaise, myalgias, and arthralgias), multivisceral involvement (lymphadenopathy, mucositis, pneumonitis, myocarditis, hepatitis, and interstitial nephritis), and hematologic abnormalities (atypical lymphocytosis and eosinophilia). The wrong statement is:
A. Abacavir hypersensitivity reaction
B. HLA-B57:01 screening
C. White patients appear to be at higher risk than African descent
D. High lymphocyte involvement in the epidermis can be found

24. The biggest reason for the beginning of opportunistic infections in HIV is:
A. Apoptosis
B. CD8 cytotoxic lymphocytes having no memory of HIV infection
C. Ineffective natural killer cells and complements
D. Loss of cell-mediated immunity

25. A 38-year-old male presents to the emergency with seizures and obtundation. His family shares a history of unprotected sex with multiple partners. In the baseline workup, an ELISA for HIV is sent that comes back as negative. You ask for a CD4 count which is 13 cells/mm^3. The next test to establish the diagnosis is:
A. Immunofluorescence assay
B. Polymerase chain reaction
C. Western blot for HIV-1
D. Nucleic acid branched sequence assay (NABSA)

26. In the same patient, the western blot test is reported as indeterminant. The most common reason for this result is:
A. Incomplete antibody response to HIV
B. Poorly reactive antigen response to HIV
C. Failure of T-cell population in HIV
D. Bone marrow suppression due to HIV

27. The chance of the false-positive result in testing for HIV in a standard two-step testing protocol, in a low risk population, is estimated to be:
A. 1 in 10,000
B. 1 in 1,00,000
C. 1 in 250,000
D. 1 in 500,000

28. A 27-year-old female presents with a condition affecting 70% of her skin to the emergency department. She was on ART for 6 years. What is this condition?

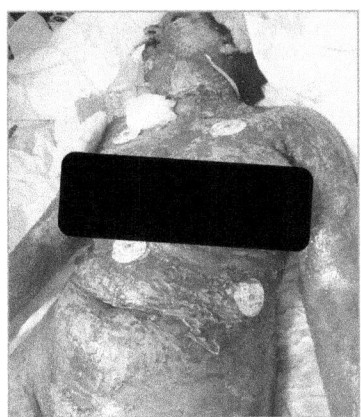

A. Pemphigus vulgaris
B. Exfoliative dermatitis
C. Stevens-Johnson syndrome
D. Toxic epidermal necrolysis

29. The same patient, mentioned in Question 28, was taking ART for 6 years and her last CD4 count was 470 cells/mm^3. She complained of giddiness, nausea, and vomiting for over 3 weeks and was advised to change to a different regimen (atazanavir, nevirapine, lopinavir/ritonavir). Three weeks after starting this regimen, she developed this reaction. The likeliest cause is:

A. Congenital ichthyosis
B. Vitamin A deficiency
C. Nevirapine-induced event
D. Hypersensitivity associated with atazanavir

30. In the same patient, the reason for this reaction is due to:

A. HLA B27 association with lopinavir toxicity
B. Uncontrolled HIV viral load
C. CD4 count of >400 in women is relative contraindication for starting nevirapine
D. Scalded-skin syndrome due to staphylococcal infection

ANSWERS WITH EXPLANATIONS

1. **Ans. C**

2. **Ans. D**
   Pyrimethamine is considered the most effective drug against toxoplasmosis and is a standard component of therapy. It is a folic acid antagonist and can cause dose-related suppression of the bone marrow, which is mitigated by concurrent administration of folinic acid (leucovorin). Leucovorin protects the bone marrow from the toxic effects of pyrimethamine. A second drug, such as sulfadiazine or clindamycin (if the patient has a hypersensitivity reaction to sulfa drugs), should also be included.
   Ref:
   1. *Centers for Disease Control and Preparation (2018). Resources for Health Professionals. [online] Available from https://www.cdc.gov/parasites/toxoplasmosis/health_professionals/index.html#tx [Last accessed February, 2020].*

3. **Ans. D**
   Miliary tuberculosis (TB) in a patient with a low CD4+ T-cell count is shown. Anteroposterior chest radiograph shows innumerable small discrete nodules 1–2 mm in diameter, diffusely distributed throughout both lungs.
   Ref:
   1. *Kisembo HN, Den Boon S, Davis JL, Okello R, William W, Cattamanchi A, et al. Chest radiographic findings of pulmonary tuberculosis in severely immunocompromised patients with the human immunodeficiency virus. Br J Radiol. 2012;85(1014):e130-9.*

4. **Ans. C**
   Miliary TB may occur in an individual organ (very rare, < 5%), in several organs, or throughout the entire body (>90%), including the brain. The infection is characterized by a large amount of TB bacilli, although it may easily be missed and is fatal if left untreated.

   Up to 25% of patients with miliary TB may have meningeal involvement. In addition, miliary TB may mimic many diseases. In some case series, up to 50% of cases are undiagnosed antemortem. Therefore, a high index of clinical suspicion is important to obtain an early diagnosis and to ensure improved clinical outcomes.

   Early empirical treatment for possible but not yet definitive miliary TB increases the likelihood of survival and should never be withheld while test results are pending. On autopsy, multiple TB lesions

are detected throughout the body in organs such as the lungs, liver, spleen, brain, and others. The most common laboratory abnormalities include anemia and other hematologic findings. Other laboratory abnormalities may include elevated acute-phase reactants, hyponatremia, hypercalcemia, and sterile pyuria. In miliary disease, the classic chest radiograph appearance is a faint, reticulonodular infiltrate distributed fairly uniformly throughout the lungs.
Ref:
1. Khan FY. Review of literature on disseminated tuberculosis with emphasis on the focused diagnostic workup. J Family Community Med. 2019;26(2):83-91.
2. Bernardo J. Clinical manifestations, diagnosis, and treatment of miliary tuberculosis, Nov 2020. In: UpToDate, Post TW (Ed), UpToDate, Waltham, MA; 2020.

5. **Ans. C**

6. **Ans. C**

Immune reconstitution inflammatory syndrome (IRIS) associated with *Mycobacterium avium* complex infection usually presents as either focal or diffuse lymphadenitis, occurring typically within 3 months of initiation of ART, and often with suppuration. *M. avium* complex-related IRIS rarely presents as focal pulmonary disease.
Ref:
1. Lawn SD, Bekker LG, Miller RF. Immune reconstitution disease associated with mycobacterial infections in HIV-infected individuals receiving antiretrovirals. Lancet Infect Dis. 2005;5:361-73.

7. **Ans. B**

Screening all patients for possible opportunistic infections before starting ART is recommended in TB-endemic areas. The timing of the start of the ART is crucial in preventing paradoxical IRIS. According to a trial that evaluated starting ART at three points in TB (SAPiT), ART initiation in TB-HIV patients should be decided based on their CD4 cell counts. If the CD4 counts are <50 cells/mm^3, ART can be started immediately after the initiation of TB treatment. If the CD4+ cell counts are ≥50 cells/mm^3, ART can be delayed.
Ref:
1. Naidoo K, Yende-Zuma N, Padayatchi N, Naidoo K, Kithoo N, Nair G, et al. The immune reconstitution inflammatory syndrome after antiretroviral therapy initiation in patients with tuberculosis: findings from the SAPiT trial. Ann Intern Med. 2012;157:313-24.

8. **Ans. C**

The World Health Organization (WHO) defines immunological failure in adults and adolescents as—CD4 count falls to the baseline (or below) or persistent CD4 levels <100 cells/mm^3; in children <5 years old—persistent CD4 levels <200 cells/mm^3 or <10%; and in children >5 years old—persistent CD4 levels <100 cells/mm^3.

The patients who come from high HIV-prevalence areas or attending their HIV care services near to high HIV-endemic settings have higher IF than patients who are attending their care in or near to low HIV-prevalence settings. The following explanations could partly justify the difference: (1) the presence of a variety of HIV-1 strains among people living with HIV in HIV-prevalent areas is very high and this could challenge the immunological response benefited from the treatment; (2) ART drug resistance is higher in high HIV-prevalence settings than in low HIV-prevalence settings, and the drug resistance diminishes the immunological benefit of the treatment; and (3) HIV-infected people who come from high HIV-prevalence settings have less access to health services, lower economic status, and lower HIV care-related knowledge and this could negatively influence the immunological benefit of ART.

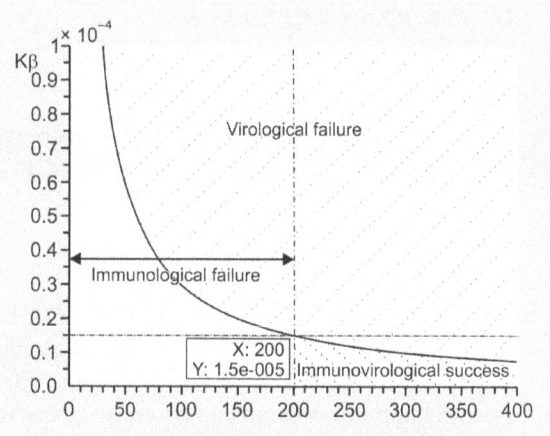

Source: Ouattara DA, Mhawej M-J, Moog CH. (2008). Clinical tests of therapeutical failures based on mathematical modeling of the HIV infection. Automatic Control, IEEE Explore Digital Library. [online] Available from https://ieeexplore.ieee.org/document/4439822 [Last accessed February, 2020].

Ref:
1. World Health Organization. [online] Available from https://www.who.int/hiv/pub/guidelines/arv2013/art/WHO_CG_table_7.15.pdf [Last accessed February, 2020]
2. Smyth RP, Davenport MP, Mak J. The origin of genetic diversity in HIV-1. Virus Res 2012;169:415-29.
3. Bhargava M, Cajas JM, Wainberg MA, Klein MB, Pant Pai N. Do HIV-1 non-B subtypes differentially impact resistance mutations and clinical disease progression in treated populations? Evidence from a systematic review. J Int AIDS Soc. 2014;17:18944.
4. Buonaguro L, Tornesello ML, Buonaguro FM. Human immunodeficiency virus type 1 subtype distribution in the worldwide epidemic: pathogenetic and therapeutic implications. J Virol. 2007;81:10209-19.

5. Li L, Lin C, Wu Z, Scott Comulada W, Ding Y. Regional differences in HIV prevalence and individual attitudes among service providers in China. Soc Sci Med. 2012;75:283-7.

9. **Ans. D**

10. **Ans. C**

    In HIV-infected patients, the common clinical manifestations of progressive disseminated histoplasmosis include fever, fatigue, weight loss, and hepatosplenomegaly. Cough, chest pain, and dyspnea occur in approximately 50% of patients. For patients whose CD4 counts are >300 cells/mm^3, histoplasmosis is often limited to the respiratory tract and usually presents with cough, pleuritic chest pain, and fever.
    Ref:
    1. Wheat LJ, Connolly-Stringfield PA, Baker RL, Curfman ME, Eads ME, Israel KS, et al. Disseminated histoplasmosis in the acquired immune deficiency syndrome: clinical findings, diagnosis and treatment, and review of the literature. Medicine (Baltimore). 1990;69(6):361-74.
    2. Baddley JW, Sankara IR, Rodriquez JM, Pappas PG, Many WJ Jr. Histoplasmosis in HIV-infected patients in a southern regional medical center: poor prognosis in the era of highly active antiretroviral therapy. Diagn Microbiol Infect Dis. 2008;62(2):151-6.

11. **Ans. B**

    Toxoplasma infection occurs by accidentally swallowing the parasite through contact with cat feces that contain toxoplasma. This occurs because cats become infected with toxoplasma through hunting and eating rodents, birds, or other small animals that are infected with the parasite.
    Ref:
    1. Centers for Disease Control and Prevention (CDC) (2018). Parasites—Toxoplasmosis (Toxoplasma infection). [online] Available from https://www.cdc.gov/parasites/toxoplasmosis/gen_info/faqs.html [Last accessed February, 2020].

12. **Ans. D**

    Salmonella is ADI.

    Arginine deiminase (ADI), carbamate kinase (CK), and ornithine transcarbamoylase (OTC) constitute the ADI system. In addition to metabolic functions, the ADI system has been implicated in the virulence of certain pathogens. The pathogenic intracellular bacterium *Salmonella enterica* serovar Typhimurium possesses the *STM4467*, *STM4466*, and *STM4465* genes, which are predicted to encode ADI, CK, and OTC, respectively.
    Ref:
    1. Choi Y, Choi J, Groisman EA, Kang DH, Shin D, Ryu S. Expression of STM4467-encoded arginine deiminase controlled by the STM4463 regulator contributes to *Salmonella enterica* serovar Typhimurium virulence. Infect Immun. 2012;80(12):4291-7.

13. **Ans. C**

    Tobacco smoking had a significantly negative effect on weight change. Up to 80% of the study population [people living with HIV (PLHIV)] reported tobacco smoking at baseline.
    Ref:
    1. Tang AM, Sheehan HB, Jordan MR, Duong DV, Terrin N, Dong K, et al. Predictors of weight change in male HIV-positive injection drug users initiating antiretroviral therapy in Hanoi, Vietnam. AIDS Res Treat. 2011;2011:890308.

14. **Ans. C**

15. **Ans. C**

    There is no benefit of postexposure prophylaxis after 72 hours.
    Ref:
    1. Siedner MJ, Tumarkin E, Bogoch II. HIV post-exposure prophylaxis (PEP). BMJ. 2018;363:k4928. doi: 10.1136/bmj.k4928.

16. **Ans. C**
    Ref:
    1. Wininger DA, Fass RJ. Impact of trimethoprim-sulfamethoxazole prophylaxis on etiology and susceptibilities of pathogens causing human immunodeficiency virus-associated bacteremia. Antimicrob Agents Chemother. 2002;46(2):594-7.
    2. World Health Organization. [online] Available from https://www.who.int/hiv/pub/guidelines/ctxguidelines.pdf [Last accessed December, 2020].

17. **Ans. C**

18. **Ans. D**

19. **Ans. C**

20. **Ans. C**

21. **Ans. B**

22. **Ans. B**

23. **Ans. D**

    This is a case of *abacavir hypersensitivity reaction*. A hypersensitivity reaction occurs in association with initiation of abacavir therapy as part of combination antiretroviral therapy in ~3.7% of patients. The reaction is possibly the result of a combination of altered drug metabolism and immune dysfunction, which is poorly understood. White patients appear to be at higher risk and patients of African descent at lower risk of abacavir hypersensitivity. Clinical management involves supportive measures and discontinuation of abacavir therapy. Rechallenge with abacavir in a hypersensitive patient should be avoided because it might precipitate a life-threatening reaction.

Patients who were hypersensitive were found to produce more IL-4 than were HIV-positive patients who were not hypersensitive. There was also a decrease in Th1 cells with an increase in the number and distribution of Th0, Th2, Tc0, and Tc2 cells. A lack of lymphocyte involvement in the epidermis distinguished the rash from Stevens-Johnson syndrome. CD8 cells predominate along with high numbers of CD4 cells.

Ref:
1. Hewitt RG. Abacavir hypersensitivity reaction. *Clin Infect Dis.* 2002;34(8):1137-42.

24. Ans. D
25. Ans. D
26. Ans. A
27. Ans. C
    Ref:
    1. Kleinman S, Busch MP, Hall L, et al. False-positive HIV-1 test results in a low-risk screening setting of voluntary blood donation. *JAMA.* 1998;280(12):1080-5
28. Ans. D
29. Ans. C
30. Ans. C

CHAPTER 16

Infections of Liver

Prasanna Shah

1. **Which of the following statements about pyogenic abscess of the liver are true?**
   A. The right lobe is more commonly involved than the left lobe
   B. Appendicitis with perforation and abscess is the most common underlying cause of hepatic abscess
   C. Mortality is largely determined by the underlying disease
   D. Mortality from hepatic abscess is currently greater than 40%

2. **Which of the following statements most accurately describes the current therapy for pyogenic hepatic abscess?**
   A. Antibiotics alone are adequate for the treatment of most cases
   B. All patients require open surgical drainage for optimal management
   C. Optimal treatment involves treatment of not only the abscess but the underlying source as well
   D. Percutaneous drainage is more successful for multiple lesions than for solitary ones

3. **Which of the following statements characterize amebic abscess?**
   A. Mortality is higher than that for similarly located pyogenic abscesses
   B. The diagnosis of amebic abscess may be based on serologic tests and resolution of symptoms
   C. In contrast to pyogenic abscess, the treatment of amebic abscess is primarily medical
   D. Patients with amebic abscess tend to be older than those with pyogenic abscess

4. **Which of the following statement(s) is/are true about benign lesions of the liver?**
   A. Adenomas are true neoplasms with a predisposition for complications and should usually be resected
   B. Focal nodular hyperplasia (FNH) is a neoplasm related to birth control pills (BCPs) and usually requires resection
   C. Hemangiomas are the most common benign lesions of the liver that come to the surgeon's attention
   D. Nodular regenerative hyperplasia does not usually accompany cirrhosis

5. **Which of the following statement(s) about malignant neoplasms of the liver is/are true?**
   A. Hepatocellular carcinoma is probably the most commom cause of death from cancers worldwide
   B. The most common resectable hepatic malignant neoplasm in the United States is colorectal metastasis
   C. Hepatoma has at least one variant that has a much more benign course than hepatomas in general
   D. Hepatomas are generally slow-growing tumor than was formerly believed
   E. All of the above

6. **Echinococcosis liver disease caused by *Echinococcus granulosus*:**
   A. Is not a neoplasm
   B. Is endemic to parts of Europe, but not the United States
   C. Is usually curable by resection
   D. Is more deadly than in its *Echinococcus multilocularis* form

7. **Which of the following explanations account(s) for the fact that hepatitis C is the most common cause of post-transfusion hepatitis?**
   A. There are more carriers of hepatitis C virus (HCV) in the normal population who serve as blood donors
   B. Blood infected with hepatitis B virus (HBV) is eliminated through routine testing, leaving only HCV as the other blood-borne pathogen
   C. Current serologic tests for HCV antigen do not exclude carriers
   D. Questions designed to eliminate risk groups for HCV from the normal donor population may not be as specific as would be desirable
   E. Hepatitis C is a more virulent form of viral hepatitis, so it is expected that more cases of post-transfusion hepatitis would occur

8. **True or false: HBV infections:**
   A. Are usually asymptomatic
   B. May not be clinically recognized but may lead to chronic hepatitis

C. Reliably protect against subsequent HBV infection regardless of the measured antibody titer to hepatitis B surface antigen (HBsAg)
D. Are completely prevented by postexposure administration of hepatitis B immunoglobulin (HBIg)
E. Preclude subsequent infection with HDV

9. Left lobe liver abscess ruptures most commonly in:
   A. Pleural cavity
   B. Peritoneal cavity
   C. Pericardial cavity
   D. Bronchus

10. True about amebic liver abscess is:
    A. Male:female > 10:1
    B. Not predisposed by alcohol
    C. More common in diabetics
    D. *Entamoeba histolytica* is isolated in >50% from blood culture

11. Which one of the following is not an indication for percutaneous aspiration in amebic liver abscess?
    A. Radiographically unresolved lesion after 6 months
    B. Suspected diagnosis
    C. Left lobe liver abscess
    D. Compression or outflow obstruction of hepatic or portal vein

12. Anti-HBc (total) is usually negative in chronic hepatitis B infection:
    A. True
    B. False

13. Extrahepatic prodromal features of hepatitis B include:
    A. Arthralgia
    B. Skin rash
    C. Polyarteritis nodosa
    D. Bleeding per rectum

14. Severe liver damage in viral hepatitis is indicated by:
    A. Aminotransferase activity over 400 U/L
    B. Raised serum bilirubin over 5 mg
    C. Alkaline phosphatase level below 250 U/L
    D. Prolongation of prothrombin time (PT)

15. Match the following:

1. Anti-HAV antibodies	A. Incubation period of hepatitis B
2. Anti-HBs only positive	B. Established viral hepatitis
3. HBsAg, IgM, and IgG positive	C. Immunization without infection
4. HBsAg + IgM positive	D. Hepatitis, transient

    Titers fall within 3 months of recovery

16. Risk group who needs hepatitis B vaccination includes all, *except*:
    A. Patient on chronic hemodialysis
    B. Newborn of infected mother
    C. Homosexual male
    D. Patient on anti-TB drugs

17. In viral hepatitis, anti-HBc implies:
    A. Previous infection—convalescence 3-9 months
    B. Previous vaccination
    C. Both 1 and 2
    D. None of the above

18. In chronic HBV infection, continued active replication of virus in liver is indicated by:
    A. HBeAg
    B. Anti-HBe
    C. HBcAg
    D. All of the above

19. Match the following:

1. Hepatitis D	A. Post-transfusional hepatitis, cause of chronic hepatitis
2. Hepatitis C	B. Spread by fecal–oral route
3. Hepatitis A	C. Dane particles contain virus
4. Hepatitis B	D. Is an RNA defective virus, which requires HBV for replication?

20. All of the following factors are contributory to mortality and poor prognosis in viral hepatitis, *except*:
    A. Preexisting chronic liver disease
    B. Old age
    C. Other coexisting diseases like carcinoma or lymphoma
    D. Level of serum alkaline phosphatase

21. Which of the following statements about immunology in liver transplantation is/are correct?
    A. Good human leukocyte antigen (HLA) matching between recipient and donor is mandatory for a good outcome for liver transplantation
    B. Hyperacute rejection is almost nonexistent following liver transplantation
    C. Acute rejection occurs in more than 50% of patients and is reversible in most patients with large doses of steroids
    D. Acute rejection is very rare later than 2 months after liver transplantation unless the patient is inadequately immunosuppressed
    E. Chronic rejection is different from acute rejection, is usually irreversible, and often requires re-transplantation

22. **Which of the following statements about hepatic artery thrombosis following liver transplantation is/are correct?**
    A. Thrombosis of the hepatic artery following liver transplantation is more common in children than in adult patients
    B. Thrombosis of the hepatic artery usually occurs several weeks after transplant as a result of arteriosclerosis
    C. Thrombosis of the hepatic artery in the early days following transplantation is a serious complication leading to death unless retransplantation can be performed within 36–72 hours
    D. Late thrombosis of the hepatic artery may present as biliary complication or intrahepatic abscesses
    E. Thrombosis of the portal vein is more frequent than hepatic artery thrombosis following liver transplantation

23. **Immunological evidence of immunity to hepatitis B is the presence of:**
    A. Hepatitis B core antibodies
    B. Hepatitis B core antigen
    C. Hepatitis B surface antibodies
    D. Hepatitis B surface antigen

24. **All are true regarding hepatitis C infection, *except*:**
    A. Serum transaminase level is a good predictor of the level of liver fibrosis
    B. Telaprevir is effective in management
    C. 3% risk of vertical transmission
    D. Sharing toothbrushes is a risk factor for transmission

25. **A 55-year-old man with established cirrhosis underwent a 6-monthly surveillance ultrasound scan. It showed a suspicious focal liver lesion. A subsequent contrast-enhanced CT scan of abdomen confirmed a 2.5 cm focal lesion in the liver. AFP was raised at 200 ng/mL. A previous AFP and USS were normal 6 months earlier. What is the most appropriate next step?**
    A. Ultrasound-guided liver biopsy
    B. Positron emission tomography (PET) scan
    C. Liver transplant referral
    D. Repeat scan in 6 weeks
    E. Repeat AFP in 6 weeks

26. **Surveillance for HCC is recommended in high-risk patients with cirrhosis. All of the following patients are considered to be at high risk, *except*:**
    A. Males and females with established cirrhosis due to hepatitis B or C
    B. Males and females with established cirrhosis due to genetic haemochromatosis
    C. Males with alcohol-related cirrhosis
    D. Males with cirrhosis due to primary biliary cirrhosis
    E. Males and females with cirrhosis due to primary sclerosing cholangitis

27. **Which one of the following statements regarding pyogenic liver abscess (PLA) is true?**
    A. Most of the PLA is monomicrobial
    B. Treatment of PLA always includes drainage of the abscess
    C. *Staphylococcus aureus* is the most common organism
    D. Colonoscopy is indicated, if biliary sepsis is excluded
    E. In 10% of cases, no obvious cause of infection can be identified

28. **Which one of the following statements regarding PLA is false?**
    A. Biliary sepsis is the most common source
    B. Blood culture identifies the organism in 50% of cases
    C. Surgery is needed for drainage in loculated abscess
    D. Usually single abscess is seen
    E. Abscess more than 5 cm usually needs some form of drainage

29. **Which of the following is true of hepatitis C infection?**
    A. Hepatitis C virus is a DNA virus
    B. Infection is a risk factor for HCC
    C. Infection is more common in women
    D. It is commonly transmitted by sexual contact
    E. Alpha-interferon is an effective treatment to cure the infection

30. **Which of the following is indication for liver transplantation?**
    A. Hemochromatosis
    B. Intentional paracetamol overdose
    C. HCC (single 9 cm lesion)
    D. Cirrhosis secondary to hepatitis

ANSWERS WITH EXPLANATIONS

1. **Ans. A and C**
   Involvement of the right lobe with abscess formation approximates 70% of pyogenic abscesses. This is thought to be due to the streaming effect of superior mesenteric venous inflow to the right lobe. In addition, the greater volume of the right lobe predisposes more tissue to seeding by bacterial organisms. While appendicitis comprised of 25-40% of cases in early series, early recognition and operative therapy for appendicitis have reduced its importance significantly. In current series, malignant or benign biliary obstruction is the underlying cause of 35-50% of cases. Recent studies have shown that the underlying disease or an immunocompromised host is more important prognostically than solitary versus multiple abscesses.

2. **Ans. C**
   The development of ultrasonography and computed tomography (CT) in the past two decades has enabled earlier diagnosis and advances in treatment of hepatic abscess. Formerly, open surgical drainage was considered necessary in essentially all cases of pyogenic abscess. Numerous recent series, however, have reported high success rates and low mortality from the percutaneous catheter drainage of abscesses under CT or ultrasonographic guidance. Optimal management of pyogenic abscess, however, involves not only treatment of the abscess, whether by percutaneous or surgical methods, but correction of the underlying source as well. All modes of therapy are more successful in treating solitary lesions than multiple ones.

3. **Ans. B and C**
   Mortality for uncomplicated amebic abscess should be less than 5%, in contrast to the 15-20% rate for pyogenic abscess. After the demonstration by radiological examination of an abscess, appropriate serologic tests and resolution of symptoms after a course of treatment with an antiamebic agent such as metronidazole constitute presumptive diagnosis of amebic abscess. Aspiration of abscess contents rarely yields amebic organisms. In contrast to pyogenic abscess, amebic abscess rarely requires surgical or percutaneous drainage, except in the case of an extremely large abscess or bacterial superinfection. Amebic abscess affects males in a 9:1 to 10:1 ratio and generally affects a younger population than pyogenic abscess.

4. **Ans. A**
   Adenomas are typically enlarge and cause symptoms, may rupture, and have a definite malignant potential. Therefore, they should generally be resected when found. FNH is not a true neoplasm and generally has an uneventful course. Both are related to BCPs, although the relationship of adenoma is more firmly established. While small bile duct hamartomas are much more common, hemangiomas are the most common lesion to come to the attention of surgeons. They should not generally be biopsied because of possible hemorrhage. By definition, nodular regenerative hyperplasia occurs in the absence of cirrhosis.

5. **Ans. E**
   Although exact comparisons are impossible, hepatoma seems to be the most common cause of cancer death worldwide, despite its relative infrequency in the United States. Colorectal metastasis is a more common indication for surgical treatment in the United States. The fibrolamellar variant and possibly the very well-differentiated tumor probably have a better prognosis than hepatomas in general. Previous studies from Africa in which there was a high incidence of rupture account for the poor prognosis that was generally attributed to hepatoma. Recent studies from Europe and the United States have shown that survival after presentation is usually measured in years.

6. **Ans. A, B, and C**
   The parasitic infection is fairly common in certain parts of Europe but very rare in the United States. Resection without peritoneal soilage is the treatment of choice. The *E. multilocularis* form, which is endemic to parts of the United States, is more likely to be fatal because it is rarely resectable. This form is more likely to resemble a malignancy than *E. granulosus*, although the natural course of the disease usually spans many years.

7. **Ans. B and D**
   The ability to specifically identify persons infected with HCV has only recently become available. Therefore, data about epidemiology are less than complete. It is very likely not true that more blood donors carry HCV because of the large preponderance of HBV in the United States. It is true, however, that successful elimination of most of the HBV carriers occurs through routine testing. Although serologic tests are available for HCV, they are tests, not of antigen, but of antibody. Therefore, this test alone may not screen out persons who are infected but have not yet developed or may never develop antibody. Risk groups for the relatively newly defined HCV may well not be comprehensively established, and therefore this explanation may be a contributor. There are no differences in virulence between these classes of hepatitis virus.

8. **Ans. True—B and C; False—A, D, and E**

   Although some types of hepatitis are more often asymptomatic than symptomatic, except for hepatitis B. Further, even if the HBV infection is asymptomatic, serious long-term side effects may occur. A prior infection with hepatitis B confers lifelong immunity even if the antibody titer wanes below the protective level of 10 mIU. HBIg is useful in reducing the incidence of postexposure HBV infection from around 30% with no intervention, to 15% with standard immune globulin, to about 5–7% with HBIg. HBV infection is required for infection with HDV and is therefore an essential step toward, rather than preventive of, HBV infection.

9. **Ans. B**

   Rupture of the abscess into the adjacent cavities (pleura, lung, pericardium or peritoneum) is an important complication. High risk of rupture in peritoneal cavity for left lobe abscess with size >5 cm.

10. **Ans. A**

    Majority of patients are young men (may be due to heavy alcohol consumption).

11. **Ans. A**

    Radiological resolution of the abscess cavity is usually delayed. The average time to radiologic resolution is 3–9 months and can take as long as years in some patients. Clinical improvement after adequate treatment with antiamebic agents is the rule.

12. **Ans. B**

    Anti-HBc should always be positive in chronic hepatitis B infection. If it is negative, it should prompt you to look at the validity of your HBsAg result.

13. **Ans. B**

    These patients may have serum sickness-like syndrome as a prodromal feature. In children, cervical lymphadenopathy and splenomegaly can occur.
    Ref:
    1. Boon NA, Colledge NR, Walker BR, Hunter JAA. Davidson's Principles and Practice of Medicine, 20th edition. London, UK: Elsevier/Churchill Livingstone; 2006. p. 963.

14. **Ans. D**

    Prolongation of PT is a feature of diffuse liver damage. It is bad prognostic sign, heralding hepatic encephalopathy.
    Ref:
    1. Boon NA, Colledge NR, Walker BR, Hunter JAA. Davidson's Principles and Practice of Medicine, 20th edition. London, UK: Elsevier/Churchill Livingstone; 2006. p. 963.

15. **Ans. 1→D; 2→C; 3→B; 4→A**

    Hepatitis A, anti-HAV antibody, which is IgG type, is positive, but its level decreases with recovery in 3 months' time. If a person has no jaundice but shows HBs antibodies implies that he has been vaccinated with HBsAg vaccine (hepatitis B) in established hepatitis B. HBsAg, IgM, and IgG are positive.
    Ref:
    1. Boon NA, Colledge NR, Walker BR, Hunter JAA. Davidson's Principles and Practice of Medicine, 20th edition. London, UK: Elsevier/Churchill Livingstone; 2006

16. **Ans. D**

    In addition to the above risk group, medical/nursing personnel such as dentists, surgeons, and obstetricians will also need hepatitis B vaccine. In general, all laboratory staff handling blood need protection.
    Ref:
    1. Boon NA, Colledge NR, Walker BR, Hunter JAA. Davidson's Principles and Practice of Medicine, 20th edition. London, UK: Elsevier/Churchill Livingstone; 2006. p. 967.

17. **Ans. C**

    With previous infection along with anti-HBs, anti-HBC is also present. If anti-HBC is absent, it means previous vaccination.
    Ref:
    1. Boon NA, Colledge NR, Walker BR, Hunter JAA. Davidson's Principles and Practice of Medicine, 20th edition. London, UK: Elsevier/Churchill Livingstone; 2006. p. 965.

18. **Ans. A**

    Hepatitis B virus active replication of virus in liver is indicated by HBeAg levels.
    Ref:
    1. Boon NA, Colledge NR, Walker BR, Hunter JAA. Davidson's Principles and Practice of Medicine, 20th edition. London, UK: Elsevier/Churchill Livingstone; 2006. p. 965.

19. **Ans. 1→D; 2→A; 3→B; 4→C**

    Hepatitis D has no independent existence. It coexists with hepatitis B. Ninety percent of post-transfusional hepatitis are due to hepatitis C. Fecal-oral route of transmission is seen in hepatitis A. There is no chronic carrier state with hepatitis A. Dane particle is virus of hepatitis B. It has chronic carrier state.
    Ref:
    1. Boon NA, Colledge NR, Walker BR, Hunter JAA. Davidson's Principles and Practice of Medicine, 20th edition. London, UK: Elsevier/Churchill Livingstone; 2006. pp. 963-8.

20. **Ans. D**

    Extreme age, other chronic debilitating illness, and chronic liver disease contribute to higher mortality rate in viral hepatitis.
    Ref:
    1. Boon NA, Colledge NR, Walker BR, Hunter JAA. Davidson's Principles and Practice of Medicine, 20th edition. London, UK: Elsevier/Churchill Livingstone; 2006. p. 986.

21. **Ans. B, C, D, and E**

    Immune-mediated reactions following liver transplantation are clearly different from those that follow other solid organ transplants. The liver is tolerated quite well, and currently donors and recipients are matched only for their ABO group. Even when the ABO barrier is not respected, survival is still over 60%. T-cell-mediated acute rejection occurs in about half of the patients within 6 weeks after liver transplantation, and acute rejection is reversed by large doses of steroids in most cases. Chronic rejection, on the other hand, is a different entity that is ill-understood and corresponds to destruction of small arteries and bile ducts. Change in the immunosuppression regimen sometimes may hinder the progression of this disease, but often retransplantation is required.

22. **Ans. A, C and E**

    Thrombosis of the hepatic artery remains one of the most serious early complications of liver transplantation. This complication is three to five times more common in children than in adults. The major cause of this complication is related to technical error, although the hypercoagulable state may play a significant role in some situations. Early thrombosis of the hepatic artery leads to rapid liver failure with a fatal outcome unless a transplant can be performed within 36–72 hours. Although thrombolytic therapy through percutaneous or surgical access can be successful, most of these patients require retransplantation. Stenosis of the hepatic artery or late thrombosis of the hepatic artery can lead to multiple intrahepatic strictures of the bile duct and/or hepatic abscesses. This complication also often requires retransplantation. Portal vein thrombosis is a rarer complication. It is a devastating condition when it occurs early, but can be tolerated well, if it develops after several months. Portal hypertension due to late portal vein thrombosis can often be treated successfully by a shunt procedure.

23. **Ans. C**

    Vaccine: + for HBV surface antibody
    Infected: + for HBV surface antigen and core antigen
    Chronic: HBV antigen but no core
    Acute: Core antigen.

24. **Ans. is A**

    Serum transaminase level is a good predictor of the level of liver fibrosis:
    - Serum transaminase level in hepatitis C is not a good predictor of the level of liver fibrosis.
    - A *liver biopsy* is required to assess the degree of liver damage.
    - There is *3% risk for acquisition of chronic hepatitis C* by *vertical transmission*.
    - *Sharing of toothbrushes and razors* is another risk factor.

25. **Ans. C**

    A raised AFP in a cirrhotic patient with a focal liver lesion confirms the diagnosis of hepatocellular carcinoma (HCC) and further investigation is only required to establish the most appropriate therapy. Biopsy of potentially operable lesions is avoided due to the risk of tumor seeding in the needle tract, which occurs in 1–3%. The only proven potentially curative therapy for HCC remains surgical, either hepatic resection or liver transplantation. Liver transplantation should be considered in any patient with cirrhosis and HCC.

26. **Ans. E**

    The risk of HCC development in cirrhosis due to autoimmune hepatitis, primary sclerosing cholangitis in both sexes, and alcoholic and primary biliary cirrhosis in women is generally low. HCC in Wilson's disease is well-described despite adequate copper chelating therapy, although the true incidence is difficult to establish. Noncirrhotic HCCs do occur in viral cirrhosis but the absolute risk is low. If surveillance is offered, it should be 6-monthly abdominal ultrasound assessments in combination with serum AFP estimation. This is based on estimated median doubling time of 6 months for HCC.

27. **Ans. D**

    PLA is mostly of polymicrobial etiology including both aerobes and anaerobes. Gram-negative bacilli and *Streptococcus milleri* group are important causes. In 40% of cases, no obvious source of infection can be identified. Liver abscesses caused by *Staphylococcus aureus* are most common in children and patients with septicemia and impaired immunity. A barium enema or colonoscopy is usually done to locate a source of infection in PLA unless a biliary or other source is apparent.

28. **Ans. D**

    Biliary source of sepsis from gallstones, biliary stricture, ERCP, and operation is the most common cause. Blood culture may identify causative organism in 50% of cases and the yield increases to 90%, if aspirated material is cultured. Surgical—open or laparoscopic drainage—may be required, if there is inadequate response to percutaneous drainage, or in situations of multiple abscesses, if the abscesses are loculated, ruptured abscess, unresolved jaundice, or renal impairment. Large pyogenic abscesses (5 cm or more) usually need drainage, in addition to antibiotics for effective resolution.

29. **Ans. B**

    Hepatitis C is an RNA virus and is a major risk factor for HCC. The major mode of transmission is by contaminated blood—before 1991 by blood transfusion, now most commonly by shared needles in drug addicts. Sexual transmission is uncommon. Although alpha-interferon in currently recommended regimens will improve liver function tests in the short term in over 50% of patients, viral clearance is achieved in only 25% of patients.

30. **Ans. C**

Indications for liver transplantation: Acute liver failure due to hepatitis A, acetaminophen, autoimmune hepatitis, hepatitis B, hepatitis C, cryptogenic, drugs, hepatitis D, Wilson's disease, Budd–Chiari syndrome, Fatty infiltration—acute fatty liver of pregnancy, Reye syndrome;

Cirrhosis from chronic liver diseases such as chronic hepatitis B virus infection, chronic hepatitis C virus infection, alcoholic liver disease, autoimmune hepatitis, cryptogenic liver disease, non-alcoholic fatty liver disease;

Malignant diseases of the liver such as hepatocellular carcinoma, carcinoid tumor, islet cell tumour, epithelioid hemangioendothelioma, cholangiocarcinoma, metabolic liver disease, Wilson's disease, Hereditary hemochromatosis, alpha-1 antitrypsin deficiency, glycogen storage disease, cystic fibrosis, glycogen storage disease I and IV, Crigler–Najjar syndrome, galactosemia, type 1 hyperoxaluria, familial homozygous hypercholesterolemia, hemophilia A and B;

Vascular diseases of the liver such as Budd–Chiari syndrome, Veno-occlusive disease, Cholestatic liver diseases, primary biliary cirrhosis, primary sclerosing cholangitis, secondary biliary cirrhosis, biliary atresia, Alagille syndrome, Byler's disease.

Miscellaneous: Adult polycystic liver disease, nodular regenerative hyperplasia, Caroli's disease, severe graft-versus-host disease, amyloidosis, sarcoidosis, hepatic trauma.

Ref:
1. *Varma V, Mehta N, Kumaran V, Nundy S. Indications and Contraindications for Liver Transplantation. International Journal of Hepatology. 2011;121862*

CHAPTER 17

Infections and Metabolic Sequelae

Rajesh Chandra Mishra, Reena Sharma

1. **What is Warburg effect in sepsis?**
   A. The anaerobic switch from oxidative phosphorylation to glycolysis
   B. The aerobic switch from oxidative phosphorylation to glycolysis
   C. The anaerobic switch from glycolysis to oxidative phosphorylation
   D. The aerobic switch from glycolysis to oxidative phosphorylation
   E. None of the above

2. **The depletion of which element is postulated for progression to septic shock?**
   A. Glutathione
   B. Hydrogen peroxide
   C. Lithium
   D. Aluminum
   E. Manganese

3. **The excess of which of the following membrane-permeable oxidizing agent is considered responsible for the pathogenesis of sepsis?**
   A. Superoxide anion
   B. Oxygen
   C. Hydrogen peroxide
   D. Nitric oxide
   E. Peroxynitrite

4. **Regarding calcium metabolism in sepsis, which one of the following statements is true?**
   A. Low intracellular calcium, increased serum calcium
   B. Increased intracellular calcium, low serum calcium
   C. Increased intracellular calcium, high serum calcium
   D. Low intracellular calcium, low serum calcium
   E. None of the above

5. **In studies, all of the following vitamin deficiencies have been associated with decreased mortality in sepsis,** *except:*
   A. Vitamin C
   B. Vitamin B1
   C. Vitamin B12
   D. Vitamin E
   E. None of the above

6. **Changes in the thyroid hormones in infection have all of the following,** *except:*
   A. Decrease in serum levels of triiodothyronine (T3)
   B. A mild increase in thyroxine (T4) levels
   C. Low TSH
   D. Increase in fT4 levels
   E. Decrease in fT4 levels

7. **Which of the following hormonal changes are associated with poor outcomes in sepsis?**
   A. Decrease in fT4 levels
   B. High GH concentrations
   C. Mean glucose concentrations
   D. High levels of precursor hormone of calcitonin
   E. All of the above

8. **Pathogens manipulate the host immune response to produce metabolic effects. Production of which of the following cytokines after infectious trigger is not associated with host hypoglycemia?**
   A. IL-17
   B. IL-6
   C. IL-1
   D. TNF-α
   E. IL-10

9. **Regarding use of L-carnitine in sepsis patients, which one of the following is true?**
   A. High-quality human trials have proven its use
   B. Its use in high doses has shown to be associated with worsening of hemodynamic parameters
   C. Lower 28-day mortality rate was shown to be associated in a phase-1 randomized controlled trial (RCT)
   D. It is used in boluses of 4 g, 6 hourly
   E. L-carnitine is involved in the rate-limiting step of β-oxidation to transport long-chain fatty acids from the mitochondria to cytoplasm

10. **Following drugs (clinically approved and candidates in clinical trials) are capable of altering host immunometabolism to improve clinical outcomes in pulmonary infections,** *except:*
    A. Aspirin
    B. Metformin
    C. Statins
    D. Rituximab
    E. Ezetimibe

11. Regarding selenium, all are true, *except:*
    A. Lower Se levels were associated with greater tissue damage and the presence of infection and organ dysfunction
    B. It is an antioxidant
    C. Recent meta-analysis found selenium to decrease mortality in ICU patients with infection
    D. ICU patients with low admission levels of Se were found to be at increased risk of nosocomial pneumonia, organ system failure, and mortality
    E. It is not recommended at the current time that Se be given to patients with sepsis

12. About adrenal insufficiency in infection, which one of the following is true?
    A. There is absolute adrenal insufficiency
    B. Major cause is inadequate synthesis of cortisol due to cellular dysfunction
    C. In septic shock, there is enhanced adrenal response to corticotropin
    D. Prevalence is about 15% in septic shock
    E. Low-dose corticosteroids in septic shock have shown to decrease mortality

13. Which of the following statements is true for liver dysfunction in sepsis?
    A. Sepsis-induced liver dysfunction does not correlate with the severity of infection
    B. Clinical jaundice is usually an early presentation in sepsis
    C. In hypoxic hepatitis, splanchnic blood flow is decreased
    D. Clinical jaundice is usually due to intrahepatic cholestasis
    E. Corticosteroids are recommended for the treatment of sepsis-induced hepatic dysfunction

14. Regarding metabolic reprogramming that happens in sepsis, which of the following statements is false?
    A. Infection-induced inflammation leads to hypoxia, which allows WBCs to produce fast ATP
    B. Glutamine and arginine play an important role in inflammatory cells
    C. There is accumulation of free fatty acids in the blood
    D. At cellular level, a strong decrease in ATP/ADP ratio is found
    E. Levels of D-lactate are significantly increased

15. Specific neuroendocrine and metabolic perturbations in sepsis include all, *except:*
    A. Dysglycemia
    B. Hyperphosphatemia
    C. Biphasic vasopressin secretion
    D. Depression of pituitary thyroid
    E. Activation and depression of HPA axis

16. A 65-year-old woman with history of fatigue; pain in the proximal interphalangeal joints, knees, and hips; and low-grade fever is evaluated during a follow-up visit after 4-weeks. She has no history of joint swelling, chest pain, or shortness of breath. Over the past 4 years, she has had progressive dryness of the eyes and mouth with a 5-month history of Raynaud phenomenon. On physical examination, she is febrile. Cardiac examination is normal, and the lungs are clear. She has bilateral parotid gland enlargement, a firm 4-cm left axillary lymph node, and a 0.3-cm left anterior cervical lymph node. Musculoskeletal examination reveals bilateral crepitus of the knees. There is no joint swelling. Laboratory studies: Hemoglobin 11.6 g/dL (116 g/L) Leukocyte count 3400/µL (3.4 m 109/L) Platelet count 120,000/µL (120 m 109/L) Rheumatoid factor 76 U/mL (76 kU/L) Antinuclear antibodies Positive, Anti-Ro/SSA antibodies Positive, Anti-La/SSB antibodies Positive, Urinalysis Normal, Blood cultures No growth, Chest radiograph and mammogram are normal. What is the likely diagnosis in the case described above?
    A. Systemic lupus erythematosus
    B. Sjögren's syndrome
    C. Systemic sclerosis
    D. Mixed connective tissue disorder (MCTD)

17. A 15-year-old male adolescent is evaluated in the emergency department for a 2-day history of persistent fever, abdominal pain, and right knee pain. During the past year, he has had three similar episodes, each lasting 2–3 days. He feels well between episodes. He takes no medications.

    On physical examination, temperature is 38.3°C (101.0°F), blood pressure is 138/82 mm Hg, pulse rate is 100 beats/min, and respiration rate is 20 breaths/min. There is diffuse abdominal tenderness without rebound and no evidence of hepatosplenomegaly or lymphadenopathy. The right knee has an effusion; flexion of the knee is limited to 105°. A well-demarcated, raised, erythematous, warm, and painful rash is noted on the right lower extremity overlying the shin.

    Laboratory studies reveal an erythrocyte sedimentation rate (ESR) of 45 mm/h and a normal serum ferritin level; antinuclear antibody test results are negative. Urinalysis reveals 1+ protein with no cells or casts.

    Which of the following is the most likely diagnosis?
    A. Adult-onset Still's disease
    B. Crohn's disease
    C. Familial Mediterranean fever
    D. Reactive arthritis

18. A 34-year-old man is evaluated in the emergency department for a 2-day history of right eye redness and pain, photophobia, and decreased visual acuity. He has a 4-year history of recurrent, painful oral ulcerations and tender nodules on his shins as well as occasional knee and ankle pain for the past 2 months. His only medication is occasional diclofenac for joint pain.

On physical examination, temperature is 99.6°F, blood pressure is 134/80 mm Hg, pulse rate is 110 beats/min, and respiration rate is 19 breaths/min. BMI is 27. On ophthalmologic examination, there is a ciliary flush around the right limbus and a constricted pupil. A slit lamp examination reveals findings consistent with anterior and posterior uveitis; retinal vasculitis is also present. Oral ulcerations varying in size from 5 mm to 1 cm are noted on the inner cheek, palate, and tongue. The lungs are clear. The abdomen is nontender. No bruits are noted. The left knee and right ankle are swollen. Peripheral pulses are normal.

Laboratory test results are pending.

Chest radiograph reveals a prominent right pulmonary artery. CT of the chest demonstrates an aneurysm of the right pulmonary artery.

Which of the following is the most likely diagnosis?

A. Behçet disease
B. Granulomatosis with polyangiitis
C. Polyarteritis nodosa
D. Sarcoidosis

19. Symptoms resembling systemic lupus erythematosus may develop in all, *except*:
   1. Parvovirus B19 infection
   2. Celiac disease
   3. Treatment with isoniazid
   4. Viral type C hepatitis
   5. Ulcerative colitis

A. Answers 1 and 3 are correct
B. Answers 1, 2, and 3 are correct
C. Answers 1, 2, 3, and 4 are correct
D. Answers 1, 3, 4, and 5 are correct
E. Answers 1, 2, 3, 4, and 5 are correct

20. A 39-year-old female presents with fever, malaise, myalgia, and weight loss. She has had a cough and recurrent hemoptysis. She has also noticed a rash. On examination, there is evidence of palpable purpura. ANCA PR3 and ANCA MPO are positive and an eosinophil count is normal. What is the most likely diagnosis?

A. Polyarteritis nodosa
B. Wegener's granulomatosis
C. Churg-Strauss syndrome
D. Goodpasture's syndrome
E. Microscopic polyangiitis

21. A 42-year-old gentleman has had chronic problems with rhinitis. He has just been recently diagnosed with asthma. He has had a few episodes of hemoptysis. He also has a purpuric rash. Bloods revealed normal eosinophils and autoantibodies revealed a positive pANCA and cANCA. Chest X-ray (CXR) shows interstitial shadowing reported as pneumonitis. What is the most likely diagnosis?

A. Wegener's granulomatosis
B. Tuberculosis
C. Polyarteritis nodosa
D. SLE
E. Churg-Strauss syndrome

22. A 38-year-old man is evaluated in the emergency department for a 2-week history of progressive pain and swelling of both ankles. He also has low-grade fever and a painful red left eye with photophobia of 2 days' duration. The patient has no other pertinent personal or family medical history. He takes no medications. On physical examination, temperature is 38.2°C (100.7°F), blood pressure is 128/26 mm Hg, pulse rate is 96. Which of the following is the most likely diagnosis?

A. Reactive arthritis
B. Sarcoidosis
C. Psoriatic arthritis
D. Ankylosing spondylitis

23. In the case discussed in Q22, which of the following is the most appropriate diagnostic test to perform next?

A. ANCA assay
B. Chest radiography
C. Colonoscopy
D. Urine polymerase chain reaction for *Neisseria gonorrhoeae*

24. A 35-year-old female presented with generalized edema, shortness of breath, and decreased urine output for 1 week, fever with joint pains for 5 days, which was associated with productive cough. She is nondiabetic normotensive. There is no any past history suggestive of pulmonary tuberculosis or rheumatic heart disease.

Clinical examination revealed anemia with anasarca. She had tachycardia and tachypnea with low-oxygen saturation. On auscultation, there was a pansystolic murmur in the mitral area with bilateral diffuse wheeze and coarse crepitations. Initially, she was diagnosed to have LRTI with acute LVF. She was treated with broad-spectrum antibiotics and diuretics. Her investigations revealed bilateral basal opacities with the possibility of bilateral pneumonitis versus CCF. 2D echo showed evidence of nodules over AML and PML. Simultaneously, patient developed oral ulcers. Investigations showed bicytopenia with normal leukocyte count and raised ESR, mild proteinuria with serum creatinine—1.9 mg/dL, normal LFT, and no growth in blood cultures. Ultrasound abdomen showed mild ascites.

What is the next suitable test to be done in this patient?
   A. Antinuclear antibody
   B. Rheumatoid factor
   C. Chikungunya IgM
   D. Complement levels

25. What is the likely cause of vegetations on the mitral valve in the patient described above?
   A. Infective endocarditis
   B. Marantic endocarditis
   C. Libman–Sacks endocarditis

26. Post-traumatic invasive fungal infection (IFI) in military patients is most often caused by the following, *except*:
   A. Candida
   B. *Mucorales*
   C. *Aspergillus*
   D. *Fusarium*

27. Risk factors associated with post-traumatic IFI development in military patients include all, *except*:
   A. Massive transfusion (>20 units/24 hours)
   B. Blast injury
   C. Penetrating wounds
   D. Dismounted status
   E. Above-knee traumatic amputation

28. Disseminated Candidiasis affects eyes in the form of:
   A. Iriditis
   B. Keratitis
   C. Chorioretinitis
   D. Uveitis

29. What is the universal mechanism that causes resistance to azoles and other systemic antifungal drugs?
   A. Target site modification
   B. Drug pump upregulation
   C. Nontarget effects
   D. Biofilm formation

30. Each of the following statements concerning mucormycosis is correct, *except:*
   A. Classically hyphae invade blood vessels and cause necrosis of tissue
   B. Acidemia and hyperglycemia in diabetic patients are a predisposing factor to mucormycosis
   C. The fungi that cause mucormycosis are transmitted by airborne asexual spores
   D. Tissue sections from a patient with mucormycosis show budding yeasts

ANSWERS WITH EXPLANATIONS

1. **Ans. B**
   Warburg effect is the aerobic switch from glycolysis to oxidative phosphorylation. It is as much a hallmark of sepsis as it is of cancer.
   One of the first lessons learned about the proinflammatory response in sepsis was that hypoxia, known to trigger glycolysis in inflammation, may contribute to this effect. However, glycolysis continues even in the presence of adequate delivery of oxygen to the affected tissues.
   Ref:
   1. *Bar-Or D, Carrick M, Tanner A II, Lieser MJ, Rael LT, Brody E. Overcoming the Warburg effect: Is it the key to survival in sepsis? J Crit Care. 2018;43:197-201.*

2. **Ans. A**
   A crucial element that can become depleted early during the progression to septic shock is glutathione. Glutathione is chiefly responsible for supplying reducing equivalents to neutralize hydrogen peroxide, a toxic oxidizing agent that is produced during normal metabolism. Without glutathione, hydrogen peroxide can rise to toxic levels in tissues and blood where it can cause severe oxidative injury to organs and to the microvasculature. Continued exposure can result in microvascular dysfunction, capillary leakage, and septic shock.
   Ref:
   1. *Pravda J. Metabolic theory of septic shock. World J Crit Care Med. 2014;3(2):45-54.*

3. **Ans. C**
   Septic shock begins with a systemic inflammatory reaction to an infection. A contemporaneous increase in metabolism is initiated, which can deplete reserves of critical nutrients such as glutathione. Glutathione is crucial for the neutralization of H_2O_2, a toxic, membrane-permeable oxidizing agent generated as a byproduct of cellular metabolism. Depletion of cellular glutathione results in elevation of H_2O_2, which can diffuse out of organ parenchymal cells and into capillary endothelium before reaching the bloodstream. Once

in the systemic circulation, excess H_2O_2 is distributed throughout the body resulting in systemic oxidative damage to plasma components, organs, and blood vessels. The net result is H_2O_2-induced coagulopathy, immunocyte apoptosis, and microvascular dysfunction leading to disseminated intravascular coagulation, immunosuppression, organ failure, and septic shock. H_2O_2 inhibits GPx and catalase, which are critical antioxidant enzymes required for H_2O_2 neutralization. This prevents restoration of normal plasma and tissue redox balance while exacerbating oxidative tissue damage. H_2O_2 can also activate nuclear factor-κB (NF-κB) contributing to the inappropriate activation of this master proinflammatory transcription factor observed in septic shock.
Ref:
1. *Pravda J. Metabolic theory of septic shock. World J Crit Care Med. 2014;3(2):45-54.*

4. **Ans. B**
Hypocalcemia in sepsis, hypothesized to be secondary to defective intracellular calcium homeostasis, is common and correlates with disease-specific scores during critical illness. Although systemic Ca^{2+} levels are reduced during sepsis, there are increased cytosolic Ca^{2+} levels. These heightened intracellular Ca^{2+} levels lead to elevated inflammatory responses, cellular dysfunction, and can even be cytotoxic. In addition, accumulation of Ca^{2+} in organs during sepsis is associated with significant organ dysfunction.
Ref:
1. *Frydrych LM, Fattahi F, He K, Ward PA, Delano MJ. Diabetes and sepsis: risk, recurrence, and ruination. Front Endocrinol. 2017;8:271.*

5. **Ans. C**
Studies have shown association between deficiencies of thiamine, vitamin C and vitamin E, and poor outcome in sepsis.

6. **Ans. D**
Patients with mild illness often show a decrease in serum levels of triiodothyronine (T3) and a mild increase in thyroxine (T4) levels, while TSH is also lowered. This condition is called the euthyroid sick syndrome or the low T3 syndrome. A decrease in fT4 levels in the course of disease may also point to adverse outcome.
Ref:
1. *Widmer A, Schuetz P. Endocrine dysfunction during sepsis—are changes in hormone levels a physiological adaptation or a therapeutic target? J Lab Precis Med. 2018;3:61.*

7. **Ans. E**
A decrease in fT4 levels in the course of disease may also point to adverse outcome. GH showed to be an independent predictor for mortality, which means that GH levels correlated with the severity of disease. There is an association between mean glucose concentrations and adverse clinical outcomes in patients without diabetes with an acute infection. The precursor hormone of calcitonin—procalcitonin (PCT)—has now emerged as an important diagnostic and prognostic marker for critically ill patients with sepsis.
Ref:
1. *Widmer A, Schuetz P. Endocrine dysfunction during sepsis—are changes in hormone levels a physiological adaptation or a therapeutic target? J Lab Precis Med. 2018;3:61.*

8. **Ans. B**
Interleukin-1 (IL-1) activates the sympathetic nervous system and causes a drop in blood glucose. Other cytokines, including IL-10, have been implicated in *Plasmodium falciparum*-induced hypoglycemia. Likewise, *Plasmodium species* elicit the production of host immunomodulators such as tumor necrosis factor-α (TNF-α) during infection, which also produces hypoglycemia. *Bordetella pertussis* infection increases host IL-1 production as well as raises levels of IL-17, which is also associated with hypoglycemia.
Ref:
1. *Freyberg Z, Harvill ET. Pathogen manipulation of host metabolism: A common strategy for immune evasion. PLoS Pathog. 2017;13(12):e1006669.*

9. **Ans. C**
L-carnitine is involved in the rate-limiting step of β-oxidation to transport long-chain fatty acids from the cytoplasm to mitochondria. The use of L-carnitine in sepsis lacks quality human trials. Two human clinical trials have evaluated the use of L-carnitine in sepsis and both showed promising results. The first, published in 1991, demonstrated early improvements in hemodynamic parameters in patients with septic shock. The second, a small phase-1 randomized control trial of 31 patients, analyzed the safety and efficacy of L-carnitine infusion in patients undergoing vasopressor-dependent septic shock. This study showed a lower 28-day mortality rate of 25 versus 60% favoring L-carnitine with no differences in significant adverse events. The dosage for L-carnitine in the later study was a 4-g bolus injection (20 mL) over 2–3 minutes followed by an 8-g infusion (8 g in 1,000 mL of 0.9% normal saline) over the following 12 hours (83 mL/h).
Ref:
1. *Belsky JB, Wira CR, Jacob V, Sather JE, Lee PJ. A review of micronutrients in sepsis: the role of thiamine, l-carnitine, vitamin C, selenium and vitamin D. Nutr Res Rev. 2018;31(2):281-90.*

10. Ans. D

Drug/chemical compound	Biological target	Description	References
Clinically approved agents			
Metformin	Activation of AMPK	Clinically approved to treat T2DM. Increases mitochondrial respiration and FA breakdown, leading to increased generation of memory CD+ T-cells. Shown to enhance immune clearance of *Mycobacterium tuberculosis (M. tb)* in murine models	Singhal et al., 2014
Bevacizumab	VEGF	Used in the treatment of glioblastoma. Corrects aberrant neovascularization in cancer tissue, allowing for oxygenation and reduction of hypoxia. Has been shown to improve vascular remodeling in TB granulomas, also increasing drug penetration. This is bound to affect immune-cell infiltration and anti-pathogen activity in situ due to an increase in oxygen, which enables aerobic glycolysis	Datta et al., 2015; Oehlers et al., 2015
Ipillmumab	CTLA-4	Both anti-CTLA-4 and anti-PD-1 are clinically approved for treating metastatic melanoma while the latter is also approved for treatment-refractory non-small cell lung cancer. Shown in the cancer setting to cause a shift to FAO from glucose metabolism, reminiscent of memory CD+ T-cells, including reduced uptake of glucose from the extracellular environment, thereby modulating the ability of T-cells to acquire effector functions and produce IFN-γ. CTLA-4, on the other hand, inhibits glycolysis without switching the cell metabolism to FAO. This might have implications in patients with diabetes and lung infections, where high blood glucose level is a characteristic; PD-1-expressing antigen-specific T-cells may be long-lived (like central memory cells) and highly amenable to therapeutic intervention.	Patsoukis et al., 2015
Nivolumab, pembrolizumab	PD-1		
Statins, i.e., atorvastatin, pravastatin, lovastatin, simvastatin	HMG-CoA reductase	Blocks the enzymatic activity of HMG-CoA reductase, which catalyzes an important intermediate step in the isoprenoid pathway: conversion of HMG-CoA to mevalonate. Downstream of this process is the synthesis of isoprenyl pyrophosphate, which is necessary for cholesterol synthesis as well as Vγ9Vδ2 T-cell activation. Statin use in the cancer setting has shown to reduce Vγ9Vδ2 T-cell-mediated tumor rejection owing to increased LDLR expression, increased LDL uptake and compromised mitochondrial function. However, statins could be useful against chronic inflammatory processes during infectious disease pathogenesis, i.e., TB	Wesch et al., 1997; Urbano et al., 2017; Rodrigues et al., 2018
Ezetimibe	Niemann-Pick-C1-Like1 (NPC1L1) protein	Ezetimibe blocks the reabsorption of cholesterol by cells, thereby reducing the amount of intracellular LDL levels. Has anti-inflammatory properties but may induce NO expression. It has been shown to reduce intracellular *M.tb* survival in macrophages while patients with T2DM taking ezetimibe have lower incidence of LTBI	Toshiyuki and Yasuchika, 2011; Tsai et al., 2017
Aspirin (potentially also other nonsteroidal anti-inflammatory drugs, NSAIDs)	Activation of NO/ROS release	NO is an important biological mediator as well as immune effector molecule, particularly against intracellular pathogens–as is the ROS hydrogen peroxide (H_2O_2). May be involved in lipid metabolism, based on observations in patients with T2DM. Aspirin-driven NO production in macrophages and dendritic cells (as well as adipocytes) may, in fact, promote eradication of local bacterial reservoirs in the case of TB without raising an exaggerated immune response	Taubert et al., 2004; Blaise et al., 2005; Niedbala et al., 2006; Tripathi et al., 2007; Morris et al., 2009; Schroder, 2009; Eisen et al., 2013; Vazquez-Meza et al., 2013; Vilaplam et al., 2013; Epperly et al., 2016; Beigier-Bompadre et al., 2017; Kroesen et al., 2017; Mishra and Mishra, 2017
Resveratrol (also metformin)	Activation of SIRT1	Sirtuin 1 (SIRT1) is an important histone deacetylase with functions in modulating lipid metabolism as well as immune regulation in myelocytic and lymphocytic cells. Treatment of obese individuals with resveratrol improved lipid metabolism and reduced circulating levels of fatty acids and glucose as well as inflammatory markers. Resveratrol-mediated SIRT1 activation results in dampened pro-inflammatory CD4+ T-cells responses as well as resolution of chronic lung inflammation and associated tissue pathology in mice infected with *M. tb*	Timmers et al., 2011; Zou et al., 2013

Contd...

Contd...

Drug/chemical compound	Biological target	Description	References
Candidates in clinical trials			
ADU-S100	Activation of STING pathway	ADU-S100 is a synthetic cyclic dinucleotide mimicking the structure of cGAMP and is currently in clinical trials as an agonist of the STING pathway. Recent evidence demonstrates that STING activation via cGAMP allows for correction of lipid/glucose metabolism dysregulation while enhancing innate and adaptive immune responses, i.e., type I interferon production and CD+ T-cell activity. This has implications for eradicating latent pathogen reservoirs, I.e., LTBI, *Cryptococcus* spp. infections, asymptomatic *Klebsiella* spp. infection in individuals, including those who suffer from metabolic conditions/diseases	(Miller et al., 1996; Weintrobe et al., 2013; Qureshi et al., 2014; Chonmaitree et al., 2015; Ohkuri et al., 2017; Desbien et al., 2018); Clinical Trials.gov identifiers: NCT02675439, NCT03172936
Dactolisib (BEZ235)	PI3K/mTOR pathway	Dactolisib inhibits the PI3K/mTOR pathway to the effect of abrogating glycolysis in exposed cells. This has shown benefit in ameliorating deleterious lung pathology in influenza A infection while extending survival (murine model). Dactolisib is currently in clinical trials for patients with cancer	Smallwood et al., 2017; National Library of Medicine, 2018

(AMPK: adenosine monophosphate-activated protein kinase; T2DM: type II diabetes mellitus; VEGF: vascular endothelial growth factor; CTIA-4: cytotoxic T lymphocyte associated antigen 4; PD-1: programmed cell death 1; FAD: fatty acid oxidation; LDI: low-density lipoprotein; NO: nitric oxide; ROS: reactive oxygen species; NSAID: nonsteroidal anti-inflammatoy drug; cGAMP: Cyclic guanosine monophosphate–adenosine monophosphate; STING: stimulator of interferon genes; LTBI: latent tuberculosis infection; PI3K: phosphatidylinositol-3-kinase; mTOR: mammalian target of rapamycin)

Ref:
1. Martin R, Ernest D, Alimuddin Z, Maeurer M. Immunometabolism and pulmonary infections: implications for protective immune responses and host-directed therapies. Front Microbiol. 2019;10:962.

11. Ans. C

Selenium is frequently referred to as an antioxidant due to its role in reversing the effects of oxidized lipids and methionine residues, and detoxifying hydrogen peroxidase. The most recent meta-analysis analyzing 21 randomized control trials found no effect of Se on mortality.

Ref:
1. Belsky JB, Wira CR, Jacob V, Sather JE, Lee PJ. A review of micronutrients in sepsis: the role of thiamine, l-carnitine, vitamin C, selenium and vitamin D. Nutr Res Rev. 2018;31(2):281-90.

12. Ans. B

In infection, there is functional/relative adrenal insufficiency (RAI). The major cause for RAI is inadequate synthesis of cortisol due to cellular dysfunction. This is often combined with peripheral glucocorticoid resistance of the target cells, which is caused by inflammatory events and aggravates the clinical course, although the absolute cortisol serum levels might be normal. In septic shock, RAI may be due to impaired pituitary corticotropin release, attenuated adrenal response to corticotropin, and reduced cortisol synthesis. Prevalence of RAI may be as high as 50–75% in septic shock. Numerous randomized controlled trials with low-dose corticosteroids in patients with septic shock also confirmed shock reversal and reduction of vasopressor support within a few days after initiation of therapy in most patients.

Ref:
1. Vincent JL, Abraham E, Moore FA, Kochanek PM, Fink MP. Textbook of critical care, 7th edition. Amsterdam, Netherlands: Elsevier; 2017.

13. Ans. D

Liver dysfunction induced by sepsis is recognized as one of the components that contribute to the severity of the disease.

Commonly during sepsis, increased bilirubin levels are a late event in the course of multiorgan dysfunction. In a large cohort of ICU patients, 11% had an "early" hepatic dysfunction defined as a bilirubin concentration of greater than 2 mg/dL (>34 µmol/L) within 48 hours of admission.

Liver histological studies in patients with bacteremic jaundice showed a predominant intrahepatic cholestasis.

In hypoxic hepatitis due to septic shock, splanchnic blood flow and cardiac output are increased but not sufficient to counterbalance the high demands for oxygen and the inability of liver cells to extract oxygen.

Corticosteroid use in septic shock is still debated, but with respect to the liver, experimental data suggest that they may have an immunomodulatory effect on sepsis-induced cholestasis through the induction of hepatobiliary transporters and restoration of bile transport. Moreover, in the CORTICUS (Corticosteroid Therapy of Septic Shock) study, hydrocortisone treated patients demonstrated a faster improvement in liver failure (SOFA hepatic score of 3 or 4) during the first week ($p < 0.0001$). However, at present, the use of corticosteroids cannot be recommended for the treatment of sepsis-induced hepatic dysfunction.

Ref:
1. Nesseler N, Launey Y, Aninat C, Morel F, Mallédant Y, Seguin P. Clinical review: the liver in sepsis. Crit Care. 2012;16(5):235.

14. Ans. E

Infection leads to direct tissue damage and to inflammation, which in turn leads to hypoxia, which is essential to allow white blood cells (WBCs) to produce fast ATP from glucose and act fast on the infectious agents.

Several amino acids are also known to play an important role in inflammatory cells. For example, glutamine is an important precursor for peptide and protein synthesis supporting cytokine production. Glutamine is also required for purine and pyrimidine and thus nucleic acid and nucleotide synthesis allowing proliferation of immune cells. Arginine can be converted into nitric oxide by nitric oxide synthase, which is then released by M1 macrophages.

There is accumulation of free fatty acids in the blood by the decreased ability of tissues to oxidize them via β-oxidation.

In biopsies of sepsis patients, a strong decrease in ATP/ADP ratio is found. A clear increase in L-lactate is usually seen directly related to poor outcome, besides signs of poor fatty acid oxidation and amino acid catabolism.

Ref:
1. Wyngene LV, Vandewalle J, Libert C. Reprogramming of basic metabolic pathways in microbial sepsis: therapeutic targets at last? EMBO Mol Med. 2018;10(8):e8712.

15. Ans. B

Specific neuroendocrine and metabolic perturbations:
- Activation and depression of HPA axis
- Biphasic vasopressin secretory response
- Hyperglycemia/dysglycemia
- Depression of pituitary thyroid
- Depression of gonadotropins and hypogonadism
- Disorders of Na/K balance, hypophosphatemia, hypocalcemia, and hypomagnesemia

Ref:
1. Khardori R, Castillo D. Endocrine and metabolic changes during sepsis: an update. Med Clin N Am. 2012;96(6):1095-105.

16. Ans. B

The Sjögren's syndrome (SS) is an autoimmune exocrine disorder with signs and symptoms of dry mouth and keratoconjunctivitis sicca, which may sometimes display a wide range of systemic, non-glandular alterations. The prevalence of this syndrome has been estimated to range between 0.5% and 1% (3), with a female:male ratio of about 9:1.

Histopathology in minor salivary gland (presence of focal lymphocytic sialadenitis with a focus score ≥1) is one out of the six diagnostic criteria set in the Revised International Classification Criteria for Sjögren's Syndrome for diagnosis of SS. It has recently become more important because of the consensus in considering only objective criteria to define a SS case, which has to meet at least two of the following three findings: (1) Positivity serum anti-SSA and/or SSB; (2) Ocular staining score >3; and (3) Presence of focal lymphocytic sialadenitis with a focus score >1 per 4 mm^2 of glandular tissue.

17. Ans. C

This 16-year-old male adolescent has familial Mediterranean fever (FMF), an autosomal recessive disorder characterized by recurrent 12- to 72-hour episodes of fever with serositis (most commonly abdominal or pleural), synovitis (most often monoarticular and affecting the lower extremities), and erysipeloid rash. Symptoms typically begin in childhood or adolescence; however, 10% of patients experience their first episode in adulthood. FMF is most prevalent in persons of Mediterranean ethnicity but is not restricted to this group. Laboratory studies are consistent with acute inflammation, and serology results for connective tissue and rheumatoid disease are negative. Proteinuria revealed on urinalysis may represent kidney amyloidosis, which can develop in untreated persons. Colchicine is standard therapy and reduces the likelihood of acute attacks and amyloidosis.

Adult-onset Still's disease (AOSD) is characterized by fever, rash, and joint pain, and serositis (usually pleuritis or pericarditis) may occur. However, fever associated with AOSD is quotidian, lasts less than 4 hours, and peaks in the early evening; rash is evanescent, salmon-colored, not painful, and appears on the trunk and proximal extremities. Abdominal pain is rare. Finally, a markedly elevated serum ferritin level occurs in most patients with AOSD.

Patients with Crohn's disease typically have progressive fatigue, prolonged diarrhea with abdominal pain, weight loss, and fever; extra-abdominal manifestations may include arthritis and skin rash (erythema nodosum or pyoderma gangrenosum). The brief episodic nature of this patient's abdominal and joint symptoms is unusual for Crohn's disease, as is the fact that he is completely well between episodes.

Monoarticular arthritis of the lower extremities may occur in patients with reactive arthritis, but fever and abdominal pain are uncommon. Patients with this disorder may have a history of conjunctivitis, oral or genital ulcers, and/or inflammatory back pain. The brief duration of this patient's episodes, with complete resolution between attacks, is not typical of reactive arthritis.

18. Ans. A

This patient most likely has Behçet's disease. Behçet's disease is a rare systemic disorder characterized by vasculitis and involvement of multiple visceral organs. The most important diagnostic clues are intermittent mucous membrane ulcerations and ocular involvement. Gastrointestinal, pulmonary, musculoskeletal, and neurological manifestations also may be present. This patient has a 2-year history of recurrent oral ulcerations, erythema nodosum, and arthritis and now presents with panuveitis, retinal vasculitis, and a pulmonary artery aneurysm, manifestations that are strongly suggestive of Behçet's disease.

Patients with granulomatosis with polyangiitis (also known as Wegener granulomatosis) can present with uveitis, retinal vasculitis, arthritis, and oral ulcers, as seen in this patient. However, the vasculitis associated with granulomatosis with polyangiitis involves small, rather than large, blood vessels, and aneurysms are not seen. Patients with granulomatosis with polyangiitis often have a history of upper airway disease such as sinusitis or epistaxis and often have glomerulonephritis, none of which is present in this patient.

Although polyarteritis nodosa can result in arterial aneurysms, it typically affects medium-sized mesenteric and renal arteries rather than pulmonary arteries and commonly results in intestinal ischemia and renovascular hypertension. Oral ulcers, uveitis, and erythema nodosum typically do not occur.

Sarcoidosis can manifest as arthritis and uveitis, and rarely can be associated with a large-vessel vasculitis. Pulmonary artery aneurysms are not typical. Chest radiograph usually demonstrates hilar lymphadenopathy with or without parenchymal lung disease.

19. **Ans. E**
Hepatitis C virus infection and SLE may share common clinical and serologic features. The extrahepatic manifestations of HCV may mimic SLE, with associated symptoms such as arthralgia, myalgia, sicca syndrome, and antinuclear antibody (ANA) positivity. Parvovirus B19 causes polyarthritis in adults. Several observers have noted a lupus-like syndrome and production of autoantibodies associated with this infection. Several drugs have been suggested to cause a lupus-like syndrome. Procainamide and hydralazine are the most common and have been shown by prospective studies to induce a mild form of a SLE like disease in 5–20% of patients treated. Isoniazid rarely induces this syndrome, with an incidence less than 1%. Drug-induced autoantibody production has been found to occur in 20% of patients receiving isoniazid, however. Celiac disease is also known to be associated with symptoms of lupus and may have positive antibodies as well. Ulcerative colitis, however, is not associated with lupus-like symptoms. ANA, however, can be falsely positive in ulcerative colitis.

20. **Ans. E**
Given the history and the positivity of ANCA-PR3 and ANCA-MPO. These autoantibodies are also observed in Churg–Strauss but there is also an associated eosinophilia. These autoantibodies are less common in Wegener's granulomatosis. Goodpasture's anti-GBM is found and the history is not indicative of PAN.

21. **Ans. A**
The most likely diagnosis is Wegener's granulomatosis. Positive ANCA-PR3 and -MPO is also very suspicious of Churg-Strauss syndrome. It affects small- and medium-sized vessels. Wegener's granulomatosis can present with rhinorrhea, cough, hemoptysis, pleuritic pain, and renal symptoms such as hematuria. Eosinophilia is not seen. The history and autoantibodies are not in keeping with SLE. Polyarteritis nodosa is ANCA negative and does not normally involve the lungs. TB is not in keeping with this.

22. **Ans. B**
Sarcoidosis is a disease involving abnormal collections of inflammatory cells that form lumps known as granulomas. The disease usually begins in the lungs, skin, or lymph nodes. Less commonly affected are the eyes, liver, heart, and brain. Any organ, however, can be affected. The signs and symptoms depend on the organ involved. Often, no, or only mild, symptoms are seen. When it affects the lungs, wheezing, coughing, shortness of breath, or chest pain may occur. Some may have Löfgren syndrome with fever, large lymph nodes, arthritis, and a rash known as erythema nodosum. So, the next step should be to do a chest radiograph.

23. **Ans. B**
As described in Question 22.

24. **Ans. A**
Patient has a multisystem involvement with joint pains, oral ulcers, ascites, proteinuria, bicytopenia, and vegetations on the mitral valve. Since blood cultures are sterile, the next step should be to rule out autoimmune conditions, most likely SLE. The best screening test for lupus is ANA.

25. **Ans. C**
In infective endocarditis, the vegetations are large, irregular, mobile with rotatory or vibratory motion, distributed along the closure of leaflets, and are homogeneous in echoreflectance. In contrast, Libman–Sacks vegetations are usually located at the basal, middle, or tip of leaflets, located on the atrial side of the mitral valve or vessel side of the aortic valve, are of variable sizes and shapes, and heterogeneous in echogenicity. Marantic endocarditis shows lesions located over the cusps and the patient usually has hypercoagulable state like APLA syndrome.

26. Ans. A

Mucorales, *Aspergillus*, and *Fusarium* species account for 34%, 31%, and 22% of IFI, respectively. Whereas in civilian patients, it is most often due to *Mucorales*. In military patients, *Mucorales*' growth is most predictive of recurrent necrosis and IFI diagnosis.

Ref:
1. Kronen R, Liang SY, Bochicchio G, Bochicchio K, Powderly WG, Spec A. Invasive fungal infections secondary to traumatic injury. Int J Infect Dis. 2017;62: 102-11.

27. Ans. C

Data derived from a case–control analysis within the TIDOS cohort focuses on the risk factors specific to military personnel. Massive transfusion (>20 U/24 hours), blast injury, dismounted status, and above-knee amputations were associated with IFI. Immunosuppression in the civilian population is well known to predispose patients to IFI. In a case–control study of patients injured during the Joplin tornado, patients with IFI had a greater number of wounds, were more likely to have penetrating wounds, and were more frequently diagnosed with rhabdomyolysis on admission compared to controls with broken skin but no evidence of IFI.

Ref:
1. Kronen R, Liang SY, Bochicchio G, Bochicchio K, Powderly WG, Spec A. Invasive fungal infections secondary to traumatic injury. Int J Infect Dis. 2017;62:102-11.
2. Neblett Fanfair R, Benedict K, Bos J, Bennett SD, Lo YC, Adebanjo T, et al. Necrotizing cutaneous mucormycosis after a tornado in Joplin, Missouri, in 2011. N Engl J Med. 2012;367(23):2214-25.

28. Ans. C

Invasive fungal infections are known to lead to hematogenous dissemination and metastatic ocular infection with potentially devastating consequences. Two distinct abnormalities are known to occur—Candida endophthalmitis with vitritis, usually presenting as fluffy balls extending into the vitreous body, and Candida chorioretinitis, with abnormalities restricted to the chorioretinal layers. It is recommended that dilated fundoscopy is performed in all patients with candidemia within a week of starting the therapy. Follow-up ophthalmological consultation with ocular candidiasis is necessary, because antifungal treatment should be continued until ocular lesions are completely resolved.

Ref:
1. Oude Lashof AM, Rothova A, Sobel JD, Ruhnke M, Pappas PG, Viscoli C, et al. Ocular manifestations of Candidemia. Clin Infect Dis. 2011;53(3):262-8.

29. Ans. D

The resistance to azoles involves several well-defined mechanisms, which include upregulation of drug transporters, overexpression or alteration of the drug target, and cellular changes caused, in some cases, by nontarget effects induced by stress responses. Biofilm formation on artificial devices, including heart valves and indwelling catheters, is another important drug-resistance mechanism that either resists drug action or promotes microbial resistance due to other mechanisms (e.g., drug pumps). The biofilm effectively reduces the concentration of the drug by trapping it in a glucan-rich matrix polymer. Mature biofilms show complex architecture with heterogeneous cell types enmeshed in extracellular matrix. Disruption of this process by genetic or chemical modulation of the β-1,3-glucan synthase decreases drug sequestration in the matrix, rendering biofilms susceptible to antifungal agents. Overall, biofilm formation is a universal mechanism that affects azole and other systemic antifungal drug classes.

Ref:
1. Perlin DS, Rautemaa-Richardson R, Alastruey-Izquierdo A. The global problem of antifungal resistance: prevalence, mechanisms, and management. Lancet Infect Dis. 2017;17:e383-92.
2. Desai JV, Mitchell AP. Candida albicans biofilm development and its genetic control. Microbiol Spectr. 2015;3:MB-0005-2014.

30. Ans. D

Mucorales, the zygomycetes class of fungi, cause mucormycosis in humans. Mucorales are obligate aerobic, nonseptate irregular hyphae with right-angled branches that measure up to 200 meter in length. The sporangiospores of the disease-causing fungi are 3–6 meter in diameter, and it is believed that human infections are caused by asexual spore formation. The predisposition of diabetics to acquire the mucormycosis infection may be related to acidosis and hyperglycemia. Acidosis disrupts iron binding of transferrin, resulting in an increased proportion of unbound iron, which may promote growth of the fungus. On histopathology, hyphae can be observed growing in and around vessels.

It is uniqueness lies in its ability to invade the vessel wall causing direct angioinvasion, which enhances hematogenous spread and results in thrombosis, ischemia, and tissue necrosis. Clinical management includes systemic antifungal therapy and surgical debridement, if possible, to remove all dead and infected tissue. Mucormycosis has an extremely high death rate even when aggressive therapy and surgical intervention are performed.

Ref:
1. Spellberg B, Edwards J Jr, Ibrahim A. Novel perspectives on mucormycosis: pathophysiology, presentation, and management. Clin Microbiol Rev. 2005;18(3):556-69.
2. Roden MM, Zaoutis TE, Buchanan WL, Knudsen TA, Sarkisova TA, Schaufele RL, et al. Epidemiology and outcome of zygomycosis: a review of 929 reported cases. Clin Infect Dis. 2005;41(5):634-53.
3. Ellis DH. Systemic zygomycosis. In: Merz WG, Hay RJ (Eds). Topley and Wilson' Microbiology and Microbial Infections. Medical Mycology. London: Arnold; 2005. pp. 659-86.

CHAPTER 18

Zoonosis

Om Shrivastav

1. A 66-year-old female presents to emergency with hemoptysis of 21 days duration. She also has fever, headache, and weakness of 4 weeks duration. She has a history of travel to Sudan where she recollects that she came in contact with the door knob of her hotel which had suspicious fluid stains. On detailed contact tracing there are seven other people quarantined with similar complains. Her most likely diagnosis is:
   A. Pulmonary tuberculosis
   B. Churg-Strauss syndrome
   C. Systemic vasculitis with polyangiitis
   D. Ebola virus disease (EVD)

2. A 16-year-old male has been treated for salmonellosis four times in the last 12 months. He has lost 23 kg of weight in the same duration and is now considered for percutaneous endoscopic gastrostomy (PEG) feeds. His *Salmonella typhi* titers both for somatic and flagellar antigens are consistently between 1:40 and 1:80. The most useful diagnostic test is:
   A. Laparoscopic exploration
   B. Biopsy of Peyer's patches
   C. Bone marrow aspirate and cultures
   D. Blood cultures

3. A 30-year-old female, migrated from Iraq has complains of fever, weight loss, diarrhea, and bone pain for last 5 months. She has a previous history of consuming meat and milk from her own farm in Iraq for several years. She cannot emphatically say if meat was fresh. She should be investigated for:
   A. *Leishmaniasis donovani*   B. Tuberculosis
   C. Tularemia   D. *Streptococcus milleri*

4. In the same patient, GeneXpert of the blood sample shows resistance to both rifampicin and isoniazid (INH) the treatment regime is expanded to six drugs. The most common cause of death in such patient is:
   A. Uterine cancer
   B. Bovine encephalopathy
   C. Pneumonia
   D. Drug-resistant colitis

5. A 31-year-old male presents with multiple joint pain, headache, back pain, and vomiting with night sweats. He describes the night sweats and the abdominal pain as progressively getting worse over last 3 weeks. He also describes contact with the sheeps and goats for work purposes. On examination, he has tender liver and multiple lymph nodes in the posterior cervical triangle, axillary, and inguinal regions. The most likely diagnosis is:
   A. Non-Hodgkin's lymphoma (NHL)
   B. Hodgkin's lymphoma
   C. Hepatocellular carcinoma with metastasis
   D. Brucellosis

6. The most useful first diagnostic modality would be:
   A. Positron emission tomography–computed tomography (PET-CT)
   B. Serology for *toxoplasma/toxocara*
   C. Liver biopsy
   D. Bone marrow aspirate and culture

7. The most optimal treatment for such patients is:
   A. Doxycycline + rifampicin for 8–12 weeks
   B. Augmentin duo twice a day for 3–4 weeks
   C. Amikacin as monotherapy
   D. Piperacillin-tazobactam + arbekacin

8. In the same patient, after 8 weeks treatment is asymptomatic for 3 months, but present with fresh complaints of severe lower back pain and MRI of spine is show in the image. The repeat immunoglobulin M (IgM) *Brucella* is positive. The most likely explanation is:

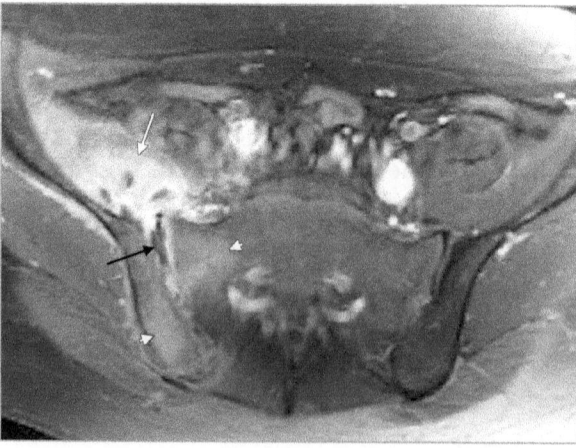

Source: Navallas M, Ares J, Beltrán B, Lisbona MP, Maymó J, Solano A. Sacroiliitis associated with axial spondyloarthropathy: new concepts and latest trends response. Radiographics. 2013;33:933-56.

   A. False positive serology
   B. *Brucella melitensis* relapse

C. Septic arthritis
D. Ankylosing spondylitis

9. Which of the following zoonotic diseases is not transmitted from dogs?
   A. Toxocariasis
   B. Brucella
   C. Scrub typhus
   D. Canine hepatitis

10. Which of the following zoonotic diseases is not transmitted from cats?
    A. Feline immunodeficiency virus (FIV) infection
    B. Cat scratch fever
    C. Toxocariasis
    D. Toxoplasmosis

11. An animal handlers looking after a sick domesticated dog presents with fever and lymphadenopathy since 6 weeks. Which of the following husbandry elements is not vitally important in reducing the risk of transmission of zoonotic disease to himself?
    A. Stopping animals from licking human faces
    B. Feeding human food to animals
    C. Having a prophylactic healthcare plan for animals
    D. Having a strict hygiene routine, especially with ill animals

12. A young male presents with urinary tract infection and a nonresolving pneumonia worsening over the last 2 weeks. He is employed a shipping company that transfers exotic birds across nations. In his work up the investigation most likely to be diagnostic is:
    A. Lymph node biopsy
    B. CT scan chest, abdomen, and pelvis
    C. Bone marrow aspirate
    D. Immunofluorescence test for *Chlamydia psittaci*

13. In the same patient the treatment of choice is?
    A. Azithromycin + rifampicin + doxycycline
    B. Amikacin + avibactam
    C. Ceftriaxone + gentamycin
    D. Crystalline penicillin + chloramphenicol

14. A 17-year-old boy presents with 5 days duration of abdominal cramps, fever, and bloody diarrhea. Two other family members have been treated for similar episodes. A third family member is hospitalized with the diagnosis of Guillain–Barré syndrome. They have an association with livestock. Stool culture and a colonoscopy are done in the foresaid patient. The most likely diagnosis is:
    A. *Entamoeba histolytica*   B. *Campylobacter*
    C. *Escherichia coli*   D. *Salmonella*

15. A 21-year-old female, laboratory technician by profession presents with a 3 months history of worsening alopecia followed by a 4 weeks history of progressively worsening lesions around her left eye. Both conditions are itchy and weeping. She has had exposure to samples from infected cattle and dogs. She has failed multiple oral and topical therapies including reported worsening with steroids. The most likely diagnosis is:

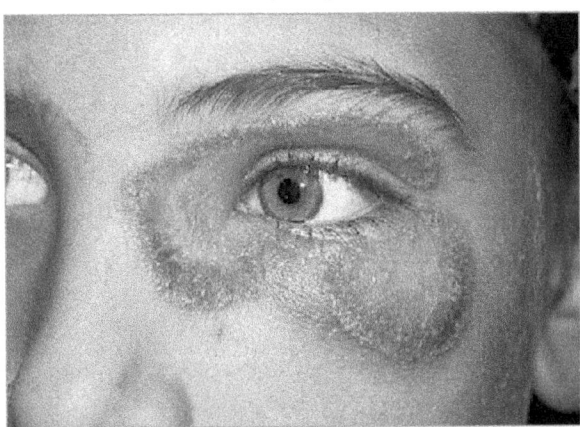

Source: Degreef H. Clinical forms of dermatophytosis (ringworm infection). Mycopathologia. 2008;166:257-65.

A. Secondary syphilis
B. Dermatophytosis
C. Cutaneous lupus
D. Dermatomyositis

16. A 46-year-old male postman by profession presents with 5 days history of painful swelling on his finger as shown in image.

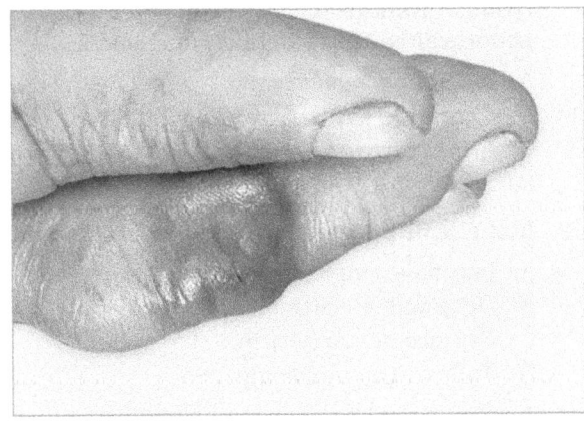

Source: Çimen C. Typical evolution of a cutaneous anthrax lesion. Infect Dis Clin Microbiol. 2020;1:27-9.

There is a significant history of a healthy pet dog that succumbed 2 weeks before without an obvious cause. Samples are taken from secretions of the patient knee and the microscopy show rod-shaped gram-positive organism.

The most likely diagnosis is:

A. *Staphylococcus aureus* osteomyelitis
B. Roundworm infestation
C. Anthrax
D. Chronic liver fluke infestation

17. A 61-year-old farmer is been investigated for 6 weeks history of fever, headache, and chills. He now reports persistent cough over last 2 weeks. His environment includes several stray goats, sheep, and dogs all apparently healthy. The most likely investigation to diagnose the infection is:

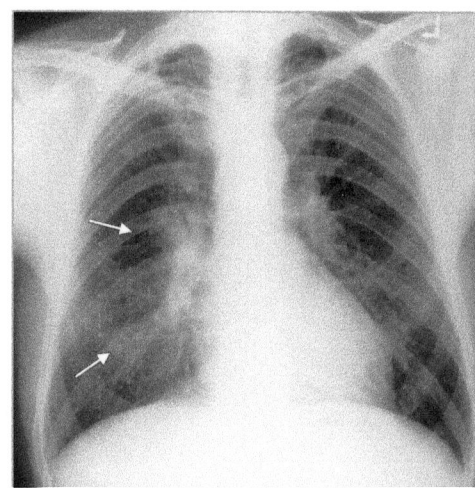

Source: Marrie TJ. *Coxiella burnetii* pneumonia. Eur Res J. 2003;21:713-9.

A. PET-CT
B. Blood culture
C. Bronchoscopy
D. Bone marrow aspiration for BioFire

18. This man now has sudden onset dyspnea, clinical examination shows bilateral pitting edema, prominent neck veins, and a loud P2 on auscultation. A transesophageal echo reveals right-sided endocarditis. The most likely diagnosis is:

A. *Mycoplasma pneumonia*
B. *Streptococcus pyogenes* septicaemia
C. *Coxiella burnetii*—Q-fever
D. *Stenotrophomonas maltophilia*

19. In the same patient, the treatment of choice is:

A. Injectable ampicillin 12 g per day
B. Doxycycline + rifampicin
C. Ceftriaxone + arbekacin
D. Amikacin monotherapy

20. A 26-year-old female presents with worsening diarrhea, vomiting, headache, and dry cough for last 5 days. She is been also investigated for a spontaneous abortion at 18 weeks of pregnancy and her history includes her third abortion in 5 years. She has been following a diet which includes fresh salads and raw milk for the last 2 years. Her most likely diagnosis is:

A. *Listeria monocytogenes*
B. *Salmonella paratyphi* carrier state
C. Chronic rotaviral infection
D. Recurrent *Vibrio cholerae* infection

21. A 21-year-old female, a professional pet trainer presents with severe abdominal pain, which her family says started after a friend gave her a hug. The emergency assessment is of an acute abdomen. An ultrasonography is done at the bedside. The ultrasound of the patient (images) is shown below. The diagnosis in this patient is:

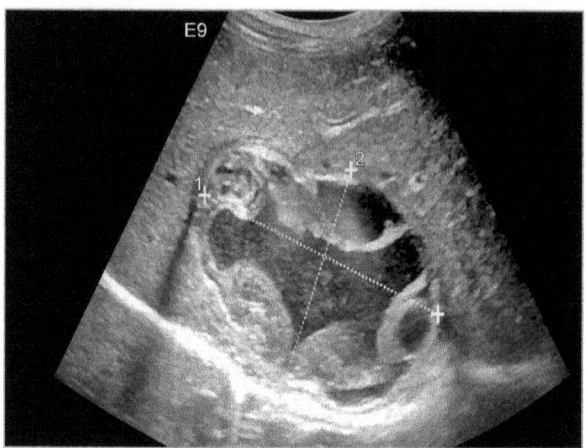

Source: Kurda D. Hepatic hydatid cyst. [online] Available from: https://radiopaedia.org/cases/hepatic-hydatid-cyst-4?lang=us [Last accessed February, 2020].

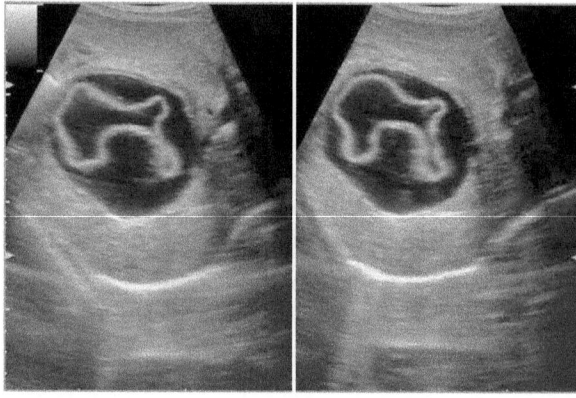

Source: Peer S. Hepatic hydatid cyst—ultrasound water lily sign. [online] Available from: https://radiopaedia.org/cases/hepatic-hydatid-cyst-ultrasound-water-lily-sign-2?lang=us [Last accessed February, 2020].

A. *Dracunculus medinensis*
B. *Loa loa*
C. Dog tapeworm—hydatid cyst
D. *Necator americanus*—roundworm

22. The treatment of choice in this patient is:

A. Laparoscopic resection of liver
B. Surgical removal/drainage of cyst using needle under albendazole cover
C. No surgical intervention
D. Pyrantel pamoate injection into the cyst

23. A 46-year-old male presents with 1 day history of fever, obtundation, and vomiting. He is transferred to intensive care unit (ICU) for control of new onset seizures. His family says the shop he works in has

multiple open drains besides nondomesticated dogs, cattle, and pigs. His first investigation strategy would be:
A. Vancomycin + ampicillin
B. Methylprednisolone 1 g twice a day for 5 days
C. CT brain with lumbar puncture
D. C + Serology for Japanese encephalitis in a reference laboratory

24. In the same patient, the treatment of choice is:
A. Mefloquine + artemether
B. Artesunate + quinine
C. Immunoglobulins and supportive care
D. Methylprednisolone

25. 26-year-old athlete by profession presents with a worsening 3 weeks history of back and leg pain. His history reveals that he consumes raw fruits and red meat. He now presents with new onset headache and weakness of both his lower limbs requiring support. The most likely diagnosis is:

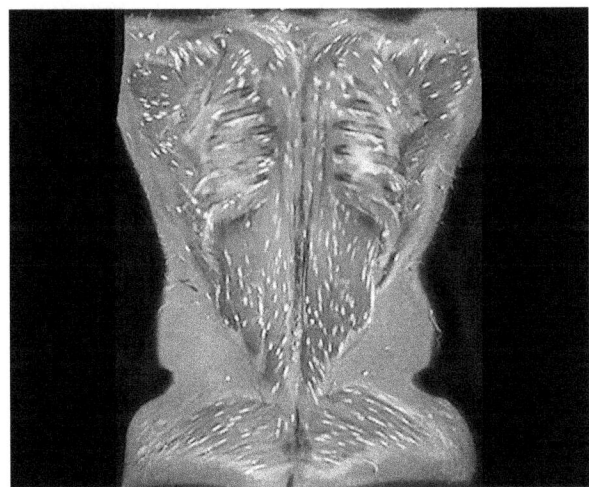

Source: Smitaman E, Flores DV, Gómez CM, Pathria MN. MR imaging of atraumatic muscle disorders. RadioGraphics. 2018;38:500-22.

A. B-cell lymphoma
B. Dermatomyositis
C. Cysticerci
D. Systemic lupus erythematosus involving muscle and bone

26. A young male farmer, with the mixed diet presents with sudden and progressive memory loss, with no significant previous or family history of any illness. On examination lack of coordination and myoclonic jerky movements are encountered. What is the likely cause?
A. Huntington disease
B. Mitochondrial encephalopathy
C. Neurocysticercosis
D. Variant Creutzfeldt-Jakob disease (vCJD)

27. A young female who was on her summer tour in Southern India, presents with fever, headache, severe muscle pain, vomiting, gastrointestinal symptoms, and bleeding problems since 3–4 days. On examination she has low blood pressure, low platelet, red blood cell, and white blood cell counts. She also gives history of contact with sick animals. What is the diagnosis?
A. Norovirus encephalitis
B. Crimean-Congo fever
C. Alkhurma hemorrhagic fever
D. Kyasanur forest disease (KFD)

28. A young male presents with severe itching, blisters, and a red growing, winding rash. He gives history of stepping barefoot and contact with droppings of his pet dog that is infected with hookworm. Which of the following is likely to occur?

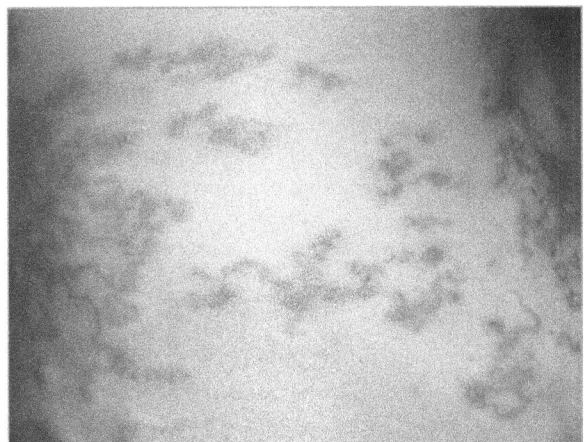

Source: Weissagung; 2009. [online] Available from: https://commons.wikimedia.org/wiki/File:Larva_Migrans_Cutanea.jpg [Last accessed September, 2020].

A. Athlete's foot
B. Creeping eruption
C. Tetanus
D. Meningococcal septicemia

29. A veterinary surgeon presents with headache, high fever, arthralgia, gastrointestinal symptoms, and redness of eyes. On examination jaundice, flushed face, sore throat, and petechiae on the palate are appreciated. In a detailed history he describes poor aseptic precaution at his center. What is the likely diagnosis?
A. Leptospirosis
B. Kawasaki disease
C. Rickettsial infection
D. *Bartonella henselae*

30. The family pet dog has a round and hairless spot on its skin. Which of the following infection members of the family are likely to acquire?
A. Tapeworm
B. Pinworm
C. Roundworm
D. Ringworm

ANSWERS WITH EXPLANATIONS

1. **Ans. D**

   Ebola virus disease is endemic in various parts of the world, especially in countries like Sudan. The disease is highly contagious and is spread through contact with infected body fluids.
   Ref:
   1. *Malvy D, McElroy AK, de Clerck H, Günther S, van Griensven J. Ebola virus disease. The Lancet. 2019; 393(10174):936-48.*

2. **Ans. C**

   While blood cultures and stool cultures may have yield of 40–60% in diagnosis of salmonella. Bone marrow is diagnostic in 90–95% patients. Treatment should be initiated after sensitivity is established. This patient is categorized now as typhoid carrier stage and will require long-term suppressive therapy.
   Ref:
   1. *Upadhyay R, Nadkar MY, Muruganathan A, Tiwaskar M, Amarapurkar D, Banka NH, Mehta KK, Sathyaprakash BS. API Recommendations for the Management of Typhoid Fever. JAPI. 2015;63 [online] Available from https://www.japi.org/q274c4b4/api-recommendations-for-the-management-of-typhoid-fever [Last accessed September, 2020].*

3. **Ans. B**

   Zoonotic transmitted tuberculosis is common in animal products which are not completely cooked. Patients' needs to be investigated for serology, IFN-γ release assays, direct microscopy for acid-fast bacilli, culture, PCR, other nucleic acid assays, combined with imaging and biopsy.
   Ref:
   1. *Spickler AR; 2019. Zoonotic Tuberculosis. [online] Available from http://www.cfsph.iastate.edu/DiseaseInfo/ factsheets.php [Last accessed September, 2020].*

4. **Ans. C**

   Bovine tuberculosis is usually resistant, and can be difficult to recognize and treat, if resistant especially to rifampicin and INH. The most potentially fatal complication is pneumonia. Patient requires backbone of a bactericidal agent such as combination of a macrolide and quinolone besides other drugs for optimal resolution.
   Ref:
   1. *Centers for Disease Control and Prevention (2012). Mycobacterium bovis (Bovine Tuberculosis) in Humans. [online] Available from https://www.cdc.gov/tb/publications/factsheets/general/mbovis.htm [Last accessed September, 2020].*

5. **Ans. D**

   The exposure to animal products especially from sheeps and goats is most likely to represents as *Brucellosis melitensis*.
   Ref:
   1. *Centers for Disease Control and Prevention (2012). Brucellosis. [online] Available from https://www.cdc.gov/brucellosis/veterinarians/host-animals.html [Last accessed September, 2020].*

6. **Ans. A**

   While bone marrow may be useful in such patients where PET-CT is inconclusive the first diagnostic tool would be PET-CT. Noninvasive modalities along with PET-CT such as blood culture and Brucella serology should be sent as noninvasive first-line investigations.
   Ref:
   1. *Centers for Disease Control and Prevention (2012). Brucellosis-Clinicians. [online] Available from https://www.cdc.gov/brucellosis/clinicians/bacterial-isolation.html [Last accessed September, 2020].*
   2. *Centers for Disease Control and Prevention (2012). Brucellosis-Clinicians. [online] Available from https://www.cdc.gov/brucellosis/clinicians/serology.html [Last accessed September, 2020].*

7. **Ans. A**

   While there are benefit of number of regimens for brucellosis, rifampicin + doxycycline is first-line therapy unless there is resistance or treatment failure.
   Ref:
   1. *Centers for Disease Control and Prevention (2012). Brucellosis. [online] Available from https://www.cdc.gov/brucellosis/treatment/index.html [Last accessed September, 2020].*

8. **Ans. B**

   About 15–25% of patients especially if immunocompromised or partially treated or having recurrent exposures will show relapse. Such patients should be treated for longer duration of time.
   Ref:
   1. *Pappas G, Akritidis N, Bosilkovski M, Tsianos E. Brucellosis. N Engl J Med. 2005;352:2325-36.*
   2. *Ariza J, Corredoira J, Pallares R, Viladrich PF, Rufi G, Pujol M. Characteristics of and risk factors for relapse of brucellosis in humans. Clin Infect Dis. 1995;20: 1241-9*
   3. *Ögredici Ö, Erb S, Langer I, et al. Brucellosis reactivation after 28 years. Emerging Infectious Diseases. 2010;16(12):2021-22.*

9. **Ans. D**

   Canine hepatitis is not a zoonotic disease. All others can be transmitted from dogs to humans.

Ref:
1. *Centers for Disease Control and Prevention (2019). Healthy Pets. [online] Available from https://www.cdc.gov/healthypets/pets/dogs.html [Last accessed September, 2020].*

10. **Ans. A**

Feline immunodeficiency virus infection cannot be passed from cats to humans but all other diseases are zoonotic.
Ref:
1. *Centers for Disease Control and Prevention (2019). Healthy Pets. [online] Available from https://www.cdc.gov/healthypets/pets/cats.html [Last accessed September, 2020].*

11. **Ans. B**

All other answers are vital elements of animal husbandry that help to reduce the risk of transmission of zoonotic disease.
Ref:
1. *Centers for Disease Control and Prevention (2019). Healthy Pets-About Pets & People. [online] Available from https://www.cdc.gov/healthypets/health-benefits/index.html [Last accessed September, 2020].*

12. **Ans. D**

This man is infected by chlamydia of urethra and genital tract. Immunofluorescence is diagnostic in active infection and should be used to guide treatment.
Ref:
1. *Stary A, Genç M, Heller-Vitouch C, Mårdh PA. Chlamydial antigen detection in urine samples by immunofluorescence tests. Infection. 1992;20(2):101-4.*

13. **Ans. A**

While several antibiotics have been shown to have partial activity against most subtype of chlamydia, a macrolide regimen boosted with rifampicin remains treatment of choice.
Ref:
1. *Goellner S, Schubert E, Liebler-Tenorio E, Hotzel H, Saluz HP, Sachse K. Transcriptional response patterns of Chlamydophila psittaci in different in vitro models of persistent infection. Infect Immun. 2006;74(8):4801-8.*
2. *Beeckman DS, Vanrompay DC. Zoonotic Chlamydophila psittaci infections from a clinical perspective. Clin Microbiol Infect. 2009;15(1):11-7.*

14. **Ans. B**

Livestock transmission of campylobacter to human beings is very common. About 40% patients have 26-35% association.
Ref:
1. *Gahamanyi N, Mboera LEG, Matee MI, Mutangana D, Komba EVG. Prevalence, Risk Factors, and Antimicrobial Resistance Profiles of Thermophilic Campylobacter Species in Humans and Animals in Sub-Saharan Africa: A Systematic Review. International Journal of Microbiology. 2020:2020;2092478.*

15. **Ans. B**

History of exposure to animal fluids, especially dogs, is highly suspicious of cutaneous lesions such as dermatophytosis. These types of skin infections from contact with cats and dogs are the most common pet-associated diseases, causing approximately more than 2 million infections each year.
Ref:
1. *Rabinowitz PM, Gordon Z, Odofin L. Pet-related infections. Am Fam Physician. 2007;76(9):1314-22.*
2. *Stehr-Green JK, Schantz PM. The impact of zoonotic diseases transmitted by pets on human health and the economy. Vet Clin North Am Small Anim Pract. 1987;17:1-15.*

16. **Ans. C**

Anthrax commonly transmitted from infected dogs to humans, presents with cutaneous and pulmonary manifestations. Cutaneous have classical appearance as described above. Symptoms can be rapidly progressive and carry 20-40% mortality even with treatment. Seen in this image is the eschar after the treatment of anthrax.

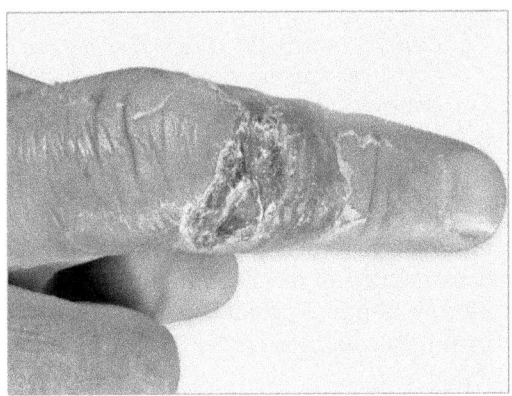

Source: Çimen C. Typical evolution of a cutaneous anthrax lesion. Infect Dis Clin Microbiol. 2020;1:27-9.
Ref:
1. *World Health Organization (2008). Anthrax [online] Available from https://www.who.int/csr/resources/publications/anthrax_web.pdf.*

17. **Ans. C**

Q fever, is a zoonotic disease, is due to *Coxiella burnetii* infection. The most common animal reservoirs are goats, cattle, sheep, cats and dogs. The clinical syndromes are, the acute form of the illness: nonspecific febrile illness, pneumonia, and hepatitis. The chronic form: Q fever is almost always involves endocarditis, but occasionally it also manifests as hepatitis, osteomyelitis or endovascular infection. The pneumonic form: the illness range from very mild-to-severe pneumonia requiring assisted ventilation. Multiple round opacities are a common finding on chest radiography. Treatment with doxycycline or a fluoroquinolone is treatment of choice. *Coxiella burnetii* pneumonia should be considered when there

is a suitable exposure history and when there are outbreaks of a pneumonic illness.
Ref:
1. Marrie TJ. Coxiella burnetii pneumonia. European Respiratory Journal. 2003;21(4):713-9.

18. **Ans. C**
The progressive nature of complains in the environment of cattle as described is classical for transmission of *Coxiella*. The organism is highly infectious in very low concentrations. It can be transported in windy conditions to long distances.
Ref:
1. Centers for Disease Control and Prevention (2019). Q Fever. [online] Available from https://www.cdc.gov/qfever/transmission/index.html [Last accessed September, 2020].

19. **Ans. B**
Drug of choice is doxycycline which along with rifampicin enhances recovery period and outcomes. In case of endocarditis treatment is for minimum 6 weeks.
Ref:
1. Cleveland KO (2019). Q Fever. [online] Available from https://emedicine.medscape.com/article/227156-overview [Last accessed September, 2020].

20. **Ans. A**
Listeriosis presents with two distinct manifestations. A milder form is listeria gastroenteritis and a chronic more severe form is listeriosis in patient's blood. The consumption of raw dairy in the above said clinical picture is pathognomonic of listeriosis. Without treatment condition carries 20–80% mortality.
Ref:
1. World Health Organization (2018). Listeriosis. [online] Available from https://www.who.int/news-room/fact-sheets/detail/listeriosis [Last accessed September, 2020].

21. **Ans. C**
A classical water lily sign which is seen on the ultrasound along with this history is diagnosed as hydatid cyst disease. Superficial hydatid cysts are known to leak fluid contents in the abdomen at very little or no trauma.
Ref:
1. World Health Organization (2020). Echinococcosis. [online] Available from https://www.who.int/news-room/fact-sheets/detail/echinococcosis [Last accessed September, 2020].

22. **Ans. B**
Superficial cysts respond well to aspiration of cyst under cover. Cyst that are in the liver parenchyma require surgical intervention. Albendazole is administered before and during procedures, to prevent the infection from spreading if the cyst's contents spill during the procedure. Albendazole is continued for 1–6 months after the procedure to reduce the likelihood that a cyst will come back or spread. Albendazole alone can kill some cysts and is also used to suppress the growth of cysts that cannot be removed surgically or drained.
Ref:
1. Pearson RD (2020). Echinococcosis (Hydatid Disease). [online] Available from https://www.msdmanuals.com/professional/infectious-diseases/cestodes-tapeworms/echinococcosis [Last accessed September, 2020].

23. **Ans. D**
The scenario described in this question makes Japanese encephalitis likely. The infectious *Culex* mosquito transmits the virus to humans which is the end stage in the life of the *Culex* mosquito.
Ref:
1. Centers for Disease Control and Prevention (2019). Japanese Encephalitis. [online] Available from https://www.cdc.gov/japaneseencephalitis/index.html [Last accessed September, 2020].

24. **Ans. C**
Japanese encephalitis virus infections carry mortality rate of (20–30%) even with the treatment. Supportive care with immunoglobulins is the option indicated in such patient. All high-risk situations should be offered with Japanese encephalitis vaccine.
Ref:
1. Centers for Disease Control and Prevention (2019). Japanese Encephalitis. [online] Available from https://www.cdc.gov/japaneseencephalitis/symptoms/index.html [Last accessed September, 2020].

25. **Ans. C**
Cysticerci often occur through poorly cooked meat while they are most likely to be a single organ, disseminated cysticerci have been described.
Ref:
1. García HH, Gonzalez AE, Evans CA, Gilman RH; Cysticercosis Working Group in Peru. Taenia solium cysticercosis. Lancet. 2003;362(9383):547-56.

26. **Ans. D**
The vCJD acquired by ingestion of beef infected with bovine spongiform encephalopathy (BSE), which is a transmissible prion disease occurring in cattle. Infection leads to vCJD in humans. BSE is also known as mad cow disease. BSE and CJD are similar but not the same. BSE which is a progressive neurological disorder in cattle similar to a disease in sheep called scrapie. It has been found primarily in cattle eating contaminated meat. BSE may be caused by feeding scrapie-infected sheep meat-and-bone meal to cattle. The new vCJD differs from CJD in that patients are typically much younger (30 versus 60) and that symptoms are more psychiatric and sensory than neurological.

The risk of contracting vCJD through any vaccine (for polio or hepatitis, for example) is remote. The concern about vaccines surfaced because some vaccines are manufactured using substances derived from cattle. Some of the bovine components have come from countries where BSE is found. There is no evidence in Europe that any vaccines have caused vCJD.

Ref:
1. *Centers for Disease Control and Prevention (2019). Variant Creutzfeldt-Jakob Disease (vCJD). [online] Available from https://www.cdc.gov/prions/vcjd/index.html [Last accessed September, 2020].*

27. **Ans. D**

Kyasanur forest disease transmission to humans may occur after a tick bite or contact with an infected animal, most importantly a sick or recently dead monkey. No person-to-person transmission has been described.

Large animals such as goats, cows, and sheep may become infected with KFD but play a limited role in the transmission of the disease. These animals provide the blood meals for ticks and it is possible for infected animals with viremia to infect other ticks, but transmission of KFD virus (KFDV) to humans from these larger animals is extremely rare. Furthermore, there is no evidence of disease transmission via the unpasteurized milk of any of these animals.

The KFD has historically been limited to the western and central districts of Karnataka state, India. However, in November 2012, samples from humans and monkeys tested positive for KFDV in the southernmost district of the state which neighbors Tamil Nadu state and Kerala state, indicating the possibility of wider distribution of KFDV. Alkhurma hemorrhagic fever virus is very similar to KFD virus and mainly occurs in Saudi Arabia.

People with recreational or occupational exposure to rural or outdoor settings (e.g., hunters, herders, forest workers, and farmers) within Karnataka state are potentially at risk for infection by contact with infected ticks. Seasonality is another important risk factor as more cases are reported during the dry season, from November through June.

There is no specific treatment available, although prevention with vaccine for KFD exists and is used in endemic areas of India. Additional preventative measures include insect repellents and wearing protective clothing in areas where ticks are endemic.

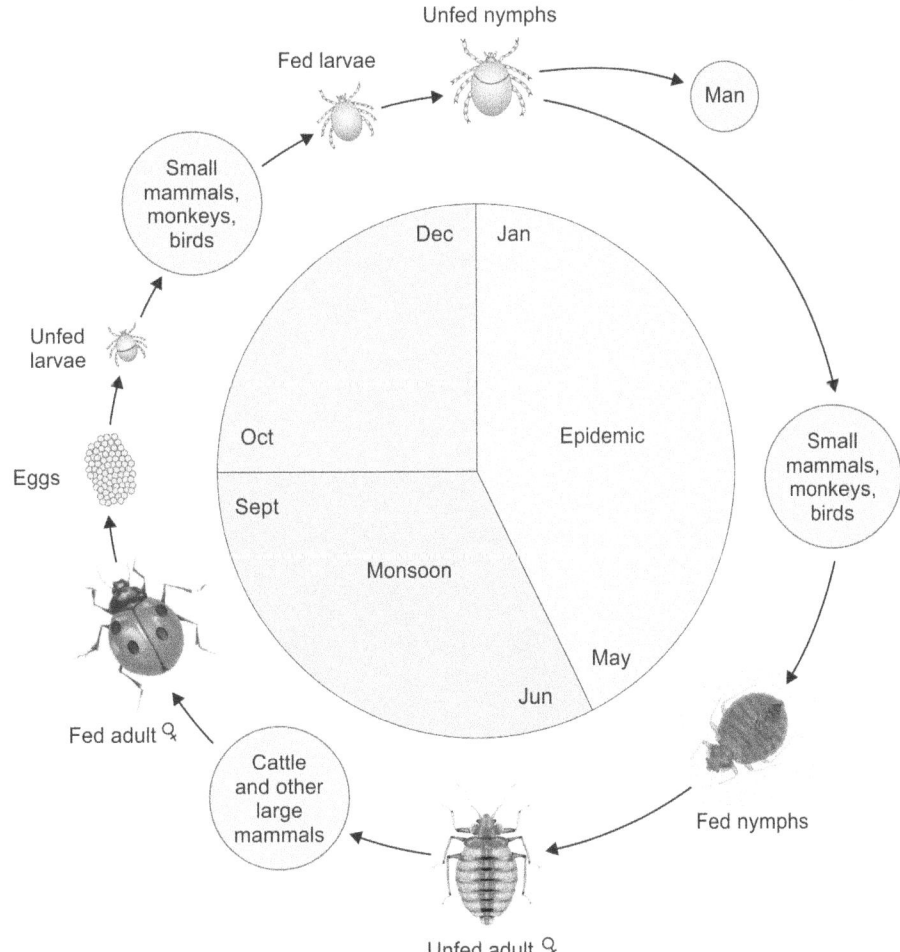

Source: John JK. Kyasanur forest disease: a status update. Adv Anim Vet Sci. 2014;2:329-36.

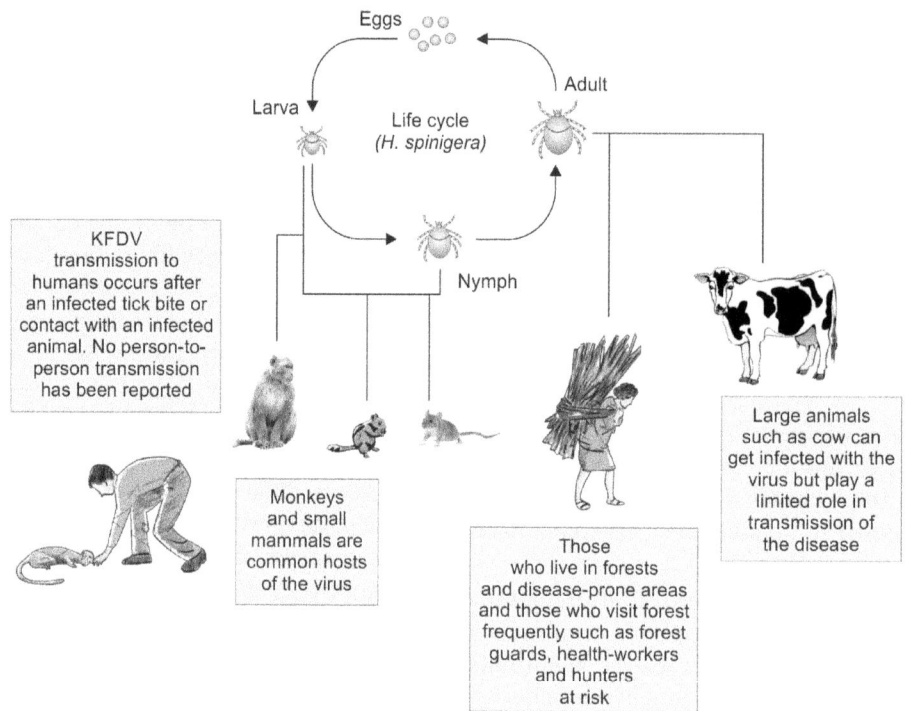

(KFDV: Kyasanur forest disease virus)

Source: Shah SZ, Jabbar B, Ahmed N, Rehman A, Nasir H, Nadeem S, et al. Epidemiology, pathogenesis, and control of a Tick-Borne disease—Kyasanur forest disease: current status and future directions. Front Cell Infect Microbiol. 2018;8:149.

Ref:
1. Centers for Disease Control and Prevention (2013). [online] Available from https://www.cdc.gov/vhf/kyasanur/exposure/index.html [Last accessed February, 2020].

28. Ans. B

This condition is caused by intestinal hookworms shed by dogs and cats in their feces. The larvae of these worms burrow into the skin and make a wandering trail just beneath the skin. According to the Centers for Disease Control and Prevention (CDC), children who play in contaminated soil are at risk of getting hookworm. Others at risk are electricians, plumbers, and others who crawl beneath raised buildings where the hookworm larvae may be found.

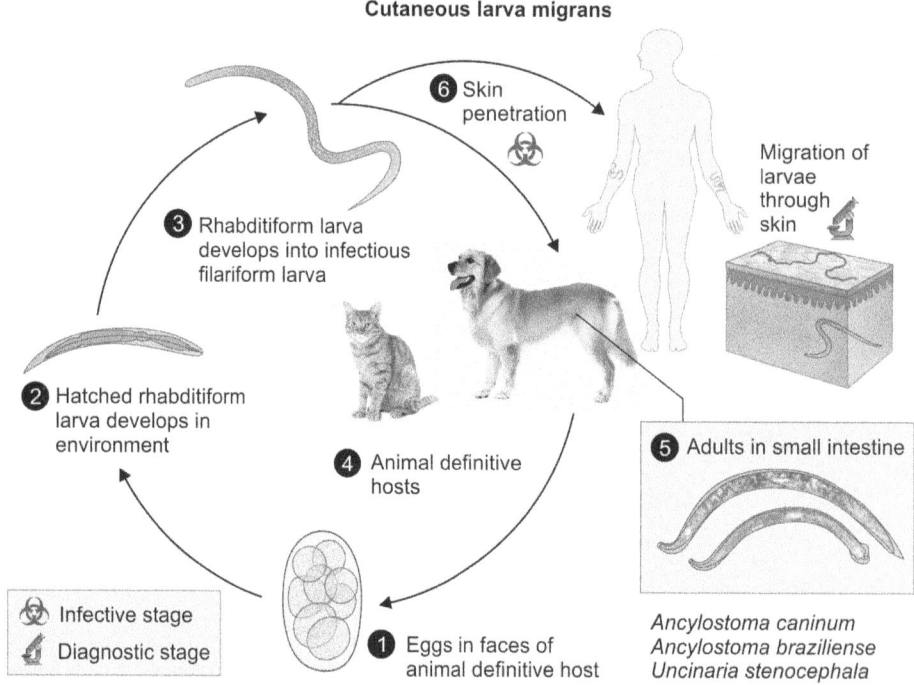

Source: Centers for Disease Control and Prevention (2019). [online] Available from https://www.cdc.gov/parasites/zoonotichookworm/biology.html [Last accessed February, 2020].

Zoonotic hookworm infections usually result in a skin condition called cutaneous larva migrans (CLM). When people walk or sit on beach sand or soil where infected dogs or cats have defecated, the dog or cat hookworm larva can penetrate the skin of the foot or body and migrate in the top layers of the skin. This migration causes severe itchiness and raised red lines can form as part of the reaction to the larva in the skin. The larva will die in the skin after several weeks without developing any further, and the itchiness and red lines will go away. Scratching at the lines can cause a bacterial infection. In rare cases, certain types of animal hookworm may infect the intestine and cause abdominal pain, discomfort, and diarrhea.

Ref:
1. *Centers for Disease Control and Prevention (2019). Biology. [online] Available from https://www.cdc.gov/parasites/zoonotichookworm/biology.html [Last accessed February, 2020].*

29. **Ans. A**

Leptospirosis is known to occur in animals domesticated or otherwise. Multiple animals can transmit multiple serovars of leptospirosis.

Ref:
1. *Azócar-Aedo L, Smits HL, Monti G. Leptospirosis in dogs and cats: epidemiology, clinical disease, zoonotic implications and prevention. Archivos de Medicina Veterinaria. 2014;46(3):337-48.*

30. **Ans. D**

Ringworm is a fungal infection that causes irritation to the scalp or skin. This makes the skin red or scaly. On the scalp, it can cause a bald patch of scaly skin. On the skin, it usually appears as a ring-shaped rash. The type of ringworm passed on from animals makes up only a small percentage of ringworm cases in people. The rest are caused by a fungus that is transmitted either from one child or an adult to another or through contaminated combs, brushes, hats, hair accessories, pillows, and bath towels. For either type of ringworm, the treatment is a topical cream or oral medication.

Animals also, get infected through touching an infected animal's skin or hair or by touching things that are infected with the fungus, like blankets and towels. Many different kinds of animals can transmit ringworm to people. Dogs and cats, especially kittens or puppies, can have ringworm that can be passed to people. Cows, goats, pigs, and horses can also pass ringworm to people. Adult animals, especially long-haired cats, do not always show signs of ringworm infection. Puppies and kittens most often have patches that are hairless, circular, or irregularly shaped areas of scaling, crusting, and redness that may or may not be itchy. The area may not be completely hairless, and instead have brittle, broken hairs. If the claws are affected, they may have a whitish, opaque appearance with shredding of the claw's surface.

Ref:
1. *Centers for Disease Control and Prevention (2014). Ringworm. [online] Available from https://www.cdc.gov/healthypets/diseases/ringworm.html [Last accessed February, 2020].*

CHAPTER 19

Parasitic Infections

Ajay Jhaveri, Om Shrivastav

1. Which of the following is not transmitted by a mosquito?
   A. *Plasmodium vivax*
   B. *Plasmodium falciparum*
   C. *Leishmania donovani*
   D. *Wuchereria bancrofti*

2. What form of plasmodia is transmitted from mosquito to humans, in case of malaria?
   A. Merozoite
   B. Hypnozoite
   C. Sporozoite
   D. Gametocyte

3. Through which of the following do the schizonts enters in human?
   A. Blood
   B. Liver
   C. Spleen
   D. None of the above

4. A 71-year-old man diagnosed with parasitic infestation involving the gut and lungs. He also had a feeling of a moving worm in his eye. Worm is removed from his eye and sent for pathological cross section. The worm is confirmed as:

   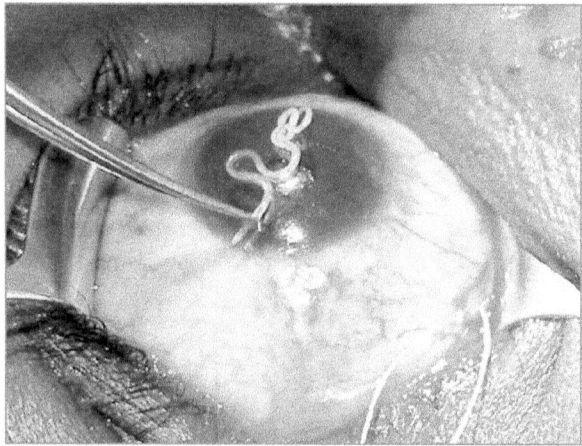

   A. *Trichuris trichiura*
   B. *Necator americanus*
   C. *Dracunculus mendelsons*
   D. *Loa loa*

5. In the same patient, ivermectin is commenced. The patient feels better in the first 2 days. On the third day there is worsening headache, poor visual acuity, and redness in the affected eye. This is most likely to represent of the following agents is contraindicated?
   A. Hypersensitivity to ivermectin
   B. Mazzotti reaction
   C. Intracranial migration of *Loa loa*
   D. Autoimmune endophthalmitis

6. A patient who is a usual resident of India presents with fever and weight loss. On examination, anemia and hepatosplenomegaly were appreciated. Laboratory evaluation suggested pancytopenia and bone marrow revealed (image):

   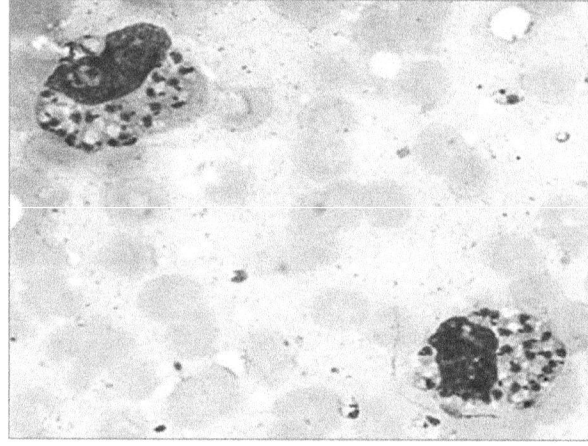

   Source: Center for Disease Control and Prevention; 2019.
   A. Hookworm infestation
   B. T-cell lymphoma
   C. Aplastic anemia
   D. Kala azar

7. A 10-year-old male brought with presentation of loose stools and fatigue. He has signs of abdominal tenderness, signs of anemia, finger clubbing, and also stunted growth. Stool microscopy is shown in the image. Which of the following is the most likely cause?

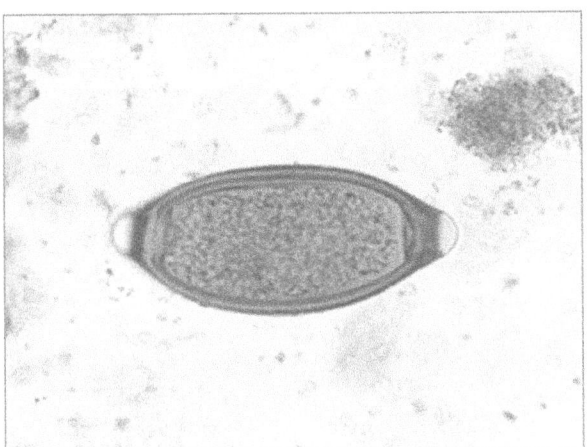

Source: Centers for Disease Control and Prevention (2017). Trichuriasis. [online] Available from: https://www.cdc.gov/dpdx/trichuriasis/index.html [Last accessed on February, 2020].

A. *Giardia lamblia*
B. *Ascaris lumbricoides*
C. *Enterobius vermicularis*
D. *Trichuris trichiura*

8. A 50-year-old female, resident of India, with history of multiple travels since last 24 months to South Africa, presented with an ulcer on the left side of the nose, fever persistent vomiting, and pain in abdomen since 8 months. On examination, painful splenomegaly was noted and ultrasound of abdomen suggested hepatosplenomegaly. What is the likely mode of transmission?

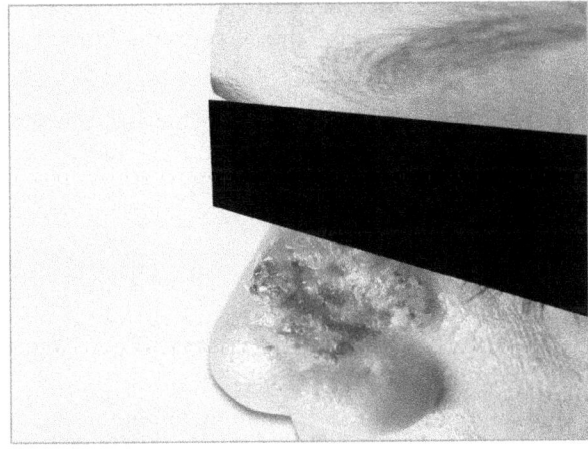

A. Rodents
B. Sand fly
C. Mosquitos
D. Contaminated water

9. A young female presents with high grade fever, periorbital edema, generalized weakness, and body ache. On examination, this is found to be splinter hemorrhages of the nail beds beneath the fingernails (image). What is the likely cause?

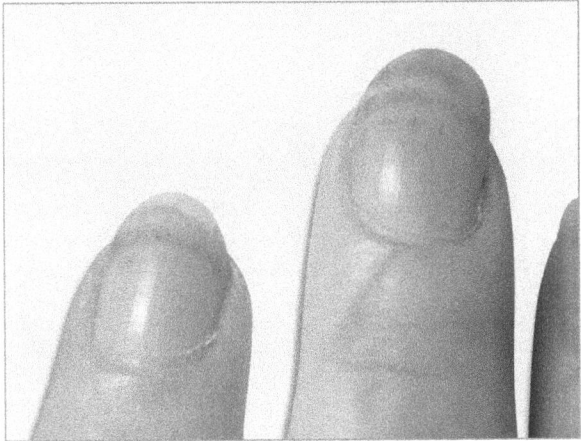

Source: Center for Disease Control and Prevention/Dr Thomas F Sellers, Emory University; 2019.

A. *Necator americanus*
B. *Ancylostoma duodenale*
C. *Trichinella spiralis*
D. *Ascaris lumbricoides*

10. A female child was presented with swelling over feet and rash. On examination, she was anemic. What is the likely diagnosis?

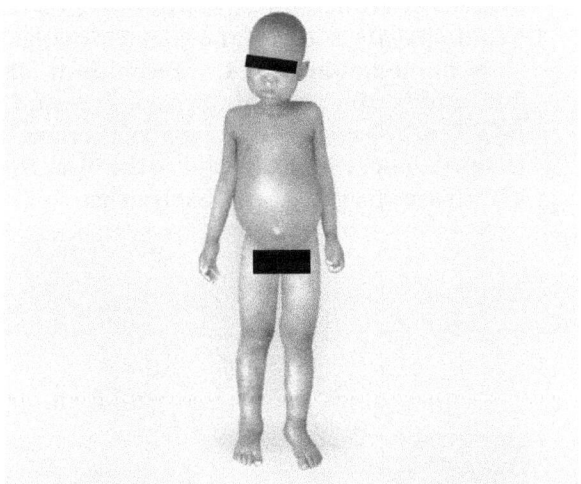

Source: Center for Disease Control and Prevention/Dr Myron G Schultz; 2019.

A. Malnutrition secondary to protein losing enteropathy
B. Autoimmune mesenteric vasculature involvement
C. Bleeding upper gastrointestinal (GI) ulceration
D. Hookworm infestation

11. A school-going child was presented with intense perianal itching and also has irritability with disturbed sleep. On microscopy from scotch tape, it demonstrated eight eggs of the human pinworm, *E. vermicularis*. What is the most likely cause?

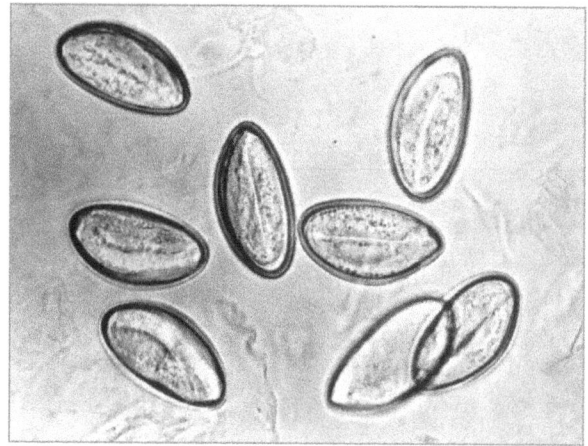

Source: Center for Disease Control and Prevention; 2019.

A. *Ascaris lumbricoides*
B. *Entamoeba histolytica*
C. *Enterobius vermicularis*
D. None of the above

12. A 37-year-old cleaner by occupation presents with 3 months history of bloating, lack of appetite, and profound weakness. He is emphatic that he is stringently careful about exposure at his work place. His clinical examination reveals tender hepatomegaly and his laboratory investigations show hemoglobin (Hb) 4, transaminitis, shot of 400, and serum glutamic pyruvic transaminase (SGPT) of 270, respectively. Besides a perianal ulcer (image), biopsy from the edge of the ulcer the cyst of the parasite, that is most likely to be:

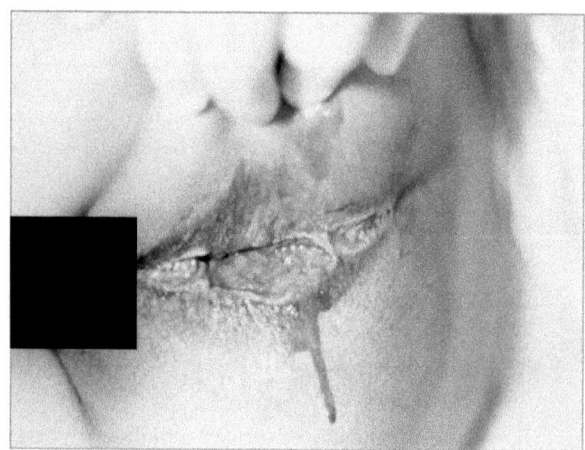

Source: Center for Disease Control and Prevention; 2019.

A. Liver fluke
B. *Entamoeba histolytica*
C. Threadworm infestation
D. *Taenia solium* (pork tapeworm)

13. A middle-aged man presents with the following. What is cause?

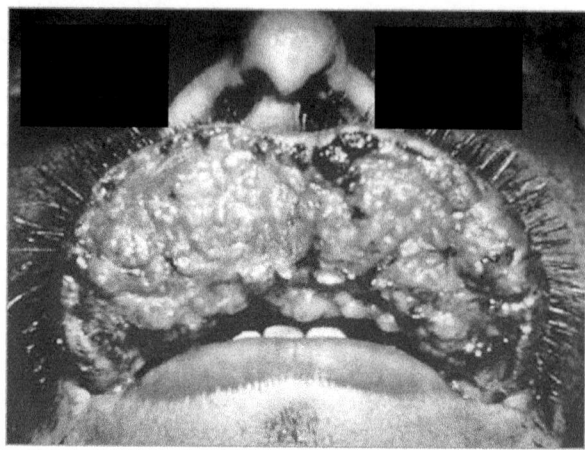

Source: Wagner KF. Infectious Diseases, Medscape; 2019.

A. *Leishmania braziliensis*
B. *Leishmania donovani*
C. *Leishmania tropica*
D. *Phlebotomus* spp.

14. A human immunodeficiency virus (HIV) positive patient with a CD4+ count 47/mm^3 presents with diarrhea. Acid-fast structures are found in the stool. Which of the following is true?

A. Even with the best treatment, the infection may be unrelenting
B. Infection will resolve with addition of Akt
C. Infection is short-lasting and self-resolving and requires no treatment
D. Treat with antibiotics and infection should resolve in 3–6 days

15. Which of the following does not have an intermediate host as part of its life cycle?

A. *Taenia solium*
B. *Ascaris lumbricoides*
C. *Toxoplasma gondii*
D. *Echinococcus granulosus*

16. Which of the following statements regarding trichinosis is not correct?

A. Eosinophilia is a prominent finding
B. Trichinosis is caused by a protozoan that has both a trophozoite and a cyst stage in its life cycle
C. Trichinosis can be diagnosed by seeing cysts in muscle biopsy specimens
D. Trichinosis is acquired by eating undercooked pork

17. Which of the following parasites is not transmitted by eating inadequately cooked fish or seafood?
    A. *Paragonimus westermani*
    B. *Clonorchis sinensis*
    C. *Diphyllobothrium latum*
    D. *Ancylostoma duodenale*

18. Trophozoites, schizonts, and gametocytes of all the malarial parasites are seen in the peripheral blood smear, *except*:
    A. *P. falciparum*
    B. *P. malariae*
    C. *P. ovale*
    D. *P. vivax*

19. Which *Plasmodium* species has longest incubation period?
    A. *P. falciparum*
    B. *P. malariae*
    C. *P. ovale*
    D. *P. vivax*

20. Mosquitoes are the vector in the following disorder(s):
    A. Onchocerciasis
    B. Visceral leishmaniasis
    C. African trypanosomiasis
    D. Bancroftian filariasis

21. Calabar swelling is seen in infections with:
    A. *Onchocerca volvulus*
    B. *Loa loa*
    C. *Brugia timori*
    D. *Wuchereria bancrofti*

22. Dog heart tape worm is the common name for:
    A. *Toxocara canis*
    B. *Dirofilaria immitis*
    C. *Mansonella streptocerca*
    D. *Toxoplasma gondi*

23. Which of the following is not a bile stained egg?
    A. *Ascaris lumbricoides*
    B. *Trichuris trichiura*
    C. *Taenia solium*
    D. *Ancylostoma duodenale*

24. Casoni's test is used for the diagnosis of:
    A. Taeniasis
    B. Hydatidiasis
    C. Trichuriasis
    D. Onchocerciasis

25. The ova that does not float in the saturated salt solution:
    A. *H. nana*
    B. *T. solium*
    C. *Ancylostoma*
    D. Fertilized *A. lumbricoides* eggs

26. Larval form of *E. granulosus* is seen in:
    A. Fox
    B. Dog
    C. Man
    D. Wolf

27. Charcot-Leyden crystals are seen in the sputum in infection with:
    A. *Paragonimus westermani*
    B. *Clonorchis sinensis*
    C. *Fasciola hepatica*
    D. *Fasciolopsis buski*

28. Primary amoebic meningoencephalitis is caused by:
    A. *Acanthamoeba*
    B. *Balamuthia* spp.
    C. *Naegleria fowleri*
    D. *Iodamoeba butschlii*

29. Congenitally transmitted parasitic infection is:
    A. *Pneumocystis carinii*
    B. *Toxoplasma gondii*
    C. Amoebiasis
    D. *Trichuris trichiura*

30. Protozoa transmitted sexually is:
    A. *Trichomonas vaginalis*
    B. *Entamoeba histolytica*
    C. *Giardia lamblia*
    D. *Balantidium coli*

ANSWERS WITH EXPLANATIONS

1. **Ans. C**

   Leishmania donovani is transmitted by the bite of infected female phlebotomine sandflies.

   Ref:
   1. https://www.cdc.gov/parasites/leishmaniasis/biology.html

2. **Ans. C**

   Discussed with the next question.

   Ref:
   1. https://www.cdc.gov/malaria/about/biology/index.html

3. **Ans. B**

   The sporozoites enter the liver and further divide into multinucleated forms which are known as schizonts.

The malaria parasite life cycle involves two hosts. During a blood meal, a malaria-infected female anopheles mosquito inoculates sporozoites into the human host (1). Sporozoites infect liver cells (2) and mature into schizonts (3), which rupture and release merozoites (4). In *P. vivax* and *P. ovale* a dormant stage (hypnozoites) can persist in the liver and cause relapses by invading the bloodstream weeks, or even years later. After this initial replication in the liver [exoerythrocytic schizogony (A)], the parasites undergo asexual multiplication in the erythrocytes [erythrocytic schizogony (B)]. Merozoites infect red blood cells (5). The ring stage trophozoites mature into schizonts, which rupture releasing merozoites (6).

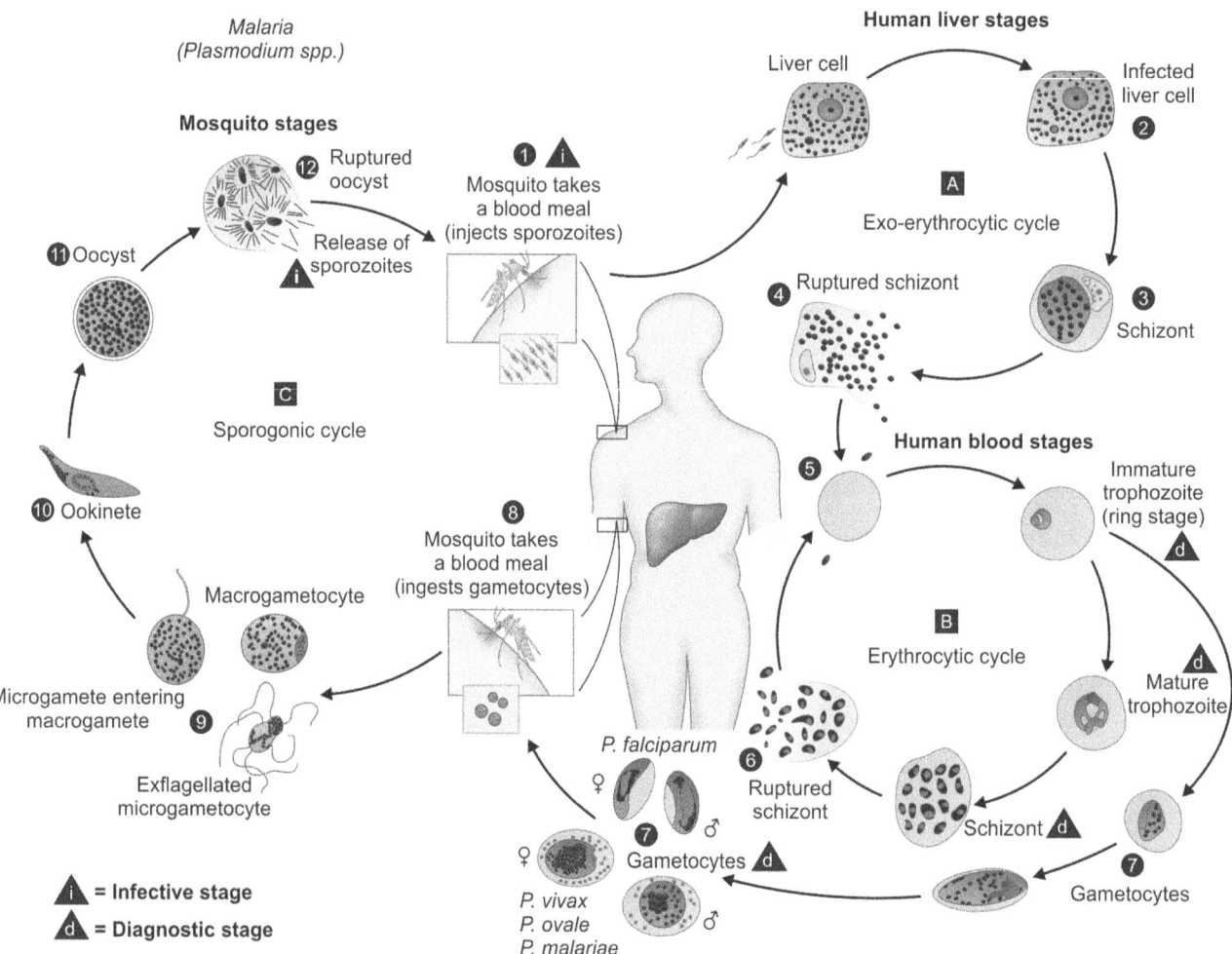

Source: Center for Disease Control and Prevention (2018). Biology. [online] Available from: https://www.cdc.gov/malaria/about/biology/ [Last accessed on February, 2020].

Some parasites differentiate into sexual erythrocytic stages (gametocytes) (7). Blood stage parasites are responsible for the clinical manifestations of the disease.

The gametocytes, male (microgametocytes) and female (macrogametocytes), are ingested by an anopheles mosquito during a blood meal (8). The parasites' multiplication in the mosquito is known as the sporogonic cycle (C). While in the mosquito's stomach, the microgametes penetrate the macrogametes generating zygotes (9). The zygotes in turn become motile and elongated (ookinetes) (10), which invade the midgut wall of the mosquito where they develop into oocysts (11). The oocysts grow, rupture, and release sporozoites (12), which make their way to the mosquito's salivary glands. Inoculation of the sporozoites (1) into a new human host perpetuates the malaria life cycle.

Ref:
1. Center for Disease Control and Prevention (2018). Biology. [online] Available from: https://www.cdc.gov/malaria/about/biology/ [Last accessed on February, 2020].

4. Ans. D

Cutaneous and migratory parasites, especially in the eye, are most likely to present as loiasis as has been confirmed in the eye by cross section. The treatment of choice is diethylcarbamazine (DEC) and albendazole with or without ivermectin.

Ref:
1. Center for Disease Control and Prevention (2015). Disease. [online] Available from: https://www.cdc.gov/parasites/loiasis/disease.html [Last accessed on February, 2020].

5. Ans. B

Mazzotti reaction occurs as a consequence of the parasite dying of the therapy leading to flare. Such therapy needs to be covered with steroids in the first 7–10 days.

Ref:
1. Padgett JJ, Jacobsen KH. Loiasis: African eye worm. T Roy Soc Trop Med H. 2008;102(10):983-9.
2. Centers for Disease Control and prevention (2017). Resources for Health Professionals. [online] Available from: https://www.cdc.gov/parasites/loiasis/health_professionals/index.html [Last accessed on February, 2020].

6. Ans. D

Light microscopic examination of a stained bone marrow specimen from a patient with visceral leishmaniasis—showing a multiple *Leishmania* amastigotes (the tissue stage of the parasite). Each amastigote has a nucleus and a rod-shaped kinetoplast. Visualization of the kinetoplast is important for diagnostic purposes, to be confident the patient has leishmaniasis.

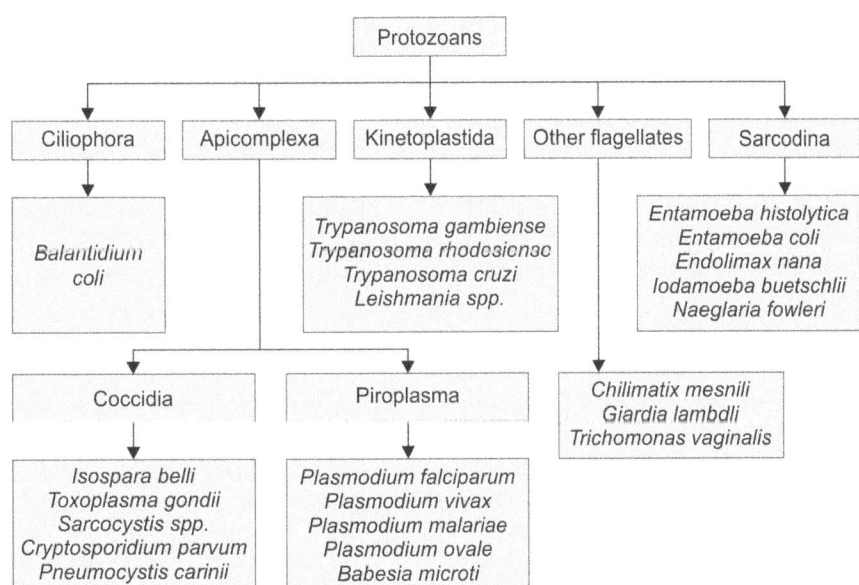

Source: Stark CG, Vidyashankar C (2020). Leishmaniasis. [online] Available from: https://emedicine.medscape.com/article/220298-overview. [Last accessed on February, 2020].

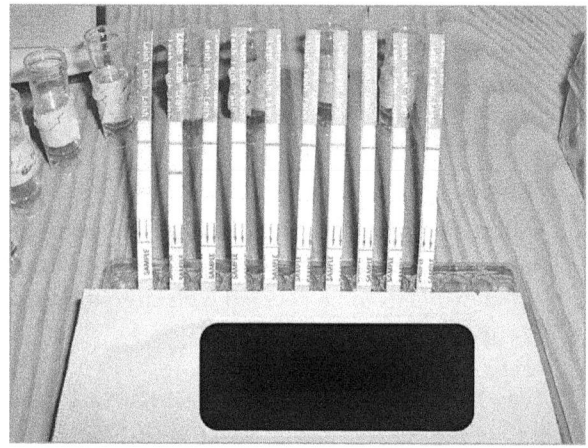

Source: Stark CG, Vidyashankar C (2020). Leishmaniasis. [online] Available from: https://emedicine.medscape.com/article/220298-overview [Last accessed on February, 2020].

Illustration of one form of the rK39 test for the serologic diagnosis of visceral leishmaniasis. It is an easy, very sensitive, and specific test for visceral disease. In this image, the dipstick second from the left shows a positive result.
Ref:
1. *Centers for Disease Control and Prevention (2018). Resources for Health Professionals. [online] Available from: http://www.cdc.gov/parasites/leishmaniasis/health_professionals/ [Last accessed on February, 2020].*
2. *Stark CG, Vidyashankar C (2020). Leishmaniasis. [online] Available from: https://emedicine.medscape.com/article/220298-overview [Last accessed on February, 2020].*

7. **Ans. D**

This image suggests stool sample with egg that is barrel shaped, with bipolar plugs.
Ref:
1. *Centers for Disease Control and Prevention (2017). Trichuriasis. [online] Available from: https://www.cdc.gov/dpdx/trichuriasis/index.html [Last accessed on February, 2020].*

8. **Ans. B**

Leishmaniasis is a disease caused by protozoan parasites of the genus *Leishmania* and spread by a bite of certain types of sand flies. The disease presents as cutaneous, mucocutaneous or visceral. This patient's clinical presentation represents less than 5% of cases documented in medical literature.
Ref:
1. *Steverding D. The history of leishmaniasis. Parasit Vectors. 2017;10(1):82.*
2. *Torres-Guerrero E, Quintanilla-Cedillo MR, Ruiz-Esmenjaud J, Arenas R. Leishmaniasis: A review. F1000Res. 2017;6:750.*

9. **Ans. C**

This image shows patient's third and fourth fingertips of her left hand with splinter hemorrhages of the nail beds beneath the fingernails, which were the result of a disease known as trichinosis. Splinter hemorrhages are one of the symptoms of trichinosis, caused by eating raw or undercooked pork infected with the larvae of roundworms from the genus *Trichinella*.
Ref:
1. *Rawla P, Sharma S. Trichinella Spiralis (Trichnellosis). StatPearls Publishing; 2019.*

10. **Ans. D**

The most common cause of anemia and pedal edema is GI track involvement and hookworm infestation. This image shows edema and rash. The hookworm uses its sharp cutting teeth to grasp firmly to the victim's intestinal wall, also ingests the host's blood, obtaining its nutrients, thus causing the sufferer to become anemic.
Ref:
1. *Ghodeif AO, Jain H. Hookworm. StatPearls Publishing; 2020.*
2. *Haburchak DR, Watson CM, Dhawan VK (2018). Hookworm Disease. [online] Available from: https://emedicine.medscape.com/article/218805-overview. [Last accessed on February, 2020].*

11. **Ans. C**

This photomicrograph depicts eight eggs of the human pinworm, *E. vermicularis*, which had been mounted on cellulose tape. Eggs are deposited on perianal folds. Self-infection occurs by transferring nematode eggs to the mouth with hands that have scratched the perianal area. Person-to-person transmission can also occur through handling of contaminated clothes or bed linens. *E. vermicularis*, a nematode (roundworm) is also called human pinworm. Although pinworm infection can affect all people, it most commonly occurs among children and institutionalized persons.

The most reliable and widely used technique for demonstrating pinworm eggs (*E. vermicularis*) is the scotch tape or cellulose tape or swube tube procedure. The adhesive part of the swube tube or tape is applied to the perianal area first thing in the morning. Specimens should be collected on three consecutive mornings prior to bathing. If an infection is present, eggs and sometimes adult worms of *E. vermicularis* will be present on the tape and can be seen under the microscope.
Ref:
1. *Center for Disease Control and Prevention (2016). Other Specimens—Cellulose Tape or Swube Tube Procedure for Demonstration of Pinworm Eggs. [online] Available from: https://www.cdc.gov/dpdx/diagnosticprocedures/other/pinworm.html [Last accessed on February, 2020].*

12. **Ans. B**

Classical appearance of *Entamoeba histolytica*. Migration of parasite occurs in both occupational and

nonoccupational exposure. Treatment is conservative. This image shows amebiasis patients who presented with tissue destruction and granulation of the anoperineal region due to an *Entamoeba histolytica* infection.
Ref:
1. Ralston KS, Petri WA Jr. Tissue destruction and invasion by Entamoeba histolytica. Trends Parasitol. 2011;27(6):254-63.

13. **Ans. A**

Mucocutaneous disease is also called espundia in South America. This condition usually is due to metastasis from disseminated protozoa rather than by local spread. Most commonly caused by New World species, although Old World *L. aethiopica* has also been reported to cause this syndrome. Secondary infection plays a prominent role in the size and persistence of ulcers. Infection by *L. (Viannia) braziliensis* may lead to mucosal involvement in up to 10% of infections, depending on the region in which it was acquired. Ulcer progression is slow and steady, after several years oral and respiratory mucosal involvement occurs which causes inflammation and mutilation of nose, mouth, oropharynx, and trachea as shown in the image, can also result in nasal obstruction and bleeding. Mucosal involvement may take approximately up to two decades from the primary lesion involvement.
Ref:
1. Stark CG, Vidyashankar C (2019). What are the clinical manifestations of mucocutaneous leishmaniasis? [online] Available from: https://www.medscape.com/answers/220298-117591/what-are-the-clinical-manifestations-of-mucocutaneous-leishmaniasis [Last accessed on February, 2020].

14. **Ans. A**

The likely infection could be *Cryptosporidium, Isospora, Microsporidia*, or *Cyclospora*, which are associated infections in acquired immunodeficiency syndrome (AIDS) patients even though they are self-resolving in normal noncompromised individuals. In AIDS patients they are most commonly unrelenting, even with treatment. They are usually acquired from water.
Ref:
1. Wang ZD, Liu Q, Liu HH, Li S, Zhang L, Zhao Y-K, et al. Prevalence of Cryptosporidium, microsporidia and Isospora infection in HIV-infected people: a global systematic review and meta-analysis. Parasit Vectors. 2018;11(1):28.

15. **Ans. B**

Ascaris lumbricoides also called "roundworm" is one of the most common intestinal parasites in humans. The lifecycle of *Ascaris lumbricoides* is passed in only one host, human. No intermediate host is required. *Toxoplasma gondii* the intermediate hosts are birds and rodents. Intermediate hosts of *Echinococcus granulosus* are sheep, cattle, goats, and pigs. Intermediate hosts of *Taenia solium* are pigs.

Ref:
1. Cox FE. History of human parasitology. Clin Microbiol Rev. 2002;15(4):595-612.

16. **Ans. B**

Trichinosis is caused by a protozoan that has both a trophozoite and a cyst stage in its life cycle.
Ref:
1. Garcia LS, Arrowood M, Kokoskin E, Paltridge GP, Pillai DR, Procop GW, et al. Laboratory diagnosis of parasites from the gastrointestinal tract. Clin Microbiol Rev. 2017;31(1):e00025-17.

17. **Ans. D**

Mode of infection for *Ancylostoma duodenale* is skin penetration by filariform larvae. When a person walks barefoot on soil containing the filariform larvae, the larvae may penetrate the skin, particularly the skin between the toes, the dorsum of the foot, and the medial aspect of the sole.
Ref:
1. Jayaram PCK. Hookworm. Textbook of Medical Parasitology, 6th edition. New Delhi: Jaypee Brothers Medical Publishers; 2007.

18. **Ans. A**

Schizogony occurs inside the capillaries of spleen, liver, and bone marrow. Therefore only the ring form is found in the peripheral blood.
Ref:
1. Franke-Fayard B, Fonager J, Braks A, Khan SM, Janse CJ. Sequestration and tissue accumulation of human malaria parasites: can we learn anything from rodent models of malaria? PLoS Pathog. 2010;6(9):e1001032.
2. Chaterjee KD. Parasitology: Protozoology and Helminthology. New Delhi: CBS Publishers; 2019.

19. **Ans. B**

Benign quartan (with a fever every third day) malaria is caused *P. malariae* whereas benign tertian (with a fever every second day) is caused by *P. vivax* and *P. ovale* and malignant tertian is caused by *P. falciparum*.
Ref:
1. Crutcher JM, Hoffman SL. Malaria. In: Baron S (Ed). Medical Microbiology, 4th edition. Galveston (TX): University of Texas Medical Branch at Galveston; 1996.
2. Chaterjee KD. Parasitology: Protozoology and Helminthology. New Delhi: CBS Publishers; 2019.

20. **Ans. D**

Vector of onchocerciasis is blackfly (*Simulium damnosum*) whereas that of visceral leishmaniasis is sand fly (*Phlebotomus argentipes*). Trypanosomiasis is transmitted by a blood sucking insect, *Tsetse fly*.
Ref:
1. Tiwary P, Kumar D, Singh RP, Rai M, Sundar S. Prevalence of sand flies and Leishmania donovani infection in a natural population of female Phlebotomus argentipes in Bihar State, India. Vector Borne Zoonotic Dis. 2012;12(6):467-72.
2. Chaterjee KD. Parasitology: Protozoology and Helminthology. New Delhi: CBS Publishers; 2019.

21. Ans. B

Loa loa causes a chronic infection in humans. It has two clinical features; Calabar swellings which are localized angioedema found predominantly on the extremities and subconjunctival migration of the adult parasites.

22. Ans. B

Dirofilaria are parasitic roundworms infecting mammals, and are transmitted by mosquito bites. Among several species, three species *D. immitis*, *D. repens*, and *D. tenuis* cause infection in humans. Hosts being dogs, foxes, wolves (*D. immitis* and *D. repens*) and raccoons (*D. tenuis*). *D. immitis* is also known as "heartworm".

Ref:
1. Cho HY, Lee YJ, Shin SY, Song HO, Ahn MH, Ryu JS. Subconjuctival Loa loa with Calabar swelling. J Korean Med Sci. 2008;23(4):731-3.
2. Chaterjee KD. Parasitology: Protozoology and Helminthology. New Delhi: CBS Publishers; 2019.

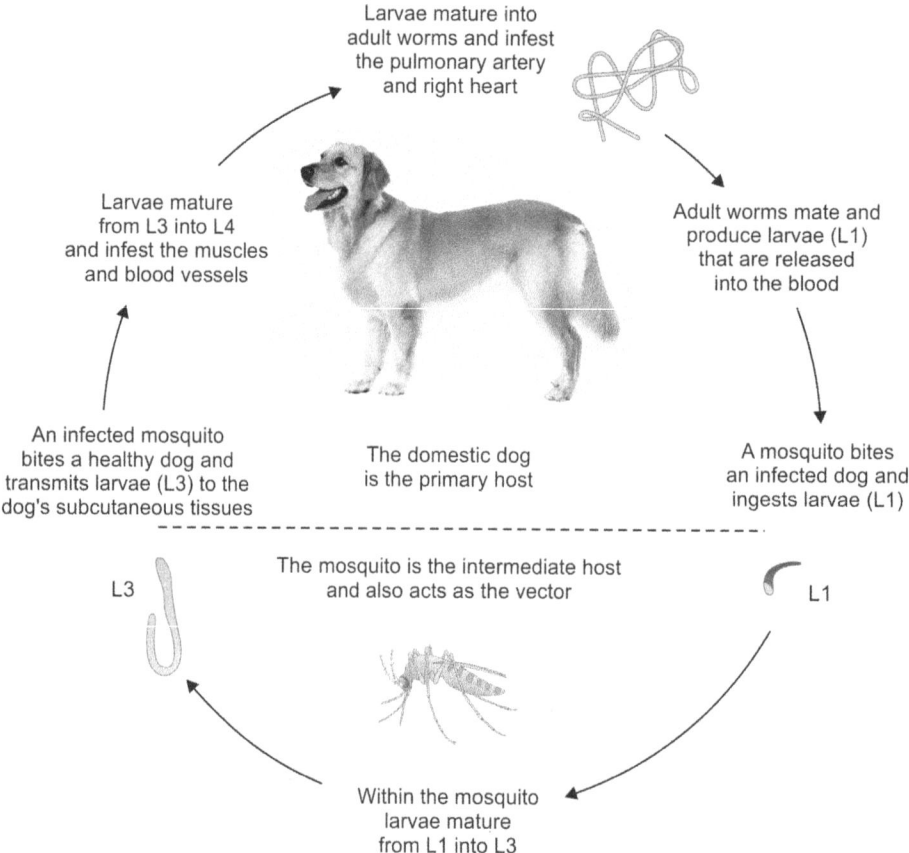

Source: Faoil C, Friedrich A. Dirofilaria immitis lifecycle; 2013.

Ref:
1. Simón F, Siles-Lucas M, Morchón R, González-Miguel J, Mellado I, Carretón E, et al. Human and animal dirofilariasis: the emergence of a zoonotic mosaic. Clin Microbiol Rev. 2012;25(3):507-44.
2. Chaterjee KD. Parasitology: Protozoology and Helminthology. New Delhi: CBS Publishers; 2019.

23. Ans. D

Nonbile stained eggs—*Ancylostoma duodenale*, *Hymenolepis nana*, *Enterobius vermicularis*, and *Necator americanus*.

Ref:
1. Kumar S. Stool/feces examination. Practical Microbiology for MBBS Students. New Delhi: Jaypee Brothers Medical Publishers; 2018.
2. Chaterjee KD. Parasitology: Protozoology and Helminthology. New Delhi: CBS Publishers; 2019.

24. Ans. B

An intradermal skin test (Casoni test) used, with sensitivity of 70% and specificity of 47%. Currently it has been replaced by newer more sensitive, specific, and safer serological tests.

Ref:
1. Dandan IS, Soweid AM, Abiad F (2019). What is the role of the Casoni test in the diagnosis of hydatid cysts? [online] Available from: https://www.medscape.com/answers/178648-69106/what-is-the-role-of-the-casoni-test-in-the-diagnosis-of-hydatid-cysts [Last accessed on February, 2020].
2. Chaterjee KD. Parasitology: Protozoology and Helminthology. New Delhi: CBS Publishers; 2019.

25. Ans. B

Helminth eggs that float in saturated salt solution are *H. nana, A. duodenale, T. trichiura, E. vermicularis,* and fertilized eggs of *A. lumbricoides*.

Ref:
1. *Chaterjee KD. Parasitology: Protozoology and Helminthology. New Delhi: CBS Publishers; 2019.*

26. Ans. C

Echinococcus granulosus is a parasitic anthropozoonosis characterized by the development of a larval tapeworm stage (metacestode) in herbivorous intermediate hosts, such as rodents and ungulates, and accidentally in humans.

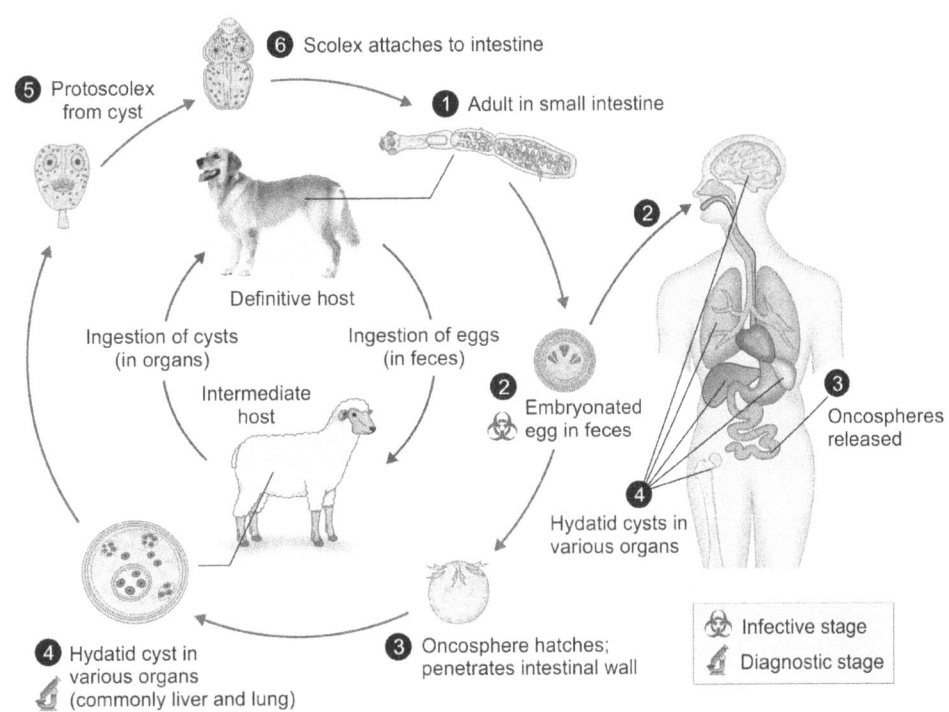

Source: Center for Disease Control and Prevention (2019). Biology. [online] Available from: https://www.cdc.gov/parasites/echinococcosis/biology.html. [Last accessed on February, 2020].

Ref:
1. *Tappe D, Stich A, Frosch M. Emergence of polycystic neotropical echinococcosis. Emerg Infect Dis. 2008;14(2): 292-7.*
2. *Chaterjee KD. Parasitology: Protozoology and Helminthology. New Delhi: CBS Publishers; 2019.*

27. Ans. A

Paragonimus ova and Charcot-Leyden crystals are demonstrated in early morning sputum specimens of patients with pleuropulmonary paragonimiasis.

Ref:
1. *Kalhan S, Sharma P, Sharma S, Kakria N, Dudani S, Gupta A. Paragonimus westermani infection in lung: A confounding diagnostic entity. Lung India. 2015;32(3):265-7.*
2. *Chaterjee KD. Parasitology: Protozoology and Helminthology. New Delhi: CBS Publishers; 2019.*

28. Ans. C

Primary amebic meningoencephalitis (PAM) is a rare and fatal disease involving central nervous system (CNS) caused by *Naegleria fowleri,* which is an amoeba found in soils and warm waters.

Ref:
1. *Gautam PL, Sharma S, Puri S, Kumar R, Midha V, Bansal R. A rare case of survival from primary amebic meningoencephalitis. Indian J Crit Care Med. 2012;16(1):34-6.*
2. *Chaterjee KD. Parasitology: Protozoology and Helminthology. New Delhi: CBS Publishers; 2019.*

29. Ans. B

The human parasites susceptible to be congenitally transferred are *Toxoplasma gondii, Trypanosoma cruzi* and *Plasmodium* spp.

Ref:
1. *Carlier Y, Truyens C, Deloron P, Peyron F. Congenital parasitic infections: a review. Acta Trop. 2012;121(2):55-70.*
2. *Chaterjee KD. Parasitology: Protozoology and Helminthology. New Delhi: CBS Publishers; 2019.*

30. Ans. A

Trichomoniasis is a very common sexually transmitted disease. It is caused by infection with a protozoan parasite called *Trichomonas vaginalis*.

Ref:
1. *https://www.cdc.gov/std/trichomonas/stdfact-trichomoniasis.htm.*
2. *Chaterjee KD. Parasitology: Protozoology and Helminthology. New Delhi: CBS Publishers; 2019.*

CHAPTER 20

Fever in the Returning Traveler

Juhi Dhar, Meghna Kabra, Raj Kumar Mani

1. Which of the following is to be considered while assessing a patient with a suspected travel-related illness?
   A. Vaccines and prophylaxis received
   B. Travel itinerary
   C. Timing of illness in relation to travel
   D. Individual exposures
   E. All of the above

2. A patient presented with loose motions, 5–10 episodes daily, with upper abdomen pain and bloating half-way during his holiday. He received some treatment which improved his condition, but symptoms persist even now, 1 month after return from his travel. What is your likely diagnosis?
   A. Bacterial infections
   B. Giardiasis
   C. Postinfectious diarrhea
   D. Tropical sprue
   E. All of the above

3. A 32-year-old computer executive from Mumbai who went trekking to Northeast India 1 month back now presented with low-grade fever which he was suffering from since 1 month. He had rash associated with itching and crampy abdominal pain on and off. His WBC was 14,000/μL, E 20%, ultrasound abdomen—normal. There was no relief on treatment received. CT scan showed a hypodense, tortuous branching lesion in the liver. Routine microscopy stool was normal. Upper GI endoscopy was done and duodenal aspirate microscopy was normal. Liver biopsy revealed eosinophilic infiltration and abscess.
   What is most likely to benefit?
   A. Praziquantel
   B. Nitazoxanide
   C. Triclabendazole
   D. Artesunate

4. A 26-year-old male presented with complaints of high-grade fever since 6 days with maculopapular rash over body and severe myalgias, some throat pain, cough, and nontender cervical lymphadenopathy. He had history of loose motions in the first few days of fever. He also had a history of travel to Thailand 2½ weeks back. History of exposure is present as well. What is the most likely diagnosis?
   A. Infectious mononucleosis (IM)
   B. Acute retroviral syndrome (ARS)
   C. Syphilis
   D. Erythema multiforme (EM)

5. In the above Question 4, which test would you do to confirm your diagnosis if ARS?
   A. HIV serology
   B. CD4
   C. HIV, RNA, and PCR viral load
   D. Western blot

6. A 40-year-old man presented with complaints of mental deterioration over the last 1 week with difficulty in coordinating. The patient is confused and sleeps poorly at night. On further enquiring, his wife said that he had been to a Safari to a game park in East Africa (Uganda) few weeks back and had developed fever and arthralgia with headache with a chancre on his right arm on reaching Delhi, but had settled with treatment from a local doctor. What is true of the disease?
   A. Serological assays are diagnostic
   B. Melarsoprol is drug of choice under prednisolone cover
   C. Eflornithine pentamidine and suramin can be used as a second-line agent
   D. All of the above

7. A 40-year-old man presented with complaints of painful swelling over his body which are intensely itchy and resolve in a week, to recur at a distant site. There is generalized swelling over the body, mainly on the abdomen with abdominal pain and rash and itching. His investigations revealed an absolute eosinophil count (AEC) of 2,500. Urine R/M revealed 15–20 RBCs/hpf. He further had a history of exposure to animals. He also gave a history of travel to Japan 1 month back where after eating sushi, he had developed signs and symptoms suggestive of gastritis which had settled with treatment.
   What is your most likely diagnosis?
   A. Gnathostomiasis
   B. Loiasis
   C. Urticaria/angioedema
   D. None of the above

8. A 26-year-old man presented with complaints of nontender swelling on the arm and legs near the joints which are associated with itching all over

the body, myalgias, and joint pain. His workup revealed Hb 12.6 g/dL, TLC 12,000, platelet count 140,000/mm^3, with 25% eosinophils, and ESR 35 mm/h. His rheumatoid arthritis (RA), anti-cyclic citrullinated peptide (anti-CCP) was negative. On further questioning, he revealed that he was on deputation for 3 months on a rubber plantation unit in western Africa and had returned home 1 month back.

What is your diagnosis?

A. Hypereosinophilic syndrome (HES)
B. Gnathostomiasis
C. Loiasis
D. Cutaneous larva migrans (CLM)

9. A 40-year-old male presented in June with fever, sore throat, myalgias, and a mild rash around the wrist and ankles for 2 days. His General Practitioner (GP) gave him paracetamol, antihistamines, and advice to drink lots of fluids. He returned 5 days later with marked worsening of symptoms. The rash was now a nodular-papular rash with central hemorrhages. There is presence of petechiae all over the body including the hands and the feet. The patient was drowsy with a heart rate (HR) of 140 beats/min and BP—80 systolic. His CBC revealed Hb 10 g/dL, TLC 6,000, and platelet count 39,000/mm^3. His prothrombin time/activated partial thromboplastin time (PT/APTT) was normal. His serum creatinine was 1.5, SGOT 550, SGPT 266, SGT 110, ALP 130, and ALB 2.5. He had a history of return from the USA 10 days back.

Drug of choice:

A. Injection ceftriaxone 2 g IV twice a day
B. Injection benzathine penicillin
C. Meropenem and teicoplanin
D. Doxycycline

10. A 40-year-old male presented with complaints of fever and nodular swelling over the left leg. He had a history of recent return from Uganda where he had gone camping. There is no history of trauma. He had a history of intense itching at the site of lesion before presentation. Then redness and swelling were noted which gradually progressed over 2 days and developed a black nodule in the center. The patient also complained of feeling of movement in the nodule. No discharge was noted.

Which statement is wrong?

A. Treatment is surgical excision
B. It is a case of cutaneous myiasis
C. Diagnosis is solely on clinical ground
D. A course of antibiotics is curative

11. A 40-year-old male presented with complaints of swelling and redness over the sole of his right foot. He had an ulcerated lesion over his foot for the last 5–6 years which had not bothered him. Recently, he had returned from Goa and now he has developed pain and redness with marked swelling. He took some local treatment but developed worsening of lesions with appearance of bullae. The patient had high fever, BP—80 mm Hg systolic and was toxic. Which is the most likely organism?

A. *Clostridium perfringens*
B. *Pseudomonas*
C. Gram-positive staphylococci or streptococci
D. *Vibrio vulnificus*

12. A 40-year-old male presented with high fever, myalgia, painful lesion on the lower limb and left inguinal bubo. The patient has recently returned from a safari in South Africa.

What is the causative agent?

A. Gram-negative bipolar staining bacilli
B. Gram-negative bacilli
C. Gram-positive bacilli
D. Gram-positive cocci

13. A 52-year-old CLD patient (alcohol induced) returned after working on an oil rig in Gulf and was in Kerala at his farmhouse during rains. He presented with fever, severe left-sided chest pain, and no improvement with a course of Amoxyclav and azithromycin. On imaging, pneumonia with pleural effusion and lymph node enlargement were seen. On further evaluation, pleural effusion showed neutrophilic predominance. CBC revealed TLC of 16,000/mm^3 with 92% polymorphs. Blood culture is positive. Urine Ag test for *Streptococcus* is negative. **What could be the causative agent?**

A. Staphylococcal pneumonia
B. *Aspergillus*
C. *Bacillus anthracis*
D. *Burkholderia pseudomallei*

14. A 35-year-old man returned from a Hajj pilgrimage 10 days back and presented with complaints of high-grade fever, headache, severe body ache, and vomiting of 1 day. The ER doctor noted a blanchable subtle rash all over the body. The patient appeared to be toxic with 103°F with PR of 130, BP of 96/60 mm Hg, and RR of 30 breaths/min. His Hb was 13.2 g/dL, TLC 17,000, platelet count 120,000/mm^3, with PT of 17.0 and APTT of 35. LFT and RFT were within normal limits. Select the wrong statement.

A. Five serogroups, A, B, C, Y, and W-135, account for majority of cases of invasive disease

B. Most common form of infection by this organism is meningitis
C. A non-blanching petechial purpuric rash may be seen in >80% of patients and in severe cases may progress to purpura fulminans
D. Chronic meningococcemia and postmeningococcal reactive disease are rare presentations of the disease

15. A 33-year-old lady resident of Delhi presented with fever on and off for 15 days, cough for 15 days, retrosternal chest pain, and breathlessness since few days. Her Hb was 8.0 g/dL, TLC 2,400, and platelet count 6,600/mm^3. Chest X-ray revealed few patchy infiltrates with hilar prominence. CT chest revealed B/L mediastinal and hilar lymph node with presence of necrosis. On further questioning, she revealed that she had returned from a 1 month trip to Ohio (USA) after a cave excavation project. There is no history of exposure to pigeon and no history of Koch's or contact with Koch's. Mantoux test is negative and her ESR is 35 mm/h. What is the best treatment for the disease?
    A. Amphotericin B
    B. Antituberculosis treatment (ATT)
    C. Steroids
    D. Antibiotics

16. A 70-year-old lady presented with complaints of fever, night sweats, cough with severe right-sided chest pain, and arthralgia of 7–8 days. The chest X-ray done was normal. She was given a course of antibiotics and sent home. She returned with worsening of symptoms. The doctor noted erythema multiforme in necklace distribution. CBC done revealed eosinophilia with an absolute count of 3,000. CT chest revealed bilateral mediastinal lymphadenopathy and no evidence of necrosis. The patient gives a history of traveling to Arizona 20 days back and had returned just recently.
    What is your likely diagnosis?
    A. Coccidioidomycosis
    B. Histoplasmosis
    C. Bacterial pneumonia
    D. Tuberculosis

17. A 24-year-old student presented with complaints of discomfort on urination with large amount of yellow-colored penile discharge. He gives history of returning from Ibiza where he had gone for a summer internship. What is your most likely diagnosis?
    A. Cystitis
    B. Genital herpes
    C. Gonorrhea
    D. Chlamydia

18. A 40-year-old male presents with a history of lesions on the left forearm for the last 4 weeks. On examination, there are two ulcers, 2.5 × 2.5 cm each, which have an erythematous base with raised edges. The patient gives a history of traveling around South America and had returned 2 days back. He had not sought any medical treatment during this time. What is your most likely diagnosis?
    A. Buruli ulcer
    B. Leishmaniasis
    C. Herpes zoster
    D. Myiasis

19. A 36-year-old international patient presented in the first week of February with complaints of high-grade fever of 102–103°F with severe headache, body aches, and malaise since 5 days, and dry cough since 3 days with marked worsening since 1 day. He had a history of some loose motions for 2 days. He gives a history of returning from Bangladesh 10 days back. A maculopapular rash is noted over her trunk and spleen is palpable. Her CBC revealed Hb 12.2 g/dL, TLC 4,500 with 75% neutrophils, and platelets of 131,000/mm^3.
    What is the choice of investigations?
    A. Malarial serology
    B. Dengue serology
    C. Blood culture
    D. X-ray posteroanterior (PA) view

20. A 30-year-old male chronic smoker, presented with complaints of worsening dyspnea, hemoptysis, and abdominal pain since few days. The patient was a soldier posted at the marshes of Bangladesh and was in India now for the last 3 weeks. He was started on inhalers, antibiotics, oral steroids, outside for his cough but there was no improvement and had now come with worsening complaint. He was febrile with a temperature of 101°F with bilateral wheeze rashes noted on his abdominal wall. His investigations revealed eosinophilia AEC 2,000 blood culture flashed gram-negative bacilli. Select the wrong statement:
    A. The organism can be detected in stool and can persist in humans for years after travel to endemic area
    B. Septicemia with enteric organism is because of translocation of bacteria from the gut by the larvae
    C. In very sick patients, one can use parenteral ivermectin which is used in veterinary practice
    D. Albendazole with steroids is the choice of treatment

21. A 44-year-old woman has returned from a 10-day vacation on a cruise ship where she developed high-grade fever with breathlessness and dry cough on her last day on the ship. Three other persons on board the ship have similar symptoms. This is the third day of fever. She also has diarrhea, with 3–4 episodes of watery loose stools daily, nausea, and 3–4 episodes of vomiting.

On examination, her pulse is 110 bpm, blood pressure is 95/50 mm Hg, and respiratory rate is 28 breaths/min. She is tachypneic. Oxygen saturation is 90% on air. Examination of the respiratory system reveals dullness to percussion and decreased breath sounds in bilateral lower zones. Her serum sodium is 125 mEq/L. Aspartate aminotransferase (AST) is 88 units/L and ALT is 78 units/L. An X-ray chest reveals bilateral lower zone nonhomogeneous opacities. Sputum Gram stain reveals numerous white blood cells. No bacteria are seen.

Which of the following is the most likely cause of the patient's symptoms?

A. *Coxiella burnetii*
B. *Legionella* pneumonia
C. *Staphylococcus aureus*
D. *Streptococcus pneumoniae*

22. A 55-year-old man presented in hospital with a history of fever for 7 days. He stayed in a refugee camp in Ethiopia till 5 days prior to presentation. Fever developed 7 days prior to the hospital visit. It was high grade and continuous. On the third day, the patient had rigors, a further elevation in temperature, and an increase in pulse and blood pressure. This was followed by profuse diaphoresis and falling temperature. The fever recurred after 4 days. It was associated with headache, myalgia, arthralgia, shaking chills, and nausea with vomiting. On examination, the patient appeared malnourished. There were insect bites on his body. A body louse was found in his clothes. His blood pressure (BP) was 100/60 mm Hg, pulse 110 bpm, respiratory rate 26 breaths/min, and temperature 101°F. Mild pallor is present. Systemic examination revealed hepatomegaly and hemoglobin 9.5 g/dL, MCV 86, WBC 5500/μL, DLC normal, platelet count 120,000/μL, AST 100 units/L, ALT 90 units/L, and ESR 74 mm/h. A Giemsa stain of peripheral blood revealed spirochetes.

Which of the following is true for this infection?

A. Penicillins and tetracyclines are the antibiotics of choice
B. Both penicillin and tetracycline can elicit the Jarisch–Herxheimer reaction
C. Coinfection with malaria may occur
D. All of the above

23. A 30-year-old woman presented with a 6-day history of high-grade fever with chills, headache, and myalgia. She was 8 weeks pregnant and had returned from a 1-week trip to Nigeria 5 days ago. She had not taken any chemoprophylaxis or immunizations prior to her trip. On examination, her temperature was 103°F, pulse 120 bpm, BP 94/50 mm Hg, and respiration rate 28 breaths/min. Icterus was present. Mild pallor was noted. There was no edema or lymphadenopathy. Chest was clear to auscultation. Examination of the cardiovascular system (CVS) revealed tachycardia. Abdominal examination revealed mild hepatomegaly. Central nervous system (CNS) examination was normal. Hemogram revealed a hemoglobin of 11.5 g/dL, hematocrit of 33%, and WBC count of 8,000/μL with normal differential. The platelet count is 152,000/μL. Renal function tests are normal. Liver function tests reveal total bilirubin of 4.2 mg/dL, indirect bilirubin of 3.2 g/dL, AST 88 units/L, ALT 70 units/L, and serum albumin 3.5 mg/dL. Urine analysis revealed trace proteinuria with 3–4 WBC/hpf and 2–3 RRCs/hpf. Random blood glucose is 110 mg/dL. A peripheral blood smear revealed *Plasmodium falciparum*. Parasitemia is 1%.

Which of the following would be appropriate management?

A. Quinine sulfate plus doxycycline
B. Quinine sulfate plus clindamycin
C. Chloroquine
D. Atovaquone-proguanil

24. A 28-year-old man presented with history of paroxysmal cough and wheezing which occurred mostly at night, weight loss of 5 kg, and low-grade fever for 3–4 months. He resided in north estern India in Bihar for 2 years and had returned from there 1 year ago.

On examination, pulse is 90 bpm, blood pressure is 120/70 mm Hg, respiratory rate is 24 breaths/min, and temperature is 98.4°F. There was no edema/icterus/pallor/clubbing. Mobile discrete 1 cm cervical and inguinal lymph nodes were palpable bilaterally.

On auscultation of the chest, he had bilateral wheezes. Cardiovascular system examination was normal. There was no organomegaly or tenderness on abdominal palpation. There was no focal deficit. Hemogram revealed a hemoglobin of 13 g/dL, WBC count of 16,000/μL, 45% neutrophils, 30% eosinophils, 30% lymphocytes, and 5% monocytes. Chest radiograph showed increased bronchoalveolar markings and diffuse interstitial lesions (1–3 mm in diameter), most prominent in the lower lung fields. The most useful initial test should be:

A. Antifilarial antibody levels in serum
B. Pulmonary function tests (PFTs)
C. Bronchoscopy with bronchoalveolar lavage
D. Serum galactomannan assay

25. A 28-year-old woman visited Borneo where she participated in recreational swimming in lakes. A week later she developed high fever with chills,

severe retro-orbital headache, nausea and vomiting, abdominal pain, and severe myalgia. Three days later, she developed dyspnea and hemoptysis and visited hospital.

On examination, pulse is 110 bpm, blood pressure 80/50 mm Hg, respiratory rate 30 breaths/min, and temperature 102°F. SpO_2 was 88% on air. Icterus was present. Conjunctival suffusion was present. Bilateral lower zone crackles were present on auscultation. CVS-S1S2 and tachycardia were present. Per abdominal examination revealed diffuse tenderness. There was no guarding or rigidity. Central nervous system examination did not reveal a focal deficit.

Investigations revealed hemoglobin 10.5 g/dL, WBC count 16,500/µL, neutrophils 90%, lymphocytes 10%, platelet count 120,000/ µL, and ESR 60 mm/h. Urine revealed 8–10 WBC/hpf and 8–10 RBC/hpf. Urine microscopy revealed granular casts and trace proteinuria. On examination, serum sodium was 130 mEq/L, serum potassium 3.3 mEq/L, urea 56 mg/dL, serum creatinine 1.8 mg/dL, total bilirubin 4.2 mg/dL, direct bilirubin 3.6 mg/dL, SGOT 190 units/L, and SGPT 180 units/L. Chest X-ray revealed bilateral lower zone infiltrates. Blood and urine cultures were sent and reports awaited. Malaria and dengue serology were negative. Other serologic studies were awaited. Which antibiotic should be started based on the clinical presentation?

A. IV ceftriaxone
B. IV gentamicin
C. IV cefuroxime
D. IV ofloxacin plus metrogyl

26. A 40-year-old woman presented with complaints of high-grade intermittent evening-rise fever with night sweats for 2 weeks. After the first week of fever, she was afebrile for 3–4 days following which the fever recurred. Fever was associated with headache, body aches, loss of appetite, and generalized weakness. She had visited a farm in northern India for a month. She drank unpasteurized goat's milk while she stayed there. Symptoms began 1 month after her return. On examination, pulse was 90 bpm, blood pressure 100/60 mm Hg, temperature 100°F, and respiratory rate 20 breaths/min. There was mild pallor. No edema, icterus, clubbing, lymphadenopathy, or cyanosis was noted. Chest was clear to auscultation. Examination of the CVS was normal. Abdominal examination revealed hepatomegaly (15 cm). Central nervous system examination was normal. Her pregnancy test was negative.

Hemoglobin was 10.8 g/dL, MCV was normal, and total leukocyte count was 4,000/µL. Differential leukocyte count was normal. Platelet count was normal. Renal and liver function tests were normal. Blood cultures (BACTEC) were positive for *Brucella*. The most appropriate treatment is:

A. Streptomycin with doxycycline
B. Streptomycin
C. Ciprofloxacin
D. Rifampicin with streptomycin

27. A 55-year-old woman visited a coastal village in Kerala during the monsoon season where she spent a fair amount of time outdoors and reported mosquito bites. Three days after returning, she developed high-grade fever with joint pain. Pain started in one or two joints, but subsequently 10 joints were involved within 24–48 hours of onset. Involvement was bilateral and symmetric. Involvement of distal joints was more than proximal joints and was associated with morning stiffness. Hands, wrists, ankles, and axial skeleton were involved. Pain was intense and disabling. She developed a maculopapular rash 3 days after the onset of fever which involved the trunk and limbs and was mildly pruritic. On examination, tenderness and synovitis of the fingers, wrist, ankles, knees, and shoulder joints was noted. Her investigations on the third day of fever revealed a hemoglobin of 12.5 g/dL and WBC count of 4,000/µL with platelet count 125,000/µL. AST was 90 units/L and ALT was 80 units/L.

For confirmation of the diagnosis, further testing should include:

A. PCR for chikungunya virus
B. Enzyme-linked immunosorbent assay (ELISA) for chikungunya immunoglobulin M (IgM)
C. ELISA for Zika virus IgM
D. Serology for *Borrelia burgdorferi*

28. A 30-year-old man presented with a 3-day history of 8–10 watery loose motions daily, vomiting, crampy abdominal pain, and fever. He had been using the local municipal swimming pool for a month. Several other swimmers had similar symptoms. On physical examination, his temperature was 100°F, pulse 100 bpm, and blood pressure 120/70 mm Hg. Mild dehydration is present. On abdominal examination, palpation elicited mild diffuse tenderness. No guarding or rigidity was present. A modified acid-fast stain of the stool showed red oocysts.

Which is the most likely cause of this patient's diarrhea?

A. *Vibrio parahaemolyticus*
B. *Norovirus*
C. Enterohemorrhagic *Escherichia coli*
D. *Cryptosporidium*

29. A 58-year-old man visited Nepal where he camped for 4 weeks. Two weeks after returning, he visited the hospital with complaints of anorexia, nausea, flatulence, fatigue, abdominal cramping, watery

diarrhea, and low-grade fever for 12 days. On examination, pulse was 100 bpm, blood pressure 110/70 mm Hg, and temperature 100°F. Chest was clear. CVS-S1S2 was normal. Per abdominal examination did not reveal tenderness, guarding or rigidity or hepatosplenomegaly. Stool microscopy revealed oocysts (diameter 8–10 μm). Using modified acid-fast staining of stool, the cysts appeared light pink to deep purple.

What is the appropriate management for this diarrhea?

- A. Praziquantel
- B. Albendazole
- C. Oral trimethoprim–sulfamethoxazole
- D. Oral metronidazole

30. A 22-year-old woman visited New Delhi in August. During the third week of her stay, she developed high-grade fever with chills, vomiting, headache, retro-orbital pain, severe myalgia, and arthralgia. On the fifth day of her illness, she visited the hospital. On questioning, she recalled being bitten by mosquitoes. There was no history of hematemesis, melena, or bleeding from any site. On examination, pulse was 100 bpm, blood pressure 95/60 mm Hg, respiratory rate 26 breaths/min, and temperature 98°F. There is no pallor, edema, icterus, lymphadenopathy, or cyanosis. Respiratory system reveals chest clear to auscultation. Cardiovascular system reveals normal S1S2. On examination, abdomen was soft, no guarding or rigidity. CNS reveals no focal neurological deficit. There are no petechiae. Mucous membranes appear dry with no rash.

Investigation reveals hemoglobin 18 g/dL, hematocrit 60%, WBC count 4,000/μL, platelet count 20,000/μL, blood urea 40 mg/dL, serum creatinine 1.4 mg/dL, AST 140 units/L, and ALT 120 units/L. Serologies for infective agents and blood cultures have been sent and reports are awaited.

Initial immediate management should include:

- A. Infusion of intravenous dextran
- B. Platelet transfusion
- C. Infusion of normal saline
- D. All of the above

ANSWERS WITH EXPLANATIONS

1. **Ans. E**
   - A. *Vaccines and prophylaxis received*: The history of vaccinations and malarial chemoprophylaxis should always be reviewed while assessing an illness in a returning traveler. Although adherence to malarial chemoprophylaxis does not rule out malaria, it reduces the risk and increases the likelihood of alternative diagnosis. Also history of vaccinations may help ruling out vaccine preventable disease and narrowing differential diagnosis.
   - B. *Travel itinerary*: The itinerary and activities in which the traveler participated are important in formulating differential diagnosis since potential exposures differ depending on region of travel and behavior. The duration of travel is also important since the risk of a travel-related illness increases with the length of the trip.
   - C. *Timing of illness in relation to travel*: Most travelers will seek medical attention within 1 month of return from their destination; most have short incubation period. Occasionally, however, infections such as schistosomiasis and leishmaniasis or TB can manifest many months or years later.
   - D. *Individual exposures*: Knowledge of the patient's exposure during travel including insect bites, contaminated foods, or water or exposure to freshwater swimming and rafting can help in differential diagnosis. Also type of accommodation, source of drinking water, ingestion of raw meat/sea food/unpasteurized dairy products, history of animal bites and scratches, body fluid exposures such as tattoos, sexual activity, and medical care while overseas such as injection transfusions all help in narrowing the differential diagnosis.
   - E. *All of the above*: Also important is underlying medical illness/immuncompromised status that can affect susceptibility to infections and severity of illness as it may help not only in triaging the patient but also help in prompting public health authorities for prevention of an epidemic or a pandemic.

   Ref:
   1. Mandell, Douglas, and Bennett's Principles and Practice of Infectious Diseases, 9th Edition, Chapters 98, 1351-1353.

2. **Ans. E**
   - A. Most cases of travelers' diarrhea are a result of bacterial infections and are short-lived and self-limited. Travelers may experience prolonged diarrhea if they are immunosuppressed, are infected sequentially with diarrheal pathogens or are infected with protozoan. Individual bacterial

infections as cause of persistent diarrhea have been reported in children infected with enteroaggregative or enteropathogenic *Escherichia coli*. Also not to forget *Clostridium difficile* associated diarrhea which may follow treatment of a bacterial pathogen with a fluoroquinolone or another antibiotic or may follow malarial chemoprophylaxis. Diagnosis of *C. difficile* diarrhea can be done by sending *C. difficile* stool toxin assay, however, now the polymerase chain reaction (PCR)-based assays are preferred. Treatment is with metronidazole, oral vancomycin or fidaxomicin.

- B. *Giardia* is by far the most likely persistent pathogen especially when upper gastrointestinal (GI) symptoms predominate. Untreated symptoms may persist for months even in immunocompetent patient. The diagnosis is often made by stool R/M, Ag detection or immunofluorescence, but PCR-based tests have become the diagnostic tool of choice. However, in view of high prevalence of *Giardia* in persistent travelers' diarrhea, empiric therapy for some is reasonable. Other rare causes include microsporidia, *Dientamoeba fragilis*, and cyclospora.
- C. In a certain number of patients, no specific cause of diarrhea would be found. Patient may experience temporary enteropathy following an acute diarrheal infection with villous atrophy decreased absorptive surface area and disaccharides deficiencies. This can lead to osmotic diarrhea particularly when large amount of lactose, sucrose, and sorbitol are consumed. Occasionally, onset of irritable bowel syndrome (IBS) can be traced to an acute bout of gastroenteritis or travelers' diarrhea. This is termed as postinfectious diarrhea or IBS.
- D. *Tropical sprue and brainerd diarrhea*: These syndromes are suspected to result from infectious diseases, but specific pathogens have not been identified. Tropical sprue is associated with deficiencies of vitamins absorbed in the proximal and distal small bowel and most commonly affect long-term travelers to tropical country. The incidence of tropical sprue has decreased over last two decades. Brainerd diarrhea persists from 7 days to 42 months and does not respond to antimicrobacterial therapy. It is one of the persistent mysteries of ongoing diarrhea.

Ref:
1. Mandell, Douglas, and Bennett's Principles and Practice of Infectious Diseases, 9th Edition, Chapters 279, 3391-3393.

3. Ans. C

- A. *Praziquantel*: The above feature suggests *Fasciola hepatica* infection but *F. hepatica* responds poorly to praziquantel.
- B. *Nitazoxanide*: Nitazoxanide 500 mg twice daily for 7 days. It can be given for treatment of *Fasciola*.
- C. *Triclabendazole*: Drug of choice for treatment of *Fasciola* is triclabendazole which is an imidazole derivative. It is effective against all stages of fascioliasis with a cure rate of >90%. Dose is 10 mg/kg orally for 1 or 2 days. The drug is well tolerated and absorption is improved by postprandial administration.
- D. *Artesunate*: Artesunate, mebendazole, and albendazole have been tried but are not effective. Fascioliasis is a trematode infection caused by *F. hepatica* or *F. gigantica*. *F. hepatica* has a worldwide distribution; *F. gigantica* occurs predominantly in the tropics. *F. hepatica* has a large ovum with an operculum. The large size (120-150 μ × 60-90 μ) distinguishes it from *Diphyllobothrium latum* and *Parogonimus* spp. Cattle and sheep are the most important definitive hosts of *F. hepatica*. Snails are intermediate hosts. Humans are incidental hosts and most often acquire infection by eating watercress grown in sheep-raising areas. Sheep, cattle or human acquire infection by eating vegetation containing metacercariae. The metacercariae exocyst in the duodenum after ingestion and migrate through the intestinal wall, peritoneal cavity and liver parenchyma into the biliary ducts, where they develop into adults in 3-4 months in human. The adult flukes reside in the large biliary ducts. Migrating metacercariae cause liver parenchymal destruction, since tracks undergo necrosis and fibrosis. In addition, adult flukes can partially obstruct the bile ducts, causing thickening, dilatation, and fibrosis of the proximal biliary tree. Acute symptoms usually begin within 6-12 weeks of metacercariae ingestion. Fever, right upper quadrant pain, and hepatomegaly are seen in early phase of migration of metacercariae through the liver. Jaundice, anorexia, nausea, vomiting, myalgia, cough, and urticaria may be seen. Marked peripheral eosinophilia is almost always present. The acute phase can be complicated by subcapsular hematomas or hemobilia of the liver. In most cases, acute symptoms generally resolve after about 6 weeks.

The diagnosis of fascioliasis should be considered in patient with abdominal pain, hepatomegaly accompanied by peripheral eosinophilia. A careful dietary history should be obtained, including a history of watercress ingestion or consumption of raw vegetables washed in potentially contaminated water.

The diagnosis can be established by identifying eggs in stool, duodenal aspirate, or bile specimens, identification of adult worms in endoscopic or surgical specimens or serology and imaging can

also help in diagnosis. Useful radiographic tools for fascioliasis include USG, CT, cholangiography, endoscopic retrograde cholangiopancreatography (ERCP), and MRI. USG, cholangiography, and ERCP may demonstrate mobile flukes in the bile ducts and gallbladder, often associated with stones. Irregular thickening of the common bile duct wall may be observed. CT scanning of the liver shows hypodense nodules or tortuous tracks due to migration of the parasite through the liver similar to that seen in this patient. Eggs of *F. hepatica* are oval, yellow-brown and measure 130–150 μm long by 60–90 μm wide. Examination of multiple specimens may be needed because egg excretion may be intermittent; negative stool examinations do not exclude the diagnosis.
Ref:
1. Mandell, Douglas, and Bennett's Principles and Practice of Infectious Diseases, 9th Edition, Chapters 288, 3459-3460.

4. **Ans. B**
   A. *Infectious mononucleosis*: The incubation period of IM in young adults is 4-6 weeks. A prodrome of fatigue, malaise and myalgias may last for 1-2 weeks before onset of fever, sore throat and lymphadenopathy. Fever is usually, low-grade and seen mostly in the first 2 weeks of illness, but may persist for >1 month, lymphadenopathy and pharyngitis are also seen mostly in the first 2 week. Enlarged nodes are bilateral symmetrical, tender but not fixed. Tonsils may be enlarged. A morbilliform or papular rash on the arm or trunks may be seen in 5% of cases. Hepatosplenomegaly may be present. There is leukocytosis with counts between 10,000 and 20,000/μL, during the second or third weeks of illness and lymphocytosis with >10% atypical lymphocytes, there is low-grade neutropenia and thrombocytopenia and mild elevated aminotransferases and alkaline phosphatase. The above case could very well be a case of infectious mononucleosis but presentation at 2½ weeks with history of travel and exposure so ARS more likely.
   B. *Acute retroviral syndrome*: Many patients with ARS will be asymptomatic. In those who are symptomatic, the diagnosis of ARS may be overlooked due to nonspecificity of symptoms. High-risk historical features in a febrile patient can give clue for diagnosis of ARS. High-risk factors are, IV drug use, high-risk sexual activity/MSM, HIV endemicity in the area from where the patient comes, presence of other sexually transmitted diseases (STDs), and genital ulcers/warts. In the above case travel to Thailand with history of exposure and onset in 2½ weeks almost clinches the diagnosis as ARS.
   C. *Syphilis*: Primary syphilis presents with a chancre at site of inoculation and persists for 4-6 weeks. Secondary syphilis presents 2-6 weeks after exposure also the rash involves palms and soles with mucosa involvement and formation of condyloma. Though fever, sore throat, and myalgias can be associated with it. The time line does not support diagnosis of syphilis.
   D. *Erythema multiforme*: In erythema multiforme (EM) the primary lesions are pink, red macules and edematous papules the centers of which may be vesicluar. Clue to diagnosis of EM is the violet color in the center of the lesion that forms the so-called target lesion. EM has been subdivided into two groups:
      i. EM minor due to herpes simplex virus (HSV).
      ii. EM major due to *Mycoplasma pneumoniae* or drugs.

Erythema multiforme major is usually associated with mucosal involvement such as fever, myalgias, malaise, sore throat, and cough which may preceed the presentation.
Ref:
1. Mandell, Douglas, and Bennett's Principles and Practice of Infectious Diseases, 9th Edition, Chapters 122, 1663-1665.

5. **Ans. C**
   A. *HIV serology*: HIV serology antibody test is usually negative at 2½ weeks. However, fourth-generation test containing p24 Ag along with antibody testing would reveal p24 Ag to be positive. In rare cases HIV-RNA may be present whereas p24 Ag still is undetectable A negative fourth-generation ELISA is as strong argument against acute HIV infection.
   B. *CD4*: It may be low but not diagnostic of ARS.
   C. *HIV, RNA, and PCR viral load* is the test of choice. The test is diagnostic of ARS and will reveal very high plasma viral load usually >100,000 copies/mL and often in millions.
   D. *Western blot*: Western blot could be negative or indeterminate. It will not help in diagnosis at 2½ weeks but later the diagnosis of acute HIV infection can be made by documenting HIV antibody conversion from a negative or indeterminate test to a positive western blot test.
   So, the right choice is C.
Ref:
1. Mandell, Douglas, and Bennett's Principles and Practice of Infectious Diseases, 9th Edition, Chapters 120, 1630-1632.

6. **Ans. B**
Sleeping sickness, or human African trypanosomiasis (HAT), is caused by flagellated protozoan parasites that belong to the *Trypanosoma brucei* complex and are transmitted to humans by tsetse flies. In untreated patients, the trypanosomes first cause a febrile illness that is followed months or years later by progressive neurologic impairment and death. The East African (*rhodesiense*) and the West African (*gambiense*) forms

of sleeping sickness are caused, respectively, by two trypanosome subspecies: *T.b. rhodesiense* and *T.b. gambiense*. These subspecies are epidemiologically and clinically distinct. Trypanotolerant antelope species in Savanna and woodland areas of Central and East Africa are the principal reservoir of *T.b. rhodesiense*. Because risk results from contact with tsetse flies that feed on wild animals, humans acquire *T.b. rhodesiense* infection only incidentally, usually while visiting or working in areas where infected game and vectors are present.

A self-limited inflammatory lesion (*Trypanosomal chancre*) may appear a week or so after the bite of an infected tsetse fly. A systemic febrile illness then evolves as the parasites are disseminated through the lymphatics and bloodstream. Systemic HAT without central nervous system (CNS) involvement is generally referred to as *stage 1 disease*. Hematologic manifestations that accompany stage 1 HAT include moderate leukocytosis, thrombocytopenia, and anemia. High levels of immunoglobulins, consisting primarily of polyclonal immunoglobulin M (IgM), are a constant feature, and heterophile antibodies, antibodies to DNA, and rheumatoid factor are often detected. *Stage 2 disease* involves invasion of the CNS. Abnormalities in cerebrospinal fluid (CSF) include increased pressure, elevated total protein concentration and pleocytosis. In addition, trypanosomes are frequently found in CSF.

Central nervous system invasion (stage 2 disease) is characterized by the insidious development of protean neurologic manifestations. A picture of progressive indifference and daytime somnolence develops (hence the designation "sleeping sickness"), sometimes alternating with restlessness and insomnia at night. A listless gaze accompanies a loss of spontaneity and speech may become halting and indistinct. Extrapyramidal signs may include choreiform movements, tremors, and fasciculations. Ataxia is frequent and the patient may appear to have Parkinson's disease. The most striking difference between the *gambiense* and *rhodesiense* forms of HAT is that the latter illness tends to follow a more acute course. Typically, in tourists with *T.b. rhodesiense* disease, systemic signs of infection, such as fever, malaise, and headache appear before the end of the trip or shortly after the return home. In general, untreated *T.b. rhodesiense* trypanosomiasis leads to death in a matter of weeks to months, often without a clear distinction between the hemolymphatic and CNS stages.

A definitive diagnosis of HAT requires detection of the parasite. Material obtained from chancre or by needle aspiration of lymph nodes. The buffy coat from 10–15 mL of anticoagulated blood can be examined directly under a microscope. It is essential to examine CSF from all patients in whom HAT is suspected. Abnormalities in the CSF that may be associated with stage 2 disease include an increase in the CSF cell count as well as increases in opening pressure and in levels of total protein and IgM. Trypanosomes may be seen in the sediment of centrifuged CSF. Any CSF abnormality in a patient in whom trypanosomes have been found at other sites must be viewed as pathognomonic for CNS involvement and thus must prompt specific treatment for CNS disease. A number of serologic assays, such as the card agglutination test for trypanosomes (CATT) for *T.b. gambiense*, are available to aid in the diagnosis of HAT. Their ease of use makes them valuable for epidemiologic surveys, but their variable sensitivity and specificity mandate that decisions about treatment be based on demonstration of the parasite.

The drugs used for treatment of HAT are suramin, pentamidine, eflornithine, and the organic arsenical melarsoprol. Therapy for HAT must be individualized on the basis of the infecting subspecies, the presence or absence of CNS disease, adverse reactions, and occasionally drug resistance. Suramin is highly effective against stage 1 *rhodesiense* HAT. Pentamidine is the first-line drug for treatment of stage 1 *gambiense* HAT. Eflornithine is highly effective for treatment of both stages of *gambiense* sleeping sickness. The arsenical melarsoprol is the drug of choice for the treatment of *rhodesiense* HAT with CNS involvement. For rhodesiense the drug should be given to adults in three courses of three doses each. The dosage is 2.0–3.6 mg/kg/day given in three divided doses and for 3 days. The later dose is repeated 7 days later. Melarsoprol is highly toxic and should be administered with great care. As noted, all patients receiving melarsoprol should be given prednisolone to reduce the likelihood of drug-induced encephalopathy. Without prednisolone prophylaxis, the incidence of reactive encephalopathy has been as high as 18% in some series. Clinical manifestations of reactive encephalopathy include high fever, headache, tremor, impaired speech, seizures, and even coma and death. Treatment with melarsoprol should be discontinued at the first sign of encephalopathy but may be restarted cautiously at lower doses a few days after signs have resolved, *so the right answers is B.*

Ref:
1. Mandell, Douglas, and Bennett's Principles and Practice of Infectious Diseases, 9th Edition, Chapters 277, 3351-3353.

7. **Ans. A**

A. *Gnathostomiasis*: Human gnathostomiasis occurs in many countries and is notably endemic in Southeast Asia and parts of China and Japan. Raw fish dishes, such as *som-fak* in Thailand and *sashimi* in Japan, account for many cases of human gnathostomiasis. Humans typically acquire the infection by eating raw or undercooked fish or poultry. There is local practice of applying frog or snake flesh as a poultice. Clinical symptoms are due to the aberrant migration of a single larva into cutaneous, visceral, neural, or ocular tissues. After invasion, larval migration may cause local inflammation, with pain, cough, or hematuria accompanied by fever and eosinophilia. Painful, itchy, migratory swellings may develop in the skin. Cutaneous swellings usually last ~1 week but often recur intermittently over many years. Cutaneous migratory swellings with marked peripheral eosinophilia, supported by an appropriate geographic and dietary history, generally constitute an adequate basis for a clinical diagnosis of gnathostomiasis. Gnathostomiasis can be prevented by adequate cooking of fish and poultry in endemic areas.

Invasion of the CNS results in eosinophilic meningitis with myeloencephalitis. Larval invasion of the eye can provoke a sight-threatening inflammatory response. Infection of human tissues with larvae of *Gnathostoma spinigerum* can cause migratory cutaneous swellings or invasive masses of the visceral organs. Surgical removal of the parasite from subcutaneous or ocular tissue, though rarely feasible, is both diagnostic and therapeutic. Albendazole or ivermectin may be helpful. At present, cerebrospinal involvement is managed with supportive measures and generally with a course of glucocorticoids.

- B. *Loiasis*: It is caused by *Loa loa* (the African eye worm). Among the indigenous population, infection may be recognized only after subconjunctival migration of an adult worm or may be manifested by episodic *Calabar swellings*, evanescent localized areas of angioedema and erythema, developing on the extremities and less frequently at other sites. In patients who are not residents of endemic areas, allergic symptoms predominate, episodes of Calabar swelling tend to be more frequent and debilitating, microfilaremia is less common, and eosinophilia and increased levels of antifilarial antibodies are characteristic.
- C. *Urticaria/angioedema*: Angioedema and urticaria may appear together or separately as evanescent self-limited eruptions and localized nonpitting edema of skin or mucosa. Urticarial eruptions are pruritic, last from 12 to 36 hours, and involve any part of body from head to foot but are mostly seen in face or extremities. Angioedema, often seen around the lips or in periorbital area, may be life threatening if causes laryngeal involvement, while gastrointestinal involvement may lead to abdominal pain with anemia and vomiting. There is absence of fever, leukocytosis, and elevated erythrocyte sedimentation rate (ESR). The rapid onset, self-limited nature and asymmetric distribution of urticarial angioedema eruption help in diagnosis.

Ref:
1. *Mandell, Douglas, and Bennett's Principles and Practice of Infectious Diseases*, 9th Edition, Chapters 290, 3476-3477.

8. **Ans. C**
    A. *Hypereosinophilic syndrome*: Eosinophilia is classified as secondary (nonneoplastic proliferation of eosinophils) and primary proliferation of eosinophils that is either neoplastic or otherwise unexplained, i.e., (idiopathic), HES a subcategory of idiopathic eosinophilia with persistent increase of the AEC to $> 1.5 \times 10^9$/L and presence of eosinophil-mediated organ damage including cardiomyopathy, gastroenteritis, cutaneous lesion, sinusitis, pneumonitis, neuritis, and vasculitis. In addition, some patients manifest hepatosplenomegaly and either cytopenia or cytosis. Bone marrow histological and cytogenetic/molecular studies should be examined before a working diagnosis of HES is made. Glucocorticoids are the mainstay of treatment. Secondary eosinophilia is by far the most frequent cause of eosinophilia and is often associated with infections, especially those related to tissue invasive helminths, an infective cause should be first ruled out before considering the diagnosis of HES.
    B. *Gnathostomiasis*: Infection of human tissues with larvae of *G. spinigerum* can cause eosinophilic meningoencephalitis, migratory cutaneous swellings, or invasive masses of the eye and visceral organs.
    C. Definitive diagnosis of loiasis requires the detection of microfilariae in the peripheral blood or the isolation of the adult worm from the eye or by PCR-based assays for the detection of *L. loa* DNA in blood. The diagnosis most often is based on a characteristic history and clinical presentation, blood eosinophilia, and elevated levels of antifilarial antibodies, particularly in travelers to an endemic region, who are usually amicrofilaremic. Other clinical findings in travelers include hypergammaglobulinemia, elevated levels of serum IgE, and elevated leukocyte and eosinophil counts.

    Diethylcarbamazine (DEC) (8-10 mg/kg/day administered orally for 21 days) is effective against both the adult and the microfilarial forms of *L. loa*. Heavy infections can be treated initially with apheresis to remove the microfilariae and with glucocorticoids (40-60 mg of prednisone per day) followed by doses of DEC (0.5 mg/kg/day). If antifilarial treatment has no adverse effects, the prednisolone dose can be rapidly tapered and the dose of DEC gradually increased to 8-10 mg/kg/day. Albendazole or ivermectin is effective in reducing microfilarial loads, although neither is approved for this purpose by the US Food and Drug Administration. Moreover, ivermectin is contraindicated in patients with >8,000 microfilariae/mL. DEC (300 mg weekly) is an effective prophylactic regimen for loiasis.

D. *Cutaneous larva migrans*: Creeping eruptions is an infectious syndrome caused by the larva of various nematode parasites of the hookworm family Ancylostomatidae. The most common species causing the disease is *Ancylostoma braziliense*. These parasites live in the intestines of dogs and cats and wild animal and should not be confused with other members of hookworm family where humans are the definitive host. Hookworm eggs are shed in the infected dog feces in the soil or sand where they then develop in 1-2 weeks into the infectious larval form. The filiform larvae can burrow through intact skin that came in contact with contaminated soil. Treatment is with albendazole.

Ref:
1. Mandell, Douglas, and Bennett's Principles and Practice of Infectious Diseases, 9th Edition, Chapters 290, 3475-3477.

9. **Ans. D**

A. *Injection ceftriaxone* 2 g IV twice a day would be initiated if meningococcal meningitis was considered as a diagnosis. However, the TLC being normal. PT/APTT normal, despite patient being in shock, though not absolute criteria for exclusion would make this diagnosis unlikely.

B. *Injection benzathine penicillin* would be indicated if secondary syphilis is the diagnosis. Secondary syphilis usually appears 6-8 weeks after exposure, does not cause petechial or hemorrhagic rash, and does not cause severe thrombocytopenia, so unlikely.

C. *Meropenem and teicoplanin* would be considered a choice if severe sepsis secondary to gram-negative or gram-positive bacteria was the diagnosis. However, TLC and PT/APTT being normal in a patient with a characteristic rash onset and progression would not make these the first choice for the management of such a case. An empirical broad spectrum antibiotic cover can be initiated at the onset before one comes to a definitive diagnosis, however, one does not need a penam and a teicoplanin for the same.

D. *Doxycycline* is the drug of choice as the case is that of Rocky Mountain spotted fever (RMSF). It is administered orally (or in presence of coma or vomiting, intravenously) at 200 mg/day in two divided doses.

Rocky Mountain spotted fever occurs in 47 states in the USA with highest prevalence in south central and southeastern states as well as in Canada, Mexico, and Central and South America. The infection is transmitted by *Dermacentor variabilis*, the American dog tick, in the eastern two-thirds of the United States and California, by *Dermacentor andersoni*, the Rocky Mountain wood tick in the western United States, by *Rhipicephalus sanguineus* in Mexico, Arizona and probably Brazil and by *Amblyomma cajennense* and *Amblyomma aureolatum* in Central and/or South America. Maintained principally by transovarian transmission from one generation of ticks to next, *Rickettsia rickettsii* can be acquired by uninfected ticks through the ingestion of a blood meal from rickettemic small mammals. Humans become infected during tick season (in northern hemisphere, from May to September), although some cases occur in winter.

The most important epidemiological factor is a history of exposure to a potentially tick-infested environment within 14 days preceding disease onset during a season of possible tick activity. However, only 60% of patients actually recall being bitten by a tick during the incubation period.

The differential diagnosis for early clinical manifestations of RMSF includes influenza, enteroviral infection, infectious mononucleosis, viral hepatitis, leptospirosis, typhoid fever, and gram-negative or gram-positive bacterial sepsis.

Thus, if a viral infection is suspected during RMSF season in an endemic area, it should always be kept in mind that RMSF can mimic viral infection early in the course, if the illness worsens over the next couple of days after initial presentation, the patient should return for reevaluation. The most common serologic test for confirmation of the diagnosis is the indirect immunofluorescence assay. Not until 7-10 days after onset, a diagnostic titer of ≥64 is usually detectable. The sensitivity and specificity of the indirect immunofluorescence IgG assay are 89-100% and 99-100%.

Ref:
1. Mandell, Douglas, and Bennett's Principles and Practice of Infectious Diseases, 9th Edition, Chapters 286, 2352-2355.

10. **Ans. B**

Myiasis refers to infestation by diverse kinds of fly larvae that invade living or necrotic tissue or body cavities and produce different clinical syndromes, depending on the species of fly. In countries where it is not endemic, myiasis is an important condition, where it can represent the fourth most common travel-associated skin disease. Physicians unacquainted with this condition can simply diagnose cases where maggots are visible. However, it is difficult to diagnose furuncular, migratory, cavitary cases and pseudomyiasis, especially for those doctors unfamiliar with myiasis and its possibilities. For the appropriate diagnosis, various aspects should be considered such as the region where the patient visited, climate conditions, and the species habitat of the region visited.

A timely accurate and diagnosis is vital not only to relieve the patient's symptoms but also to forestall the establishment of myiasis-causing flies in regions where they are not endemic, a phenomenon that is already happening with the movement of farm animals. In many cases, the patient receives unnecessary oral antibiotics, increasing the development of bacterial resistance. The African tumbu fly (*Cordylobia anthropophaga*) deposits its eggs on sand or drying laundry contaminated with urine or sweat. Larvae hatch on contact with the body, penetrate the skin, and produce boils from which they emerge 9–10 days later. The penetration of *C. anthropophaga* into the skin is usually asymptomatic, although the area of penetration can be slightly itchy for up to 2 days after the infestation. In a few days, a reddish papule develops and takes on a boil-like appearance when fully developed. An intense inflammatory reaction in the surrounding tissue of the lesions develops over a period of 6 days. Some lesions may develop a central pustule, similar to that of pyoderma. The mature third-instar maggot leaves the host in about 12 days. Furuncular myiasis is suggested by uncomfortable lesions with the central breathing pore that emits bubbles when submerged in water, a sensation of movement under the patient's skin may lead to severe emotional distress.

Agitation and insomnia can also occur in cases of tumbu fly infestations. Furuncle-like lesions are commonly seen in some cases. These changes can be very intense, mimicking soft-tissue bacterial infections such as cellulitis. Numerous lesions can lead to formation of large plaques of coalescing furuncles. A clear fluid, occasionally stained with blood or larval feces, may ooze from the boil. The posterior spiracles will be seen sometimes in the central pore after development of the third instar. The *C. anthropophaga* discharge may become purulent, crusted and odoriferous or may be serosanguineous, other findings such as regional lymphadenopathy or malaise may be seen with multiple lesions. People are most commonly parasitized in the rainy season, when the natural sylvan hosts approach human settlement. Adult flies tend to oviposit on soiled clothing, which explains the distribution of the lesions on covered sites such as trunk, buttocks, and thighs and also the elevated number of lesions.

Ref:
1. Mandell, Douglas, and Bennett's Principles and Practice of Infectious Diseases, 9th Edition, Chapters 294, 3492-3493.
2. https://www.cdc.gov/parasites/myiasis/.

11. **Ans. D**
    A. *Clostridium perfringens, C. histolyticum, C. septicum, C. sordellii,* and *C. novyi* cause necrotizing clostridial infections resulting in aggressive necrotizing infections of skin and soft tissues which are rapidly progressive and are characterized by marked tissue destruction, gas in tissues, shock, severe pain, crepitus, brawny skin induration and bullae with marked tachycardia.
    B. *Pseudomonas* causes pyoderma gangrenosum in neutropenic patient and can also cause folliculitis and papular or vesicular lesions. Infections have been linked to exposure to whirlpools, spas, and swimming pools where its growth can be controlled by proper chlorination. Patient in question is neither neutropenic nor has history of exposure to whirlpools or pools or spa, so it is unlikely to be causative agent.
    C. Infection by *staphylococci or streptococci and group A streptococci* can cause cellulitis. These infections are characterized by pus-containing blisters. It can spread or involve contiguous musculoskeletal planes causing necrotizing fasciitis. There is leukocytosis with raised ESR. Blood culture is usually positive. Metastatic infections can be seen. Patient may develop shock but course is more prolonged over days to weeks. The source of infection is either the skin with organisms introduced in tissue through trauma or bowel flora, or organisms released in abdominal surgery or an enteric source like diverticular abscess. The onset is usually acute and is marked by severe pain at site of involvement, malaise, fever, chills, and a toxic appearance. Skin changes become more evident with worsening of symptoms. The presentation is usually subacute but a fulminant form has been described in association with severe systemic toxicity, bacteremia, and high mortality rate. Treatment is by early surgical debridement and high dose of penicillin.
    D. *Vibrio vulnificus* is a gram-negative bacterium that can cause serious and fatal infection. It can cause three distinct syndromes:
        i. An overwhelming primary septicemia caused by consumption of contaminated sea food especially raw oysters with 25% mortality especially in patient with chronic liver disease (CLD) or hemochromatosis

ii. Gastrointestinal limited infection
iii. Wound infections leading to necrotizing fasciitis when open wound is exposed to sea waters.

Vibrio vulnificus infection should be considered in patients with sepsis and severe skin lesions. These patients should be asked about raw oyster consumption, sea water exposure and history of liver disease and intense pain around the lesion followed by cellulitis which spread rapidly and is accompanied by vesicular bullous or necrotic lesions. *V. vulnificus* can be cultured from blood and cutaneous lesion. It can infect either fresh old wound that comes in contact with sea water and becomes symptomatic after a period of 4 hours to 4 days. Treatment should be initiated immediately because antibiotics improve survival. Aggressive attention should be given to the wound site as fasciotomy or amputation of the infected limbs is sometimes needed to save the life of the patient. Antibiotic of choice is doxycycline 100 mg twice a day for 7–14 days, and a third-generation cephalosporin such as ceftazidime 1–2 g given 8 hourly is recommended.

Ref:
1. *Mandell, Douglas, and Bennett's Principles and Practice of Infectious Diseases, 9th Edition, Chapter 215.*

12. Ans. B

A. *Gram-negative bipolar staining bacilli* mean *Yersinia pestis*, which causes plague. Fever with chills and simultaneous onset of intensely painful bubo are clinical features seen in bubonic plague. Eschar and travel history is not seen in plague.

B. *Gram-negative bacilli* suggest rickettsia. Features of African tick-bite fever caused by *Rickettsia africae* are headache, fever, myalgia, and eschar with regional lymphadenitis draining the eschar which is characteristic. It is prevalent in sub-Saharan Africa, where vectors *Amblyomma* spp. are present.

C. *Gram-positive bacilli* mean *Bacillus anthracis*. The cutaneous lesion of *B. anthracis* starts as pruritic papule and becomes vesicular and involves face, arms, neck, and back. There is painless central necrotic lesion with congestion and nonpitting edema in the area with several satellite lesions.

D. *Gram-positive cocci*: There was no response to antibiotics and clinical presentation does not suggest staphylococcal and streptococcal infection, so not, a gram-positive cocci.

Ref:
1. *Mandell, Douglas, and Bennett's Principles and Practice of Infectious Diseases, 9th Edition, Chapters 229A, 2779–2780.*

13. Ans. D

A. Risk factors for *staphylococcal pneumonia* such as diabetes mellitus (DM), head injury, coma > 24 hours, renal failure, or IV drug abuse are absent, so staphylococcal pneumonia is less likely.

B. Although new risk factors are emerging, the patient did not have the classical risk factors for *Aspergillus*, so fungus is not the likely cause. Also it is very rare to grow *Aspergillus* from blood.

C. *Bacillus anthracis* may be considered. Inhalational *B. anthracis* results from inhalation of *B. anthracis* spores. It enters into alveoli aerosolized through either industrial processing, working with the animal products such as wool, hair or hides that are contaminated with anthrax spores or intentional release such as bioterrorism event. Inhalational anthrax presents with nonspecific symptoms such as fever, myalgia, and malaise that mimic those of influenza. Later the patient develops hypoxemia. On chest X-ray (CXR), mediastinal widening and pleural effusion are the most accurate predictors of inhalational anthrax. Other CXR findings include hilar abnormalities, pulmonary infiltrates or consolidation and pleural effusion. Hemorrhagic meningitis and submucosal gastrointestinal lesions can occur if hematogenous spread occurs. Blood culture or pleural fluid culture will reveal the organism. It is unlikely to be the causative agent.

D. *Burkholderia pseudomallei* (a gram-negative bacilli) infection presents with cavitary pneumonia in persons with risk factors such as alcoholism, DM, and exposure to paddy fields in early monsoon season. Infection is acquired predominantly through inhalation of contaminated aerosols, dusts or droplets. In view of the history melioidosis caused by *Burkholderia* is the right answer.

Ref:
1. *Mandell, Douglas, and Bennett's Principles and Practice of Infectious Diseases, 9th Edition, Chapters 221, 2709–2715.*

14. Ans. B

The most common form of infection with *Neisseria meningitidis* is asymptomatic carriage of the organism in the nasopharynx. Upper respiratory tract symptoms are common prior to the presentation with invasive disease. After acquiring the organism, susceptible individuals develop disease manifestations in 1–10 days, usually within 4 days, although colonization for 11 weeks has been documented.

Most common clinical syndromes are meningitis and meningococcal septicemia. In fulminant cases, death may occur within first hour of the symptoms. A non-blanching rash (petechial or purpuric) develops in more than 80% of cases of meningoccal disease. However, the rash is often absent early in the illness. Usually initially blanching in nature and indistinguishable from more common viral rashes, the rash of meningococcal infection becomes petechial or frankly purpuric over the hours after onset. In the most severe cases, large purpuric lesions develop (Purpura fulminans). Some patients including those with overwhelming sepsis may not have rash. While 30-50% of patients present with meningitis syndrome alone, up to 40% of meningitis patients also present with some features of septicemia. Most deaths from meningococcal meningitis alone (that is without septicemia) are associated with raised intracranial pressure presenting as a reduced level of consciousness, relative bradycardia and hypertension, focal neurological signs, abnormal posturing and signs of brainstem involvement such as unequal dilated or poorly reactive pupils, abnormal eye movements, and impaired corneal responses.

Ref:
1. Mandell, Douglas, and Bennett's Principles and Practice of Infectious Diseases, 9th Edition, Chapters 211, 2593-2595.

15. **Ans. A**
    A. Histoplasmosis can cause asymptomatic to life-threatening disease signs and symptoms of acute histoplasmosis develops 1-4 weeks after exposure with flu-like illness with fever, chills, headache, myalgia, cough, chest pain. On evaluation chest radiography usually shows sign and symptom of pneumonitis with prominent hilar and mediastinal lymphadenopathy. Affected hilar or mediastinal lymphadenopathy can undergo necrosis and coalesce to form large mediastinal mass. Histoplasmosis is endemic in Mississippi valley of North America, Asia, Africa, and parts of Central and South America. Soil enriched with bird and bat droppings promote growth of *Histoplasma*, disruption of soil leads to aerosolization and exposure to human beings. Diagnosis depends on *Histoplasma* antigen on BAL fluid, serum, urine, and fungal culture of BAL fluid. Histopathology on transbronchial biopsy (TBB) may show structure resembling *Histoplasma*. The treatment of choice is *amphotericin B* for 15 days followed by oral itraconazole for 12 weeks.
    B. *Antituberculosis treatment* would be indicated if tuberculosis is the diagnosis, this could be a possible diagnosis but histoplasmosis more likely in view of historical details.
    C. *Steroids* would be indicated if sarcoidosis is the diagnosis, unlikely in view of historical details.
    D. *Antibiotics* not indicated in view of historical details.

Ref:
1. Mandell, Douglas, and Bennett's Principles and Practice of Infectious Diseases, 9th Edition, Chapters 236, 3116, 3174-3175.

16. **Ans. A**
    A. Clues suggesting a diagnosis of coccidioidomycosis include eosinophilia, hilar adenopathy marked with fatigue, failure to response after a course of antibiotics, and visit to Arizona. Coccidioidomycosis is confined to the western hemisphere between latitude of 40° North and 40° South and is endemic in south central Arizona and San Joaquin Valley of California (so the name "valley fever"). Serology plays an important role in diagnosis. On tube precipitation, IgM and IgG are seen in serum. An antigen test also been developed but it cross reacts with histoplasmosis and blastomycosis. PCR-based assay also are available. *Coccoides* can be grown from sputum and often respiratory fluids and tissue. Treatment in most cases are not needed and antifungal therapy is indicated in patients who are immunocompromised or have prolonged symptom persisting >2 months, night sweats >3 weeks, weight loss of >10%, excessive pulmonary involvement seen in chest radiography or a serum complement fixation (CF) antibody level titer of >1:16. Treatment of choice is amphotericin B/azole group of antifungal drugs.
    B. *Histoplasmosis* is endemic in Mississippi Valley of North America, Asia, Africa, and parts of Central and South America. Soil enriched with bird and bat droppings promote growth of *Histoplasma*, disruption of soil leads to aerosolization and exposure to human beings. Diagnosis depends on *Histoplasma* antigen on BAL fluid, serum, urine, and fungal culture of BAL fluid. Histopathology on TBB may show structure resembling *Histoplasma*. Treatment of choice is amphotericin B for 15 days followed by oral itraconazole for 12 weeks, unlikely in view of the historical details.
    C. *Bacterial pneumonia* unlikely as patient did not respond to course of antibiotics.
    D. *Tuberculosis* could be but unlikely to be the first choice in view of the historical details.

Ref:
1. Mandell, Douglas, and Bennett's Principles and Practice of Infectious Diseases, 9th Edition, Chapters 265, 3193-3198.

17. **Ans. C**
    A. *Cystitis*: It usually presents with fever and dysuria may present without fever with discomfort on urination and increased frequency but is unlikely to cause a urethral discharge so cystitis is not the right answer.
    B. *Genital herpes*: It presents with a sudden outbreak of painful vesicular rash over the genitalia. Urethral discharge may or may not be there. There may also be a prodrome of fever and malaise. However, there is absence of the classical rash in the above patient, so genital herpes is not the right choice.
    C. *Gonorrhea*: It is caused by *Neisseria gonorrhoeae*. In men it presents with dysuria and profuse purulent urethral discharge. Women may present with vaginal discharge, pelvic pain, intermenstrual bleeding,

and dysuria. Infections may be asymptomatic in both men and women. Local complications such as salpingitis, endometritis, and tubo-ovarian abscess in females, and periurethritis and epididymitis in males can develop if not treated. A rapid diagnosis can be made by detection of gram-negative intracellular monococci and diplococci on Gram stain of urethral discharge or cervical smears (poor sensitivity) single endocervical culture is 80–90% sensitive. Increasingly, nucleic acid amplification tests (NAATs) are being substituted for culture for direct detection of *N. gonorrhoeae* in urogenital specimens. Treatment is by injection ceftriaxone 250 mg IM single dose or cefixime 400 mg single dose.
   D. *Chlamydia*: It is the most common sexually transmitted disease in the United Kingdom. It is usually asymptomatic in both men and women. Symptomatic men may present with dysuria and urethral discharge. This is similar to the features seen in our patient but the presence of large amount of purulent penile discharge makes gonorrhea more likely. However, as coinfection of both gonorrhea and chlamydia occur frequently, initial treatment must include agents effective against chlamydia such as azithromycin or doxycycline.
   Ref:
   1. Mandell, Douglas, and Bennett's Principles and Practice of Infectious Diseases, 9th Edition, Chapters 212, 2619-2624.

18. **Ans. B**
   A. *Buruli ulcer*: It is caused by *Mycobacterium ulcerans*, an environmental bacterium, and mode of transmission is unknown. It is a chronic debilitating disease that affects mainly the skin and sometimes the bone and can lead to permanent disfigurement and long-term disability. Buruli ulcer has been seen in countries with tropical, subtropical, and temperate climates such as Africa, South America, Western pacific region, and Australia. Buruli ulcer often starts as a painless nodule or plaque-like lesion or arms legs and face. A toxin, mycolactone, which is produced by the organism inhibits the immune response and causes tissue damage. The nodule or plaque will ulcerate within 4 weeks with the classical undermined border. Diagnosis clinically depends on the patient's age, geographical area, location of lesion, and extent of pain. It is a diagnosis of exclusion. Direct microscopy cultures and PCR-based tests can help in diagnosis. Also detection of mycolactone by fluorescent chromatography may help in rapid diagnosis. Treatment is combination of rifampicin and clarithromycin.
   B. *Leishmaniasis*: It is the most likely diagnosis considering the history. Leishmaniasis is caused by a protozoa, *Leishmania*, and is transmitted by bites of sandflies. It is seen in Africa, Europe, Asia, and Central and South America. In cutaneous leishmaniasis there is development of an itching papule at the site of bite of the sandfly which then develops into any erythematous ulcer with raised edges. The protozoa may spread from this lesion to the reticuloendothelial system via the lymphatics and progress to visceral leishmaniasis, or mucocutaneous leishmaniasis which occurs when primary cutaneous lesion spread to the mucosa of the nose, palate, pharynx or larynx.
   C. *Herpes zoster*: It produces a vesicular rash which has a dermatomal distribution with significant pain and would show settling trend over 4 weeks.
   D. *Myiasis*: It refers to infestation by diverse kinds of fly larvae that invade living or necrotic tissue or body cavities and produce different clinical syndromes, depending on the species. Furuncular myiasis is suggested by uncomfortable lesions with the central breathing pore that emits bubbles when submerged in water, a sensation of movement under the patients skin which may lead to severe emotional distress. Topically, symptoms develop within the first 2 days of infestation and can range from a mild or a "prickly heat" sensation to severe pain. A clear fluid occasionally stained with blood or larval faces, may ooze from the boil. People are most commonly parasitized during the rainy season, when the natural sylvan hosts approach human villages. Adult flies tend to oviposit on soiled clothing, which explains the distribution of the lesions on covered sites such as trunk, buttocks, and thighs and also the elevated number of lesions. Historical details do not match, so it is unlikely.
   Ref:
   1. Mandell, Douglas, and Bennett's Principles and Practice of Infectious Diseases, 9th Edition, Chapters 275, 3323-3325.

19. **Ans. C**
   A. *Malaria serology*: Malaria should be considered in travelers with pyrexia and thick and thin blood films sent. However, the maculopapular rash is not seen in malaria, thus making this answer incorrect.
   B. *Dengue serology*: It should be considered in patient with fever with rash returning from a tropical country. However, dengue fever in usually not seen in the month of February and is seen after rains mainly in August and September.
   C. *Blood culture*: The case in this question describes the presentation of a patient with typhoid, so blood culture is the right answer. This is caused by infection with *Salmonella typhi*. The features in the question that should alert the diagnosis of typhoid are the patchy maculopapular rash (known as rose spots), which occur in approximately 40%

of cases, and the low white cell count, due to a leukopenia. Complications of disease include meningitis, pneumonia, osteomyelitis, and intestinal perforation. Diagnosis of typhoid is confirmed on culture of blood, bone marrow, and urine or stool. The rash on the trunk, splenomegaly, and low cell count are all features, which point toward the diagnosis of enteric fever, so blood culture is the right choice.

D. *X-ray PA view:* It is warranted as an initial workup of fever. In the above patient viral fever is a differential diagnosis, influenza cannot be ruled out but first choice of investigation would remain blood culture.

Ref:
1. *Mandell, Douglas, and Bennett's Principles and Practice of Infectious Diseases, 9th Edition, Chapters 223, 2732-2733.*

20. Ans. D

It is a case of strongyloidiasis. Strongyloides stercoralis can replicate in humans producing infective larvae leading to autoinfection and can persist for decade in immunocompromised hosts. It can disseminate widely and can be fatal. Humans acquire infection when infective filiform larvae in fecally contaminated soil penetrate the skin or mucous membrane. The larvae reach the alveolar spaces in lung via the blood stream and then ascend the bronchial tree. They are swallowed and reach the small intestine. The larvae now mature in the intestinal wall and adult female reproduces by pathogenesis, eggs hatch into rhabditiform larvae which pass in feces or mature to produce filiform larvae. These larvae penetrate the colonic wall to enter the circulation and establish ongoing internal reinfection. Patient may be asymptomatic or have mild cutaneous and abdominal symptoms. Recurrent urticaria involves the buttocks and the wrists. Serpiginous eruptions larvae currens may be seen. Nausea, diarrhea bleeding, weight loss, bowel obstruction may develop and eosinophilia is common. Immunosuppression especially with glucocorticoids can lead to disseminated strongyloidiasis which can be fatal. Larvae may invade brain, peritoneum, liver, and kidneys. Gram-negative sepsis may develop due to passage of enteric flora through disrupted mucosal barrier. Diagnosis is by finding larvae in stool or in duodenal aspirate and biopsy or in BAL and lung biopsy. Ivermectin is preferred over albendazole.

Ref:
1. *Mandell, Douglas, and Bennett's Principles and Practice of Infectious Diseases, 9th Edition, Chapter 286, 3440-3441.*

21. Ans. B

Legionnaires' disease may often present with the following features:
- Diarrhea
- High fever (>40°C; >104°F)
- Numerous neutrophils but no organisms revealed by Gram's staining of respiratory secretions
- Hyponatremia (serum sodium level < 131 mEq/dL)
- Failure to respond to β-lactam drugs (penicillins or cephalosporins) and aminoglycoside antibiotics
- Occurrence of illness in an environment in which the potable water supply is known to be contaminated with *Legionella*
- Onset of symptoms within 10 days after discharge from the hospital (hospital-acquired legionellosis manifesting after discharge).

Legionella can survive under a wide range of environmental conditions. The organisms can live for years in refrigerated water samples. Once the organisms enter human constructed aquatic reservoirs (such as drinking-water systems), they can multiply. *Legionella* is transmitted through aerosolization, aspiration, and direct instillation into the lungs. Clustering of cases may be seen in institutions with contaminated water supply.

The differential diagnosis of atypical pneumonia should include *Legionella, Chlamydia pneumoniae, Chlamydia psittaci, Mycoplasma pneumoniae, C. burnetii,* and some viruses. Atypical pneumonias may present with nonproductive cough or infrequently grossly purulent sputum. The clinical manifestations of Legionnaires' disease are usually more severe than those of most atypical pneumonias. Patients with community-acquired Legionnaires' disease are more likely than patients with pneumonia of other etiologies to require admission to an intensive care unit on presentation. The incubation period for Legionnaires' disease is usually 2–10 days. Fever is almost always present. The presenting features may range from a mild cough and a slight fever to altered sensorium with widespread pulmonary infiltrates and multiorgan dysfunction. Sometimes the sputum is streaked with blood. Chest pain and shortness of breath may also occur. Gastrointestinal symptoms are often present with abdominal pain, nausea, and vomiting affecting 10–20% of patients. Diarrhea, which is frequently watery, is reported in 25–50% of cases. Neurologic abnormalities such as confusion and changes in mental status may occur. Patients may also present with headache, lethargy, and encephalopathy. Almost all patients with Legionnaires' disease have abnormal chest radiographs showing pulmonary infiltrates at the time of clinical presentation. Radiologic findings are nonspecific. Pleural effusion is seen in 28–63% of patients on hospital admission.

Pneumonia is treated with levofloxacin or azithromycin.

The typical symptoms of *Legionella* along with the clustering of cases in an area with a common water supply make *Legionella* the most likely cause of infection.

Ref:
1. Mandell, Douglas, and Bennett's Principles and Practice of Infectious Diseases, 9th Edition, Chapters 298, 3535-3536.

22. **Ans. D**

Relapsing fever is an infection caused by spirochetes of the genus *Borrelia*. It is an arthropod-borne infection that occurs in two forms. They are tick-borne relapsing fever (TBRF) and louse-borne relapsing fever (LBRF). LBRF is caused by *Borrelia recurrentis*. It is mostly seen in the developing world or among refugees from developing countries. It is spread from person-to-person by the body louse. It can result in epidemics. Clinical manifestations are recurrent episodes of fever, during phases of spirochetemia. Relapsing fever presents with the abrupt onset of fever interspersed with an intervening afebrile period, and then recurrent fevers. The temperature is usually above 39°C, and may be as high as 43°C. The incubation period is between 3 and 12 days. Other symptoms include headache, neck stiffness, arthralgia, myalgia, nausea, and abdominal pain. On physical examination, the patient may be delirious or apathetic. There may be body lice in the patient's clothes or signs of insect bites. Splenomegaly or spleen tenderness is common in both forms of relapsing fever. The majority of patients with LBRF and approximately 10% of patients with TBRF have hepatomegaly.

Laboratory studies may be nonspecific. Mild-to-moderate normocytic anemia is common. Leukocyte counts are usually in the normal range or only slightly elevated, and leukopenia can occur during the crisis. Platelet counts can fall below 50,000/μL. Laboratory evidence of hepatitis can be found with elevated serum concentrations of unconjugated bilirubin and aminotransferases; the prothrombin and partial thromboplastin times may be moderately prolonged. A characteristic fever pattern and a history of recent exposure, within the previous 2 weeks, to body lice, soft-bodied ticks, or *Ixodes* species, hard-bodied ticks, in geographic areas where the disease is known to be prevalent should raise suspicion for relapsing fever. Manual differential counts of white blood cells by Wright or Giemsa stain usually reveal spirochetes in thin blood smears if their concentration is ≥105/mL and several oil-immersion fields are examined. Lower concentrations of spirochetes may be revealed by a thick blood smear that is either directly stained with acridine orange and then examined by fluorescence microscopy or treated with 0.5% acetic acid before Giemsa or Wright staining. Penicillins and tetracyclines are the antibiotics of choice for relapsing fever. Erythromycin is a second choice. There is no evidence of acquired resistance to these antibiotics. *Borrelia* species are also susceptible to most cephalosporins and chloramphenicol. *Borreliae* are relatively resistant to rifampicin, sulfonamides, fluoroquinolones, and aminoglycosides. Spirochetes are no longer detectable in the blood within a few hours after the first dose of an effective antibiotic.

The Jarisch–Herxheimer reaction during treatment of relapsing fever can be severe or even fatal. Rigors, fever, and hypotension occur within 2–3 hours of initiation of antibiotic treatment. The incidence of this reaction is approximately 80% in LBRF and approximately 50% in TBRF. Both penicillin and tetracycline can elicit the Jarisch–Herxheimer reaction. Coinfections with malaria, typhus, typhoid, or Lyme disease may complicate relapsing fever.

Ref:
1. Mandell, Douglas, and Bennett's Principles and Practice of Infectious Diseases, 9th Edition, Chapters 240, 2906-2909.

23. **Ans. B**

Malaria is most frequently acquired by travel to Africa and parts of Asia. Chloroquine-resistant *Plasmodium falciparum* malaria is endemic in sub-Saharan Africa. A high degree of parasitemia (5–10%) with parasitized erythrocytes revealing ring forms is seen. Schizonts are seldom seen in *P. falciparum* infection. *P. falciparum* infection is a potentially severe and life-threatening infection. Pregnant women are at increased risk of severe disease and mortality. Pregnant women with chloroquine-resistant *P. falciparum* should receive quinine sulfate plus clindamycin.

Detection of parasites on Giemsa-stained blood smears by light microscopy is the standard tool for diagnosis of malaria. In expert hands, the sensitivity of microscopy is high, with detection of malaria parasites at densities as low as 20 parasites/μL of blood. However, it is time and labor intensive and requires experience and training. The diagnosis may be missed in cases with lower densities of parasites. The species of *Plasmodium* as well as quantification of parasitemia can be achieved with microscopy. It also helps diagnose other infectious diseases such as filariasis, trypanosomiasis, and babesiosis. Rapid, simple, sensitive, and specific antibody-based diagnostic stick or card tests can detect *Plasmodium falciparum* specific, histidine-rich protein 2 (PfHRP2), lactate dehydrogenase, or aldolase antigens in finger-prick blood samples. These are commonly used. Some of these rapid diagnostic tests carry a second antibody to help distinguish falciparum malaria from other malarias. PfHRP2-based tests may remain positive for several weeks after acute infection. A disadvantage of rapid tests is that they do not quantify parasitemia.

Malaria in early pregnancy causes fetal loss. In areas of high malaria transmission, falciparum malaria is associated with low birth weight and increased infant mortality rates. In areas with unstable transmission of malaria, pregnant women may develop severe infections. They develop high parasitemias with anemia, hypoglycemia, and acute pulmonary edema. The treatment below is based on the World Health Organization (WHO) 2015 guidelines and Centers for Disease Control and Prevention (CDC) guidelines for oral treatment for uncomplicated chloroquine-resistant *P. falciparum* malaria in pregnancy.

Ref:
1. *Mandell, Douglas, and Bennett's Principles and Practice of Infectious Diseases, 9th Edition, Chapters 274, 3301, 3310-3312.*

First Trimester
Quinine PLUS Clindamycin

Artemisinin combination therapy can be used as alternate therapy in first trimester if quinine + clindamycin is unavailable or treatment failure.

Second or Third Trimester
Artemisinin Combination Therapy

One of the following:
- Artemether-lumefantrine
- Artesunate-amodiaquine
- Artesunate-mefloquine
- Dihydroartemisinin-piperaquine

Severe malaria is acute malaria with major signs of organ dysfunction and/or high level of parasitemia. Initial treatment of severe malaria consists of parenteral therapy. Intravenous artesunate (in areas where intravenous artesunate of reliable quality is readily available) rather than intravenous quinine is preferred.

This approach is warranted for adults and children (including infants, pregnant women in all trimesters, and lactating women). Doxycycline would not be preferred as treatment in a pregnant woman. Since chloroquine-resistant falciparum malaria is prevalent in Africa. Chloroquine would not be an effective choice.

24. **Ans. A**

Tropical pulmonary eosinophilia (TPE) is caused by *Wuchereria bancrofti*, a parasitic infection caused by nematodes (roundworms) that involve the lymphatics and bloodstream. TPE is caused by an immune hyper-responsiveness to microfilariae that are trapped in the lungs. TPE can occur in any tropical area where filariasis occurs and is most common among young adults. It is more common in individuals from the Indian subcontinent.

The onset of clinical manifestations is usually gradual. Symptoms include a dry, hacking, nonproductive cough that is frequently paroxysmal and nocturnal. Asthma-like attacks are associated with breathlessness and wheezing. Other symptoms include weight loss, fatigue, and malaise.

The cardinal laboratory finding in TPE is blood eosinophilia usually above 3,000/μL. Increased serum immunoglobulin E level is observed, often above 1,000 units/mL. The diagnosis can be confirmed by raised serum filarial antibody titers.

Similar hyper-responsive pulmonary syndromes may occur with other helminthic infections.

The differential diagnosis of TPE includes asthma, Löffler syndrome, allergic bronchopulmonary aspergillosis (ABPA), allergic granulomatosis with polyangiitis, other systemic vasculitides, chronic eosinophilic pneumonia, and the hypereosinophilic syndrome.

Pulmonary function tests would reveal obstructive airway disease, but would not confirm the diagnosis. Bronchoscopy with BAL and biopsy is an invasive test and may be performed if noninvasive tests are unrevealing. Serum galactomannan assay is used to detect fungal infections, but given the patient's age, immunocompetent state, and recent residence in an area where filariasis is commonly seen, testing for filariasis would be more useful.

Ref:
1. *Mandell, Douglas, and Bennett's Principles and Practice of Infectious Diseases, 9th Edition, Chapters 287, 3448-3449.*
2. *https://www.cdc.gov/parasites/lymphaticfilariasis/disease.html.*

25. **Ans. A**

This patient had recently participated in recreational freshwater activities. Transmission of leptospirosis occurs through skin or mucous membranes, especially the conjunctival or oral mucosa. This patient presented with symptoms of severe leptospirosis also known as Weil's syndrome which consists of the triad of hemorrhage, jaundice, and acute kidney injury. A definitive diagnosis can be based on isolation of the organism from blood by blood cultures or by a polymerase chain reaction (PCR). It can also be diagnosed by seroconversion or a fourfold rise in antibody titers. Treatment of leptospirosis should be with intravenous penicillin or intravenous ceftriaxone or intravenous doxycycline. Since this patient is critically ill, antibiotics should be started empirically while awaiting confirmatory results.

Leptospirosis is a zoonosis caused by pathogenic spirochetes of the genus *Leptospira*. It occurs in both temperate and tropical regions. Human infection occurs from exposure to animal urine, contaminated water or soil, or infected animal tissue. The organism enters through cuts or abraded skin, mucous membranes, or conjunctivae. The infection may also occur by the ingestion of food contaminated with urine or by aerosols.

The spectrum of disease ranges from mild and self-limited, subclinical, or severe and fatal. The illness often manifests with the abrupt onset of fever, rigors, myalgias, and headache. The incubation period is of 2-26 days (average 10 days). Conjunctival suffusion, with conjunctival redness, is an important sign. This finding should raise the possibility of leptospirosis. Subconjunctival hemorrhages also occur. Other features are nonproductive cough, nausea, vomiting, and diarrhea. Muscle tenderness, splenomegaly, lymphadenopathy, pharyngitis, hepatomegaly, muscle rigidity, or skin rash may occur.

Complications seen are jaundice and renal failure, pulmonary hemorrhage, acute respiratory distress syndrome (ARDS), uveitis, optic neuritis, peripheral neuropathy, myocarditis, and rhabdomyolysis. A history of epidemiologic exposure and consistent clinical findings suggest the possibility of leptospirosis. The diagnosis is made most often by serologic testing. Molecular techniques are promising for rapid diagnosis but are not widely available. Blood cultures during the bacteremic phase and urine cultures after the first week may confirm the diagnosis but growth may take several weeks.

When clinical suspicion for leptospirosis is high, administration of empiric treatment is appropriate especially in a seriously ill patient, even in the absence of confirmatory laboratory tests.

Malaria, dengue, chikungunya, scrub typhus, typhoid, and hantavirus may present in a similar fashion.

Ref:
1. Mandell, Douglas, and Bennett's Principles and Practice of Infectious Diseases, 9th Edition, Chapters 239, 2900-2904.

26. **Ans. A**

Important principles of treatment for brucellosis are the use of antibiotics with activity in the acidic intracellular environment (e.g., doxycycline, rifampicin), use of combination regimens, and prolonged duration of treatment. It is important to prevent complications, relapses, and sequelae.

There are three major regimens for the treatment of nonpregnant adults with uncomplicated brucellosis (e.g., not having spondylitis, neurobrucellosis, or endocarditis).

 i. Doxycycline 100 mg orally twice daily for 6 weeks, with streptomycin 1 g intramuscularly once daily for the first 14-21 days. This is the gold standard of treatment.
 ii. Doxycycline orally plus Rifampicin orally daily. Both drugs are administered for 6 weeks.
 iii. Doxycycline orally for 6 weeks plus gentamicin parenterally for the first 7-10 days.

Fluoroquinolones (ciprofloxacin 500 mg twice daily or ofloxacin 200 mg twice daily) are not appropriate as first line agents against *Brucella* as they are less effective due to low intravacuolar pH. They can be used in combination with doxycycline or rifampin. They may be useful in cases of drug resistance, antimicrobial toxicity, and relapse.

Ref:
1. Mandell, Douglas, and Bennett's Principles and Practice of Infectious Diseases, 9th Edition, Chapters 226, 2275-2276.

27. **Ans. A**

Chikungunya virus is an alphavirus transmitted by mosquitoes. It causes high fever, polyarthralgia and inflammatory arthritis. It also causes a maculopapular rash. Chikungunya virus has spread from West Africa to Asia, Europe, islands in the Indian and Pacific Oceans, and in the Americas. Infected travelers can spreads into new areas, where local transmission can occur if the mosquito vector is present. The incubation period is 3-7 days (range 1-14 days). High fever and malaise are associated with pain in multiple joints. Polyarthralgia often develops 2-5 days after onset of fever and commonly involves multiple joints. Arthralgia is usually bilateral and symmetric. Distal joints are often involved more than proximal joints. Morning stiffness is often present. A macular or maculopapular rash is often seen. It usually appears on the third day or later after onset of illness and lasts 3-7 days. The duration of acute illness is usually 7-10 days. Severe complications can occur, more frequently in patients older than 65 years and with chronic diseases. Complications include meningoencephalitis, cardiopulmonary decompensation, acute renal failure, and death.

Reverse transcription polymerase chain reaction (RT-PCR) is done for detection of chikungunya virus. It should be performed for patients who present in the first 7 days following the onset of symptoms. A positive result confirms a diagnosis of chikungunya virus. RT-PCR during the first 5 days following onset of symptoms has a high sensitivity and specificity.

For individuals presenting >8 days following onset of symptoms, chikungunya virus serologic testing with ELISA or indirect fluorescent antibody (IFA) should be performed. A positive result confirms the diagnosis of chikungunya virus infection.

Dengue fever and Zika virus may also present like chikungunya. However, dengue fever is more typically presents with hemoconcentration, leukopenia, severe thrombocytopenia, and abdominal pain with acalculous cholecystitis, hypotension, and bleeding. Zika virus also presents with fever, myalgia, arthralgia, headache, rash, and conjunctivitis. Both these infections should be investigated and ruled out. Zika virus IgM is positive after the second week of illness. *B. burgdorferi* is spread by the *Ixodes* tick and is prevalent in North America.

Ref:
1. *Mandell, Douglas, and Bennett's Principles and Practice of Infectious Diseases, 9th Edition, Chapters 151, 2004-2005.*

28. Ans. D

Cryptosporidium is an intracellular protozoan parasite that causes gastrointestinal disease in humans. *Cryptosporidium* species have been identified in every continent except Antarctica and are an important cause of diarrhea in both children and adults.

Cryptosporidiosis outbreaks have been associated with drinking water supplies, animal contact, travel, swimming pools, and recreational water facilities. *Cryptosporidium* oocysts passed in stool are ingested and cause infection. Transmission of cryptosporidiosis occurs via spread from an infected person or animal or from a fecally contaminated source, such as a food or water. *Cryptosporidium* oocysts are present in a large percentage of surface waters and are difficult to eradicate. The oocysts are resistant to many disinfectants such as chlorine, are not effectively removed by many filtration systems, and can survive in the environment for months.

Foodborne outbreaks are less common than waterborne outbreaks. Person-to-person transmission is common, particularly among household members, sexual partners, children in daycare centers and their caretakers, and healthcare workers.

Cryptosporidium infection can cause an asymptomatic infection, mild diarrhea, or severe enteritis with or without biliary tract involvement. *Cryptosporidium* may give rise to a secretory diarrhea and malabsorption. Fecal blood or leukocytes are unusual unless there is coinfection with another enteric pathogen. The incubation period is usually 7-10 days (range 2-28 days). The diarrhea associated with cryptosporidiosis may be acute or chronic. It may be intermittent. It may be of small volume or profuse, with up to 25 L/day of watery stool. There may also be malaise, nausea, and anorexia, crampy abdominal pain, and low-grade fever. The infection may be severe in the elderly and in immunocompromised patients causing electrolyte imbalances and dehydration.

The diagnosis of cryptosporidiosis can be established by microscopy, PCR, or enzyme immunoassays (EIAs). Organisms may be detected in stool, duodenal aspirates, bile secretions, and biopsy specimens from affected gastrointestinal tissue.

In stool samples, the most sensitive tests are visualization of the parasites through direct immunofluorescent antibody (DFA) testing or through the use of a multiplex PCR. Routine examination for ova and parasites usually does not detect cryptosporidia spores.

With the modified Ziehl–Neelsen (MZN) acid-fast stain, fresh or formalin fixed specimens can be examined by light or phase-contrast microscopy. The oocysts stain red or pink and are usually 4-6 μm in diameter. The accuracy of the MZN acid-fast stain depends upon the number of stool specimens examined, since the number of oocysts shed in feces is not constant.

Nitazoxanide, a nitrothiazole benzamide, is the preferred agent for all patients ≥1 year of age.

Ref:
1. *Mandell, Douglas, and Bennett's Principles and Practice of Infectious Diseases, 9th Edition, Chapters 282, 3419-3421.*

29. Ans. C

Cyclospora cayetanensis is the cause of foodborne and waterborne parasitic diarrheal illness in children and adults. *Cyclospora* can occur as a locally acquired infection or in travelers or in patients with HIV. The organism is most frequently reported in Latin America, the Indian subcontinent, and Southeast Asia.

Risk factors for infection in endemic areas include contaminated water or food and poor sanitation. Small bowel biopsies in symptomatic patients have revealed developmental forms of the parasite within epithelial cells. There is jejunal inflammation with increased intraepithelial lymphocytes and degrees of villous atrophy. The incubation period is around 7 days following ingestion (range 2-14 days).

Infected patients may have a single self-limited episode or a prolonged course with persistent diarrhea, anorexia, and upper gastrointestinal symptoms lasting for weeks to months. The diagnosis of *Cyclospora* infection is confirmed with stool microscopy and detection of oocysts in the stool of a symptomatic patient. *Cyclospora cayetanensis* oocysts can be detected by modified acid-fast staining of stool. They have a diameter of 8-10 μm. Recommended treatment of *Cyclospora* infection in immunocompetent adults consists a combination of two antibiotics trimethoprim–sulfamethoxazole.

Ref:
1. *Mandell, Douglas, and Bennett's Principles and Practice of Infectious Diseases, 9th Edition, Chapters 283, 3422-3423.*

30. Ans. C

Dengue fever is a mosquito-borne infection. It is caused by dengue viruses and transmitted by *Aedes aegypti* or *Aedes albopictus* mosquitoes. There are four serotypes of dengue virus. Plasma leakage due to increased vascular permeability results in intravascular volume depletion and shock in severe dengue. Severe dengue manifests with hemoconcentration, pleural effusion, or ascites. There may be a 20% rise in hematocrit above baseline. Patients present with fever, thrombocytopenia, and hemorrhagic manifestations. Platelet transfusion has not been shown to be effective at preventing or controlling hemorrhage and therefore is not advised for most patients with thrombocytopenia. Platelet transfusion may be warranted in patients with severe thrombocytopenia (<10,000/mm^3) or those with active bleeding. There is no indication for prophylactic platelet transfusion in patients with thrombocytopenia in the absence of active bleeding. The initial fluid for resuscitation should be crystalloid. There is no advantage of colloid over crystalloid. Dextran is associated with more hypersensitivity reactions and renal dysfunction. Plasma leakage should be managed with intravascular volume repletion to prevent or reverse hypovolemic shock. Administration of intravenous fluid is warranted in patients with intravascular volume depletion. Blood transfusion is indicated in patients with significant bleeding or low hematocrit and failure to improve with fluid resuscitation. It is critical to assess the adequacy of both blood and fluid repletion. A decrease in hematocrit may reflect volume repletion or blood loss. Intravenous colloid solution is indicated for patients with intractable shock resistant to crystalloid resuscitation.

Ref:
1. *Mandell, Douglas, and Bennett's Principles and Practice of Infectious Diseases, 9th Edition, Chapters 153, 2013-2014.*
2. *https://www.cdc.gov/dengue/healthcare-providers/testing/index.html.*

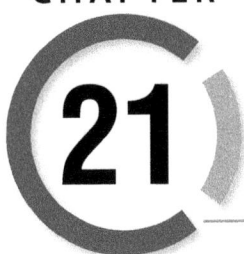

CHAPTER 21

Pyrexia of Unknown Origin

Altaf Patel, Hasnain Patel

1. **Increased body temperature is mediated by:**
   A. Altered hypothalamic function
   B. Upward shift in values of thermogenesis
   C. Inhibition of heat dispersion
   D. Pyrogens
   E. All of the above
   F. None of the above

2. **Pyrexia of unknown origin (PUO) must have the following, *except*:**
   A. Fever above 38.3°C
   B. Measured on several occasions for 2 weeks
   C. At least 3 days of intensive diagnostic evaluations
   D. Neutropenic < 500 neutrophils/mm^3

3. **Classic PUO is defined as: which is wrong?**
   A. Febrile illness > 21 days
   B. Temperature > 38.3°C
   C. Uncertain diagnosis despite 7 days of observation/investigation
   D. Presence of immunocompromised state

4. **Nosocomial PUO is defined as:**
   A. Fever occurring in a hostel
   B. Fever occurring in a hospital
   C. Fever occurring in a school
   D. Fever occurring with a bad nose cold

5. **Human immunodeficiency virus (HIV)-associated fever is defined as: which statement is wrong?**
   A. Confirmed HIV infection
   B. Fever 38.3°C on many occasions
   C. Duration of 4 weeks in outpatient
   D. Duration 7 days in inpatient
   E. All reports and cultures are negative

6. **Important causes of PUO are:**
   A. Multisystem disease
   B. Giant cell arteritis
   C. Tuberculosis (TB)
   D. Babesia
   E. Androgenic's syndrome
   F. A, B, D, and E
   G. A, B, C, and D

7. **Malignancies associated with PUO are:**
   A. Non-Hodgkin's lymphoma
   B. Carcinoma colon
   C. Castleman's disease
   D. All of the above
   E. None of the above

8. **Leading diagnosable cause of PUO is:**
   A. Epstein-Barr (EB) virus
   B. TB
   C. Amebic liver abscess
   D. HIV
   E. Diabetic peripheral neuropathy
   F. All the above
   G. A, B, C, and E
   H. A, B, C, and D

9. **Prolonged mononucleosis syndromes are caused by:**
   A. *Mycobacterium tuberculosis*
   B. *Streptococcus pyogenes*
   C. *Staphylococcus*
   D. *Leishmania*
   E. All of the above
   F. None of the above

10. **Renal malakoplakia which submucosal plaques or nodules affecting urinary tract (804)?**
    A. Responds to fluoroquinolones
    B. TMP
    C. Amoxicillin
    D. Steroids
    E. A and B
    F. B and D

11. **What % of PUO remains undiagnosed?**
    A. 10–15%   B. 12–20%
    C. 25–30%   D. 20–30%

12. **Most common malignancy in PUO is:**
    A. Hodgkin's disease
    B. Non-Hodgkin's lymphoma
    C. Leukemia
    D. Colon carcinoma
    E. Carcinoma of the esophagus
    F. A, B, C, and D

13. The following are uncommon in drug-induced fever:
    A. Tachycardia
    B. Bradycardia
    C. Hypotension
    D. Hypertension
    E. Both A and C
    F. Both B and C

14. The following may be causes of drug-induced fever:
    A. Phenytoin
    B. Beta-lactam antibiotics
    C. Quinidine
    D. All of the above
    E. None of the above

15. Factitious fever is defined as:
    A. Habitual hyperthermia
    B. Temperature < 38.3°C
    C. None of the above
    D. All of the above

16. Factitious fever is commonly seen in:
    A. Jail inmates
    B. Men
    C. Young women
    D. Medical professionals
    E. Both A and B
    F. Both C and D

17. Febrile agglutinins (FA) are seen in:
    A. *Salmonella*
    B. *Brucella*
    C. Rickettsial's disease
    D. None of the above
    E. All of the above

18. Tests for Rocky Mountain spotted fever (RMSF) are:
    A. Immunofluorescence assay (IFA) assay for immunoglobulin G
    B. IFA assay for immunoglobulin M (IgM)
    C. PCR from DNA in whole blood
    D. Culture from skin
    E. None of the above
    F. All of the above

19. Blood culture fever should be supplemented with which of the following to assist isolation of nutritionally variant *Streptococci*?
    A. L-cysteine
    B. Pyridoxal
    C. Blood agar
    D. Marijuana
    E. A and C
    F. Both A and B
    G. All of the above
    H. None of the above

20. Liver biopsy and bone marrow are in PUO despite liver function test (LFT) being normal (Y/N):
    A. No
    B. Yes

21. Still's disease is characterized by which of the following:
    A. Elevated erythrocyte sedimentation rate (ESR)
    B. Anemia
    C. Leukocytosis
    D. Splenomegaly
    E. Rash
    F. Hepatitis
    G. A, B, C, D, and E

22. Purified protein derivative (PPD) tests are negative in the following types of TB:
    A. Miliary TB
    B. Pulmonary TB
    C. Abdominal TB
    D. Glandular TB

23. Noninvasive tests for PUO are:
    A. Barium meal with FT
    B. Barium enema
    C. Pulmonary function test (PFT)
    D. CO diffusing capacity
    E. A, B, and C
    F. All of the above

24. 2D echo is beneficial in PUO in which of the following?
    A. Bacterial endocarditis
    B. Pericarditis
    C. Nonbacterial thrombotic endocarditis
    D. Atrial myxoma
    E. ACD
    F. All of the above

25. Noninfectious causes of PUO are:
    A. Acalculous cholecystitis
    B. Deep vein thrombosis (DVT)
    C. Pulmonary embolism
    D. Pancreatitis
    E. All of the above
    F. B, C, D, and F

26. Features of familial Mediterranean fever are all, *except*:
    A. Swollen tender scrotum
    B. Swollen joints
    C. Rash on legs
    D. Muscle aches
    E. Coryza

27. If PUO is prolonged for more than 6 months, the prognosis is:
    A. Good
    B. Poor
    C. Intermediate
    D. None of the above

28. Of the noninfectious inflammatory diseases (NIIDs), common causes of PUO are:
    A. Still's disease
    B. Familial Mediterranean fever
    C. Sarcoid
    D. TB
    E. Large vessel vasculitis
    F. A, B, C, and D
    G. A, B, C, and E

29. **Drug-induced fever can occur with:**
    A. Nevirapine
    B. Phenytoin
    C. Allopurinol
    D. Furosemide
    E. Clopidogrel
    F. All of the above
    G. A, B, C, and D

30. **Granulomatous causes of PUO are:**
    A. Sarcoid
    B. Apical granuloma
    C. Idiopathic granulomatous hepatitis
    D. All the above

31. **Features of factitious fever are:**
    A. Generally young men
    B. Artificially induced by injecting contaminated Coca Cola
    C. Standing in sun for hours
    D. All of the above
    E. None of the above

ANSWERS WITH EXPLANATIONS

1. **Ans. E**
   Fever is mediated by altered hypothalamic function, upward shift in values of thermogenesis, inhibition of heat dispersion, pyrogens, tumor necrosis factor (TNF), interleukin (IL)-1, IL-6, and interferons.
   Ref:
   1. Szolcsányi J. Effect of capsaicin on thermoregulation: an update with new aspects. Temperature (Austin). 2015;2(2):277-96.

2. **Ans. B**
   Pyrexia of unknown origin: (1) Temperature >38.3°C on multiple occasions, (2) duration of illness of >3 weeks, and (3) exclusion of patients who are currently immune compromised or have been recently immune compromised.
   Ref:
   1. Agarwal PK, Gogia A. Fever of unknown origin. J Assoc Physicians India. 2004:52;314-8.

3. **Ans. D**
   Pyrexia of unknown origin: (1) temperature >38.3°C on multiple occasions; (2) duration of illness of >3 weeks, and (3) exclusion of patients who are currently immune compromised or have been recently immune compromised.
   Ref:
   1. Beresford, RW, Goshell IB, Pyrexia of unknown origin: causes, investigation and management. Intern Med J. 2016;46:1011-16.

4. **Ans. B**
   Nosocomial PUO: Fever occurring on several occasions in a patient who has been hospitalized for at least 24 hours and has not manifested an obvious source of infection that could have been present before admission.
   Ref:
   1. Durack DT, Street AC. Fever of unknown origin—reexamined and redefined. Curr Clin Top Infect Dis. 1991;11:35-51.

5. **Ans. D**
   Human immunodeficiency virus fever: Temperature above 100.4°F or 38°C, sore throat, headache, and muscle and joint pain. These symptoms last approximately 2 weeks.
   Ref:
   1. uptodate.com

6. **Ans. G**
   Bacterial:
   - Occult abscess
   - Complicated urinary tract infection
   - Culture negative endocarditis
   - Osteomyelitis
   - Tuberculosis (TB)
   - *Coxiella burnetii* (Q fever)
   - Rickettsial infections
   - Enteric fever
   - Brucellosis

   Viral:
   - Epstein–Barr (EB) virus
   - Cytomegalovirus
   - HIV

   Parasitic:
   - Malaria
   - Toxoplasmosis
   - Babesiosis

   Fungal:
   - Histoplasmosis

   Inflammatory:
   - Giant cell arteritis
   - Adult-onset Still's disease
   - Systemic lupus erythematosus
   - Polyarteritis nodosa
   - Granulomatosis with polyangiitis (Wegener granulomatosis)
   - Familial Mediterranean fever (FMF)

Neoplastic:
- Non-Hodgkin lymphoma
- Leukemia
- Renal cell carcinoma
- Hepatocellular carcinoma
- Metastatic lesions (commonly hepatic metastasis from adenocarcinomas)

Miscellaneous:
- Drugs
- Cirrhosis
- Pulmonary embolism
- Inflammatory bowel disease
- Sarcoidosis
- Hyperthyroidism
- Factitious fever.

Ref:
1. Beresford RW, Gosbell IB, Pyrexia of unknown origin: causes, investigation and management. Intern Med J. 2016;46(9):1011-6.
2. Harrison's Principles and Practice of Medicine. 19th Edition; 2015. pp. 123-6.

7. **Ans. D**

Pyrexia of unknown origin-related malignancies are as follows:
- Atrial myxoma
- Colonic cancer
- Hepatic carcinoma
- Metastatic disease
- Pancreatic cancer
- Renal cell carcinoma
- Leukemia
- Lymphoma
- Multiple myeloma
- Myeloproliferative disorders.

Ref:
1. Fernandez C, Beeching NJ. Pyrexia of unknown origin. Clin Med (Lond). 2018;18(2):170-4.
2. Harrison's Principles and Practice of Medicine. 19th Edition; 2015. pp. 123-6.

8. **Ans. H**

Infections such as TB, bacterial endocarditis, localized abscesses, and HIV were frequently the causes of PUO.

Ref:
1. Kejariwal D, Sarkar N, Chakraborti SK, Agarwal V, Roy S. Pyrexia of unknown origin: a prospective study of 100 cases. J Postgrad Med. 2001;47(2):104-7.
2. Onal IK, Cankurtaran M, Cakar M, et al. Fever of unknown origin: What is remarkable in the elderly in a developing country? Journal Of Infection. 2006;52(6):399-404.
3. Hot A, Revue NJ. Unexplained prolonged fevers: the paradox of a diagnostic becoming more and more difficult. Revue de Medecine Interne. 2006;27(Suppl 3):S255-8.

9. **Ans. F**

Prolonged mononucleosis syndromes are caused by EB virus (EBV).

Ref:
1. Harrison's Principles and Practice of Medicine. 19th Edition; 2015.

10. **Ans. E**

Therapy with antibiotics that concentrate in macrophages such as quinolones, trimethoprim-sulfamethoxazole.

Ref:
1. Elbendary AM, Elston DM. Malakoplakia Treatment and Management. Dermatology. Medscape; 2019. HYPERLINK http://reference.medscape.com/guide/dermatology.

11. **Ans. C**

Despite advanced modalities of investigations up to 27% of PUO patients remain undiagnosed.

Ref:
1. Kumar DP, Kumar DA, Rajeshwari K, et al. Fever of unknown origin (FUO): evolution of case definition, changing aetiological spectrum. Journal of Clinical and Scientific Research. 2016;5(1):33-9.

12. **Ans. F**

Leukemia, lymphoma, sarcoma, atrial myxoma, renal cell carcinoma, and colon and liver metastases are the most common culprits are common malignancies in PUO.

Ref:
1. Bodel P. Generalized perturbations in host physiology caused by localized tumors. Tumors and Fever. Ann NY Acad Sci. 1974;230:6-13.
2. Browder AA, Huff JW, Petersdorf RG. The significance of fever in neoplastic disease. Annals of Internal Medicine. 1961;55(6):932-42.
3. Boggs DR, Frei E. Clinical studies of fever and infection in cancer. Cancer. 1960;13(6):1240-53.

13. **Ans. F**

Fever can be the sole manifestation in drug-induced fever in 3–5% of cases.

Ref:
1. Roush MK, Nelson KM. Understanding drug-induced febrile reactions. Am Pharm. 1993;NS33(10):39.
2. Tabor PA. Drug-induced fever. Drug Intell Clin Pharm. 1986;20(6):413.
3. Jugtawat S, Daulatabadkar B, Pande S. Drug-induced fever versus infection-induced fever. Indian J Drugs Dermatol. 2016;2:115-6.

14. **Ans. D**

Causes of drug-induced fever are antimicrobials, anticonvulsants, and antiarrhythmic agents.

Ref:
1. Jugtawat S, Daulatabadkar B, Pande S. Drug-induced fever versus infection-induced fever. Indian J Drugs Dermatol. 2016;2:115-6.

2. Tisdale JE, Miller DA. *Drug-induced Diseases: Prevention, Detection, and Management.* Bethesda, MD: American Society of Health-Systems Pharmacists; 2005.
3. Mackowiak PA, LeMaistre CF. Drug fever: A critical appraisal of conventional concepts. An analysis of 51 episodes in two Dallas hospitals and 97 episodes reported in the English literature. *Ann Intern Med.* 1987;106:728-33.

15. Ans. C
Factitious fever is a false disease. It can be secondary to psychiatric illness or can be malingering.
Ref:
1. Rumans LW, Vosti KL. Factitious and fraudulent fever. *Am J Med.* 1978;65(5):745-55.

16. Ans. F
Factitious fever is more common amongst medical and paramedical staff, e.g., nurses, pharmacists, bacteriologist, laboratory technicians, and medical students, because of their familiarity with the hospital and easy access to thermometers and drugs.
Ref:
1. Qureshi H. Factitious fever. *JPMA.* 1983;33(8).

17. Ans. E
The use of FA serologic tests in the diagnosis of *Salmonella* (*typhi and paratyphi*), *Rickettsia*, *Brucella*, and *Francisella* infections.
Ref:
1. Zuerlein TJ, Smith PW. The diagnostic utility of the febrile agglutinin tests. *JAMA.* 1985;254(9):1211-4.

18. Ans. F
The standard serologic test for diagnosis of RMSF is the indirect immunofluorescence antibody (IFA) assay for immunoglobulin G (IgG) using *Rickettsia rickettsii* antigen. IgG IFA assays should be performed on paired acute and convalescent serum samples collected 2-4 weeks apart to demonstrate evidence of a fourfold seroconversion. IgM IFA assays are available through some reference laboratories; however, results might be less specific than IgG IFA assays for diagnosing a recent infection. Polymerase chain reaction (PCR) amplification is performed on DNA extracted from the whole blood. Culture and immunohistochemistry (IHC) assays also performed on skin biopsies of a rash lesion or postmortem tissue specimens.
Ref:
1. uptodate.com

19. Ans. B
The isolate failed to grow on unsupplemented blood agar, but grew as small α-hemolytic colonies on sheep blood agar supplemented with l-Cysteine (100 µg/mL) and pyridoxal hydrochloride (10 µg/mL). The organism was optochin resistant. Susceptibility testing was done on Mueller Hinton sheep blood agar supplemented with l-cysteine and pyridoxal hydrochloride. These findings were suggestive of growth of nutritionally variant *Streptococci*.
Ref:
1. Ray M, Subramanian C, Ray P, Singhi P. Infective endocarditis in a child due to Abiotrophia defectivus. *Indian Pediatrics.* 2002;39:388-92.

20. Ans. A
More invasive diagnostics, such as bone marrow biopsy, temporal artery biopsy, and transesophageal biopsy (TOE), should not be performed routinely and only be performed, if indicated by previous history, examination, or investigations. Factors such as suspicion of hematological malignancy, thrombocytopenia, and anemia will increase the likelihood of a bone marrow biopsy.
Ref:
1. Beresford RW, Gosbell IB. Pyrexia of unknown origin: causes, investigation and management. *Intern Med J.* 2016;46:1011-6.

21. Ans. G
Still's disease has clinical features such as the abruptness of onset, fever patterns, transient nature of the rash, almost equal female-to-male ratio, arthritis, and neutrophilia. The erythrocyte sedimentation rate (ESR) is raised in almost all patients, with C-reactive protein (CRP). Common hematological abnormalities include leukocytosis, anemia, and thrombocytosis.

Viruses such as hepatitis B and hepatitis C have been implicated in cases. Less common manifestations include pleuritis (26.4%), pericarditis (23.8%), and splenomegaly (43.9%).
Ref:
1. Efthimiou P, Paik PK, Bielory L. Diagnosis and management of adult onset Still's disease. *Ann Rheum Dis.* 2006;65(5):564-72.

22. Ans. A
About 10-25% of people with newly diagnosed TB of the lungs will have a negative result, due to poor immune function, poor nutrition, accompanying viral infection, or steroid therapy. Over 50% of patients with widespread, disseminated TB or miliary TB will also have a negative TB test.

Tuberculin anergy is more common in miliary TB than in pulmonary and extrapulmonary TB.
Ref:
1. Sharma SK, Mohan A, Sharma A. Challenges in the diagnosis and treatment of miliary tuberculosis. *Indian J Med Res.* 2012;135(5):703-30.

23. Ans. F
Noninvasive procedures for PUO: Complete blood count, biochemical tests [liver and kidney function tests, lactate dehydrogenase (LDH), creatine phosphokinase (CPK), thyroid-stimulating hormone (TSH),

free thyroxine (FT4), and ferritin], urine analysis, immunological and viral serological tests, cultures of blood and other body fluids, molecular studies, imaging studies [chest X-ray, ultrasonography (USG), computed tomography (CT), magnetic resonance imaging (MRI), fluorodeoxyglucose positron emission tomography (FDG-PET)/CT, and barium meal], and CO diffusion capacity study.

24. **Ans. F**

It is recommended to perform echocardiography when there is a possibility of culture-negative endocarditis, pericarditis, and atrial myxomas. Transesophageal echocardiography has a higher sensitivity than transthoracic echocardiography.
Ref:
1. *Jitendranath L, Slim J. Work-up of fever of unknown origin in adult patients. Hosp Phys. 2005;41:9-15.*
2. *Mourad O, Palda V, Detsky AS. A comprehensive evidence-based approach to fever of unknown origin. Arch Intern Med. 2003;163:545-51.*

25. **Ans. E**

Inflammatory disorders:
- Behçet's disease
- FMF
- Felty's syndrome
- Giant cell arteritis and temporal arteritis
- Gout and pseudogout
- Granulomatosis with polyangiitis (Wegener's disease)
- Polyarteritis nodosa
- Polymyositis
- Rheumatoid arthritis
- Sarcoidosis
- Still's disease
- Systemic lupus erythematosus
- Takayasu's arteritis

Solid tumors:
- Atrial myxoma
- Colonic cancer
- Hepatic carcinoma
- Metastatic disease
- Pancreatic cancer
- Renal cell carcinoma

Hematological malignancy:
- Leukemia
- Lymphoma
- Multiple myeloma
- Myeloproliferative disorders

Miscellaneous:
- Drug fever
- Factitious fever
- Hypoadrenalism
- Hypothalamic dysfunction
- Inflammatory bowel disease
- Thyroiditis
- Cholecystitis
- Deep vein thrombosis (DVT)
- Pulmonary embolism
- Pancreatitis.

26. **Ans. E**

Familial Mediterranean fever is a hereditary autosomal recessive disorder, characterized by recurrent, self-limiting episodes of fever, serositis, abdominal pain, chest pain, painful and swollen joints, rash on legs, myalgia, and swollen and tender scrotum.
Ref:
1. *Manna R, Cerquaglia C, Curigliano V, Fonnesu C, Giovinale M, Verrecchia E. Clinical features of familial Mediterranean fever: an Italian overview. Eur Rev Med Pharmacol Sci. 2009;13(Suppl 1):51-3.*

27. **Ans. A**

Pyrexia of unknown origin has a good long-term prognosis and resolves within a year.
Ref:
1. *Gompf SG. Fever of unknown origin (FUO). Infectious Diseases. Medscape; 2018.*

28. **Ans. G**

Noninfectious inflammatory disease causes for PUO are as follows:
- Behçet's disease
- FMF
- Felty's syndrome
- Giant cell arteritis and temporal arteritis
- Gout and pseudogout
- Granulomatosis with polyangiitis (Wegener's disease)
- Polyarteritis nodosa
- Polymyositis
- Rheumatoid arthritis
- Sarcoidosis
- Still's disease
- Systemic lupus erythematosus
- Takayasu's arteritis.

Ref:
1. *Fernandez C, Beeching NJ. Pyrexia of unknown origin. Clin Med (Lond). 2018;18(2):170-4.*

29. **Ans. G**

The causes of drug-induced fever are antimicrobials, anticonvulsants, and antiarrhythmic agents.
Ref:
1. *Jugtawat S, Daulatabadkar B, Pande S. Drug-induced fever versus infection-induced fever. Indian J Drugs Dermatol. 2016;2:115-6.*

2. Tisdale JE, Miller DA. Drug-induced Diseases: Prevention, Detection, and Management. Bethesda, MD: American Society of Health-Systems Pharmacists; 2005.
3. Mackowiak PA, LeMaistre CF. Drug fever: A critical appraisal of conventional concepts. An analysis of 51 episodes in two Dallas hospitals and 97 episodes reported in the English literature. Ann Intern Med 1987;106:728-33.

30. Ans. D

Granulomatous diseases:
- Sarcoidosis
- Crohn's disease (the most common gastrointestinal cause)
- Granulomatous hepatitis
- Apical granuloma

Idiopathic granulomatous hepatitis (IGH) is a rare cause of pyrexia of unknown origin (PUO).

Ref:
1. Holla RG, Gupta A, Dubey AK. Idiopathic Granulomatous Hepatitis. Indian Pediatrics. 2004;41: 610-3.
2. Harrison's Principles and Practice of Medicine. 19th Edition; 2015.

31. Ans. E

Factitious fever is more common amongst medical and paramedical staff, e.g., nurses, pharmacists, bacteriologist, laboratory technicians, and medical students, because of their familiarity with the hospital and easy access to thermometers and drugs.

Ref:
1. Qureshi H. Factitious fever. JPMA. 1983;33(8).

CHAPTER 22

Outbreaks

Laxman Jessani

1. Peritoneal fluid of three different patients who underwent paracentesis on the same day but in different hospital locations showed growth of *Klebsiella oxytoca*. The microbiology laboratory calls with results of positive *Klebsiella oxytoca* cultures and is concerned. What is going on?
   A. Outbreak
   B. Pseudo-outbreak
   C. Any of the above
   D. None of the above

2. Record review of above cases indicates that clinical presentation is not consistent with spontaneous bacterial peritonitis for any of the cases. Molecular typing demonstrates that isolates are genetically related. What is going on?
   A. Outbreak
   B. Pseudo-outbreak
   C. Any of the above
   D. None of the above

3. A 35-year-old male with acute myeloid leukemia (AML) having continuous fever for 5 days and on meropenem and vancomycin. *Past history*—he was treated with R-CHOP chemotherapy and had two episodes of neutropenic sepsis in past and recovered. Subsequently, he underwent allogeneic hematopoietic stem cell transplant 20 days back. He has received nearly 4 weeks of broad-spectrum antibiotic treatment earlier and bone marrow function had not recovered. At present—blood cultures from Hickman line had been negative to date. He was getting hypoxic, so a chest X-ray was performed, which showed some haziness in the right upper lobe. Blood was also tested for galactomannan. A CT scan of the chest, abdomen, and pelvis was done. Two other AML patients with prolonged inpatient stay in the same bone marrow transplant (BMT) unit had behaved similarly and both were now being treated for invasive pulmonary aspergillosis. There were no cases of invasive aspergillosis in the unit for several months.

   What do you suspect in this case?
   A. Gram-negative sepsis
   B. Invasive aspergillosis
   C. Other mold infection
   D. None of the above

4. Pseudo-outbreaks occur when:
   A. Increased number of laboratory-positive tests that do not correlate with clinical findings
   B. Enhanced surveillance systems
   C. Improvement in laboratory diagnostic methods
   D. All of the above

5. A new renal dialysis unit is scheduled to be built on the site of an earlier recreation club, which will have to be demolished first. The site is next to the block containing the hospital's hematology inpatient and outpatient units. Which of the following is true?
   A. Oppose the development, as it is highly likely to put immunosuppressed patients at increased risk of *Aspergillus*-related conditions
   B. Ensure that ventilation ducts, windows, and water pipes are isolated from areas where demolition is taking place and draw up an assessment of all at-risk groups on the hospital site
   C. Insist that contractors use external waste disposal chutes when gutting the upper floors of the building to be demolished
   D. There is no specific need to discuss and plan measures to reduce exposure to *Aspergillus* and other potential pathogens with the contractor and clinical teams affected

6. A 44-year-old female presented to the emergency department with a left-sided hemiparesis and was admitted to the hospital. CT scan of her brain showed a space-occupying lesion. 5 days into her admission, the patient had a brain biopsy of her space-occupying lesion. Her condition deteriorated, and she required a decompressive craniotomy and admission to ICU, where she was intubated and required mechanical ventilation, central venous access and intracranial pressure probe (ICP) was inserted. Her methicillin-resistant *Staphylococcus aureus* (MRSA) screening swabs on admission to the ICU were negative. The patient required further surgical interventions, and a ventriculoperitoneal (VP) shunt was inserted. She remained in the ICU for 3 weeks and was later shifted to the general ward. On admission to the ward, a repeat MRSA screening swab was reported as being positive. Then, 48 hours later, the patient spiked a temperature of 39°C and further dropped her Glasgow Coma Scale (GCS). Her examination was unremarkable for the cardiovascular and respiratory system, but he noted small blistering on the right forearm at the peripheral vascular access site.

What is the most likely cause of fever?
- A. *Streptococcus*
- B. MRSA
- C. MSSA
- D. None of the above

7. Regarding invasive aspergillosis and hematopoietic stem cell transplant (HSCT) recipients, which of the following is true?
   - A. National Institute for Health and Clinical Excellence (NICE) guidance recommends positive-pressure, high-efficiency particulate air (HEPA)-filtered side rooms for all patients undergoing HSCT and those who have received a HSCT
   - B. Recipients of allogeneic stem cell transplants are deemed lower risk for hospital-acquired and other infections than autologous HSCT patients
   - C. Refractory hematological malignancy is associated with poorer response to antifungal treatment of invasive aspergillosis
   - D. Invasive pulmonary aspergillosis is most likely to occur immediately after HSCT

8. Regarding invasive pulmonary aspergillosis, which one of the following is true?
   - A. Most cases are caused by *Aspergillus flavus*
   - B. Voriconazole is the first choice antifungal therapy
   - C. Diagnosis can only be made on the basis of positive culture
   - D. A positive culture of *Aspergillus* from bronchiolar lavage always indicates infection

9. Which one of the following is not associated with MRSA?
   - A. Screening
   - B. Nasal carriage
   - C. Petting zoo
   - D. Dialysis

10. Medical head of tertiary care hospital was informed of the absence from work of 15 staff with symptoms of gastroenteritis. There were unconfirmed reports that additional workers not scheduled to be on shift or scheduled to be in later were also affected. The following day, a further 10 cases had been reported, of whom three had required attendance at the hospital for rehydration. There was suspicion of non-*Salmonella typhi* (NST) outbreak since one of stool cultures was positive. In order to prevent further outbreak of nontyphoidal *Salmonella* (NTS), which of preventive measures undertaken is correct?
    - A. Consumption of meat does not cause nontyphoidal *Salmonella*
    - B. Dry or cracked eggs need not be discarded
    - C. Food handler infected with NTS should stay away from work until he/she has been diarrhea-free for 48 hours
    - D. All of the above are correct

11. An outbreak is:
    - A. An increase in the number of cases of a particular disease greater than is expected for a given time and place
    - B. Two or more cases of a similar illness among individuals who have had a common exposure
    - C. Both of the above
    - D. None of the above

12. What is a virus pandemic?
    - A. A sharp and rapid epidemic involving more than one country
    - B. An outbreak, which recurs again and again
    - C. A rapid global outbreak starting from a single focus
    - D. A characteristic of common cold virus and HIV

13. Which of the following is a primary goal for undertaking foodborne disease outbreak investigations?
    - A. To study the natural history of the causative agent
    - B. To train staff
    - C. To stop the current outbreak by implementing effective control measures
    - D. To respond to public concerns

14. Purpose of developing hypotheses in outbreak investigation is:
    - A. To give a working diagnosis
    - B. To help to direct immediate control measures
    - C. To help to narrow the focus of subsequent studies and to determine if others need to be involved in the investigation
    - D. All of the above

15. Among the given options, knowledge and skills from all of the following disciplines should be represented on every foodborne outbreak investigation team, *except*:
    - A. Environmental health
    - B. Epidemiology
    - C. Laboratory
    - D. Molecular diagnostics

16. All of the following are true of pathogen-specific surveillance, *except*:
    - A. Detects all types of foodborne illness
    - B. Relies on reports from physicians and clinical laboratory staff
    - C. Is the primary means to detect widespread outbreaks such as multistate outbreaks
    - D. Has an inherent lag in reporting due to time necessary to confirm pathogen through laboratory testing

17. Investigation of a restaurant named in a foodborne illness complaint is most likely to identify a food safety problem for which of the following?
    A. One person reported becoming ill after eating at the restaurant
    B. Family members are at the restaurant and developed diarrhea 6 hours later
    C. Three friends became ill with vomiting within 4 hours of eating fried rice at the restaurant
    D. Two people became ill (one with a migraine headache and one with diarrhea) after eating at the restaurant

18. Why is it important to identify as many cases associated with an outbreak as possible?
    A. To determine true magnitude of outbreak
    B. To characterize outbreak accurately
    C. To increase the ability of epidemiologic studies to link illness with true cause of outbreak
    D. All of the above

19. Which of the following can improve the accuracy of a food history solicited during a foodborne illness complaint?
    A. Have case look at a calendar and identify key events to jog memory
    B. Have case review credit card or cash register receipts to identify where or what they ate
    C. Enlist help of dining partners
    D. All of the above

20. A case definition might include all of the following, except:
    A. Symptoms of the illness
    B. Laboratory test results
    C. Food that is the suspected source of the outbreak
    D. Date of illness onset

21. Which of the following statements is true about contributing factors?
    A. An outbreak will occur, if a contributing factor is present
    B. The three major categories of contributing factors are contamination, survival (lack of inactivation), and proliferation
    C. Contributing factors in an outbreak depend on the causative agent but not the food vehicle or processing method
    D. Correction of the contributing factor will correct the food safety problem and prevent it from occurring again

22. All of the following activities might be performed during an environmental health assessment of the implicated facility in an outbreak, except:
    A. Interview of the manager of the implicated facility
    B. Walk through of the facility
    C. Collection of information from ill food workers
    D. Observation of all food preparation processes undertaken at the facility

23. Which of the following causative agents tend to have the longest incubation period?
    A. Preformed toxins
    B. Viruses
    C. Bacteria
    D. Parasites

24. Subtyping of isolates from cases of the same disease can be used for all of the following, except:
    A. Link cases together
    B. Link outbreaks in different geographic locations
    C. Link foods with cases
    D. As sole proof of an outbreak

25. Which of the following should be undertaken during an outbreak investigation to improve communication between team members?
    A. Introduce team members to each other
    B. Hold regular meetings
    C. Create a list of persons and agencies who should be contacted in the event of an outbreak
    D. Develop formal communication processes for team member agencies

26. The following are true statements about stool specimens collected during a foodborne disease outbreak, except:
    A. Stool is the specimen of choice for most causative agents
    B. Routine stool cultures cover the most common foodborne disease causative agents
    C. The method of collection and handling depends on the suspected causative agent
    D. Freezing of stool specimens can interfere with detection of some causative agents

27. The purpose of writing a final report from an outbreak investigation includes all of the following, except:
    A. Facilitates implementation of prevention and control measures
    B. Identifies team members who did not complete the tasks assigned to them
    C. Allows investigators to learn from the experience
    D. Justifies program resources

28. A patient presented to emergency room with profuse bloody diarrhea. The diarrhea occurred more than 10 times a day and had started suddenly. An initial diagnosis of inflammatory bowel disease was made and he was admitted to an open ward. Initial laboratory investigations included CBC and biochemistry and a specimen of diarrhea was sent to the microbiology laboratory for culture of fecal

gastrointestinal bacterial pathogens and detection of relevant viruses by polymerase chain reaction (PCR). 3 days later, the ward received a report from the laboratory that *Campylobacter jejuni* had been isolated from the feces. The patient was then isolated and because of the severity of the attack he was started on treatment with erythromycin. 2 days later, two additional patients on the ward developed severe diarrhea, and they also were isolated and specimens sent to the laboratory. There was no evidence of direct contact between the index (initial) case and the new cases in that ward. The following day, a patient in a separate ward developed diarrhea and subsequently a patient in a third ward also developed diarrhea. In all cases, *C. jejuni* was isolated from the feces.

All of the following are true statements about the epidemiology of *Campylobacter* gastroenteritis, *except*:

A. It is a zoonosis
B. The organism can be acquired from companion animals
C. The infectious dose is believed to be approximately 10^2 organisms
D. The most frequent multilocus sequence typing (MLST) type in the UK is ST 21 for *C. jejuni*

29. Prevention of further cases of gastroenteritis involves all of the following, *except*:

A. Separate processing lines for different meats
B. Vaccination of slaughterhouse staff
C. Separate storage of cooked and uncooked food in a kitchen
D. Veterinary inspection of carcasses

30. Which of the following would be reasonable to include in the final report from a foodborne outbreak investigation?

A. Notes from interviews with food workers at implicated establishment
B. Individual laboratory reports
C. Summary of findings from case-control or cohort studies
D. Names of patients

ANSWERS WITH EXPLANATIONS

1. **Ans. C**
Three culture-positive cases from three different hospitals suggest a possible outbreak. But, it is very much possible that this could have been a laboratory error and possible pseudo-outbreak. It merits further investigation.
Ref:
1. Perez F, Deshpande A, Kundrapu S, Hujer AM, Bonomo RA, Donskey CJ. Pseudo-outbreak of Klebsiella oxytoca spontaneous bacterial peritonitis attributed to contamination of multidose vials of culture medium supplement. Infect Control Hosp Epidemiol. 2014;35(2):139-43.

2. **Ans. B**
This pseudo-outbreak was related to the hospital's laboratory procedures. The blood cultures used for peritoneal fluid were supplemented with a culture medium of yeast extract and dextrose from a multidose vial. Once the culture medium supplementation was discontinued, the incidence of contaminated peritoneal fluid cultures decreased dramatically (14.3% vs. 0.9%; $p < 0.001$).
Ref:
1. Perez F, Deshpande A, Kundrapu S, Hujer AM, Bonomo RA, Donskey CJ. Pseudo-outbreak of Klebsiella oxytoca spontaneous bacterial peritonitis attributed to contamination of multidose vials of culture medium supplement. Infect Control Hosp Epidemiol. 2014;35(2):139-43.

3. **Ans. B**
Considering clinical and radiological findings and in view of recent cases of invasive aspergillosis in the same BMT, possibility of invasive aspergillosis needs to be kept in mind. Other options are also possible but since other patients in same BMT had presented earlier with invasive aspergillosis, a possible outbreak of aspergillosis needs to be ascertained. This case merited further investigation by the infection control team (ICT). It was noted that extensive emergency building work had been carried out over the past 3 months in the vicinity of BMT. Outbreaks of nosocomial aspergillosis are generally related to construction work or renovation without adequate infection control precautions and failure to control spread of contaminated dust or debris.
Ref:
1. Alberti C, Bouakline A, Ribaud P, Lacroix C, Rousselot P, Leblanc T, et al. Relationship between environmental fungal contamination and the incidence of invasive aspergillosis in haematology patients. J Hospl Infect. 2001;48(3):198-206.

4. **Ans. D**
Pseudo-outbreaks occur when there is an artifactual increase in disease incidence, without an actual increase in clinical disease, which can occur in laboratory or secondary to enhanced surveillance programs.

Ref:
1. Perez F, Deshpande A, Kundrapu S, Hujer AM, Bonomo RA, Donskey CJ, et al. Pseudo-outbreak of Klebsiella oxytoca spontaneous bacterial peritonitis attributed to contamination of multidose vials of culture medium supplement. Infect Control Hosp Epidemiol. 2014;35(2):139-43.

5. **Ans. B**

Ensure that ventilation ducts, windows, and water pipes are isolated from areas where demolition is taking place.

A. False: The development is likely to go ahead in any case. They should focus on working with the hospital architect, management, and contractors to put proper infection control measures in place and ensure the layout of the unit meets operational and infection control standards.

C and D. False: Disposal chutes disperse fungal spores and other contaminants over a wide area. Waste should be removed in sealed bags along a designated route that is screened off as far as possible from the hospital's clinical areas. Need to discuss and plan measures to reduce exposure to *Aspergillus* and other potential pathogens with the contractor and clinical teams affected.
Ref:
1. Oren I, Haddad N, Finkelstein R, Rowe JM. Invasive pulmonary aspergillosis in neutropenic patients during hospital construction: before and after chemoprophylaxis and institution of HEPA filters. Am J Hematol. 2001;66(4):257-62.

6. **Ans. B**

Even though in this patient MRSA swab on admission was negative, given her prolonged stay in ICU, her clinical presentation of skin soft tissue infection with presence of VP shunt and central lines in situ, possibility of nosocomial infection related to MRSA is always possible. Methicillin-sensitive *Staphylococcus aureus* (MSSA) as cause of nosocomial infection is less likely.

Blood cultures were taken from the patient and she was started on vancomycin for a possible cellulitis caused by MRSA. In the next morning, the microbiologist called, informing the clinical team that the patient's blood culture was growing Gram-positive cocci in clusters in both the aerobic and anaerobic bottles indicative of MRSA.
Ref:
1. Hidron AI, Kourbatova EV, Halvosa JS, Terrell BJ, McDougal LK, Tenover FC, et al. Risk factors for colonization with methicillin-resistant Staphylococcus aureus (MRSA) in patients admitted to an urban hospital: emergence of community-associated MRSA nasal carriage. Clin Infect Dis. 2005;41(2):159-66.

7. **Ans. C**

A and B. False: Many regimens have a significant outpatient component. NICE recommends that such patients are managed in specialist units with appropriate measures to avoid air contamination and not all patients.

D. False: More and more cases are seen many months after transplantation and relate to the use of corticosteroids for graft-versus-host disease.
Ref:
1. Oren I, Haddad N, Finkelstein R, Rowe JM. Invasive pulmonary aspergillosis in neutropenic patients during hospital construction: before and after chemoprophylaxis and institution of HEPA filters. Am J Hematol. 2001;66(4):257-62.

8. **Ans. B**

Voriconazole is the first choice antifungal therapy. Other alternatives include liposomal amphotericin. Echinocandins have been used with reported success. Refractory disease may warrant dual antifungal therapy.

A. False: Aspergillus fumigatus accounts for most cases worldwide.

C. False: Obtaining invasive samples may not be possible, as for instance in profoundly neutropenic patients requiring platelet support.

D. False: Unless the patient has underlying lung disease or is immunosuppressed, it is likely to represent a contaminant. However, if fungal hyphae were seen on initial microscopy or an isolate is repeatedly isolated, the patient should be investigated further including screening for acquired and genetic immunosuppressive conditions.
Ref:
1. Gayet-Ageron A, Iten A, van Delden C, Farquet N, Masouridi-Levrat S, Von Dach E, et al. In-hospital transfer is risk factor for invasive filamentous fungal infection among hospitalized patients with hematological malignancies: a matched case-control study. Infect Control Hosp Epidemiol. 2015;36(3):320-8.

9. **Ans. C**

Staphylococcus aureus is found in the nose, axilla, and groin (carrier sites), and screening is an important method of controlling infection and onward transmission of MRSA by giving an appropriate suppression regimen to the colonized patient and isolating the patient in a single room. Risk factors for MRSA are residence in a long-term care facility, admission to hospital, prior use of antibiotics, hemodialysis, and HIV infection. Petting zoos are a risk factor for infection with verotoxin-producing organisms, leading in some cases to the hemolytic uremic syndrome.

Ref:
1. Hidron AI, Kourbatova EV, Halvosa JS, Terrell BJ, McDougal LK, Tenover FC, et al. Risk factors for colonization with methicillin-resistant Staphylococcus aureus (MRSA) in patients admitted to an urban hospital: emergence of community-associated MRSA nasal carriage. Clin Infect Dis. 2005;41(2):159-66.

10. **Ans. C**

   People infected with NTS should stay away from childcare, school, or work until they have been diarrhea-free for 24 hours. If working as a food handler, then this should be 48 hours.
   Ref:
   1. Jackson BR, Griffin PM, Cole, Walsh KA, Chai SJ. Outbreak-associated Salmonella enterica serotypes and food commodities, United States, 1998-2008. Emerg Infect Dis. 2013;19(8):1239-44.

11. **Ans. B**

   An outbreak is two or more cases of a similar illness among individuals who have had a common exposure. A cluster is the occurrence of more cases of a particular disease than expected for a given place and time.

12. **Ans. C**

   A pandemic is an epidemic of disease that has spread across a large region, for instance multiple continents, or even worldwide. A widespread endemic disease that is stable in terms of how many people are getting sick from it is not a pandemic.

13. **Ans. C**

   To stop the current outbreak by implementing effective control measures. The primary goals for undertaking foodborne disease outbreak investigations are to stop the current outbreak as soon as possible by implementing effective control measures and prevent similar outbreaks in future.

14. **Ans. D**

   Development of a hypothesis early in an outbreak helps to direct subsequent steps of an outbreak investigation and should involve all investigation team members.

15. **Ans. D**

   The knowledge and skills represented on an outbreak investigation team are configured to meet the needs of the particular outbreaks. However, the team always needs knowledge and skills in environmental health, epidemiology, laboratory, food regulations, public health education, and communications.

16. **Ans. A**

   For pathogen-specific surveillance, cases of interest are specific laboratory-confirmed diseases or well-defined syndromes selected by the state or local health department.

17. **Ans. C**

   Investigation of a restaurant named in a foodborne illness complaint is most likely to identify a food safety problem in the following situations:
   - The complainant observed specific food preparation or serving procedures likely to lead to a food safety problem at the establishment.
   - Two or more persons reported a similar illness and shared a food or meal at the establishment, and had no other shared exposure. The illness should be consistent with the foods eaten and the incubation period.

   The only scenario meeting these criteria is the three friends who developed a similar illness after eating fried rice at a restaurant.

18. **Ans. D**

   It is important to actively search for additional cases associated with each outbreak to:
   - Get a sense of the true magnitude of the outbreak.
   - Characterize the outbreak (and its cause) accurately.
   - Have sufficient power (statistically speaking) to make inferences from epidemiologic studies.

19. **Ans. D**

   To improve the completeness and accuracy of food, histories obtained during foodborne illness complaints have the complainant:
   - Look at a calendar
   - Describe each meal in time period
   - Identify key events to jog memory
   - Review receipts or menus
   - Enlist help of dining partners
   - Consider a list of foods
   - Think about food preferences
   - Rule out or rule in specific foods.

20. **Ans. C**

   Never include the suspected source of an outbreak in the case definition. If you include the suspected source in the case definition, all of your cases will have exposure to that source and you will not be able to test your hypothesis.

21. **Ans. B**

   Contributing factors can be classified into three major categories—contamination, survival (or failure to inactivate), and proliferation. Presence of a contributing factor alone is not sufficient to cause foodborne illness. Not all contributing factors have relevance with all causative agents, foods, or settings. Correction of contributing factors alone will not prevent the food safety problem from occurring again.

Identification (and correction) of underlying factors that led to the occurrence of contributing factors is necessary.

22. **Ans. D**

    The environmental health assessment will focus on the food vehicle implicated in an outbreak. The investigator will observe procedures used to make the implicated food during the period of interest, not all food preparation processes undertaken at the facility.

23. **Ans. D**

    Illnesses due to preformed toxins have short incubation periods, often measured in terms of minutes or hours. Illnesses due to infections have incubation periods that are relatively long, often measured in terms of days as compared to hours or minutes for intoxications. Gastrointestinal illnesses due to parasites, in general, have the longest incubation periods, ranging from 1–4 weeks.

24. **Ans. D**

    In a foodborne outbreak, subtyping of isolates from cases and food can be used to link cases together, link outbreaks in different geographic locations, link foods with outbreaks, and refine the case definition. Matching of subtypes, however, should not be considered proof of a common exposure among cases, merely that the isolates share a common ancestry. An epidemiologic investigation is necessary to demonstrate that there is a common source of exposure.

25. **Ans. B**

    To improve communications among team members, the team should hold regular meetings to share information, interpret findings, and decide on activities. The other activities in this question should be undertaken before an outbreak occurs.

26. **Ans. B**

    In most laboratories, "routine stool cultures" are limited to screening for *Salmonella* and *Shigella* species and *Campylobacter jejuni/coli*. Some laboratories now routinely test for Shiga toxin-producing *Escherichia coli* (STEC). Routine stool cultures do not cover viruses (the most common cause of outbreaks of foodborne illness), selected bacteria, or parasites.

27. **Ans. B**

    The purpose of the final report includes the following:
    - Documents what actually happened during the investigation and the results.
    - Records and clarifies recommended control and prevention measures.
    - Documents health department activities and performance and as such can help to justify necessary staffing and other resources for the future.
    - Acts as a public record that documents information in writing.
    - Allows investigators and others to learn from the experience.

    Although identifying what went well and what did not go well allows investigators to learn from the experience, there are better ways to deal with individual team members who did not complete their assigned tasks than identifying them in a public document.

28. **Ans. C**

    Campylobacter is a zoonosis, which can be acquired from several different animal sources, including food-source animals and companion animals. Although milk can be a source, it is not the main route of infection. The infectious dose is considered to be more than 10^4; although in immunocompromised individuals, it can be much less. The three most common MLST types in the UK are 21, 42, and 61.

    Ref:
    1. Olsen SJ Hansen GR, Bartlett L, Fitzgerald C, Sonder A, Manjrekar R, et al. An outbreak of Campylobacter jejuni infections associated with food handler contamination: the use of pulsed-field gel electrophoresis. J Infect Dis. 2001;183(1):164-7.

29. **Ans. B**

    Contamination can occur at any stage in meat production from source (e.g., *C. jejuni* is found in chickens commonly as part of their microbiome) to food preparation in the kitchen. The principles of preventing meat contamination are to stream the production process to prevent cross-contamination and personal hygiene particularly handwashing. Vaccines are being developed for poultry and sheep and a human vaccine is also in development.

    Ref:
    1. Wagenaar JA, French NP, Havelaar AH. Preventing Campylobacter at the source: why is it so difficult? Clin Infect Dis. 2013;57(11):1600-6.

30. **Ans. C**

    The report should be concise, but include the information necessary for the reader to draw the same conclusions as the investigators. Include summaries of the various investigations and both positive and negative findings, as appropriate. Do not include detailed data analyses, transcripts of interviews, or technical reports. If appropriate, they may be included as appendices.

CHAPTER 23

Nosocomial Infections

Ayesha J Sunavala, Indraneel Raut, Krutarth Kanjiya

Case 1

A 73-year-old diabetic lady was admitted with a cerebrovascular accident. During hospitalization, she was catheterized. 3 weeks later; her relatives noticed turbid urine in the urometer bag. Routine urine examination showed plenty of pus cells. There was repeated isolation of *Escherichia coli* with worsening resistance pattern on culture despite escalating antibiotic courses.

CULTURE AEROBES	URINE CULTURE ESCHERICHIA COLI	COLONY COUNT MIC µg/mL
Ampicillin	Resistant	>=32.0
Amox+Clavulanic Acid	Resistant	>=32.0
Piperacillin+Tazobactam	Resistant	>=128.
Cefuroxime	Resistant	>=64.0
Ceftriaxone	Resistant	>=64.0
Cefaperazone+Sulbactam	Resistant	>=64.0
Cefepime	Resistant	>=64.0
Ertapenem	Resistant	>=8.0
Imipenem	Resistant	>=16.0
Meropenem	Resistant	>=16.0
Amikacin	Resistant	>=64.0
Gentamicin	Resistant	>=16.0
Nalidixic Acid	Resistant	>=32.0
Ciprofloxacin	Resistant	>=4.0
Nitrofurantoin	Resistant	>=512.
Trimethoprim/Sulfamethoxa	Resistant	>=320.
SPECIMEN	URINE	

1. **How would you treat this patient?**
   A. Colistin
   B. Fosfomycin
   C. Change the Foley catheter
   D. None of the above

2. **If this patient developed fever with chills, leukocytosis and you suspected urosepsis, how would you manage this case?**
   A. Colistin/fosfomycin after checking minimum inhibitory concentrations (MICs)
   B. Change of Foley catheter only
   C. Repeat urine cesarean section (C/S) from a freshly placed catheter prior to commencing treatment
   D. Look for other source of infection as this is a catheterized sample and a likely colonizer

Case 2

A 42-year-old farmer from rural Maharashtra presented elsewhere with bilateral obstructive ureteric calculi. He underwent a lithotripsy procedure with bilateral DJ stent insertion. 6 days postprocedure, he developed sepsis with acute kidney injury (serum creatinine 22 mg%) for which he was transferred to our hospital.

He had received multiple antibiotics and was presently on meropenem and colistin.

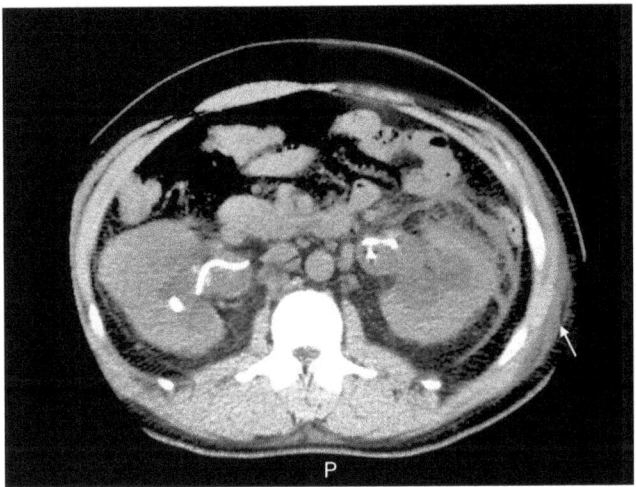

Computed tomography (CT) abdomen: Bilateral bulky kidneys with significant perinephric fat stranding. Obstructive calculus is noted involving the right pelvi-ureteral junction causing resultant right-sided moderate hydronephrosis. Multiple obstructive calculi are noted in the left lower ureter causing resultant upstream moderate hydronephrosis and hydroureter. DJ stent is seen in situ bilaterally.

The patient underwent right pyelolithotomy with bilateral DJ stent removal. Urine was collected for culture intraoperatively which grew *Candida* species.

3. **What are the indications for treating candiduria in general?**
   A. Neutropenic host
   B. Recent urinary instrumentation
   C. Low birth weight neonates
   D. All of the above

4. **Given that this is candidemia of a urinary tract source, what antifungal will you choose for treatment?**
   A. 5-flucytosine
   B. Voriconazole
   C. Micafungin
   D. Amphotericin B bladder wash

Case 3

A 79-year-old gentleman with advanced chronic obstructive pulmonary disease (COPD) was admitted to intensive care unit (ICU) in severe respiratory distress. He was intubated, ventilated, and required initial inotropic support for 48 hours. There was no growth on tracheal cultures sent during intubation; however, piperacillin tazobactam, azithromycin, and steroids were started empirically on admission for exacerbation of COPD. There was initial clinical improvement in symptoms; extubation was planned when he started spiking fever. The blood culture report sent from the central line is shown below. No peripheral percutaneous culture was sent.

The patient has had multiple access failures and the nephrologist is keen to preserve the line.

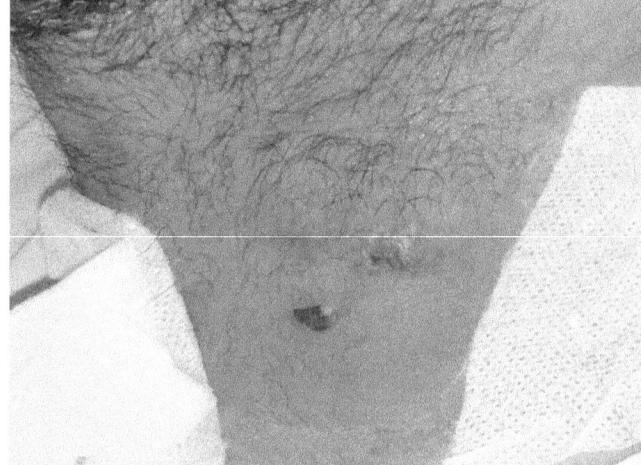

5. **What would you do?**
   A. Start vancomycin/teicoplanin
   B. Resend simultaneous culture samples from central line and percutaneous collection
   C. Remove central line and send the tip for culture
   D. Ignore the report, as this organism is a colonizer. Look for other sources of infection

Case 4

A 47-year-old gentleman with end-stage renal disease was on maintenance hemodialysis (HD) thrice weekly through a HD catheter placed in the right internal jugular vein. He complained of fever with chills post dialysis for the past 2 weeks, for which he received tablet cefixime clavulanate on an OPD basis. He was admitted with persistence of fever and severe lower back pain for the past 2 days.

On examination you notice purulence at the HD catheter exit site.

Simultaneously collected paired culture samples drawn from the catheter and left hand grow methicillin-susceptible *Staphylococcus aureus* (MSSA) with a positive DTP of 5 hours.

6. **How will you manage this case?**
   A. The HD catheter has to be removed in this case. Investigate for metastatic spread of infection—2D Echo, magnetic resonance imaging (MRI) spine and start appropriate culture-based antibiotics
   B. In view of difficult access, the HD catheter may be replaced over a guidewire by a new catheter at the same site
   C. Appropriate culture-based antibiotic systemically and as antibiotic lock therapy (ALT) may be attempted to salvage the catheter
   D. Appropriate culture-based antibiotic systemically and as ALT may be attempted to salvage the catheter plus investigate for metastatic spread of infection—2D Echo, MRI spine

7. **Of the following, what would be the most appropriate choice of antibiotic and duration of treatment in this case?**
   A. Vancomycin/teicoplanin for 14 days
   B. Vancomycin/teicoplanin for 14 days followed by oral linezolid for 1 month
   C. Vancomycin/teicoplanin for 6–8 weeks
   D. Cloxacillin/cefazolin for 14 days
   E. Cloxacillin/cefazolin for 6–8 weeks

Case 5

A 62-year-old diabetic lady with diverticulitis underwent a laparotomy for a sealed diverticular perforation.

16 days postoperative; she developed fever, leukocytosis, and seropurulent discharge from the surgical site.

She was started on empirical cefoperazone-sulbactam after which the symptoms resolved completely.

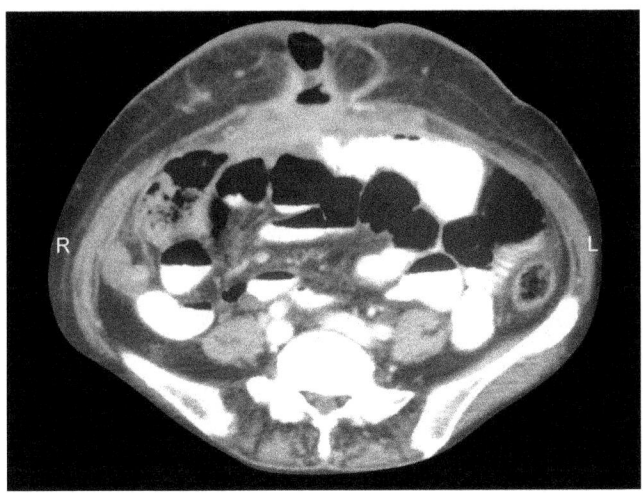

Contrast-enhanced CT (CECT) abdomen: Intestinal loop adherent to the abdominal wall but no evidence of contrast leak.

Enterococcus spp. was isolated on wound swab Culture & Sensitivity (C/S).

8. What is your treatment plan?
   A. Change to ampicillin/linezolid
   B. Switch to ampicillin + gentamicin
   C. Continue cefoperazone-sulbactam (since the patient responding)
   D. Escalate to meropenem

Case 6

A 56-year-old gentleman underwent laparoscopic inguinal hernioplasty. He presented 4 months later with wound gape and multiple purulent discharging sinuses. Surgical debridement with removal of hernioplasty mesh is performed. Intraoperative Culture & Sensitivity (C/S) are as:
- AFB smear positive
- *GeneXpert: Mycobacterium tuberculosis* (MTB) not detected.

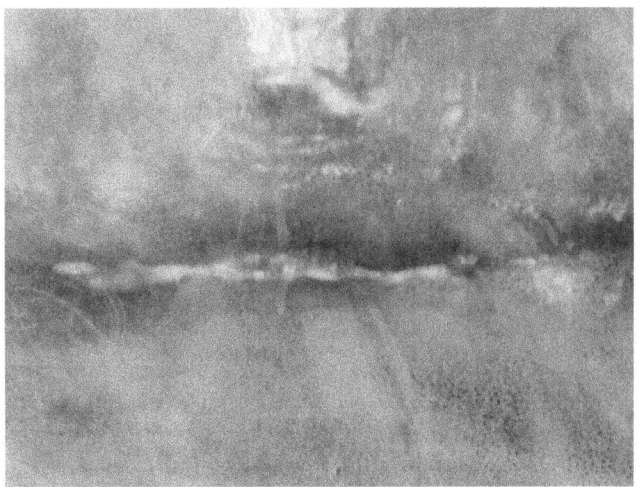

9. What will you do next?
   A. Ignore the report, wait for culture
   B. Start rifampicin isoniazid ethambutol and pyrazinamide
   C. Collect additional pus/tissue and repeat gene Xpert test
   D. None of the above

10. The infection control measures to prevent NTM contamination of endoscopes are all, *except*:
   A. Laparoscopes/arthroscopes should be completely disassembled, immersed in an enzymatic detergent and meticulously flushed and cleaned to manually remove all organic debris
   B. Disinfection with glutaraldehyde 2% for 10 minutes
   C. Disinfection with orthophthalaldehyde for 12 minutes
   D. Autoclaving or plasma sterilization

Case 7

A 72-year-old diabetic with a history of chronic alcohol abuse is on oral and inhaled steroids for chronic obstructive airway disease. He is recently diagnosed with carcinoma lung and has completed 6 cycles of chemotherapy.

He is now admitted with progressive lower back pain, paresthesiae and weakness in the lower limbs. MRI shows a prolapsed intervertebral disk and the patient is posted for decompressive laminectomy.

A reference is given to decide on appropriate perioperative surgical prophylaxis in view of his numerous comorbidities.

11. **What will you choose?**
    A. Cefoperazone-sulbactam
    B. Vancomycin
    C. Cefazolin (first-generation cephalosporin)
    D. Cefotaxime (third-generation cephalosporin)
    E. Something else

12. **What will you advise?**
    A. No change in prophylaxis
    B. Change to vancomycin/teicoplanin
    C. Cefazolin plus vancomycin
    D. Defer surgery

Case 8

A 24-year-old female suffered an open comminuted, displaced fracture of the left tibial condyle due to a tractor injury on a farm. She underwent surgical debridement and fixation elsewhere. No intraoperative culture was sent. On the 10th postoperative day, redness and purulence were noted at the surgical site followed by fever and leukocytosis 48 hours later. A surgical wound swab was collected and sent for culture which grew below organism.

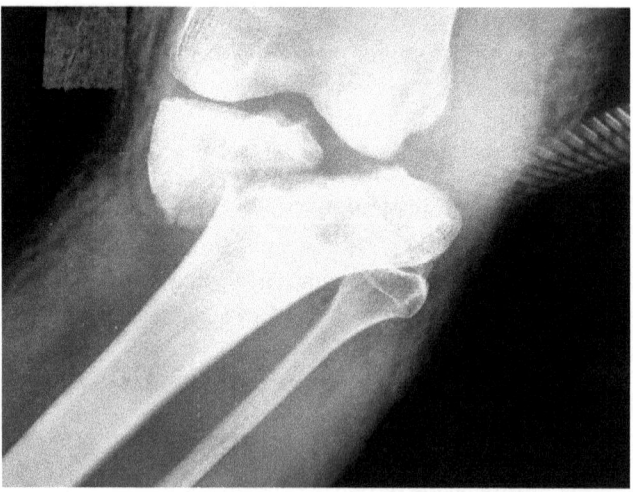

WOUND SWAB CULTURE	
GRAM STAIN (PRIMARY)	
Organisms	NOT APPARENT
ZIEHL NIELSON STAIN (AFB)	
Acid Fast Bacilli	NOT SEEN
CULTURE AEROBES	COAGULASE NEGATIVE STAPHYLOCOCCI
Ampicillin	Resistant
Methicilin / Oxacillin	Resistant
Amox+Clavulanic Acid	Resistant
Cefazolin	Resistant
Cefuroxime / Cefaclor	Resistant
Cefotaxime	Resistant
Ceftriaxone/Cefixime	Resistant
Erythromycin / Azithromyci	Susceptible
Clindamycin	Susceptible
Tetracycline / Doxycycline	Susceptible
Co-trimoxazole	Susceptible
Chloramphenicol	Susceptible
Gentamicin	Susceptible
Netilmicin	Susceptible
Amikacin	Susceptible
Ciprofloxacin / Ofloxacin	Susceptible
Rifampicin	Susceptible
Vancomycin/Teicoplanin	Susceptible
Linezolid	Susceptible

13. **How will you treat this patient?**
    A. Broad-spectrum gram-negative and positive cover as this was a contaminated soil injury and the patient is in impending sepsis
    B. Clindamycin/linezolid for SSI due to CoNS
    C. Insist on redebridement with intraoperative cultures followed by empiric broad-spectrum cover
    D. Repeat a wound swab and start empiric broad spectrum cover

Case 9

A 54-year-old male underwent permanent pacemaker insertion (PPI) for sick sinus syndrome. 3 weeks later, he is admitted with intermittent fever with chills and malaise. He has no other symptoms. The PPI site has minimal overlying inflammation with no discharge. However, there is minimal tenderness over the area.

An ultrasonography (USG) of the local area is done which reveals a pocket collection 2 × 3 cm.

USG-guided aspiration of the collection shows growth of *P. aeruginosa*.

Organisms CULTURE AEROBES	CULTURE BILE NOT APPARENT PSEUDOMONAS AERUGINOSA	MIC µg/mL
Ticarcillin/Clavulanic Acid	Resistant	>=128.
Piperacillin+Tazobactam	Resistant	>=128.
Ceftazidime	Resistant	>=64.0
Cefaperazone+Sulbactam	Resistant	>=64.0
Cefepime	Resistant	>=64.0
Aztreonam	Resistant	=32.0
Doripenem	Resistant	>=8.0
Imipenem	Resistant	>=16.0
Meropenem	Resistant	=8.0
Amikacin	Susceptible	<=2.0
Gentamicin	Susceptible	<=1.0
Ciprofloxacin	Susceptible	<=0.25
Levofloxacin	Susceptible	=1.0

SPECIMEN: BILE
Comments: Rich growth

14. **How will you manage this case?**
    A. Start appropriate antibiotics
    B. 2D Echo to rule out infective endocarditis (IE)
    C. Early removal of PPI with insertion of new pacemaker if required at another site
    D. All of the above

Case 10

A 51-year-old gentleman, known case of osteoarthritis underwent right total knee replacement. On follow-up, 2 weeks postoperatively, wound gape was noted. He was treated with multiple courses of oral antibiotics over the next few months for persistent pain and surgical site inflammation. 5 months postoperative, a USG-guided aspiration of the knee joint isolated carbapenem-resistant *Klebsiella pneumoniae*, susceptible to colistin alone.

CULTURE AEROBES	KLEBSIELLA PNEUMONIAE	MIC µg/mL
Ampicillin	Resistant	>=32
Amox+Clavulanic Acid	Resistant	>=32
Piperacillin+Tazobactam	Resistant	>=128
Cefuroxime	Resistant	>=64
Ceftriaxone	Resistant	>=64
Cefaperazone+Sulbactam	Resistant	>=64
Cefepime	Resistant	>=64
Ertapenem	Resistant	>=8
Imipenem	Resistant	>=16
Meropenem	Resistant	>=16
Amikacin	Resistant	>=64
Gentamicin	Resistant	>=16
Nalidixic Acid	Resistant	>=32
Ciprofloxacin	Resistant	>=4
Nitrofurantoin	Resistant	=128
Trimethoprim/Sulfamethoxa	Resistant	>=320
Colistin	Resistant	>=16

15. **What is the most appropriate management option for this patient?**
    A. No surgical procedure, chronic suppressive antibiotic therapy alone
    B. Debridement and retention of implant with appropriate antibiotics
    C. One stage joint revision with appropriate antibiotics
    D. Two stage joint revision with appropriate antibiotics
    E. Removal of prosthetic implant, arthrodesis

16. **The surgeon seeks your opinion on the duration of antibiotics and plan for joint revision:**
    A. 6 weeks of antibiotic followed by 2 weeks antibiotic free interval followed by joint revision
    B. 4 weeks of IV antibiotic followed by joint revision
    C. 2 weeks of antibiotic followed by joint revision followed by 2 weeks of antibiotic
    D. 6 weeks of antibiotic followed by 2 weeks antibiotic free interval followed by aspiration and culture

Case 11

67-year-old male; K/C/O Ca gallbladder (GB)-inoperable as GB mass was adherent to liver and extending to involve the duodenum. The patient underwent a percutaneous trans biliary drainage procedure with internalization of the stent. Chemotherapy was started. 6 weeks later, he presented with fever with chills, abdominal pain, dyspepsia, nausea, and cholestatic jaundice.

The patient was started on empiric meropenem and biliary stent was changed. Blood culture sent on admission was sterile.

He improved for 48 hours followed by recurrence of high grade fever with chills, leukocytosis and increase in bilirubin.

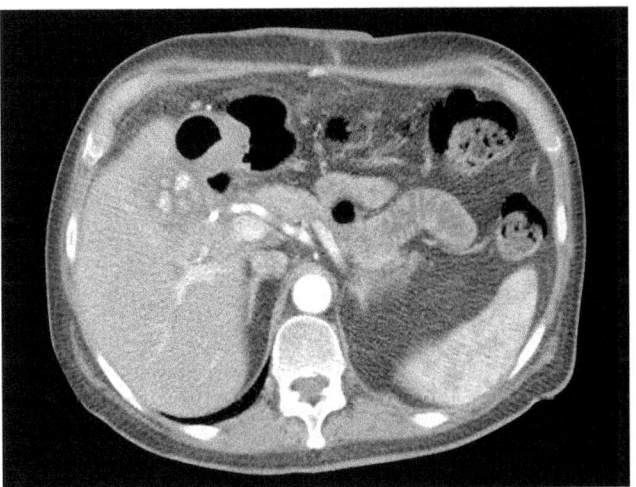

17. **What organisms can be expected in this case of biliary sepsis with a biliary stent in situ?**
    A. *Klebsiella pneumoniae*
    B. MRSA
    C. *Pseudomonas aeruginosa*
    D. *Candida* species
    E. All of the above

18. **How will you further treat this patient?**
    A. Add teicoplanin to meropenem
    B. Add teicoplanin and caspofungin to meropenem
    C. Change to tigecycline in view of broad spectrum cover and excellent biliary penetration
    D. None of the above

Case 12

A 63-year-old male; DM/HTN/old CVA admitted with sudden onset vomiting followed by loss of consciousness.

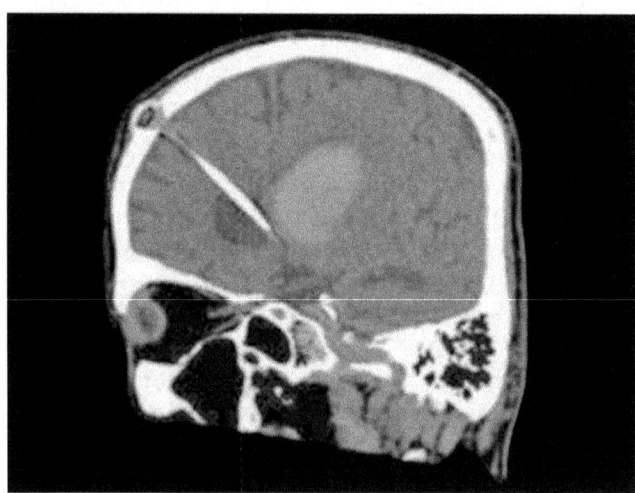
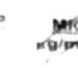

A CT brain revealed IC bleed with intraventricular hemorrhage and hydrocephalus. An emergency craniotomy was performed with insertion of Ommaya reservoir and external ventricular drain (EVD). He remained unconscious but stable in ICU postoperatively.

On the 8th postoperative day; he developed fever spikes. Cerebrospinal fluid (CSF) analysis showed neutrophilic leukocytosis.

19. **What is true about this organism?**
    A. It is a gram-positive bacillus
    B. It is usually a culture contaminant and should be ignored
    C. It has been isolated in the hospital environment in water supplies, disinfectants, and medical devices
    D. It is an opportunistic pathogen and only causes infections in neonates and immunocompromised hosts

20. **What is true regarding intrathecal/intraventricular antibiotic administration for meningitis?**
    A. Although not routinely recommended for treatment of bacterial meningitis, it is an option for adjunctive therapy to IV antibiotics in infections due to multidrug-resistant organisms (MDROs), refractory infections, and device-associated nosocomial meningitis
    B. Intrathecal/intraventricular β-lactams are avoided due to risk of seizure
    C. When administered through the EVD, the ventricular drain should be clamped for at least 1 hour after instillation to allow the drug to equilibrate throughout the CSF
    D. Drug dosages and intervals should be adjusted based on CSF antimicrobial concentrations, to 10–20 times the MIC of the causative microorganism, ventricular size, and daily output from the ventricular drain
    E. All of the above

Case 13

A 68-year-old female; Uncontrolled DM, CHF, CLD presented elsewhere with a gluteal abscess.

She received multiple antibiotics on an OPD basis (FQNs, linezolid, and cefixime), finally underwent an I&D as there was no clinical response to antibiotics.

She was admitted to ICU a few days later with high grade fever, leukocytosis 23,000/cmm, hypotension and respiratory distress. She had bilateral crackles on auscultation and chest X-ray was suggestive of pulmonary edema. Tenderness and induration were appreciable at the local site.

Blood cultures were sent on admission and the patient was started on empiric meropenem and teicoplanin.

MRI revealed a gluteal abscess with ileosacral osteomyelitis. After hemodynamic stabilization, the patient was taken up for surgical debridement. Intraoperative cultures as well as blood C/S were sterile, hence, meropenem and teicoplanin were continued.

On the 8th postoperative day, the patient developed fever and white blood cell (WBC) started rising once again. She also complained of 7–8 episodes of watery stools in the past 24 hours.

Given, the history of multiple broad-spectrum antibiotics, you suspect *Clostridium difficile*-associated diarrhea (CDAD).

21. **How will you confirm the diagnosis of CDAD?**
    A. Stool glutamate dehydrogenase (GDH)
    B. Stool *C. difficile* nucleic acid amplification test (NAAT)
    C. Stool toxin assay
    D. GDH + toxin/NAAT
    E. Both B and D

22. **It seems difficult to stop antibiotics at this stage, how will you treat this patient?**
    A. Oral vancomycin
    B. Fidaxomicin
    C. Oral metronidazole
    D. Oral vancomycin + IV metronidazole

Case 14

The infection control team of your hospital has been alerted in view of three cases of CDAD in the general ward over the past week.

23. **What practical measures can the team take to contain the outbreak?**
    A. Evacuate the patients from the affected ward, close, and fumigate
    B. Screen all patients in the ward-rectal swab for *C. difficile* toxin and offer prophylaxis to positive contacts
    C. Healthcare workers (HCW) to follow hand hygiene protocols with (chlorhexidine hand rub) before and after contact with the patient or his/her surroundings
    D. None of the above

Case 15

A 54-year-old male diabetic, renal transplant recipient presented 4 years post-transplant with dry cough for several days followed by fever. He was on triple immunosuppressants—mycophenolate mofetil (MMF), tacrolimus and steroids. WBC count on admission was 10,600/cmm. Chest X-ray showed multiple bilateral dense nodules.

Detailed history revealed that he had received pulse methylprednisolone for acute cellular rejection followed by increase in maintenance steroids. No chemoprophylaxis was given following this.

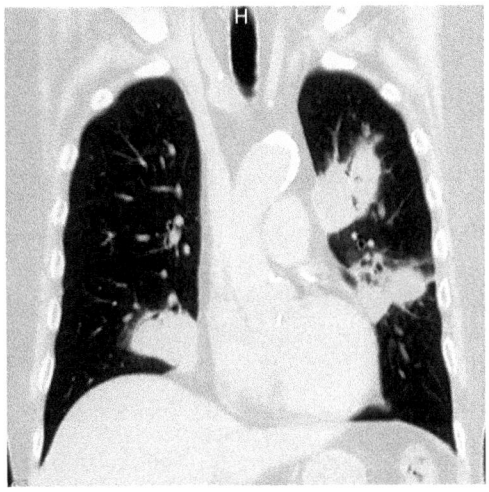

24. **What empiric treatment would you start?**
    A. Piperacillin tazobactam, and vancomycin
    B. First-line antitubercular treatment
    C. Ceftriaxone, linezolid, and TMP SMX
    D. Voriconazole
    E. None of the above

25. **What is true regarding this organism?**
    A. Slow growing, ubiquitous organism found in the environment and water sources
    B. Unlike MTB, drug-susceptibility testing need not be done to guide antimicrobial therapy
    C. May be a pathogen or an environmental contaminant especially in respiratory secretions. Nosocomial pseudoinfections related to contaminated bronchoscopes are known
    D. All of the above

Case 16

A 45-year-old homemaker, known case of multiple myeloma, was admitted for allogeneic bone marrow transplant (on acyclovir and posaconazole prophylaxis).

D+17 post-transplant, she developed abdominal pain, loose motions followed by fever 2 days later. She was empirically commenced on meropenem and teicoplanin and shifted to ICU due to clinical deterioration and hypotension. Her blood pressure normalized with a fluid challenge. Blood and urine cultures were sterile and *S. procalcitonin* was negative. Multiplex PCR on a stool sample was positive for *Giardia lamblia* which was treated with metronidazole. The diarrhea gradually resolved, neutrophil count normalized indicating engraftment;

however, fever persisted. Fever chart and USG abdomen are given below.

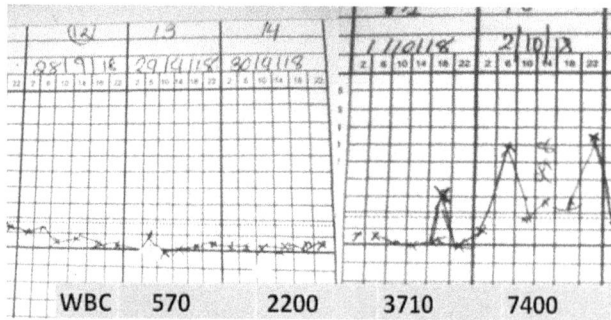

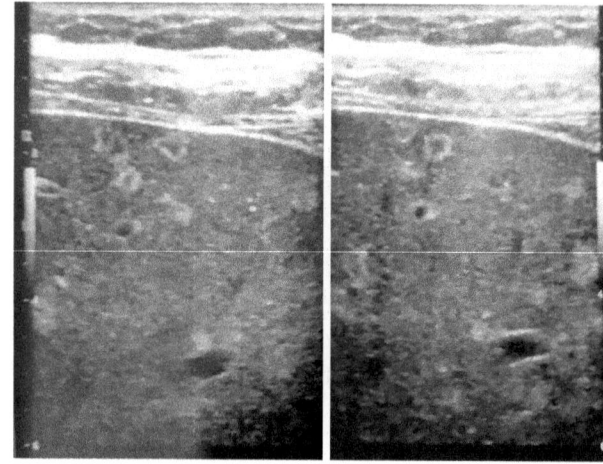

26. **What is the most likely cause for fever?**
    A. Gram-negative bacterial sepsis
    B. Disease-related fever
    C. Intestinal giardiasis
    D. Hepatosplenic candidiasis

27. **Patient was on syrup posaconazole antifungal prophylaxis. What is the most likely cause of failure of prophylaxis in this case?**
    A. Resistant *Candida* spp.
    B. Missed doses
    C. Diarrhea causing reduced drug concentrations
    D. Drug interactions with cyclosporine

28. **What is the duration of treatment for hepatosplenic candidiasis?**
    A. Until resolution of fever and negative blood culture reports
    B. Three months
    C. Complete resolution of radiological findings
    D. 6 months

Case 17

A 44-year-old female C/O AML on induction chemotherapy developed febrile neutropenia with severe mucositis and diarrhea. She was started on empiric meropenem and vancomycin. Blood C/S from the chemotherapy port and periphery were sterile.

Fever spikes initially subsided, though she remained profoundly neutropenic and diarrhea persisted.

5 days later, fever spikes recurred and she was shifted to ICU with breathlessness and hypotension. Polymyxin B was added and blood cultures were repeated. Catheterized urine and sputum culture grew *C. albicans*.

SENSITIVITY ATB SPECIMEN	URINE
CULTURE AEROBES	CANDIDA ALBICANS
Flucytosine	* (<=1) mcg/ml
Amphotericin B	* (<=0.25) mcg/ml
Fluconazole	Susceptible(<=0.5) mcg/ml
Voriconazole	Susceptible(<=0.12)mcg/ml
Caspofungin	Susceptible(<=0.12)mcg/ml

29. **How would you interpret her reports?**
    A. Ignore them, *Candida* species isolated from catheterized urine or sputum are always colonizers
    B. Calculate candida colonization score and treat accordingly as candida prediction scores have high positive predictive value
    C. Start empirical antifungal in view of multiple risk factors in this patient
    D. Await blood culture reports

30. **Blood culture from chemo port and percutaneous collection grow the same organism after which the chemo port is removed. How will you further manage this case?**
    A. Continue antifungal treatment for 14 days after the 1st positive blood culture report
    B. Step up from fluconazole to echinocandin and continue echinocandin for the entire duration of treatment
    C. Advise a 2D Echo and fundoscopy to rule out metastatic complications
    D. All of the above

31. **The patient improves. 2D Echo is normal. Fundoscopy performed during recovery from neutropenia reveals bilateral retinal deposits with macular involvement. How will you manage this complication?**
    A. Bilateral vitrectomy
    B. Intravitreal amphotericin B administration
    C. Intravitreal amphotericin B and systemic fluconazole
    D. Any of the above

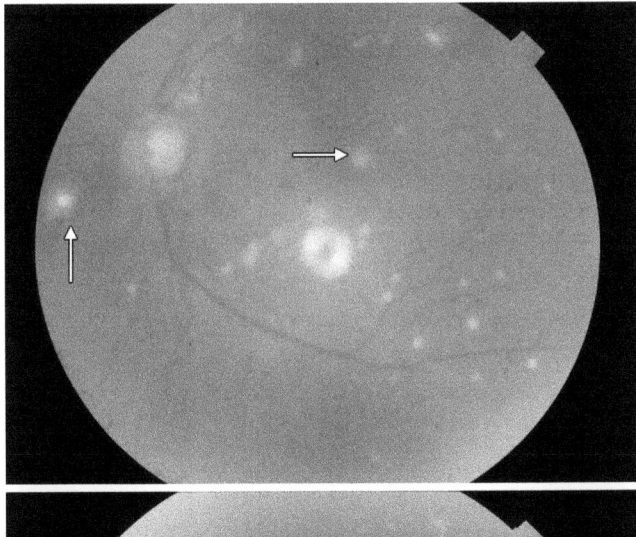

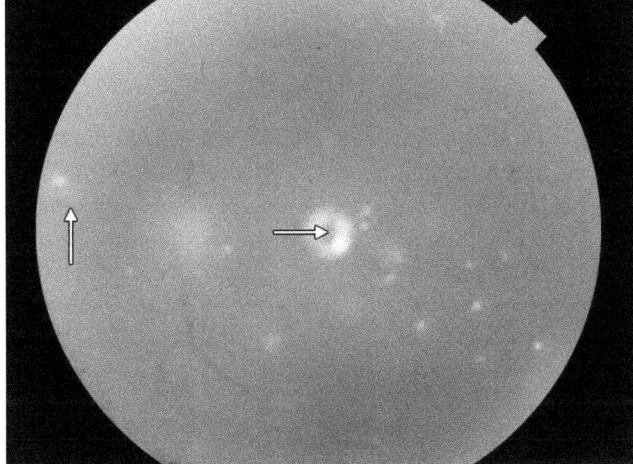

Case 18

A 65-year-old male; K/C/O DM, COPD on inhaled steroids and short course of oral steroids for exacerbation was admitted to ICU with high grade fever, cough with purulent expectoration and respiratory distress. WBC—19,500/cmm. The patient was intubated and ventilated.

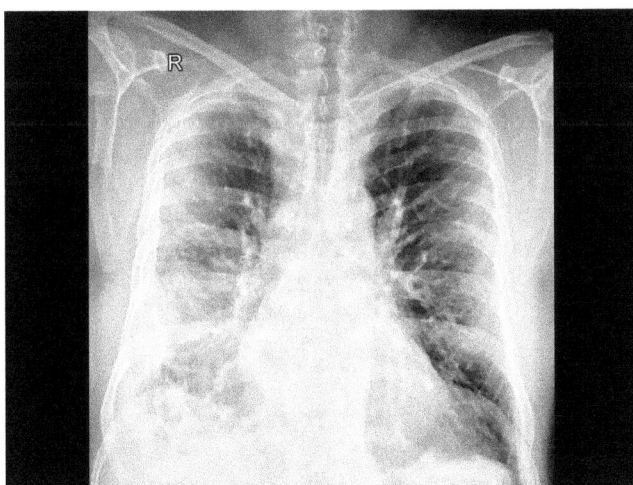

Blood and sputum C/S grew carbapenem-resistant *K. pneumoniae* (CRKP) for which he was started on colistin and minocycline.

Fever spikes started reducing but the patient failed multiple weaning attempts and on day 7, a chest X-ray showed new bilateral consolidates.

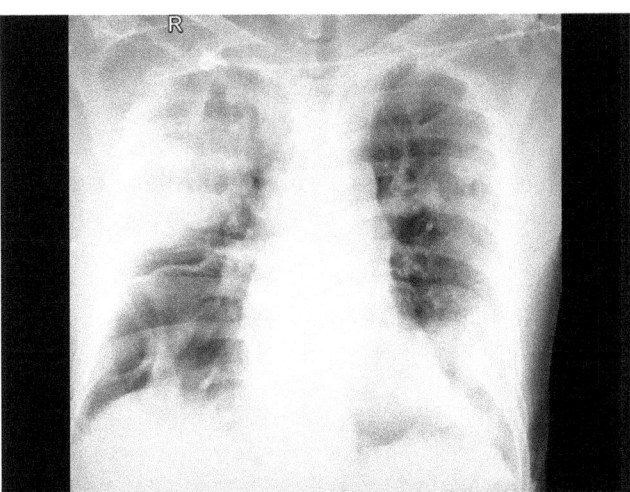

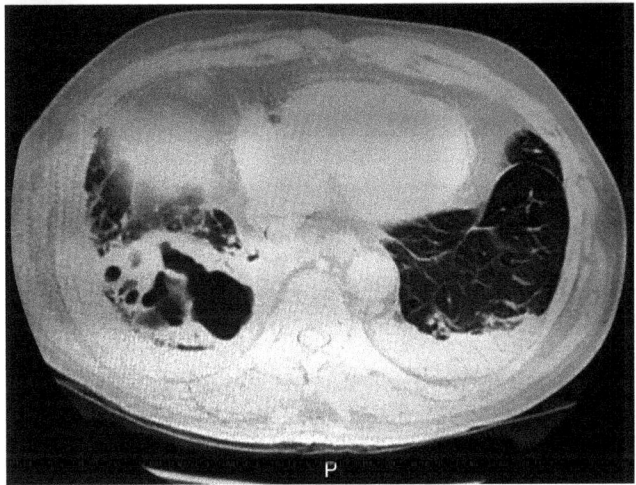

CT chest and pulmonary angiography: Irregular cavitating lesion in right lower lobe, pleural effusions.

Scattered irregular nodules bilaterally? Necrotizing pneumonia.

Bronchoalveolar lavage is performed.

ASPERGILLUS GALACTOMANNAN			
Sample : BRONCHIAL ALVEOLAR LAVAGE			
Test	Result	Units	Significant Titre
ASPERGILLUS GALACTOMANNAN	5		
Patients value	5.743		Negative < 0.500
			Positive >= 0.500
Results	POSITIVE		

Comments Test Method: Immunoenzymatic sandwich microplate assay
Comments Limitations of the test
1. A negative test cannot rule out the diagnosis of Invasive Aspergillosis.
2. Patients at risk for Invasive Aspergillosis should be tested twice a week
3. The concomitant use of mold-active anti-fungal therapy in some patients with invasive Aspergillosis may result in reduced sensitivity
4. Other molds such as Penicillium, Alternaria and Paecilomyces may give false positive results.
5. False positives may also occur with dietary cereals, humanized milk, pasta and antibiotics such as Piperacillin/Tazobactam and Amoxycillin/Clavulanic Acid

32. **Which statement is true regarding pulmonary aspergillosis?**
    A. IPA is unlikely in the absence of characteristic radiological features like halo sign and cavitating nodules
    B. IPA only occurs in patients with neutropenia and malignancy
    C. Galactomannan (GM) is found in cell wall of *Aspergillus* species
    D. Serum GM is more useful than BAL for diagnosis of IPA in non-neutropenic patients

33. **Which of the following is not correct about diagnosis of SSI?**
    A. Superficial incisional SSI includes event occurring within 30 days after any National Healthcare Safety Network (NHSN) operation procedure
    B. Superficial incisional SSI involves infection of skin and subcutaneous tissue
    C. Stitch abscess alone (minimal inflammation and confined to the point of suture penetration) also is a superficial SSI
    D. Criteria for of deep incisional SSI requires the event to occur within 30 days of procedure or within 6 months if implant is inserted

34. **Which of the following statement about coagulase-negative *Staphylococcus* (CoNS) infection is true?**
    A. *Staphylococcus epidermidis* is one of the common causes of native valve endocarditis
    B. *S. epidermidis* is a common pathogen in UTI
    C. *S. saprophyticus* is a common cause of prosthetic valve endocarditis
    D. *S. lugdunensis* and *S. schleiferi* are CoNS species which are known to produce more serious infection like native valve endocarditis and osteomyelitis

35. **Which of the following is untrue about *Clostridium difficile* infection?**
    A. Majority of humans first develop antibody to *C. difficile* when colonized asymptomatically during the first year of life or after CDI in childhood
    B. Discontinuation of any ongoing antimicrobial administration is recommended as first step in treatment of CDI
    C. Negative examination of pseudomembranous colitis (PMC) on colonoscopy does not rule out CDI
    D. IV vancomycin is an effective treatment of *C. difficile* in fulminant episodes of CDI

36. **A 56-year-old female presented with history of fever with cough since 1 week and severe weakness and purulent sputum. She has history of bronchial asthma and takes SOS inhalers for the same. She was admitted to ICU in view of tachypnea and hypoxemia on background of bronchial asthma. Patient was conscious, alert. No headache. X-ray showed nodular infection and sputum sent for microscopy and AFB.**
    Sugar was 446 mg/dL. Not a known diabetic but gave history of diabetes in family. Sputum culture reported growth of gram positive filamentous bacilli. Treatment of initial choice in patient care:
    A. IV Amikacin
    B. IV Ceftriaxone
    C. IV (trimethoprim + SMX) + amikacin + ceftriaxone or imipenem initially
    D. Doxycycline + amikacin

37. **Following statements regarding control of MRSA are true, *except*:**
    A. Active surveillance cultures appear to be the most useful in the setting of hospital outbreaks and among patients at risk of MRSA carriage
    B. Active surveillance strategies involved a multifaceted approach including surveillance contact isolation, HCWs screening with decolonization and closing units for comprehensive screening and cleaning when warranted
    C. Decolonization regimen for reducing likelihood of subsequent MRSA infections postdischarge indicates 0.5% rinse of chlorhexidine for daily bath and showering
    D. Decolonization strategy in outpatient setting includes (for both patient and household members) nasal application of 2% mupirocin and topical body decolonization with either chlorhexidine (2% or 4%) daily washes for 14 days or dilute bleach baths for 15 minutes twice weekly for approximately 3 months

38. **A 62-year-old male patient was on chemotherapy for NHL. After her second cycle of chemotherapy patient presented with high grade fever, weakness, and breathlessness. Patient was found to be tachypneic and in hypertension. ABG showed severe metabolic acidosis. Patient had developed a black necrotic lesion on the face where he gave history of being nicked while shaving. Blood culture grew GNB.**
    What would be the treating strategy?
    A. Carbapenem + aminoglycosides
    B. Ceftazidime alone
    C. Aminoglycosides alone
    D. IV colistin alone

39. **Which of the following is true about *C. auris*?**
    A. *Candida auris* is associated with high mortality rates

B. *Candida auris* requires specialized methods for identification of as it is often misidentified as another yeast commonly *C. haemulonii* or *C. famata*
C. Initial treatment of choice is echinocandin
D. If patient does not respond to an echinocandin or has persistent candidemia for 5 days the patient should be switched to amphotericin B

40. A 60-year-old gentleman was recovering from a spine surgery for which he was catheterized. On day 4 developed high grade fever with chills and by day 5 developed hypotension and shock. Patient was shifted to ICU. Meanwhile, urine showed 60–70 pus cells/cmm and urine culture had growth of gram positive diplococci which are nonhemolytic. Meanwhile, blood culture also reported growth of similar organism. The growth were then confirmed as ampicillin and vancomycin-resistant *E. faecium*. What is treatment of choice?
    A. Removal of catheter. No antibiotics
    B. Removal of catheter plus IV Linezolid 600 mg 12 hourly
    C. IV daptomycin 5-6 mg/kg with ampicillin
    D. Oral fosfomycin 3 g per orally one dose

41. Which of the following about treatment of enterococcal infection is not true?
    A. Linezolid IV 600 mg 12 hourly ± another CSF penetrating active agent (fluoroquinolone or rifampicin), if susceptible is one of the regimen in meningitis due to VRE *E. faecium*
    B. Dose of ampicillin for *E. faecium* UTI is 2 g IV or orally 6 hourly
    C. Daptomycin can be used for pulmonary infections due to *E. faecalis*
    D. Resistance of enterococci to linezolid is usually due to mutation in 23S *rRAA* genes or the presence of rRNA

42. A 58-year-old farmer from Karnataka was brought to casualty with tachypnea, history of fever since 2 days with RASH and severe pain, myalgia, and headache. He complains of severe nausea and vomiting. A papule with necrosis was seen on the trunk. On examination, patients investigation revealed leukocytosis, deranged liver functions, and raised serum creatinine. Patient has fever of 101°F but her heart rate was 88 beats/min. There was history of similar illness in many workers who were working in his farm. Along with other investigation biopsy from the papule with necrosis showed lymphohistiocytic vasculitis. What would be the treatment of choice?
    A. Doxycycline 100 mg twice a day for 7–15 days
    B. Tetracycline 100 mg daily
    C. IV tigecycline
    D. Chloramphenicol 500 mg 6 hourly

43. Which of the following statement is true about treatment of seasonal influenza likely H1N1?
    A. Children 6 months to 18 years on chronic aspirin therapy are considered high-risk group
    B. Salicylate/aspirin is strongly contraindicated to be given in any influenza patient due to its potential to cause Reye's syndrome
    C. High-dose corticosteroids have been found to be helpful in patients of septic shock and MODS with H1N1
    D. Suspected case not having pneumonia does not require antibiotic therapy

44. Which of the following statement about *Acinetobacter* infections is correct?
    A. *Acinetobacter* usually does not cause community-acquired infections
    B. *Acinetobacter baumannii* is the least resistant of genospecies
    C. *Acinetobacter junii* has been described as an opportunistic pathogen in the setting of prior antimicrobial therapy, invasive procedures, and malignancy
    D. *Acinetobacter* species are gram-negative coccobacilli, strictly aerobic, ferment glucose, and oxidase positive

ANSWERS WITH EXPLANATIONS

1. **Ans. D**
   Catheter-associated urinary tract infection (CA-UTI) in patients with indwelling urethral, indwelling suprapubic, or intermittent catheterization is defined by the presence of symptoms or signs compatible with UTI with no other identified source of infection along with 1,000 colony forming units (cfu)/mL of ≥1 bacterial species in a single catheter urine specimen or in a midstream-voided urine specimen from a patient whose urethral, suprapubic, or condom catheter has been removed within the previous 48 hours.
   Signs and symptoms compatible with CA-UTI include new onset or worsening of fever, rigors, altered mental status, malaise, and lethargy with no other identified

cause. Additionally, flank pain, costovertebral angle tenderness, acute hematuria, or pelvic discomfort is also considered as positive signs. The presence of cloudy urine or pyuria alone, as seen in this patient is not considered diagnostic of CA-UTI.

Catheter-associated asymptomatic bacteriuria (CA-ASB) in patients with indwelling urethral, indwelling suprapubic, or intermittent catheterization is defined by the presence of 100,000 cfu/mL of ≥1 bacterial species in a single catheter urine specimen in a patient without symptoms compatible with UTI. In patients with an indwelling catheter, urine should not be routinely screened as patients with urinary catheters often have multiple organisms isolated from the urine due to the universal formation of a biofilm along the indwelling catheter. Acquisition of bacteriuria is 3–5% per catheter day. Antimicrobials can temporarily suppress the bacteriuria, but often recurrence occurs with the same or different species, often with organisms of increased antimicrobial resistance. Hence, it is advisable not to treat ASB from catheterized urine samples.

Ref:
1. Hooton TM, Bradley SF, Cardenas DD, Colgan R, Geerlings SE, Rice JC, et al. Diagnosis, prevention, and treatment of catheter-associated urinary tract infection in adults: 2009 International Clinical Practice Guidelines from the Infectious Diseases Society of America. Clin Infect Dis. 2010;50(5):625-63.

2. **Ans. C**

As discussed above, isolated organisms likely represent contamination of the urine specimen from organisms present in the biofilm along the device rather than true bacteriuria. In such cases, if CA-UTI is suspected in a symptomatic patient, urine culture should be obtained following insertion of a fresh indwelling catheter prior to the initiation of antimicrobial therapy.

Ref:
1. Nicolle LE, Gupta K, Bradley SF, Colgan R, DeMuri GP, Drekonja D, et al. Clinical practice guideline for the management of asymptomatic bacteriuria: 2019 Update by the Infectious Diseases Society of America. Clin Infect Dis. 2019;68(10)e83-e110.

3. **Ans. D**

Patients who are elderly, female, diabetic, have indwelling urinary devices, broad-spectrum antibiotics or recent surgical procedures are at the greatest risk for candiduria. In the asymptomatic patient, candiduria usually represents colonization. Elimination of underlying risk factors, such as indwelling catheters, is often adequate to eradicate candiduria and treatment is not routinely warranted in these patients.

Definite indications to treat candiduria are:
- Neutropenic patients
- Very low birth weight infants (<1,500 g)
- Patients who will undergo urologic manipulation.

Ref:
1. Pappas PG, Kauffman CA, Andes DR, Clancy CJ, Marr KA, Ostrosky-Zeichner L, et al. Clinical practice guideline for the management of candidiasis: 2016 Update by the Infectious Diseases Society of America. Clin Infect Dis. 2016;62(4):e1-e50.

A blood culture sent on admission suggests:

Test	Result
SENSITIVITY ATB SPECIMEN	BLOOD
CULTURE AEROBES	CANDIDA AURIS
Flucytosine	* (>=64) µg/mL
Amphotericin B	* (8) µg/mL
Fluconazole	* (32) µg/mL
Voriconazole	* (4) µg/mL
Caspofungin	* (0.25) µg/mL
Micafungin	* (0.12) µg/mL
Comments	* Guidelines not defined for interpretation.

4. **Ans. C**

Candida auris is considered a *Candida* superbug, causing healthcare-associated outbreaks across the world. It is usually multidrug resistant and may be misidentified with standard laboratory methods, hence inappropriately treated.

There are currently no established susceptibility breakpoints *for C. auris*. Therefore, breakpoints are defined based on those established for closely related *Candida* species and on expert opinion.

In April 2019, Centers for Disease Control and Prevention (CDC) published the following guide to interpret antifungal susceptibility of *C. auris*. There is no known correlation between microbiologic breakpoints and clinical outcomes, hence this information should be considered as a general guide and not as definitive breakpoints for resistance.

Drugs	Tentative MIC breakpoints (µg/mL)	Comment
Fluconazole	≥32	Modal minimum inhibitory concentration (MIC) to fluconazole among isolates tested at CDC was ≥ 256; isolates with MICs ≥ 32 were shown to have a resistance mutation in the *Erg11* gene, making them unlikely to respond to fluconazole.

Contd...

Contd...

Drugs	Tentative MIC breakpoints (µg/mL)	Comment
Voriconazole and other second generation triazoles	N/A	Consider using fluconazole susceptibility as a surrogate for second generation triazole susceptibility assessment. However, isolates that are resistant to fluconazole may respond to other triazoles occasionally. The decision to treat with another triazole will need to be made on case-by-case basis
Amphotericin B	≥2	Recent pharmacokinetic/ pharmacodynamic analysis of *C. auris* in a mouse model of infection indicates that under standard dosing, the breakpoint for amphotericin B should be 1 or 1.5, similar to what has been determined for other *Candida* species. Therefore, isolates with an MIC of ≥2 should now be considered resistant. If using E-test for amphotericin B and an MIC of 1.5 is determined, that value should be rounded up to 2
Anidulafungin	≥4	Tentative breakpoints are based on the modal distribution of echinocandin MICs of approximately 100 isolates from diverse geographic locations
Caspofungin	≥2	
Micafungin	≥4	

In this case, we require an antifungal agent with fungicidal activity (blood culture positive), good renal parenchymal concentration (pyelonephritis), good urinary penetration, and biofilm activity (stent in situ).

Echinocandins are fungicidal, have excellent biofilm activity, and achieve higher parenchymal concentrations. Among the echinocandins, micafungin achieves better urinary levels. Hence micafungin is correct antifungal agent in the given clinical scenario.

5 FC has excellent concentrations in the urine, but resistance tends to developed if used alone and MIC is higher for *C. auris*.

Voriconazole is a static drug, it lacks biofilm activity, has minimal excretion in urine and has higher MICs for *C. auris*.

Irrigation of the bladder with AmB deoxycholate has been found to be useful only for isolated cystitis. Although it resolves candiduria in 80–90% of patients, several studies have shown recurrence of candiduria within several weeks. In this patient, with associated candidemia, and pyelonephritis it would not be an appropriate choice.

Ref:
1. CDC (2020). Antifungal Susceptibility Testing and Interpretation. [online] Available from www.cdc.gov/fungal/candida-auris/c-auris-antifungal.html [Last accessed February, 2020].
2. Pappas PG, Kauffman CA, Andes DR, Clancy CJ, Marr KA, Ostrosky-Zeichner L, et al. clinical practice guideline for the management of candidiasis: 2016 Update by the Infectious Diseases Society of America. Clin Infect Dis. 2016;62(4):e1-e50.

5. **Ans. B**

Blood samples collected through catheters are associated with a higher rate of false-positive results due to colonization as compared with cultures of percutaneous blood samples.

For suspected catheter-related blood stream infection (CRBSI), blood samples from the catheter as well as the peripheral vein should be collected simultaneously and cultured before initiation of antimicrobial therapy. Appropriate labeling of culture bottles should be done to identify the site of collection.

CRBSI may be diagnosed from the differential time to positivity (DTP), i.e., growth of microbes from blood drawn from a catheter hub at least 2 hours before microbial growth is detected in blood samples obtained from a peripheral vein. DTP of 120 minutes or more was associated with 81% sensitivity and 92% specificity for short-term catheters and 93% sensitivity and 75% specificity for long-term catheters.

Coagulase-negative staphylococci (CoNS) as isolated in the culture report shown above, are colonizers of human skin. If a catheterized patient has a single positive blood culture that grows *CoNS* species, then additional cultures of blood samples obtained through the suspected catheter and from a peripheral vein are warranted before the initiation of antimicrobial therapy and/or catheter removal.

Ref:
1. Raad I, Hanna HA, Alakech B, Chatzinikolaou I, Johnson MM, Tarrand J. Differential time to positivity: a useful method for diagnosing catheter-related bloodstream infections. Ann Intern Med. 2004;140(1):18-25.
2. Mermel LA, Allon M, Bouza E, Craven DE, Flynn P, O'Grady NP, et al. Clinical practice guidelines for the diagnosis and management of intravascular catheter-related infection: 2009 update by the Infectious Diseases Society of America. Clin Infect Dis. 2009;49(1):1-45.

6. **Ans. A**

When alternative access is difficult, indwelling catheters have been salvaged with systemic and ALT.

This involves instilling a high concentration of an antibiotic into the catheter lumen for a prolonged period of time.

Contraindications for ALT:
- Tunnel infections, port abscesses, or exit site infections
- Hemodynamic instability
- Complicated CRBSI (suppurative thrombophlebitis, endocarditis, osteomyelitis, or other metastatic infection)
- Infections caused by *Staphylococcus aureus*, *Pseudomonas aeruginosa*, fungi, or mycobacteria
- Short-term central venous catheters (indwelling < 14 days)
- Persistent bacteremia despite 72 hours of antibiotic therapy to which the infecting organism is susceptible

This patient had purulence at the exit site and MSSA was isolated from central as well as peripheral line with DTP of 5 hours, indicating a CRBSI. Additionally, the presence of acute onset lower back pain may indicate metastatic focus of infection in the spine. Given the above contraindications in this case, ALT is not recommended and thus the catheter must be removed.

In patients with *S. aureus* bacteremia (SAB), clinical assessment must be done to identify the source and extent of the infection and every attempt must be made to eliminate and/or debride metastatic sites of infection whenever possible.

Detailed history regarding potential portals of entry including recent skin or soft tissue infection and presence of indwelling catheters/prosthetic devices should be taken. Patient should be questioned regarding symptoms that indicate metastatic spread of infection, such as back pain (vertebral osteomyelitis), protracted fever and/or sweats (endocarditis), left upper quadrant pain (splenic infarction), costovertebral angle tenderness (renal infarction or psoas abscess), and headache (septic emboli).

Additional blood cultures 2–4 days after initial positive cultures and as needed thereafter are recommended to document clearance of bacteremia. Echocardiography is recommended for all adults with bacteremia.

Ref:
1. Mermel LA, Allon M, Bouza E, Craven DE, Flynn P, O'Grady NP, et al. Clinical practice guidelines for the diagnosis and management of intravascular catheter-related infection: 2009 Update by the Infectious Diseases Society of America. Clin Infect Dis 2009;49(1)1-45.
2. Fowler VG, Holland TL, Uptodate (2018). Clinical approach to Staphylococcus aureus bacteremia in adults. [online] Available from https://www.uptodate.com/contents/clinical-approach-to-staphylococcus-aureus-bacteremia-in-adults [Last accessed February, 2020].

MRI spine of the patient revealed bilateral paravertebral collection with spondylodiscitis. Surgical debridement was avoided in view of the absence of neurodeficit and multiple comorbid conditions.

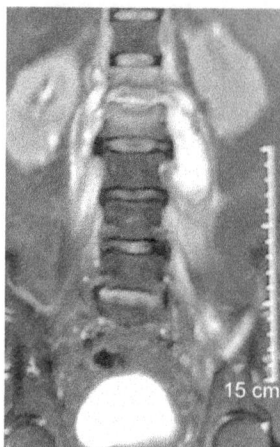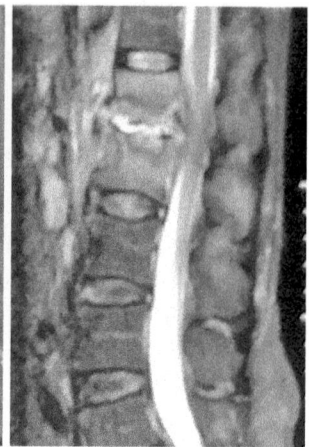

7. **Ans. E**

Glycopeptides have been found to be inferior (lower bactericidal effect), to cloxacillin/cefazolin for the treatment of MSSA infection with studies reporting higher mortality in MSSA bacteremia in patients receiving glycopeptides as definitive therapy.

Treatment of MSSA bacteremia generally consists of a beta-lactam agent such as nafcillin (2 g IV every 4 hours), oxacillin (2 g IV every 4 hours), or flucloxacillin (2 g IV every 6 hours). In patients who are allergic to penicillin, cefazolin (2 g IV every 8 hours) is an acceptable alternative. Although cefazolin has been observed to demonstrate an inoculum effect (increase in MIC with high inoculum infections); studies to examine the impact of this effect have been conflicting.

For adults, the recommended minimum duration of therapy for uncomplicated SAB is 2 weeks, as defined by: (1) exclusion of endocarditis, (2) no implanted prostheses (e.g., prosthetic valves, cardiac devices, and arthroplasties), (3) sterile follow-up cultures of blood samples drawn 2–4 days after commencement of treatment, (4) defervescence within 72 hours of therapy, and (5) no evidence of metastatic sites of infection.

If the above criteria are not met, 4–6 weeks of therapy is recommended for complicated bacteremia depending on the extent of infection. For osteomyelitis, 6–8 weeks treatment is recommended.

Ref:
1. Lambert M. IDSA guidelines on the treatment of MRSA infections in adults and children. Am Fam Physician. 2011;84(4):455-63.
2. Fowler VG, Holland TL. Uptodate (2018). Clinical approach to Staphylococcus aureus bacteremia in adults. [online] Available from https://www.uptodate.com/contents/clinical-approach-to-staphylococcus-aureus-bacteremia-in-adults [Last accessed February, 2020].

8. Ans. C.

Enterococcus species are normal inhabitants of the large bowel, oropharynx, and vaginal secretions. They are selected by altered dynamics of colonization; broad spectrum antibiotics (cephalosporins) and biofilm on catheters, etc.

Intra-abdominal and pelvic infections need not be treated if they are part of a mixed flora (unless repeatedly isolated):

- *Ampicillin/linezolid:* Will offer static cover for *Enterococcus species* but will not cover aerobic and anaerobic gram-negative bacilli (GNB) (other pathogens involved in intra-abdominal sepsis).
- *Ampicillin + gentamicin: This combination is* cidal for *Enterococcus* species. However, cidality is not required in this case.
- *Continue cefoperazone-sulbactam:* Enterococci are intrinsically resistant to cephalosporins. However, it will cover other gut pathogens, thus may be continued if the patient is improving.
- *Escalate to meropenem:* Enterococci are resistant to carbapenems (except imipenem). Meropenem would work against other gut pathogens, but is not indicated if patient improving.

Ref:
1. *Murray B, Miller WR. Uptodate (2019). Treatment of Enterococcal Infections. [online] Available from https://www.uptodate.com/contents/treatment-of-enterococcal-infections [Last accessed February, 2020].*

9. Ans. D

For smear positivity, >100,000 AFB/mL of isolate is required. The gene Xpert can detect as few as 131 AFB/mL of isolate. Hence, if a smear is AFB positive indicating heavy organism burden, but Xpert is negative, nontuberculous mycobacteria (NTM) infection should be strongly suspected.

NTM is an acid fast organism and has identical morphology to MTB complex, hence smear microscopy is unable to distinguish MTB from NTM.

The Xpert MTB/RIF assay is a cartridge-based NAAT capable of simultaneously detecting MTBC and RIF resistance within 2 hours; It amplifies an MTB-specific sequence of the rpoB gene. As it targets only MTB-specific rpoB gene, it is always negative in NTM infection.

Among the NTM, rapidly growing mycobacteria (RGM) are most commonly implicated in nosocomial infections. The three most common clinically relevant species are: *Mycobacterium fortuitum* complex, *Mycobacterium chelonae,* and *Mycobacterium abscessus.*

They are widely distributed in nature and have been isolated from soil, dust, natural surface, and municipal water. The use of quaternary ammonium disinfectant solution, (glutaraldehyde) which is an inadequate mycobactericidal agent, and tap water in the processing of the surgical equipment (laparoscope and arthroscope) are often factors in these nosocomial infections.

RGM are resistant to standard antituberculous drugs (rifampin, ethambutol, and isoniazid). Antibiotic susceptibility testing is important to determine appropriate therapy in view of significant resistance rates to various drugs such as quinolones, tetracyclines, and trimethoprim/sulfamethoxazole (TMP SMX).

In a study by Gupta et al., >95% RGM isolates were sensitive to amikacin, linezolid, and clarithromycin. Hence, inclusion of these three drugs in empiric regimen may help to improve patient outcome when drug-susceptibility testing (DST) is awaited or not available.

Ref:
1. *Helb D, Jones M, Story E, Boehme C, Wallace E, Ho K, et al. 2010. Rapid detection of Mycobacterium tuberculosis and rifampin resistance by use of on-demand, near-patient technology. J Clin Microbiol. 2010;48:229-37.*
2. *Rice JP, Seifert M, Moser KS, Rodwell TC . Performance of the Xpert MTB/RIF assay for the diagnosis of pulmonary tuberculosis and rifampin resistance in a low-incidence, high-resource setting. PLoS One. 2017;12(10):e0186139.*
3. *Phillips MS, von Reyn CF. Nosocomial infections due to Nontuberculous Mycobacteria. Clin Infect Dis. 2001;33(8):1363-74.*
4. *Soman R, Gupta N, Suthar M, Sunavala A, Shetty A, Rodrigues C. Intravascular stent-related endocarditis due to rapidly growing mycobacteria: a new problem in the developing world. J Assoc Physicians India. 2015;63(1):18-21.*

10. Ans. B

Glutaraldehyde 2% (Cidex) although widely used for disinfection of scopes has slow or variable antimycobacterial activity. A minimum disinfection time of at least 20 minutes is required for reliable killing.

Ortho-phthalaldehyde is now recommended for scope disinfection, for its superior mycobacterial and sporicidal activity.

Regardless of the method of sterilization/disinfection, meticulous manual cleaning of the instrument is a must. Thorough drying of the instrument is recommended to prevent contamination with water-borne organisms.

Ref:
1. *Mathur P. Cleaning, disinfection and sterilization. hospital acquired infections–prevention and control. India: Wolters Kluwer Health; 2010.*

11. Ans. C

Laminectomy for herniated disk is classified as a clean surgery. Although this patient has multiple risk factors including diabetes, systemic steroids, recent chemotherapy, and alcohol abuse; surgical prophylaxis should be effective against the "most likely" organisms at the surgical site:

Clean surgery:	Skin flora:
• Uninfected, no inflammation	• GPCs (Streptococcal spp., Staphylococcus aureus, CONS)
• Respiratory, GI, GU tracts not entered	
• Closed primarily	

First-generation cephalosporin (cefazolin):
- Active against most likely pathogens [*Streptococcal* spp., *Staphylococcus aureus*, and coagulase-negative staphylococci (CoNS)]
- Achieves good tissue levels
- Adequate half-life (2 hours)
- Does not significantly alter indigenous flora.

Third-generation cephalosporin/β-Lactam/β-lactamase inhibitor (BLBLI):
- Less effective than first-generation cephalosporins against *S. aureus*
- Needless activity against organisms not commonly encountered in elective, clean surgery
- Widespread use for prophylaxis encourages emergence of resistance.

The surgeon asks for a preoperative methicillin-resistant *S. aureus* (MRSA) screen which comes positive.

12. Ans. C

World Health Organization surgical site infection (WHO SSI) prevention guidelines 2016 recommend that "patients undergoing cardiothoracic and orthopedic surgery with known nasal carriage of *Staphylococcus aureus* should receive perioperative intranasal applications of mupirocin 2% ointment with or without a combination of chlorhexidine body wash.

In patients with positive MRSA screen, preoperative prophylaxis should be changed to glycopeptides. Teicoplanin 400 mg should be given within 1 hour OR vancomycin 15 mg/kg should be given within 120 minutes of skin incision and continued for 24 hours postoperatively. Furthermore, surgical duration of greater than 4 hours or estimated blood loss over 1,500 mL necessitates repeat intraoperative dosing of antibiotics. When vancomycin is used, single dose is enough due to its long half-life.

As the glycopeptides are less effective than cefazolin for preventing SSIs caused by MSSA, in such cases vancomycin should be used in combination with cefazolin for prevention of SSI due to MRSA and MSSA. So In this case, prophylaxis should be changed to cefazolin plus vancomycin.

Ref:
1. Finkelstein R, Rabino G, Mashiah T, Bar-El Y, Adler Z, Kertzman V, et al. Vancomycin versus cefazolin prophylaxis for cardiac surgery in the setting of a high prevalence of methicillin-resistant staphylococcal infections. J Thorac Cardiovasc Surg. 2002;123(2):326.
2. Berríos-Torres SI, Umscheid CA, Bratzler DW, Leas B, Stone EC, Kelz RR, et al. Centers for Disease Control and Prevention Guideline for the Prevention of Surgical Site Infection, 2017. JAMA Surg. 2017;152(8):784-91.
3. Iqbal HJ, Ponniah N, Long S, Rath N, Kent M. Review of MRSA screening and antibiotics prophylaxis in orthopaedic trauma patients; The risk of surgical site infection with inadequate antibiotic prophylaxis in patients colonized with MRSA. Injury. 2017;48(7):1382-7.

13. Ans. C

Contamination of a surgical wound with soil organisms must be suspected in open injuries.

Potential soil pathogens include:
- Enterobacteriaceae
- *Pseudomonas/Aeromonas* species
- *Acinetobacter* species
- Anaerobes
- *Nocardia* species
- *Actinomyces*
- NTM
- Environmental molds.

Bacterial contamination of wounds is a serious problem in the hospital, especially in surgical practice where the site of a sterile operation can become contaminated and subsequently infected. This patient had an open fracture in farm hence there is a higher chances of getting polymicrobial infection. CoNS is a part of normal skin flora and its isolation in wound swab culture may represent just colonization of skin rather than true pathogen. Hence, intraoperative specimen or deep tissue culture is must to find and hit the right bug.

Ref:
1. Baumgardner DJ. Soil-related bacterial and fungal infections. J Am Board Fam Med. 2012;25(5):734-44.

14. Ans. D

Clinical diagnosis of this patient is local pocket site infection. It is defined as an infection limited to the pocket of the cardiac device and is clinically suspected in the presence of local signs of inflammation at the generator pocket, including erythema, warmth, fluctuance, wound dehiscence, erosion, tenderness, or purulent drainage.

In such cases every effort should be made to rule out cardiac device related IE (CDRIE) defined as an infection extending to the electrode leads, cardiac valve leaflets, or endocardial surface.

Echocardiography and blood cultures should be performed. Echocardiography is useful for the diagnosis of lead vegetations and tricuspid involvement, quantification of tricuspid regurgitation, sizing of vegetations, and follow-up after lead extraction. A normal echographic examination does not rule out CDRIE. In difficult cases, other modalities such as radiolabelled leukocyte scintigraphy389 and fluorodeoxyglucose F 18 positron emission tomography/CT (18F-FDG PET/CT) scanning have been described as additive tools in the diagnosis of CDRIE and related complications.

CDRIE must be treated by prolonged antibiotic therapy associated with complete hardware removal. The duration of therapy is 4–6 weeks in most cases.

In the case of definite CDRIE, medical therapy alone has been associated with high mortality and risk of recurrence. For this reason, cardiac implantable electronic device (CIED) removal is recommended in all cases of proven CDRIE and should also be considered when CDRIE is only suspected in the case of occult infection without any apparent source other than the device.

Ref:
1. *Habib G, Lancellotti P, Antunes MJ, Bongiorni MG, Casalta JP, Del Zotti F, et al. 2015 ESC Guidelines for the management of infective endocarditis: The Task Force for the Management of Infective Endocarditis of the European Society of Cardiology (ESC). Endorsed by: European Association for Cardiothoracic Surgery (EACTS), the European Association of Nuclear Medicine (EANM). Euro Heart J. 2015;36:3075-123*

15. Ans. D

Different modalities for management of prosthetic joint infections (PJI) are:

- *A two-stage exchange strategy:*
    - It is indicated in relatively younger, medically fit patients who a have chronic PJI with skin and soft tissue involvement and resistant or difficult to treat pathogens such as the patient described above. This approach involves removal of prosthetic material, debridement of periprosthetic tissue, appropriate systemic +/- local antibiotic spacers for several weeks followed by reimplantation of prosthesis after a successful antibiotic free interval.
    - Synovial fluid examination and joint aspirate cultures prior to reimplantation have been recommended in selected cases when there is concern about persistent infection.
- *Debridement and implant retention (DAIR):* Patients diagnosed with a PJI who meet the criteria for joint retention:
    - Well-fixed prosthesis without a sinus tract
    - Early postoperative PJI within 30 days of prosthesis implantation
    - <3 weeks of onset of infectious symptoms in hematogenous infections
    - Susceptibility to oral antimicrobial agents
    - In patients who do not meet these criteria such as the patient discussed above, relapse of infection is more likely.
- *One-stage exchange or revision procedure:* It involves removal of all prosthetic components, debridement of devitalized bone and soft tissues, and implantation of a new prosthesis. This procedure is typically reserved for patients without a sinus tract, provided the infecting organism has been identified prior and is easily treatable with oral antibiotics.
- *Permanent resection arthroplasty:* It is reserved for patients who are medically unfit to undergo revision surgery, nonambulatory patients with limited bone stock, poor soft tissue coverage, or infections due to highly resistant organisms for which there is no or limited medical therapy.

Ref:
1. *Osmon DR, Berbari EF, Berendt AR, Lew D, Zimmerli W, Steckelberg JM, et al. Diagnosis and management of prosthetic joint infection: Clinical Practice Guidelines by the Infectious Diseases Society of America. Clin Infect Dis. 2013;56(1):e1-e25.*

A two stage revision is planned for this patient. He is started on IV colistin. He undergoes removal of prosthesis with insertion of a colistin impregnated cement spacer.

16. Ans. D

This patient is planned for two stage revision, an overview of two-stage revision is given in chart below. 4–6 weeks of antibiotic should be given followed by 2 weeks of antibiotic free interval followed by aspiration and culture. If any signs of infection or culture positive, revision surgery should be deferred and debridement and treatment of infection must be done based on culture reports.

First surgery:
- Debridement and implant removal
- Obtain tissue culture
- Put antibiotic impregnated spacer (it provides mechanical support and local antimicrobial therapy)

↓

Pathogen-directed antimicrobial therapy is usually given intravenously for 4–6 weeks

↓

Two or more weeks antibiotic-free time period evaluate patient for:
- Signs of ongoing infection
- Inflammatory markers
- Synovial fluid aspiration, if there is evidence of ongoing infection, a repeat debridement procedure may be performed

↓

Second surgery:
- Biopsy, spacer removal and prosthetic implantation
- Continue perioperative antibiotics until intraoperative cultures negative

Ref:
1. *Tande AJ, Patel R. Prosthetic joint infection. Clin Microbiol Rev. 2014;27(2):302-45.*

17. Ans. E

This patient presented with cholangitis most probably due to stent infection. The most common causative organisms involved in biliary stent infections include gram-negative pathogens such as *Escherichia coli*, *Klebsiella*, *Enterobacter*, *Pseudomonas*, and *Citrobacter* species. The most common gram-positive bacteria are *Enterococcus* species. *Candida species may* also frequently be encountered in such patients. Anaerobes, such as *Bacteroides* and *Clostridia*, are usually present as part of a mixed infection.

Ref:
1. *Basioukas P, Vezakis A, Zarkotou O, Fragulidis G, Themeli-Digalaki K, Rizos S, et al. Isolated microorganisms in plastic biliary stents placed for benign and malignant diseases. Ann Gastroenterol. 2014;27(4):399-403.*

18. Ans. D

The most important step in the management of this patient is source control. Thus, every attempt should be made to look for any localized collection, stent obstruction, stricture, or intrahepatic bile duct (IHBD) dilatation. Percutaneous or endoscopic retrograde cholangiopancreatography (ERCP)-guided drainage of collection should be done and bile must be send for bacterial and fungal culture to identify causative organism and drug sensitivity pattern, which will help to choose appropriate antimicrobial treatment.

Ref:
1. *Solomkin JS, Mazuski JE, Bradley JS, Rodvold KA, Goldstein EJ, Baron EJ, et al Diagnosis and management of complicated intra-abdominal infection in adults and children: IDSA guideline. Clin Infect Dis. 2010;50(2):133-64.*

19. Ans. C

Flavobacterium meningosepticum, now known as Elizabethkingia meningoseptica, is a gram-negative bacillus. It has been isolated from hospital water supplies, sinks, taps, saline solution used for flushing procedures, disinfectants, and medical devices, including feeding tubes, arterial catheters, and respirators. It has been reported to cause neonatal meningitis associated with nosocomial outbreaks. In adults, most infections due to *E. meningoseptica* are nosocomial, particularly affecting immunocompromised individuals. However, device-associated infections have been known to occur in nonimmunosuppressed adults as described above.

Although gram-negative, this organism shows resistance to most antimicrobial classes commonly used to treat gram-negative bacteria (aminoglycosides, B-lactam agents including carbapenem) but displays susceptibility to agents used to treat infections caused by gram-positive bacteria (rifampicin, quinolones, vancomycin, and trimethoprim-sulfamethoxazole).

Ref:
1. *Ratnamani MS, Rao R. Elizabethkingia meningoseptica: emerging nosocomial pathogen in bedside hemodialysis patients. Indian J Crit Care Med. 2013;17(5):304-7.*

The patient receives IV vancomycin with monitoring of serum concentrations. However, CSF culture repeated on day 7 grows the same organism. Intraventricular vancomycin administration through the EVD is considered.

20. Ans. E

Direct instillation of antimicrobial agents into the ventricles through either an external ventriculostomy or shunt reservoir is occasionally necessary in patients who have nosocomial or device-associated infections that are difficult to eradicate.

The main advantage of this route of administration is that it provides larger effective concentration of antibiotics at the infected site with reduced systemic toxicity by direct antibiotic delivery to local site bypassing the blood-brain barrier.

Intrathecal/intraventricular beta-lactams are avoided in view of seizurogenic potential of these agents.

After administration of the first intraventricular dose, the drain should be clamped for 15–60 minutes to allow the agent to equilibrate throughout the CSF.

Additional doses can be determined by calculation of the "inhibitory quotient." Prior to administration of the next intraventricular dose, a sample of CSF is withdrawn to obtain the trough CSF concentration. The inhibitory quotient is then determined by taking the trough CSF concentration divided by the MIC of the agent for the isolated bacterial pathogen; it should exceed 10–20 for consistent CSF sterilization.

Ref:
1. *Tunkel AR, Hasbun R, Bhimraj A, Byers K, Kaplan SL, Scheld WM, et al. 2017, Infectious Diseases Society of America's Clinical Practice Guidelines for Healthcare-Associated Ventriculitis and Meningitis. Clin Infect Dis. 2017;64(6):e34-e65.*

21. **Ans. E**

Testing for *Clostridium difficile* infection (CDI) should be performed in patients with unexplained and new-onset of ≥3 unformed stools in 24 hours. In such patients, highly sensitive tests such as a NAAT alone or multistep algorithm (i.e., GDH plus toxin; GDH plus toxin, arbitrated by NAAT; or NAAT plus toxin) may be best.

Test	Sensitivity	Specificity	Substance detected
NAAT	High	Low/moderate	*C. difficile* nucleic acid
GDH assay	High	Low	*C. difficile* common antigen
Toxin A and B enzyme immunoassay	Low	Moderate	Free toxins

Molecular tests/NAATs detect DNA from *C. difficile* organisms capable of producing toxin (also referred to as toxigenic *C. difficile*) found in stool. Polymerase chain reaction (PCR) is one type of NAAT. The sensitivity of detection of toxigenic *C. difficile* organism by GeneXpert has been reported to be 94-99% and correlated well with a clinical diagnosis of *CDI*. Because they are very sensitive, molecular tests can be used to "rule out" *C. difficile* in the majority of patients.

Not all patients testing positive for *C. difficile* with PCR-based assays should be treated. Only patients who meet the clinical criteria for CDI should be treated; patients who test positive by PCR who do not meet those criteria may be colonized. The decision to administer antibiotic therapy should be based on disease severity, history of prior CDI, and the individual patient's risk of recurrence.

Ref:
1. *McDonald LC, Gerding DN, Johnson S, Bakken JS, Carroll KC, Coffin SE, et al. Clinical practice guidelines for clostridium difficile infection in adults and children: 2017 Update by the Infectious Diseases Society of America (IDSA) and Society for Healthcare Epidemiology of America (SHEA). Clin Infect Dis. 2018;66(7):e1-e48.*
2. *Berry N, Sewell B, Jafri S, Puli C, Vagia S, Lewis AM, et al. Real-time polymerase chain reaction correlates well with clinical diagnosis of Clostridium difficile infection. J Hosp Infect. 2014;87:109-14.*
3. *Bagdasarian N, Rao K, Malani PN. Diagnosis and treatment of Clostridium difficile in adults: a systematic review. JAMA. 2015;313(4):398-408.*

22. **Ans. A**

CDI is strongly associated with increasing cumulative dose and duration of antibiotic exposure. Inciting antibiotics should be discontinued as soon as possible as their continued use has been shown to decrease clinical response and increase recurrence rates. Any antibiotic can cause CDI but drugs such as fluoroquinolones, clindamycin, and cephalosporins are the most commonly implicated and should be avoided as far as possible.

Therapy for CDI should be started empirically if a substantial delay in laboratory confirmation is expected (e.g., >48 hours) or if a patient presents with fulminant CDI.

Either vancomycin or fidaxomicin is recommended over metronidazole for an initial episode of CDI. When vancomycin or fidaxomicin is not available, metronidazole can be used for an initial episode of nonsevere CDI only.

For fulminant CDI (hypotension or shock, ileus, or megacolon), vancomycin administered orally is the regimen of choice. If ileus is present, vancomycin can also be administered per rectum. Intravenous metronidazole should be administered together with oral or rectal vancomycin, particularly if ileus is present.

In above described case, the patient does not fit the criteria for fulminant CDI, hence, oral vancomycin should be started.

Ref:
1. *McDonald LC, Gerding DN, Johnson S, Bakken JS, Carroll KC, Coffin SE, et al. Clinical practice guidelines for Clostridium difficile infection in adults and children: 2017 Update by the Infectious Diseases Society of America (IDSA) and Society for Healthcare Epidemiology of America (SHEA). Clin Infect Dis. 2018;66(7):e1-e48.*

23. **Ans. D**

An infection control "bundle" strategy has been used to successfully control major CDI outbreaks. The "bundle" approach involves measures such as hand hygiene, isolation measures, environmental disinfection, and antibiotic stewardship.

Patients with CDI should be placed in a private room as far as possible to decrease transmission to other patients. If it is not possible than it is advisable to cohort infected patients in a single ward.

Healthcare personnel must adhere to strict contact isolation precautions. Gloves and gowns should be worn on entry to a room of a patient with CDI and while caring for patients with CDI.

There is a possibility for alcohol-based hand hygiene products to increase the incidence of CDI because of their inability to eliminate *C. difficile* spores from the hands. Therefore, before and after providing care for a patient with CDI, it is recommended to preferentially use soap and water over alcohol-based products alone for hand hygiene in CDI-hyperendemic (sustained high rates) or outbreak settings. Contact precautions should be continued for at least 48 hours after diarrhea has ceased.

Patients should wash hands and shower regularly to reduce the burden of spores on the skin. Disposable patient equipment should be used when possible and reusable equipment must be thoroughly cleaned and disinfected, preferentially with a sporicidal disinfectant that is equipment compatible.

Terminal room cleaning with a sporicidal agent should be considered in conjunction with other measures to prevent CDI during endemic high rates or outbreaks, or if there is evidence of repeated cases of CDI in the same room.

Ref:
1. Wenzler E, Mulugeta SG, Danziger LH. The antimicrobial stewardship approach to combating Clostridium difficile. Antibiotics. 2015;4(2):198-215.

24. Ans. E

Causes of nodular shadows in patients with cellular immunosuppression:
- *Bacteria*: *Staphylococcus*, *Rhodococcus*, GNB, *Nocardia* and *Mycobacterium* (tuberculous and nontuberculous).
- *Invasive mold infections*: Invasive pulmonary aspergillosis (IPA), *Mucor*, *Cryptococcus*, and endemic mycoses.
- *Protozoa and parasites*: *Toxoplasma* and *Strongyloides stercoralis*

This patient is postrenal transplant, on triple immunosuppression plus recently pulsed with high dose of steroid and now presented with cough and fever. Due to the heightened immunosuppression, this patient is at risk for diverse opportunistic infections, hence empiric treatment for such patients may be disastrous and every attempt must be made to obtain tissue for microbiological diagnosis.

Ref:
1. Kohno S. Pneumonia in immunosuppressed patients. Respirol. 2004;9:S25-S9.

Bronchoscopy with acid-fast bacilli (BAL) was done. Bronchoalveolar lavage (AFB) was identified on smear.

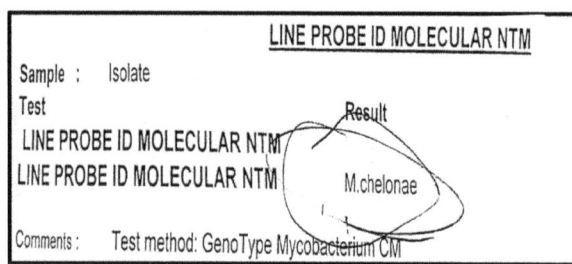

25. Ans. C

Mycobacterium chelonae is a NTM, which is classified as rapidly growing mycobacterium (RGM). It is a gram-positive, acid-fast bacillus, ubiquitous in soil, water, and aquatic animals.

Identification of species and drug susceptibility is a must as resistance to commonly used drugs is well known and varies as per mycobacterial species.

In immunocompetent patients, it commonly presents as localized skin infections after an invasive procedure, or catheter-related infection. Pulmonary infections due to *M. chelonae* are rare, but colonization is common in cystic fibrosis patients. Disseminated and invasive infections are seen in immunocompromised patients.

M. chelonae can be a contaminant in endoscopes. Pseudo outbreaks of *M. chelonae* have been reported due to contaminated bronchoscopes and endoscopes.

Criteria for diagnosis of NTM lung infection:
- *Clinical:* Pulmonary symptoms.
- *Radiological:* Nodular or cavitary opacities on chest radiograph or a high-resolution CT (HRCT) scan that shows multifocal bronchiectasis with multiple small nodules.
- *Microbiologic*:
  - Positive culture results from at least two separate expectorated sputum samples.
  - Positive culture results from at least one bronchial wash or lavage.
  - Transbronchial or other lung biopsy with mycobacterial histopathologic features (granulomatous inflammation or AFB) and positive culture for NTM or biopsy showing mycobacterial histopathologic features (granulomatous inflammation or AFB) and one or more sputum or bronchial washings that are culture positive for NTM.

All criteria must be met to make a diagnosis of NTM lung disease plus appropriate exclusion of other diagnosis.

This patient described above fulfills all three criteria (symptomatic + CT findings + BAL culture positive) for NTM lung disease hence warrants appropriate treatment for the same.

Ref:
1. Akram SM, Anjum F, StatPearls. (2019). Mycobacterium chelonae. [online] Available from https://www.statpearls.com/as/eyes/25417/ [Last accessed February, 2020].
2. Saeed DK, Shakoor S, Irfan S, Hasan R. Mycobacterial contamination of bronchoscopes: challenges and possible solutions in low resource settings. Int J Mycobacteriol. 2016;5(4):408-11.

3. Griffith DE, Aksamit T, Brown-Elliott BA, Catanzaro A, Daley C, Gordin F, et al. An official ATS/IDSA Statement: diagnosis, treatment, and prevention of nontuberculous mycobacterial diseases. Am J Respir Crit Care Med. 2007;175(4):367-416.

26. Ans. D

In this case, fever started a few days after abdominal symptoms. Routine fever work-up, blood cultures, and PCT were negative and hypotension responded to fluid challenge. The above is not consistent with gram-negative bacterial sepsis.

Myeloma related fever was unlikely in this patient in remission, postautologous HSCT.

Intestinal giardiasis can cause fever but diarrhea had settled down with metronidazole.

Temporal association of fever and neutrophil recovery is very classical of hepatosplenic candidiasis. In this case, the onset of fever coincided with neutrophil recovery and USG abdomen showed multiple targetoid bull's eye lesions which is characteristically seen in hepatosplenic candidiasis.

27. Ans. C

Azole resistant *Candida* species is a possibility, however, apart from *C. glabrata*, other *Candida* species generally remain susceptible to voriconazole and posaconazole.

Missed posaconazole doses were unlikely as the patient was hospitalized during this time and drug administration would be under medical supervision.

Posaconazole exhibits variable pharmacokinetics and the absorption and bioavailability of the suspension is significantly affected by factors such as raised gastric pH, mucositis, diarrhea, and coadministration of interacting drugs.

Breakthrough infections due to subtherapeutic drug levels are common in patients with diarrhea and therapeutic drug monitoring (TDM) is recommended.

Posaconazole is an inhibitor of CYP3A4 as a result of which it has numerous drug-drug interactions. The calcineurin inhibitors such as cyclosporine and tacrolimus are CYP3A4 substrates and coadministration with posaconazole will lead to increased plasma concentration of these drugs and potential toxicity. The concentration of posaconazole, however, is not affected by coadministration with calcineurin inhibitors. Hence, drug interaction with cyclosporine is wrong answer.

Ref:
1. Dekkers BGJ, Bakker M, van der Elst KCM, Sturkenboom MGG, Veringa A, Span LFR, et al. Therapeutic drug monitoring of posaconazole: an update. Curr Fungal Infect Rep. 2016;10:51-61.
2. Moore JN, Healy JR, Kraft WK. Pharmacologic and clinical evaluation of posaconazole. Expert Rev Clin Pharmacol. 2015;8(3):321-34.

28. Ans. C

For hepatosplenic candidiasis, antifungal therapy be continued until radiological resolution of all lesions in order to prevent relapse.

Ref:
1. Pappas PG, Kauffman CA, Andes DR, Clancy CJ, Marr KA, Ostrosky-Zeichner L, et al. Clinical practice guideline for the management of candidiasis: 2016 Update by the Infectious Diseases Society of America. Clin Infect Dis. 2016;62(4):e1-e50.

29. Ans. C

The isolation of *Candida* species from the respiratory or urinary tract is commonly encountered among patients who are in the ICU, intubated with chronic indwelling catheters. This almost always reflects colonization and not infection. Pneumonia due to *Candida* species is generally limited to severely immunocompromised patients who develop infection following hematogenous spread to the lungs.

Candiduria in the febrile neutropenic host, however, may represent indicate invasive candidiasis and should be treated aggressively.

Multiple scoring systems have been proposed for patients who are at higher risk of developing candidemia, mostly critically ill patients in the ICU. However, these scores have all been found to have a high specificity but low sensitivity, thus missing many patients with candidiasis. Moreover, most of these studies targeted ICU patients, with very little data on other risk groups such as neutropenics, hence their accuracy and usefulness in these patients is unknown.

This patient described above is neutropenic with mucositis and diarrhea, hence she is at higher risk for candida gut translocation. Other risk factors are presence of a chemotherapy port, broad-spectrum antibiotics, candida colonization at two different sites and septic shock.

The overall sensitivity of blood cultures for diagnosing invasive candidiasis is roughly 50%. They may be negative in cases of low-level candidemia, intermittent candidemia and deep-seated candidiasis. The utility of cultures are limited by slow turnaround times (1 to ≥7 days), and the fact that they may become positive relatively late in the disease course. Hence, in high-risk patients, the use of risk stratification scores and nonculture-based fungal biomarkers has aided in initiation of timely preemptive and empiric treatment.

Ref:
1. Pappas PG, Kauffman CA, Andes DR, Clancy CJ, Marr KA, Ostrosky-Zeichner L, et al. Clinical practice guideline for the management of Candidiasis: 2016 Update by the Infectious Diseases Society of America. Clin Infect Dis. 2016;62(4):e1-e50.

30. Ans. C

Duration of therapy for candidemia without obvious metastatic complications is for 2 weeks after documented clearance of *Candida* species from the bloodstream and resolution of symptoms. Blood cultures should be performed every day or alternate day to establish blood clearance. Echocardiography and ophthalmological examination must be done in all patients with candidemia within the first week after diagnosis or during neutrophil recovery in neutropenic patient to rule out metastatic sites of infection.

Selection of antifungal agents is based on prior azole exposure, risk factor, hemodynamic status, and source of infection or metastasis.

An echinocandin is the agent of choice as initial therapy in candidemia. Fluconazole may be used as an initial therapy in hemodynamically stable patients with no prior azole exposure.

Transition from an echinocandin to fluconazole can be done within 5-7 days for patients who are:
- Clinically stable
- Isolates that are susceptible to fluconazole
- Negative repeat blood cultures following initiation of antifungal treatment.

Ref:
1. Pappas PG, Kauffman CA, Andes DR, Clancy CJ, Marr KA, Ostrosky-Zeichner L, et al. Clinical practice guideline for the management of Candidiasis: 2016 Update by the Infectious Diseases Society of America. Clin Infect Dis. 2016;62(4):e1-e50.

31. Ans. C

For *Candida* chorioretinitis without vitritis, oral/IV azole should be started depending on sensitivity.

Drug	Loading dose	Maintenance dose
Fluconazole	12 mg/kg OD	6–12 mg/kg OD
Voriconazole	6 mg/kg BD	4 mg/kg BD

For azole resistant isolates, liposomal AmB, 3–5 mg/kg intravenous daily, with or without oral flucytosine, 25 mg/kg four times daily should be given.

Patient with macular involvement antifungal agents as above PLUS intravitreal injection of either AmB deoxycholate or voriconazole should be given.

The duration of treatment is at least 4–6 weeks, with the final duration depending on resolution of the lesions as determined by repeated ophthalmological examinations.

Vitrectomy is recommended only in patients with vitritis.

Ref:
1. Pappas PG, Kauffman CA, Andes DR, Clancy CJ, Marr KA, Ostrosky-Zeichner L, et al. Clinical practice guideline for the management of Candidiasis: 2016 Update by the Infectious Diseases Society of America. Clin Infect Dis. 2016;62(4):e1-e50.

32. Ans. C

Galactomannan is a polysaccharide antigen that found primarily in the cell walls of *Aspergillus* species. It can be released into the blood and other body fluids in the early stages of *Aspergillus* invasion.

IPA is commonly seen in neutropenic patients, however, there has been increasing evidence of infection in non-neutropenic hosts with emerging risk factors such as COPD, bronchiectasis, critical illness, chronic liver disease, chronic kidney disease, HIV, and patients on immunosuppressants.

Non-neutropenic patients with IPA may present with nonspecific radiological findings like pulmonary infiltrates and micronodules.

In nonneutropenic patient, serum GM has poor sensitivity as neutrophils in the serum may eliminate GM antigens via the mannan-binding receptor. Hence, BAL GM is more valuable than serum GM for the early diagnosis of IPA in nonneutropenic patients.

Ref:
1. Zhou W, Li H, Zhang Y, Huang M, He Q, Li P, et al. Diagnostic value of galactomannan antigen test in serum and bronchoalveolar lavage fluid samples from patients with nonneutropenic invasive pulmonary aspergillosis. J Clin Microbiol. 2017;55(7):2153-61.

33. Ans. C

A wound is not considered superficial SSI if stitch abscess is present; if the infection is at an episiotomy, a circumcision site, or a burn wound; or if the SSI extends into fascia or muscle.

Ref:
1. CDC guidelines for diagnosis of SSI.

34. Ans. A

Staphylococcus epidermidis is the CoNS species most often associated with prosthetic device following colonization. It is part of normal human flora and is found on skin as well as in oropharynx and vagina. It is uniquely adapted to colonize these devices because of its capacity to elaborate the extracellular polysaccharide that facilitates formation of a protective biofilm on device surface.

Staphylococcus saprophyticus is a common pathogen in UTI. Its capacity to cause UTI in young women appears to be related to its enhanced capacity to adhere to uroepithelial cells.

The basis of enhanced virulence of *Staphylococcus lugdunensis* and *Staphylococcus schleiferi* to cause serious infection is not known but they all known to share more virulent determinants with *S. aureus*.

Ref:
1. Lowy FD. Staphylococcal infection. In: Jameson JL, Fauci AS, Kasper DL, Hauser SL, Longo DL, Loscalzo J (Eds). Harrisons Principles of Internal Medicine, 20th edition. United States of America: McGraw-Hill Education; 2018.

35. Ans. D

In initial fulminant episode of CDI treatment recommended is vancomycin 500 mg PO or via NG tube plus metrogyl IV 500 mg 8 hourly plus consider retention enema of vancomycin 500 mg in 100 mL of NS.

IV vancomycin is ineffective for *C. difficile.*

IV metrogyl has failed in adynamic ileus.

Pseudomembranous colitis is more advanced form of *C. difficile* and is visualized at endoscopy in 50% of patient who have a positive stool culture and for assay for *C. difficile.*

Endoscopy is a rapid diagnostic tool in seriously ill patient with suspected PCMC and acute abdomen but a negative result does not rule out CDI.

Infants are thought not to develop symptomatic CDI because they lack suitable mucosal receptors to toxin that develops later in life.

In adults, serum level of IgG antibody to toxin A increases more in response to infection in includes which becomes asymptomatic carriers than in those who develop CDI. For persons who develop CDI increasing level of antitoxin A during treatment correlate with a lower risk of recurrence.

Ref:
1. Gerding DN, Johnson S. Clostridium Difficile infection including pseudomembranous colitis. In: Jameson JL, Fauci AS, Kasper DL, Hauser SL, Longo DL, Loscalzo J (Eds). Harrisons Principles of Internal Medicine, 20th edition. United States of America: McGraw-Hill Education; 2018.

36. Ans. C

The infection is most likely to be *Nocardia* as *Nocardia* species are gram-positive branching, beaded and acid fast. Usually, majority of causes of pulmonary nocardias occur in people with a host defense defect. Pneumonia is a common presentation of nocardial infection. *Nocardia* grows relatively slowly on media and may take up to 2 weeks to appear. Treatment of choice is TMZ + SMX

In severe pulmonary disease without central nervous system (CNS) disease initial regimen is TMZ SMX + amikacin + IV ceftriaxone or IV imipenem.

After definite clinical improvement therapy can be continued with single oral drug especially TMZ SMX.

Treatment duration for pulmonary or systemic disease with intact host defense is 6-12 months.

With defective host defenses 12 months and with CNS disease 12 months.

37. Ans. C

For hospitalized patients with MRSA infection or MRSA colonization initiating a decolonization regimen at time of hospital discharge reduces likelihood of subsequent MRSA. The optimal regimen and durations of colonization are variable. The best studied regimen consists of 4% rinse of chlorhexidine for daily bathing and showering. 0.12% chlorhexidine mouth wash twice daily and 2% nasal mupirocin twice daily all administered 5 days per month for 6 months.

Ref:
1. Huang SS, Singh R, McKinnel JA, Park S, Gombosev A, Eells SJ, et al. Decolonization to reduce postdischarge infection risk among MRSA carrier. N Engl J Med. 2019;380:638-650.
2. Creech CB, Al-Zubedi DN, Fritz SA. Prevention of recurrent staphylococcal skin infections. Infet Dis Clin North AM. 2015;29:429.
3. Peterson LR, Hacek DM, Robicsek A. 5 Million Lives Campaign on MRSA. Case study: Intervention at Northwestern Healthcare. Jt Corm J Qual Patient Saf. 2007;33:732-8.
4. Siegel JD, Rhinehar E, Jackson M, Chiarello L, the Healthcare Infection Control Practices Advisory Committee (2006). Management of multidrug resistant organisms in health care settings 2006. [online] Available from https://www.cdc.gov/infectioncontrol/pdf/guidelines/mdro-guidelines.pdf [Last accessed February, 2020].
5. Kluytmans-Vandenbergh MF, Kluytmans JA, Voss A. Datch guidelines for preventing nosocomial transmission of highly resistant microorganisms (HRMO). Infection. 2005;33:309-13.

38. Ans. A

Patient lesions seem to be ecthyma gangrenosum, which is most commonly associated with *Pseudomonas*. Patient already has grown GNB which is most likely to be *Pseudomonas*. Also patient is in shock with neutropenia.

Use of two agents from different classes with in vitro activity against *P. aeruginosa* is suggested for *Empiric* treatment of serious infections known or suspected to be caused by *P. aeruginosa* or in hosts for whom inappropriate antibiotic therapy would likely to be associated with high mortality. Such circumstance would include:

- Signs of severe sepsis or septic shock
- Neutropenic patient with bacteremia
- Burns patient with severe infections
- Where incidence of resistance to chosen antibiotic class is high (e.g., more than 10-15%).

Rational for use of combination therapy is to provide initial broad spectrum of activity whom there is risk of MDR *Pseudomonas* so that if *P. aeruginosa* is resistant to one, it may be susceptible to other. Delays in active antimicrobial therapy of *P. aeruginosa* have been possible resistant pathogen when resistant rates to primary agent are high.

Ref:
1. Tamma PD, Cosgrove SE, Maragakis LL. Combination therapy for treatment of infection with gram negative bacteremia. Clinical Microbial Rev. 2012;25(3):450-70.

39. Ans. D

Candida auris develops resistance quickly. Patient requiring antifungal therapy should be carefully monitored with follow-up cultures.

If patient does not respond clinically to echinocandin or has persistent candidemia > 5 days, patient can be switched to amphotericin B lipid formulation 5 mg/kg IV daily.

Ref:
1. CDC (2018). Recommendations for treatment of Candida auris infection. [online] Available from https://www.cdc.gov/fungal/candida-auris/c-auris-treatment.html [Last accessed February, 2020].
2. Tsay S, Kallen A, Jackson BR, Chiller TM, Vallabhaneni S. Approach to the investigation and management of patients with candida auris, an Emerging Multidrug resistant Yeast. Clin Infect Dis. 2018;66(2):306-11.

40. Ans. B

Enterococci are gram-negative diplococci usually nonhemolytic. Though *E. faecalis* is the most commonly reported enterococcus causing nosocomial infection *E. faecium* is now almost as common as *E. faecalis* as a cause of nosocomial infections. More than 80% *E. faecium* are resistant to vancomycin and more than 90% are resistant to ampicillin. vancomycin-resistant *Enterococcus* (VRE) colonization of GI tract is a critical step in development of enterococcal disease and that a substantial proportion of patients admitted with VRE remain colonized for a prolonged period over >1 year and are more likely to develop enterococcal-related illnesses (e.g., bacteremia) than those without colonization. VREs can survive exposure to heat and disinfectants and have been found on numerous inanimate objects in the hospital excluding bed rails, medical equipment, door knobs, telephones, and computer keyboards. Thus HCW and the environment play pivotal roles in enterococcal transmission from patient to patient and infection control measures are crucial in breaking the chain of transmission. General analysis of vancomycin resistant *E. faecium* in different parts of would suggest that the emergence and dissemination of these organisms worldwide are due to success of hospital associated genetic lineages that acquired the genes responsible for vancomycin resistance as well as other antibiotic resistant determinants. Bacteremia without endocarditis is one of most common presentation of enterococcal disease. Intravascular and other devices are commonly associated with these bacteremic episodes. Other well-known causes of enterococcal bacteremia are GI and hepatobiliary tracts, pelvic and intra-abdominal foci and less frequently UTI, and wound infections.

For nonendovascular VRE bacteremia treatment recommended is high-dose daptomycin (10–12 mg/kg) ± another agent (ampicillin or ceftaroline or tigecycline) + an aminoglycoside.

Linezolid 600 mg IV 12 hourly.

In UTI without bacteremia:
- Fosfomycin 3 g one dose only for uncomplicated UTI
- Nitrofurantoin 100 mg orally 6 hourly
- Ampicillin or amoxicillin 2 g IV 4–6 hourly.

Concentrations of ampicillin and amoxicillin urine far exceed those in serum.

In selected cases of catheter-associated bacteremia removal of catheter and a short course of antibiotics (5–7 days) may be sufficient. A single routine blood culture that is likely to be associated with a catheter in a patient who is otherwise doing well may not require therapy after removal of catheter.

Ref:
1. Arias CA, Murray BE. Enterococcal infection. In: Jameson JL, Fauci AS, Kasper DL, Hauser SL, Longo DL, Loscalzo J (Eds). Harrisons Principles of Internal Medicine, 20th edition. United States of America: McGraw-Hill Education; 2018.

41. Ans. C

Daptomycin is not useful against pulmonary infection because the pulmonary surfactant inhibits its antibacterial activity. Ampicillin dose in complicated UTI is 2 g IV or orally 4–6 hourly. Concentration achieved in urine is much more than in blood hence can be used against isolation with high MIC as well. Dose up to 12 g/day for MIC ≥ 64 µg/mL.

Treatment for *E. faecium* meningitis includes linezolid 600 mg IV 12 hourly ± another CSF penetrating active agent (fluoroquinolone or rifampicin if susceptible).

High-dose daptomycin (10–12 mg/kg) + intraventricular daptomycin ± another CSF penetrating active agent (fluoroquinolone or rifampicin if susceptible).

Quinupristin-dalfopristin (Q/D) 22.5 mg/kg per day in divided doses 8 hourly + intraventricular Q/D ± another active agent (fluoroquinolone or rifampicin if susceptible).

42. Ans. A

The diagnosis here is most likely to be rickettsial disease (scrub typhus). *Rickettsia* due to scrub typhus may present as an acute febrile illness with intense headache and myalgias. Approximately, one-half of all patients develop a characteristically nonpruritic macular or maculopapular rash. A painless papule often appears at site of infecting chigger bite with subsequent central necrosis which in turn leads to formation of eschar with a black crust. Other signs and symptoms of scrub typhus are a localized or generalized lymphadenopathy, acute kidney injury, nausea, vomiting and diarrhea respiratory complications, meningitis, and encephalitis syndromes; relative bradycardia occurs in scrub typhus.

No laboratory test is diagnostically reliable in early phase of scrub typhus. Patient with scrub typhus may develop following laboratory abnormalities, thrombocytopenia elevated creatinine and hepatic enzymes and bilirubin, leukopenia or leukocytosis but usually normal WBC.

The indirect fluorescent antibody (IFA) test remains one of mainstay of serologic diagnosis. A conclusive diagnosis of acute scrub typhus using the IFA assay should be based on upon at least fourfold increase in titer in paired sample drawn at least 14 days apart. When single measurement is presented the most common cut off titer is 1:50.

Ref:
1. Aronott DM, Nat G. Prevalence of relative bradycardia in Oriental tsutsugamushi infection. Am J Trop Med Hyg. 2003;68(4):477-9.
2. Blacksell SD, Bryant NJ, Paris DH, Doust JA, Sakoda Y, Day NPJ. Scrub typhus serological testing with indirect immunofluorescent method as a diagnostic standard: a lack of consensus leads to lot of confusion. Clinical Infect Dis. 2007;44(3):391-401.
3. Doxycycline 100 mg orally or IV twice daily is drug of choice. Azithromycin is advised as an alternate agent. Chloramphenicol can also be used. Optimal duration of therapy is uncertain.

43. Ans. D

Immunomodulating drugs have not been found to be beneficial in treatment of acute respiratory distress syndrome (ARDS) or sepsis associated with multiorgan failure. High-dose corticosteroids in particular have no evidence of benefit and there is potential for harm.

Low-dose corticosteroids in particular hydrocortisone 200–400 mg/day may be useful in persisting shock.

Suspected case not having pneumonia does not require antibiotic therapy. Antibacterial agents should be used as per locally accepted clinical practice guidelines. Patient on mechanical ventilation should be administered antibiotics prophylactically to prevent hospital-acquired infections.

Ref:
1. Ministry of Health and Family Welfare (2019). Clinical management protocol for seasonal influenza. [online] Available from https://ncdc.gov.in/WriteReadData/l892s/66872871241561442115.pdf [Last accessed February, 2020].

44. Ans. C

Acinetobacter has been seen to cause community-acquired pneumonia. *A. Baumannii* is the most resistant of the genospecies. *A. junii* is usually seen in patients having a malignancy. *Acinetobacter* species are gram-negative coccobacilli, strictly aerobic, nonfermenters of glucose and oxidase negative.

Ref:
1. Chuang YC, Sheng WH, Li SY, Lin YC, Wang JT, Chen YC, et al. Influence of genospecies of Acinetobacter baumannii complex on clinical outcomes of patients with acinetobacter bacteremia; Clin Infect Dis. 2011;52(3):352-60.
2. Hung YT, Lee YT, Huang LJ, Chen TL, Yu KW, Fung CA, et al. Clinical characteristics of patients with Acinetobacter junii infection. J Microbial Immuno Infect. 2009;42(1):47-53.

CHAPTER 24

Hematological Disorders and Infections

VP Antia, Dipsha Kriplani

1. A child of 5 years of age presented with severe anemia, reticulocytopenia, and febrile illness associated with typical cutaneous eruptions, arthralgia, and arthritis. Bone marrow shows giant pronormoblasts. Most likely etiological agent is?
   A. Hepatitis B virus infection
   B. Cytomegalovirus (CMV) infection
   C. Parvovirus B19 infection
   D. Marrow failure syndrome

2. Which of the following is not a risk factor for disseminated intravascular coagulation (DIC)?
   A. Amniotic fluid embolism
   B. Snake bite
   C. Abruptio placentae
   D. Major orthopedic surgery

3. Which of the following is not seen in DIC?
   A. Prolonged prothrombin time (PT) and activated partial thromboplastin time (aPTT)
   B. Thrombocytopenia with schistocytes in peripheral blood
   C. High levels of fibrinogen degradation product (FDP) with D-dimer
   D. Increased fibrinogen levels

4. A young lady presented with purpura all over the body with gum bleeding and having platelet count of 15,000/mm^3. She was given steroid to which she responded and again the platelets dropped to 40,000/mm^3 after which tapering of steroids was done. At this time, she was found to be human immunodeficiency virus (HIV) positive. What treatment should be given to this patient?
   A. Anti-D
   B. High-dose intravenous immunoglobulin (IVIg)
   C. Highly active antiretroviral therapy
   D. No treatment

5. Epstein-Barr virus (EBV) is not associated with:
   A. Nasopharyngeal carcinoma
   B. Hairy cell leukemia
   C. Oral hairy leukoplakia
   D. Leiomyosarcoma in young people with acquired immunodeficiency syndrome (AIDS)

6. Which of the following findings is not true in visceral leishmaniasis?
   A. Lymphadenopathy
   B. Positive leishmanin test in most cases
   C. Thrombocytopenia
   D. Splenomegaly

7. A 30-year-old man has had a sore throat with fever for 5 days. On physical examination, he has mildly tender generalized cervical lymphadenopathy. Laboratory findings include hemoglobin 13 g/dL, platelet count 277,000/mm^3, white blood cell (WBC) of 12,670/mm^3 with differential of 75 neutrophils, 10 band forms, and 15 lymphocytes. Which of the following is the most likely diagnosis?
   A. Lymphocytic lymphoma
   B. Hodgkin's lymphoma
   C. Group A streptococcal infection
   D. HIV

8. A 17-year-old adolescent has malaise for past 3 weeks. He has mild pharyngitis on physical examination, as well as tender axillary and inguinal lymphadenopathy. Spleen is palpable. Hemogram shows: Hb 14 g/dL, hematocrit (Hct) 42.2%, mean corpuscular volume (MCV) 90 fL, platelet count 301,000/mm^3, and WBC 8,100/mm^3 with atypical lymphocytes on peripheral blood smear. His illness is most likely acquired via following mechanisms:
   A. Congenital genetic abnormality
   B. As a result of insect bite
   C. From close contact on a date
   D. Through environmental exposure at work

9. A 10-year-old girl is noted to have increasing facial distortion for past 8 months from a lesion involving her jaw. On examination, she has a right mandibular mass. A biopsy is performed and microscopic examination reveals monotonous pattern of small noncleaved lymphocytes. Cytogenetic analysis shows t(8;14). Infection with which of the following organisms is likely to be associated with this?
   A. Adenovirus   B. CMV
   C. EBV   D. Hepatitis C virus

10. Monocytosis is seen in all, *except*:
    A. Leishmaniasis
    B. Parvovirus infection
    C. Acute bacterial infection
    D. Poststeroid therapy

11. Reactive eosinophilia is seen in all, *except*:
    A. Hodgkin's lymphoma
    B. Acute lymphoblastic leukemia (ALL)
    C. Filariasis
    D. CMV

12. Parvovirus B19 infection is associated with:
    A. PRCA
    B. Essential thrombocythemia (ET)
    C. Polycythemia vera
    D. Myelodysplastic syndrome (MDS)

13. Which of the following is not true in *Plasmodium vivax* malaria?
    A. Maybe complicated by severe anemia
    B. Maybe complicated by jaundice
    C. Is always sensitive to chloroquine
    D. May coexist with falciparum malaria in same patient

14. Which statement concerning septic shock is accurate?
    A. Abnormal activation of normal pathways appears to be the mechanism of toxic effect of gram-negative endotoxins
    B. The urinary tract is the second most common source of gram-negative bacteremia
    C. Leukopenia is not seen in septic shock
    D. Gram-negative organisms lacking cell wall endotoxins do not cause septic shock

15. How is interleukin 6 (IL-6) best described?
    A. Analogue of interferon
    B. Inflammatory cytokines
    C. Another form of tumor necrosis factor
    D. Platelet-activating factor

16. All of the following conditions are associated with increased platelet destruction, *except*:
    A. ITP
    B. Thrombotic thrombocytopenic purpura (TTP)
    C. HIV
    D. Hemolytic uremic syndrome (HUS)

17. Which surface marker is often found on natural killer cells?
    A. CD4
    B. CD8
    C. CD56
    D. CD21

18. Which of the following is true about Parvovirus B19 infection?
    A. Most adults are immune to the virus
    B. A patient with initial infection is infectious until the rash clears
    C. The virus spreads by fecal-oral contamination
    D. The virus can cause anemia

19. How often should IVIg be given for humoral immunodeficiency?
    A. Every 2 weeks
    B. Every 2 months
    C. Every 4 weeks
    D. Every 4 months

20. What usually causes post-transplant lymphomas?
    A. CMV
    B. EBV
    C. Herpes
    D. HIV

21. Myeloperoxidase (MPO) stains granules of all, *except*:
    A. Neutrophils
    B. Eosinophils
    C. Basophils
    D. Monocytes

22. Treatment of CMV pneumonia is:
    A. High-dose acyclovir
    B. Ganciclovir
    C. Valganciclovir
    D. Foscarnet

23. Mycophenolate mofetil is:
    A. Antibacterial
    B. Antifungal
    C. Immunosuppressant
    D. All of the above

24. Which viral infection is most likely to be responsible for a clinical picture of fever and pulmonary infiltration 6 weeks after allogenic stem cell transplant (SCT)?
    A. CMV
    B. Varicella zoster virus
    C. Herpes simplex virus
    D. *Pneumocystis jirovecii*

25. Antifungal prophylaxis is not required in:
    A. Acute myeloid leukemia (AML) patient on chemotherapy
    B. Autologous SCT with mucositis
    C. Autologous SCT without mucositis
    D. Must be given to all

26. *Plasmodium vivax* infects which of the following?
    A. Mature red blood cells (RBCs)
    B. Young RBCs
    C. RBCs of all ages
    D. None of the above

27. Which of the following statements is correct about postsplenectomy infection?
    A. Prophylaxis with oral penicillin 250 mg is recommended for life
    B. Patient should not travel to malaria endemic areas
    C. Inactivated vaccines are not useful in preventing infections
    D. Patient should be monitored for viral infection, particularly herpes

28. True regarding angioimmunoblastic lymphoma are all, *except*:
    A. Elderly population is affected
    B. Caused by virus
    C. Autoimmune features are present
    D. Autologous transplant should be considered early

29. The following are EBV-associated lymphomas in HIV positive patients, *except*:
    A. Burkitt lymphoma
    B. Diffuse large B-cell lymphoma (DLBCL)
    C. Primary central nervous system (CNS) lymphoma
    D. Marginal zone lymphoma

30. The following viruses are implicated in the pathogenesis of non-Hodgkin lymphoma (NHL), *except*:
    A. EBV
    B. Human T-cell lymphotropic virus 1 (HTLV-1)
    C. Human herpes virus 8 (HHV-8)
    D. Hepatitis B virus

ANSWERS WITH EXPLANATIONS

1. **Ans. C**
   A child is most likely having pure red cell aplasia (PRCA) secondary to Parvovirus B19 infection. Usually, this infection causes PRCA, transient aplastic crisis in younger children who are chronically anemic, hereditary spherocytosis, sickle cell disease, or other hemolytic anemia.
   Ref:
   1. *Brown KE, Young NS. Parvoviruses and bone marrow failure. Stem Cells. 1996;14(2):151-63.*

2. **Ans. D**
   The risk factors for DIC are: Infections, solid tumors, leukemia, trauma, brain injury, burns, liver disease, snake bite, transfusion reaction, abruptio placentae, amniotic fluid embolism, preeclampsia and eclampsia, and HELLP (hemolysis, elevated liver enzyme levels, and low platelet levels) syndrome.
   Ref:
   1. *Kramer J, Otten HM, Levi M, ten Cate H. The association of disseminated intravascular coagulation with specific diseases. Réanimation. 2002;11:575-83.*

3. **Ans. D**
   Fibrinogen levels are decreased and not increased in DIC.
   Ref:
   1. *Moake JL. Disseminated Intravascular Coagulation (DIC). MSD Manuals; 2018.*

4. **Ans. C**
   What was initially described as HIV-associated idiopathic thrombocytopenic purpura (ITP) is changed to primary HIV-associated thrombocytopenia (PHAT). PHAT is the most common cause of thrombocytopenia in people with HIV.
   Highly active antiretroviral therapy (HAART) is an important treatment modality in patients with PHAT and should be the initial treatment of choice.
   Ref:
   1. *O'Bryan TA, Okulicz JF, Bradley WP, Ganesan A, Wang X, Agan BK. Impact of the highly active antiretroviral therapy era on the epidemiology of primary HIV-associated thrombocytopenia. BMC Res Notes. 2015;8:595.*

5. **Ans. B**
   Epstein-Barr virus is associated with nasopharyngeal carcinoma in both low and high incidence areas. EBV is present in every anaplastic nasopharyngeal carcinoma.
   Oral hairy leukoplakia is an unusual disease of the lingual squamous epithelium and is a mucocutaneous manifestation of EBV.
   Epstein-Barr virus is associated with leiomyosarcoma of gastrointestinal (GI) tracts, liver, spleen, and lung in young people with AIDS.
   Ref:
   1. *Khammissa RA, Fourie J, Chandran R, Lemmer J, Feller L. Epstein-Barr virus and its association with oral hairy leukoplakia: a short review. Int J Dent. 2016;2016:4941783.*

6. **Ans. B**
   The intradermal leishmanin test (Montenegro test) becomes positive in majority cases of cutaneous or mucosal leishmaniasis. Skin test is negative in progressive visceral leishmaniasis.
   Ref:
   1. *Magill AJ, Hill DR, Solomon T, Ryan ET. Leishmaniasis. Hunter's Tropical Medicine and Emerging Infectious Disease, 9th edition. Philadelphia: Saunders Elsevier; 2012.*

7. **Ans. C**

   Tender lymphadenopathy is not seen in malignancy, so lymphocytic lymphoma and Hodgkin's lymphoma are ruled out.

   Group A streptococcal infection presents with high-grade fever and cervical adenopathy. It commonly accompanies exudative pharyngitis. HIV lymphadenopathy is usually generalized.

   Ref:
   1. *Mohseni S, Shojaiefard A, Khorgami Z, Alinejad S, Ghorbani A, Ghafouri A. Peripheral lymphadenopathy: approach and diagnostic tools. Iran J Med Sci. 2014;39(Suppl 2):158-70.*

8. **Ans. C**

   The clinical features of the patient suggest mononucleosis syndrome (kissing disease). Hematological abnormalities include peripheral blood lymphocytosis and >10% leukocytes are atypical, also called Downey cells. The routine test for infectious mononucleosis is Paul-Bunnell test proving heterophilic antibodies.

   Ref:
   1. *Balfour HH Jr, Dunmire SK, Hogquist KA. Infectious mononucleosis. Clin Transl Immunology. 2015;4(2):e33.*

9. **Ans. C**

   Presence of mandibular mass, small noncleaved cells and t(8;14) points toward the diagnosis of Burkitt lymphoma which is always associated with EBV.

   Ref:
   1. *Dozzo M, Carobolante F, Donisi PM, Scattolin A, Maino E, Sancetta R, et al. Burkitt lymphoma in adolescents and young adults: management challenges. Adolesc Health Med Ther. 2017;8:11-29.*

10. **Ans. A**

    Monocytosis is seen in *Parvovirus* infection, acute bacterial infection, and can be seen poststeroid therapy.

    Ref:
    1. *Stock W, Hoffman R. White blood cells 1: non-malignant disorders. Lancet. 2000;355(9212):1351-7.*
    2. *Lynch DT, Hall J, Foucar K. How I investigate monocytosis? Int J Lab Hem. 2018;40:107-14.*

11. **Ans. D**

    Eosinophilia is seen in Hodgkin lymphoma, ALL, and filariasis.

    Ref:
    1. *Singh V, Gomez VV, Swamy SG, Vikas B. Approach to a case of eosinophilia. IJASM. 2009;53(2):58-64.*
    2. *Montgomery ND, Dunphy CH, Mooberry M, Laramore A, Foster MC, Park SI, et al. Diagnostic complexities of eosinophilia. Arch Pathol Lab Med. 2013;137(2):259-69.*

12. **Ans. A**

    Acquired PRCA are mostly idiopathic, others are associated with underlying conditions such as thymoma, myelodysplastic syndromes, lymphoma, leukemia, systemic autoimmune disorders, and viral infection (Parvovirus B19).

    Ref:
    1. *Frickhofen N, Chen ZJ, Young NS, Cohen BJ, Heimpel H, Abkowitz JL. Parvovirus B19 as a cause of acquired chronic pure red cell aplasia. Br J Haematol. 1994; 87(4):818-24.*

13. **Ans. C**

    The occurrence of severe vivax malaria in many parts of the world is linked to declining efficacy of chloroquine.

    Ref:
    1. *Jain V, Agrawal A, Singh N. Malaria in a tertiary health care facility of Central India with special reference to severe vivax: implications for malaria control. Pathog Glob Health. 2013;107(6):299-304.*

14. **Ans. A**

    Both gram-negative and gram-positive organisms cause septic shock.

    Although the urinary tract is the third most common site of infection, it is the most common source of bacteremia. Endotoxin activates the normal complement, coagulation, and inflammatory pathways.

    Leukopenia or leukocytosis may be seen and are a part of the diagnostic criteria for sepsis.

    Ref:
    1. *Ramachandran G. Gram-positive and gram-negative bacterial toxins in sepsis. Virulence. 2014;5(1):213-8.*

15. **Ans. B**

    - IL-6 is a proinflammatory cytokine and stimulates lymphocytes and macrophages.
    - IL-6 is elevated during infections and after trauma and osteoblasts secrete IL-6 to stimulate osteoclasts formation.
    - IL-6 is an important cause of fever and an acute phase reactant.
    - IL-6 is thought to mediate disease process in atherosclerosis, lupus, and rheumatoid arthritis.

    Ref:
    1. *Tanaka T, Narazaki M, Kishimoto T. IL-6 in inflammation, immunity, and disease. Cold Spring Harb Perspect Biol. 2014;6(10):a016295.*

16. **Ans. C**

    Human immunodeficiency virus causes thrombocytopenia as a result of reduced platelet production. ITP, TTP, and HUS cause thrombocytopenia as a result of increased platelet destruction.

    Ref:
    1. *Chosamata BI. The management of immune thrombocytopenic purpura. Malawi Med J. 2015;27(3): 109-12.*

17. Ans. C
- CD4 and CD8 are T-cell markers.
- NK cells express CD16 and CD56.
- CD21 is a B-cell marker.

Ref:
1. Angelo LS, Banerjee PP, Monaco-Shawver L, Rosen JB, Makedonas G, Forbes LR, et al. Practical NK cell phenotyping and variability in healthy adults. Immunol Res. 2015;62(3):341-56.

18. Ans. D
- Only 50% of adults are immune to parvovirus.
- Once the rash associated with Parvovirus B19 appears, the patient is no longer infectious.
- The virus is spread by droplets.
- Complications of Parvovirus B19 include anemia, inflammatory arthritis, pneumonia, and encephalitis.

Ref:
1. Barah F, Whiteside S, Batista S, Morris J. Neurological aspects of human Parvovirus B19 infection: a systematic review. Rev Med Virol. 2014;24(3):154-68.

19. Ans. C
- Based on immunoglobulin half-life, IVIg should be given every 3–4 weeks
- In case where severe deficiencies occur; it can be given every 2 weeks.

Ref:
1. Prasad AN, Chaudhary S. Intravenous immunoglobulin in pediatrics: a review. Med J Armed Forces India. 2014;70(3):277-80.

20. Ans. B
Single most important risk factor of post-transplant lymphomas is EBV.

Ref:
1. Al-Mansour Z, Nelson BP, Evens AM. Post-transplant lymphoproliferative disease (PTLD): risk factors, diagnosis, and current treatment strategies. Curr Hematol Malig Rep. 2013;8(3):173-83.

21. Ans. C
Myeloperoxidase stains primary and secondary granules of cells of neutrophil lineage, eosinophil granules, granules of monocytes, and Auer rods. Granules of normal mature basophil do not stain with MPO.

Ref:
1. Bain BJ. The Nature of Leukaemia, Cytology, Cytochemistry and the Morphological Classification of Acute Leukaemia. Leukaemia Diagnosis, 5th edition. Hoboken: John Wiley and Sons Ltd; 2017.

22. Ans. B
Treatment of CMV pneumonia is ganciclovir in combination with IVIg.

Ref:
1. Alexander BT, Hladnik LM, Augustin KM, Casabar E, McKinnon PS, Reichley RM, et al. Use of cytomegalovirus intravenous immune globulin for the adjunctive treatment of cytomegalovirus in hematopoietic stem cell transplant recipients. Pharmacotherapy. 2010;30(6):554-61.

23. Ans. D
Mycophenolate mofetil has antibacterial, antifungal, antiviral, antitumor, and immunosuppressive properties.

Ref:
1. Park H. The emergence of mycophenolate mofetil in dermatology: from its roots in the world of organ transplantation to its versatile role in the dermatology treatment room. J Clin Aesthet Dermatol. 2011;4(1):18-27.

24. Ans. A
Cytomegalovirus is an important complication after postallogenic SCT. Its reactivation is common in the first 3 months after transplant.

Ref:
1. Azevedo LS, Pierrotti LC, Abdala E, Costa SF, Mara T, Strabelli V, et al. Cytomegalovirus infection in transplant recipients. Clinics (Sao Paulo). 2015;70(7):515-23.

25. Ans. C
According to National Comprehensive Cancer Network (NCCN) guidelines, AML and MDS patients with neutropenia should be given antifungal prophylaxis with posaconazole. SCT recipients should get fluconazole prophylaxis. Severe mucositis is a risk factor for candidemia in patients with hematological malignancies.

Ref:
1. Vazquez L. Antifungal prophylaxis in immunocompromised patients. Mediterr J Hematol Infect Dis. 2016;8(1):e2016040.

26. Ans. B
Plasmodium vivax invades only young RBCs whereas *Plasmodium falciparum* attacks both young and old RBCs.

Ref:
1. McQueen PG, McKenzie FE. Age-structured red blood cell susceptibility and the dynamics of malaria infections. Proc Natl Acad Sci USA. 2004;101(24):9161-6.

27. Ans. A
Postoperatively lifelong antibiotics should be advocated in all cases but if not possible, at least 2 years and for children up to 16 years of age.

Ref:
1. Salvadori MI, Price VE, Le Saux N, Lebel M, Moore D, Top K, et al. Preventing and treating infections in children with asplenia or hyposplenia. Canadian Paediatric Society; 2019.

2. *Gulbin A, Murat D, Aybar TM, Guzel TO. Cases of Opsi syndrome still candidate for medical ICU. Braz J Infect Dis. 2008;12(6):549-51.*

28. Ans. B

Angioimmunoblastic lymphoma is difficult to diagnose and treat because of the presence of B-cell and T-cell clones. It is a disease of the elderly, most common in sixth and seventh decade. Patient usually presents with fever, hepatosplenomegaly, lymphadenopathy, and autoimmune features. Autologous SCT should be considered early.

Ref:
1. *Sachsida-Colombo E, Barbosa Mariano LC, Bastos FQ, Rassi AB, de Pádua Covas Lage LA, Barreto A, et al. A difficult case of angioimmunoblastic T-cell lymphoma to diagnose. Rev Bras Hematol Hemoter. 2016;38(1):82-5.*

29. Ans. D

Epstein-Barr virus-associated lymphomas in AIDS are Burkitt lymphomas, DLBCL with immunoblastic morphology, primary CNS lymphoma, Kaposi's sarcoma, and primary effusion lymphoma.

Ref:
1. *Cesarman E. Pathology of lymphoma in HIV. Curr Opin Oncol. 2013;25(5):487-94.*

30. Ans. D

Lymphocyte transforming virus includes EBV linked to Burkitt lymphoma, HHV-8—primary effusion lymphoma, and HTLV-1—adult T-cell leukemia/lymphoma.

Ref:
1. *Ramos JC, Lossos IS. Newly emerging therapies targeting viral-related lymphomas. Curr Oncol Rep. 2011;13(5):416-26.*

CHAPTER 25

Infections in Renal Transplants

Rushi Deshpande, Rishit K Harbada, Sukanya Verma

TIME TABLE OF INFECTIONS AND RISK FACTORS

1. **A 42-year-old male patient underwent renal transplant with donor being uncle. His postoperative course was uneventful with nadir creatinine of 1.3 mg/dL. He, however, developed fever in 7th postoperative day. There were no other signs and symptoms. Which of the following will NOT be the cause of his fever?**
   A. Urinary tract infection (UTI)
   B. Line related sepsis
   C. Wound infections
   D. BK virus infection

2. **A post solid organ transplant (SOT) recipient has an increased susceptibility to various infections as compared to the general population. Which of the following statements is incorrect with respect to the risk of infections in postrenal transplant recipients?**
   A. Uncontrolled diabetes, uremia and other metabolic derangements are associated with increased risk of infections
   B. Hypogammaglobinemia is not associated with an increased risk of infections
   C. Surgical instrumentation, wound, abdominal fluid collections, and devitalized tissues are associated with increase chance of infections in post-transplant recipients
   D. Routine pretransplant vaccination is ideal to reduce the post-transplant risks of infections

BACTERIAL INFECTIONS

3. **A 39-year-old female underwent renal allograft transplant for her ESRD. Patient was on routine triple immunosuppressive medications and was put on prophylaxis with sulfamethoxazole-trimethoprim and valganciclovir and insulin for her new onset diabetes after transplant (NODAT). Two months after transplant, she presented with fever and dysuria of 1 week duration. Fever was high-grade, intermittent associated with chills. Investigations revealed a neutrophilic leukocytosis with 24,000 cells/mm³ and creatinine had increased to 2.73 mg/dL from a baseline of 1.4 mg/dL. The only source of infection was urine which on routine microscopy revealed 45 pus cells with culture being positive. What is the most likely organism?**
   A. *Escherichia coli (E. coli)*
   B. *Mycobacterium tuberculosis (MTB)*
   C. *Candida* spp.
   D. *BK virus*

4. **Which of the following statements is true with regard to UTI in postrenal transplant recipients?**
   A. Asymptomatic bacteriuria requires no treatment in transplant recipients
   B. Routine screening for UTI with periodic urine cultures at 2, 4, 8, and 12 weeks post-transplant is not recommended
   C. Complicated UTI requires treatment with injectable antibiotics for 14–21 days
   D. Six or more incidences of UTI in a year are called recurrent UTI

5. **A 34-year-old female patient underwent renal transplant for ESRD 5 months back. Her post-transplant period was uneventful. She was on routine triple immunosuppression of prednisolone, mycophenolate mofetil, and tacrolimus. She presented to the outpatient department with complaints of cough without expectoration, dyspnea, and fever since 6–7 days. Clinically, she appeared tachypneic with respiratory rate being 22 breaths/min and pulse 102 beats/min. Her oxygen saturation by pulse oximetry was 88% on room air. Chest X-ray revealed reticulonodular lesions with ground-glass opacity as shown below.**

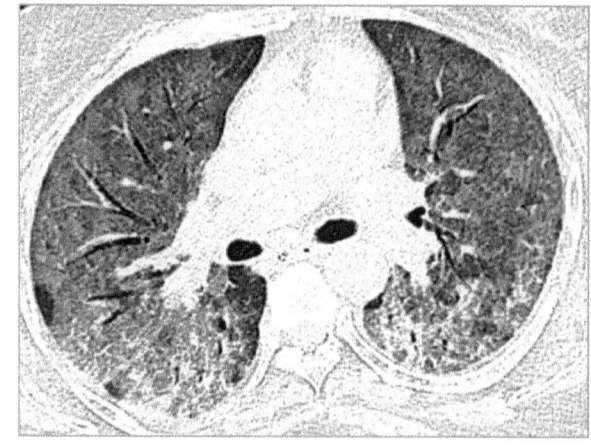

A bronchoscopy was performed. Bronchoscopic fluid was sent for evaluation that showed the following finding of acid fast branching filaments on modified Zeil–Neelson (ZN) stain.

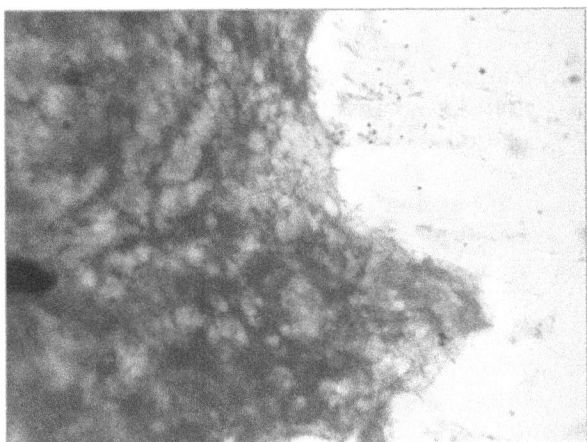

A diagnosis of nocardiosis was made. What is the treatment of choice in this patient?

A. Ampicillin
B. Cefotaxime
C. Levofloxacin
D. Trimethoprim-sulfamethoxazole (TMP-SMX)

6. A 44-year-old female underwent renal transplant for ESRD due to diabetic nephropathy. She was on routine triple immunosuppressive therapy. Third month post-transplant she underwent a kidney biopsy for increase in serum creatinine which revealed acute cellular rejection. Hence she was treated with methylprednisolone pulse therapy and antithymocyte globulin (ATG). Two months later she developed fever since 1 week, dyspnea on exertion and dry cough. No expectoration or hemoptysis. Her chest X-ray revealed patchy infiltrates in both lungs. CT scan revealed subcentrimetric nodules in the lungs with 1–2 cm paratracheal lymph node enlargement. As she did not produce sputum she underwent a bronchoalveolar lavage (BAL), reports of which were awaited.
What is the most likely diagnosis in this case?

A. *Mycobacterium avium* complex
B. Fungal pneumonia
C. *Mycobacterium tuberculosis*
D. *Histoplasma capsulatum*

7. A 38-year-old male underwent renal transplant 3 years back. He is on triple immunosuppression consisting of tacrolimus and mycophenolate mofetil, and he is admitted for complains of fever, cough, and weight loss. Chest X-ray showed infiltrates. Bronchoscopy was performed. BAL fluid showed AFB on ZN staining. TB culture is awaited. A diagnosis of primary TB was made and treatment is to be commenced. Which of the following is the most preferred treatment regimen in this patient?

A. Isoniazid (INH), rifampicin, ethambutol and pyrazinamide
B. INH, ofloxacin, ethambutol and pyrazinamide
C. INH, streptomycin, levofloxacin
D. Pyrazinamide, ethambutol, capreomycin and moxifloxacin

8. A 35-year-old female underwent a renal transplant 4 years back due to diabetic nephropathy. Her course post-transplant was uneventful except uncontrolled diabetes. She was on maintenance triple immunosuppressive therapy. Four years later she developed fever, oliguria, dysuria, and increased frequency of micturition. She was admitted and a working diagnosis of UTI was made. After sending all appropriate investigations including a urine culture she was started on injectable piperacillin and tazobactam. The urine culture showed *E. coli* and it was sensitive to the antibiotic and hence she received it for 14 days. Her symptoms were resolved and she was discharged. However, 4 days later she presented to the emergency with symptoms of multiple episodes of diarrhea and diffuse abdominal pain. On examination she looked mildly dehydrated. Laboratory reports revealed that she had marked leukocytosis (18,500 cells/mm^3), lactic acidosis and elevated serum creatinine (2.5 mg/dL). What is the most likely diagnosis in this case?

A. Giardiasis
B. *Cryptosporidium parvum* infection
C. Noninfective colitis
D. *Clostridioides difficile* infection

9. In the above case a clinical diagnosis of *C. difficile* diarrhea is made. What is the investigation of the choice in this case?

A. Detection of toxin A and B from stool
B. Detection of toxin A and B from blood
C. Detection of enzyme glutamate dehydrogenase (GDH) from stool
D. Detection of both GDH and toxin A, B from stool

10. A 53-year-old lady underwent renal transplant 8 years back. She was admitted to the hospital for a cholecystectomy. However, postoperatively she developed fever and hence the treating surgical team continued IV antibiotics for 8 days empirically. Three days later she developed diarrhea and was evaluated for the same. Stool for *Clostridium difficile* toxin A and B and GDH came positive. A diagnosis of *C. difficile* diarrhea was made. What is the treatment of choice?

A. Oral metronidazole 500 mg thrice daily for 10–14 days

B. Oral metronidazole 250 mg thrice daily for 10–14 days
C. Oral metronidazole 500 mg thrice daily for 7 days
D. Oral vancomycin (125 mg every 6 hours)

11. All of the following are implicated in the prevention of *C. difficile* infection, *except*:
    A. Judicious use of antibiotics
    B. Contact precaution
    C. Adequate environmental cleaning
    D. Droplet precaution

VIRAL INFECTIONS

12. A 38-year-old man presents to the emergency with increasing frequency of diarrhea over the last 4 days. He is a known case of renal transplant 5 years ago who is well managed on azathioprine 100 mg, tacrolimus 5 mg and prednisolone 5 mg. He had increase in serum creatinine 1 year back and received high dose immunosuppression after which his creatinine remained stable at 2.1 mg/dL. He also has ulcerative colitis with the last flare 2 years back. Presently, he is passing up to 10 watery stools a day associated with fecal urgency and nocturnal episodes. He has cramping pain in the left iliac fossa. There is no blood or mucus in the stools. On examination he is febrile at 38.2°C. His blood pressure is 120/70 mm Hg and his heart rate is 100 beats/min. He is underweight with a BMI of 18.5 and appears dehydrated. His abdomen is soft but he has tenderness in the left iliac fossa. He refuses a per rectal examination. Respiratory and cardiovascular examinations are normal.

    Laboratory investigations:
    Hemoglobin: 11.g/dL, platelets: 189 × 10^9/L, WBC: 3200 cells/mm^3 (Neutrophils: 40%) Creatinine: 2.8 mg/dL. Liver function tests and electrolytes were within normal limits. He was started on IV hydrocortisone 100 mg and IV fluids. Stools specimens were negative for routine microscopy and *C. difficile* toxin. Blood CMV PCR was awaited. He undergoes a flexible sigmoidoscopy the next day which shows widespread left-sided colitis. The biopsy results show the presence of inclusion bodies in the colonic mucosa. What is the diagnosis for this gentleman?
    A. Fungal colitis
    B. Acute exacerbation of ulcerative colitis
    C. CMV colitis
    D. *C. difficile* colitis

13. A 46-year-old lady was admitted in the nephrology ward with complaints of feeling generally unwell with headache, generalized aches and pains, lethargy and fever. She had a previous medical history of ESRD and had undergone kidney transplant 10 months prior, during the same post-transplant period she had neutropenia which had led to early cessation of her valganciclovir prophylaxis and a reduction in her immunosuppression. Her medications comprised of tacrolimus, prednisolone, mycophenolate, amlodipine, and aspirin. On examination she appeared pale, lethargic, and unwell. She had a laparotomy scar in the right iliac fossa with palpable renal transplant. Her temperature was 39.4°C, her pulse was 115 beats/min and regular, her blood pressure was 102/59 mm Hg, her respiratory rate was 22 breathes/min, and her oxygen saturation was 95% on room air. Investigations revealed anemia with hemoglobin of 9 g%, total leukocyte count of 3,500 cells/mm^3 and creatinine was 1.9 mg/dL, alanine transaminase 72 IU/L, aspartate transaminase 62 IU/L, and CRP-101 mg/L. Chest radiograph showed clear lung fields. What is the next best investigation in this patient?
    A. Plasma CMV PCR quantitative
    B. Urine culture
    C. CT scan abdomen
    D. Plasma BK virus PCR quantitative

14. Miss S, a 33-year-old female, underwent a live-related ABO compatible renal transplant with donor being mother. She received 3 mg/kg of ATG as induction. She was on routine immunosuppression with tacrolimus, mycophenolate mofetil, and prednisolone. The donor (D) and recipient (R) CMV serostatus (IgG antibody titer) was not known. She is started on valganciclovir prophylaxis. Which of the following statements is correct with respect to CMV prophylaxis?
    A. CMV-seropositive donors and negative recipient (D+/R–) are at the lowest risk
    B. Transplantations among seronegative recipients and donors (D–/R–) have the lowest risk
    C. Transplantations among D+/R+ or D–/R+ are considered to be high risk
    D. Induction with ATG does not warrant CMV prophylaxis

15. A 44-year-old female underwent renal transplant surgery 8 months back and was on maintenance immunosuppression with low dose tacrolimus, mycophenolate mofetil, and prednisolone. She underwent a kidney biopsy for increase in serum creatinine which was suggestive of acute cellular rejection. She was treated with methylprednisolone pulse and ATG and was discharged with creatinine reducing to 1.4 mg/dL. After 1 month she presented with multiple episodes of loose motions and pain

in abdomen with pancytopenia. Blood CMV PCR quantitative was done which showed 15,000 copies/mL. A diagnosis of CMV disease was made. What will be the ideal treatment in this situation?

A. Reduction in immunosuppression
B. IV Ganciclovir
C. IV Ganciclovir plus reduction in immunosuppression
D. Tab valganciclovir

16. A 30-year-old male postrenal transplant patient is being treated for CMV disease for lower respiratory tract infection (LRTI). The X-ray shown below:

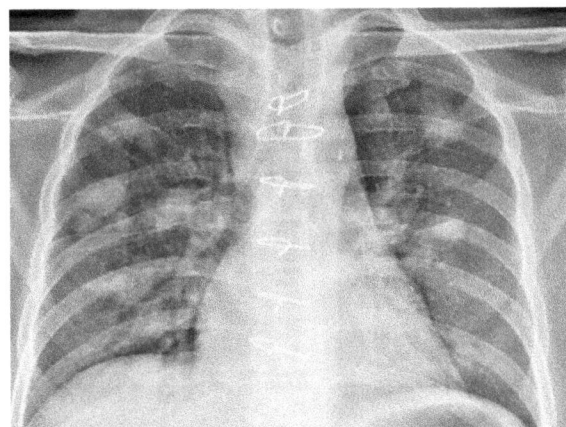

The initial starting viral load CMV PCR was 5,200 copies/mL. He was diagnosed as CMV pneumonia and he was commenced on injection ganciclovir at 5 mg/kg twice a day. However, he continued to have fever and other symptoms and CMV viral load by PCR increased to 25,000 copies/mL. A clinical diagnosis of DR CMV disease was made. What will be the next best drug to be started in this case?

A. Valganciclovir   B. Foscarnet
C. Cidofovir   D. Maribavir

17. A 60-year-old male underwent kidney transplant from a deceased donor 1 year ago. He was on triple immunosuppression (tacrolimus, mycophenolate mofetil, and prednisolone). He got admitted with complaints of low-grade fever and reduced urine output gradually since a few days. His serum creatinine levels also increased from baseline of 1.2–1.9 mg/dL. After admission he was adequately hydrated; however, his creatinine level did not decline. Urine analysis revealed 3–4 RBC/HPF with trace proteinuria (1+). Total proteinuria in 24 hours was 100 mg/24 hours.
What could be the likely cause of acute kidney injury (AKI) in this case?

A. Prerenal   B. BK viruria and viremia
C. Acute tubular necrosis D. All of the above

18. As a part of routine screening and prevention of BK virus nephropathy when should the screening for BK virus be ideally done?

A. First month of transplantation and then monthly for 6 months
B. On increase in serum creatinine
C. 6 monthly for 2 years
D. After 1 year of transplant

19. A young male aged 27 years underwent renal transplant 9 months ago with donor being his grandfather. He, however, developed gradually increasing serum creatinine. The nephrologist suspects a BK virus nephropathy. A renal biopsy is performed to detect the cause of nephropathy with a likely suspicion of BK virus nephropathy. What is the likely histopathological finding you expect which could be suggestive of BK virus nephropathy?

A. Early nephropathy with minimal injury to tubular epithelium
B. Interstitial nephritis with infiltration of mononuclear cells
C. Enlarged tubular epithelial cells with recognition of viral nuclear inclusions
D. The presence of simian virus (SV) 40 T antigen by immunohistochemistry
E. All of the above

20. A 34-year-old lady postrenal transplantation 1 year back with creeping creatinine was evaluated for her graft dysfunction. She was evaluated and allograft biopsy was suggestive of BK virus nephropathy. Considering her clinical diagnosis of BKVN what is the first step in the treatment of this case?

A. Reduction of immunosuppressive agents
B. Ciprofloxacin
C. Cidofovir
D. IV immunoglobulin

21. A 42-year-old female patient underwent renal transplant for ESRD due to hypertensive nephropathy. She was on routine triple immunosuppression (tacrolimus, mycophenolate, and prednisolone). Her immediate postoperative period was uneventful. Three years later she developed gradual onset quadriparesis. A neurology opinion was sought and a CT scan performed revealed enhancing multifocal lesions in the basal ganglia. A diagnosis of progressive multifocal leukoencephalopathy (PML) was made. Which of the following is a causative agent of PML?

A. Epstein–Barr virus
B. Cytomegalovirus
C. John Cunningham (JC) polyomavirus
D. BK polyomavirus

22. A 37-year-old gentleman underwent living donor related renal transplant with donor being father (age 62 years). He had good graft function postsurgery with baseline creatinine remaining around 1.1 mg/dL. His therapeutic regimen of immunosuppression included tacrolimus (4 mg daily) prednisolone (5 mg daily), and mycophenolate mofetil (1,500 mg daily).

After 11 months he presented to the emergency with fatigue on minimal exertion, nonspecific arthralgia and malaise for 10–15 days. On examination he had cutaneous mucosa paleness with other examination being unremarkable. Levels of hemoglobin and hematocrit were 5.6 g/dL and 16.8%, respectively. Other reports being leukocytes $5,200/mm^3$ and platelet $232,000/mm^3$, serum creatinine was 2.15 mg/dL. He also had reticulocytopenia with counts being $5,700/mm^3$. Serum iron studies and Vitamin B_{12}/folate levels were well within normal range which did not suggest a nutritional or iron deficient anemia. Also the anemia was resistant to erythropoietin (levels being 1,525 mUI/mL). Other laboratory investigations revealed he was seropositive for CMV (IgG positive) but viral load was undetectable and serology was negative for antihepatitis B, antihepatitis C, anti-HIV antibodies and Epstein–Barr antibodies. In this case, what would be the next best test for the diagnosis?

    A. Tissue transglutaminase antibody (TTG Ab)
    B. Soluble transferrin receptor antibody
    C. Parvovirus immunoglobulin M (IgM) and IgG assay
    D. Parvovirus RT-PCR

23. A 24-year-old female patient presented to the nephrology OPD with vesicular rash on the right side of the chest since 2 days which was associated with severe burning sensation. There was no history of fever. She had undergone a renal transplant 2 years back and was on routine triple drug immunosuppression. She gave a history of having chicken pox when she was 10 years old. On examination, the rash was vesicular with no scarring, excoriation or evidence of secondary bacterial infection. The rash was confined to the T2 and T3 dermatomal area. No similar lesion was present in any other site of the body. The patient was not on CMV prophylaxis. A Tzanck smear was sent for microscopic examination.
What is the likely picture seen on Tzanck smear?

    A. Multinucleated giant cells
    B. Henderson–Patterson bodies
    C. Guarneri bodies
    D. Acantholytic cells

FUNGAL INFECTIONS

24. A 44-year-old woman represents with new skin lesions.

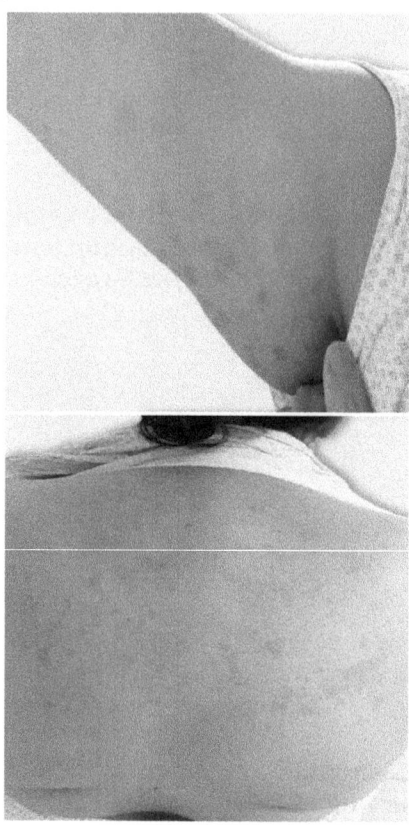

She is a kidney transplant recipient 3 years ago following IgA nephropathy. After several modifications to her immunosuppressive therapy her graft function is stable with a baseline creatinine of 0.9 mg/dL. She also has a past history of hypothyroidism for which she takes levothyroxine. She had first noticed the lesions 3 months ago. She had noted them a few years previously but on occasion they had disappeared of their own. The lesions are not itchy. On examination she has well demarcated depigmented patches on her arms, her shoulders, and her upper back. These lesions produce a yellow green fluorescence on Wood's lamp examination. What is the most likely diagnosis?

    A. Vitiligo
    B. Pityriasis alba
    C. Idiopathic guttate hypomelanosis
    D. Pityriasis versicolor (PV)

25. A 40-year-old female patient presented to the OPD with pain and difficulty on swallowing, sore throat and loss of appetite. These symptoms were present since past 10 days and symptoms worsened over time. Swallowing water resulted in burning sensation in the throat. She had undergone renal

transplant 2 years back and was on maintenance triple immunosuppression with prednisolone, mycophenolate mofetil, and tacrolimus. On examination of the oral cavity there is diffuse erythema associated with white patches on the throat, soft palate, and posterior part of tongue. The same findings of diffuse erythema and white patches were seen on the upper GI endoscopy as shown in the image.

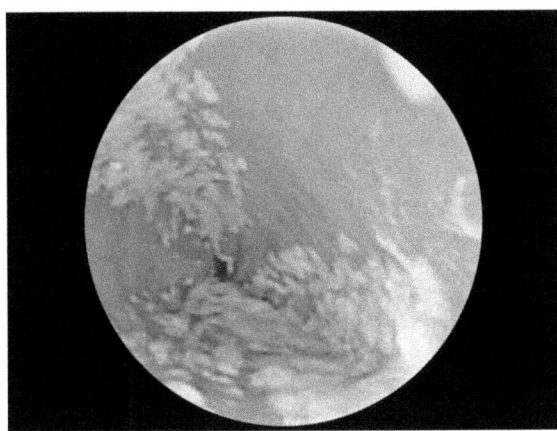

What is the likely diagnosis?
A. Herpes simplex esophagitis
B. Vincent angina
C. Oropharyngeal candidiasis
D. Cytomegalovirus esophagitis

26. A 15-year-old boy underwent renal transplant 15 days ago with donor being mother. He was on triple immunosuppression. Post period was uneventful. Two weeks later he developed fever. Urinary catheter was still in place due to voiding difficulty. On evaluation,

Laboratory parameters	Patient value
Hemoglobin	13.2 g%
Total leukocyte count	21,100 cells/mm^3
Blood urea nitrogen	62 mg/dL
Serum sodium	148 mEq/L
Serum potassium	4.6 mEq/L
Serum creatinine	2.9 mg/dL
Urine R/m	Pus cells 10–15/hpf
	RBC 6–10/hpf, Yeast cells

The child was started on IV antibiotic meropenem. However, after 2 days of treatment the urine culture grew *Candida glabrata* (*C. glabrata*) and the blood culture was also positive for *C. glabrata*.
Which of the following statements about treatment of *Candida* urosepsis is true?
A. Antifungal treatment of candiduria with indwelling catheter should be reserved for those patients who have solid clinical evidence of infection of the kidney or collecting system or disseminated candidiasis

B. Fluconazole is the drug of choice for treating lower UTI irrespective of the *Candida* species
C. 5-Flucytosine is the drug of choice for treating UTI in cases where *Candida* strain is resistant to fluconazole
D. Echinocandin cannot be used in disseminated candidiasis because of its inability to completely eradicate resultant lower urinary tract foci of infection

27. A 51-year-old male was admitted with worsening difficulty of breathing since 1 week. He has undergone kidney transplant 5 months back. He is on triple immunosuppressive regimen consisting of tacrolimus, mycophenolate, and prednisone 5 mg once daily.
On arrival he was afebrile and his vital signs were stable except for hypoxia to a saturation of 78% at room air. Chest auscultation revealed bilateral crackles with a chest X-ray showing bilateral mild interstitial and alveolar opacities as below.

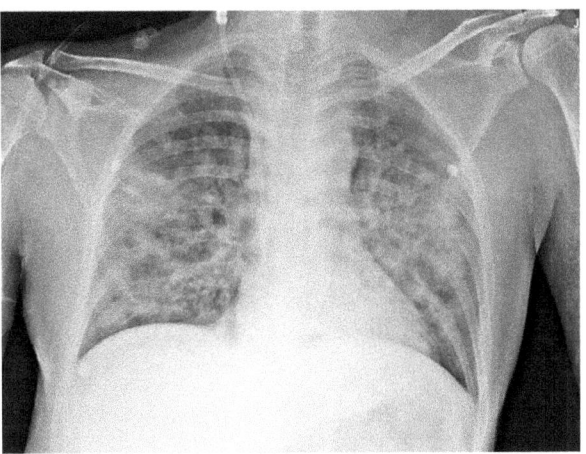

His arterial blood gas (ABG) on an FiO$_2$ 35% showed a pH of 7.41 and a pO$_2$ of 64 mm Hg. He was initially started on treatment for community acquired pneumonia with ceftriaxone and azithromycin. However, there were no signs of improvement. A BAL done on day 3 of hospital stay showed following.

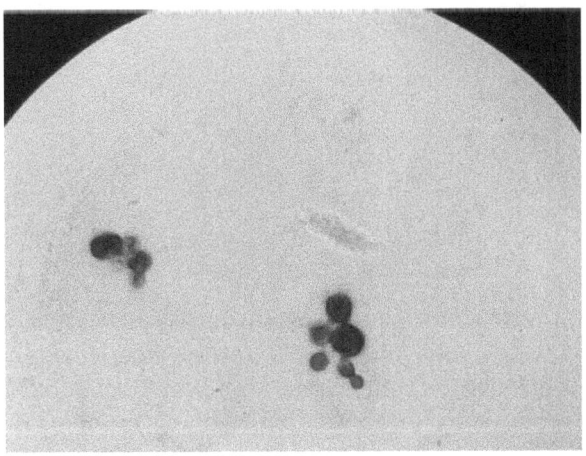

What is the likely diagnosis and treatment of choice?
A. Histoplasma and amphotericin B
B. *Mycoplasma* and azithromycin
C. *Pneumocystis jirovecii* [*Pneumocystis carinii* pneumonia (PCP)] and trimethoprim-sulfamethoxazole
D. Blastomyces and itraconazole

28. A 47-year-old male patient, known case of diabetes and hypertension, underwent allogenic renal transplant for ESRD with wife as the donor. He received heavy immunosuppression due to acute cellular rejection. Also his diabetes was uncontrolled. He presented to the emergency department 4 months later with complaints of severe headache and blurring of vision in the right eye. Blood investigations revealed leukocytosis with elevated glucose levels of 348 mg/dL and creatinine of 3.63 mg/dL.
Computed tomography scan revealed soft tissue opacification of left anterior ethmoid sinus and inflammatory changes in the apex of the left orbit with extension into the cerebrum as shown below.

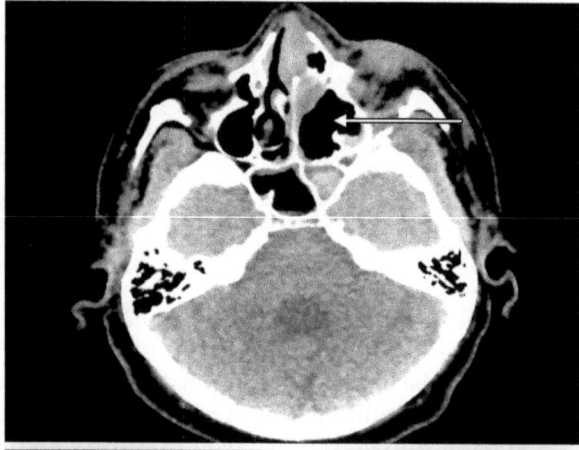

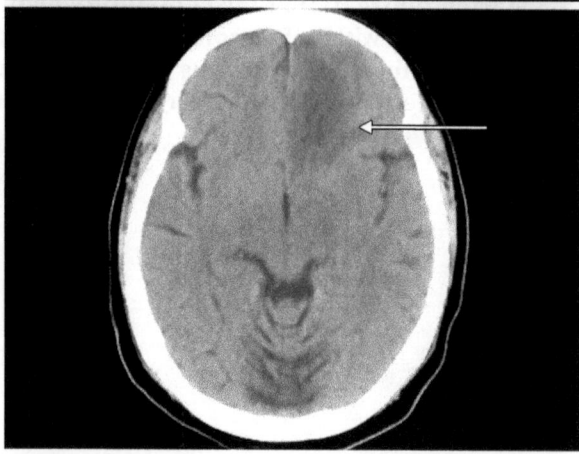

Two days later his condition deteriorated and movement of his right eye was restricted. Fundoscopy revealed central retinal artery occlusion on the left side with edema, posterior pole retinal edema, and arteriolar sclerosis. A nasal endoscopy was performed that showed necrotic tissue in the left middle meatus and the middle turbinate.
What is the likely diagnosis?
A. Histoplasmosis
B. Aspergillosis
C. Pneumocystis pneumonia
D. Mucormycosis

29. A 45-year-old female patient with chronic glomerulonephritis and ESRD underwent renal transplant 1 year ago. She presented with 3–4 episodes of loose motions and cough with mucoid expectoration since 1 month. She had low-grade fever with dyspnea on exertion since 10 days. Her routine hematological and biochemical investigations were within normal limits.
Chest X-ray, CT scan of chest and bronchoscopy revealed a large mass nodular lesion in right upper lobe of lung which was increasing in size and destroying ribs and vertebrae.
Her sputum and BAL fluid for AFB and routine biochemical, microbiological, and culture were negative.
Sputum cytology showed round to ovoid capsulated yeast-like organisms with giant cell mixed inflammatory reaction. These organisms had thick capsule which was confirmed on India Ink preparation.

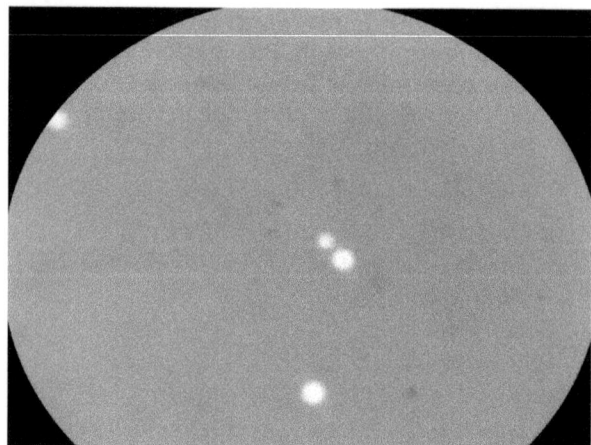

What is the likely diagnosis?
A. *Candida* pneumonia
B. Histoplasmosis
C. Blastomycosis
D. Cryptococcosis

30. A 45-year-old patient underwent postrenal transplant 2 years ago, was admitted 15 days back for increased creatinine. Empirically he received a high dose of pulse methylprednisolone therapy. Also he received a single dose of 500 mg of

injection rituximab. The patient now presents with a progressive cough, rigors and fever up to 39.4°C on his home thermometer. His physician tried two courses of antibiotics that had no beneficial effect on his symptoms. He attended the emergency services after a particularly bad episode of coughing having blood stained sputum with symptoms of fever and generalized weakness.

Investigations are as follows:

Hemoglobin: 10.4 g/dL	Platelet count: 460 × 10⁹/L	Total leukocyte count: 16,400 cells/mm³ (neutrophils: 13,500 cells/mm³)
Creatinine: 2.8 µg/dL	CRP: 135	Procalcitonin: 2.2 ng/mL

Blood culture: No growth after 48 hours of incubation.

Chest X-ray showed cavitation in right upper zone with no evidence of pleural effusion. No other focal consolidation. CT thorax—cavitation with halo sign. Sputum routine and microscopy—no organism seen on Gram stain and no AFB seen and aseptate thin branching hyphae seen.

What is the most likely diagnosis?

A. Invasive aspergillosis
B. Allergic bronchopulmonary aspergillosis (ABPA)
C. Tuberculosis
D. Lung abscess

ANSWERS WITH EXPLANATIONS

1. **Ans. D**

   Infections in the postrenal transplant follow a time table pattern. The post-transplantation period has been divided into three time frames on the basis of type and incidence of infections. In the 1st month post-transplantation, infections are mostly due to UTIs, line sepsis, wound infections, and bacterial and fungal pneumonia. Anatomic or surgical technical problems such as lymphocele, urinary leak or perigraft hematoma may increase the risk of infection. Herpes virus types 1 and 2 can get reactivated during the 1st month. Other infections that can occur in this period are untreated infections in the recipient that may be exacerbated by immunosuppression.

   Opportunistic infections are most common in the 2nd to the 6th month post-transplantation. *Cytomegalovirus (CMV), Pneumocystis jirovecii, Nocardia, Listeria* are quite common. Latent infections present in the recipient or transmitted from the donor may become reactivated or become clinically apparent like viral hepatitis or tuberculosis (TB).

   The allograft function and the degree of immunosuppression dictate the risk of infections beyond the 6th month of transplantation. The risk is increased in patients with poor allograft function and those with repeated episodes of acute rejection requiring increased immunosuppressive therapy with methylprednisolone pulses. Varicella zoster virus (VZV) reactivation is commonly seen during this period manifesting as herpes zoster. Chronic viral infections such as hepatitis B virus (HBV), hepatitis C virus (HCV), human immunodeficiency virus (HIV), Epstein–Barr virus (EBV) and CMV chorioretinitis also become apparent in this time period.

Time frame	Source of infection/ Cause of infection	Infective organism
Less than 4 weeks (Nosocomial, Donor derived, Recipient derived)	Wounds, central and peripheral lines, Aspiration pneumonia, UTI	*Nosocomial* • Multidrug-resistant organisms (MDRO)—methicillin-resistant *Staphylococcus aureus* (MRSA), extended spectrum β-lactamases (ESBL), carbapenem-resistant Enterobacteriaceae (CRE), vancomycin-resistant enterococcus (VRE) • *Clostridioides difficile* colitis • *Candida* spp. *Donor derived* HSV, HIV, *Trypanosoma cruzi* *Recipient derived-* *Aspergillus* spp.
1–6 months (Opportunistic, relapse; Reactivation of latent infection)	Immunosuppression	Bacteria: *Mycobacterium tuberculosis, Listeria, Nocardia* Virus: HSV, CMV, HBV, HCV, VZV, EBV, BK virus Parasite: *Toxoplasma gondii, Leishmania donovanii, Strongyloides stercoralis*
More than 6 months (Community acquired)	Cancers namely skin, post-transplant lymphoproliferative disorder (PTLD), anogenital	• Community acquired pneumonia • UTI • Late viral infections such as CMV, HBV, HCV, HSV, John Cunningham (JC)

(CMV: cytomegalovirus; EBV: Epstein–Barr virus; HBV: hepatitis B virus; HCV: hepatitis C virus; HIV: human immunodeficiency virus; HSV: herpes simplex virus; UTI: urinary tract infection; VZV: varicella zoster virus)

Ref:
1. Khoury JA, Brennan DC. Infectious complications in kidney transplant recipients: review of the literature. Saudi J Kidney Dis Transpl. 2005;16(4):453-97.
2. Karuthu S, Blumberg EA. Common infections in kidney transplant recipients. Clin J Am Soc Nephrol. 2012;7(12):2058-70.

2. Ans. B

In SOT patients, the risk of infection is determined by the synergy between the epidemiologic exposures of the individual and the net state of immunosuppression.

Risk factors for post-transplant infectious complications include:

Epidemiological exposure	Net state of immunosuppression
Reactivation of latent infections such as CMV, tuberculosis	Type, dose, duration, and temporal sequence of immunosuppressive therapies
Contact with potential community pathogens such as influenza, parainfluenza, respiratory syncytial virus (RSV), bacterial, viral, and parasitic gastrointestinal pathogens	Underlying diseases or comorbid conditions such as diabetes, uremia or concomitant infection with immunomodulating viruses including CMV, EBV, HBV, HCV or HIV
Geographic exposure to endemic fungi, e.g., *Histoplasma capsulatum*, *Coccidioides* spp.	Presence of devitalized tissues or fluid collections
Nosocomial infections such as *Legionella*, multidrug-resistant organisms, *Aspergillus*, azole-resistant *Candida* spp.	Invasive devices such as vascular access or urinary catheters, surgical drains, and ventricular assist devices
Donor-derived infections	Other host factors affecting immune function including neutropenia, hypogammaglobulinemia, protein-calorie malnutrition

(CMV: cytomegalovirus; EBV: Epstein–Barr virus; HBV: hepatitis B virus; HCV: hepatitis C virus; HIV: human immunodeficiency virus)

The general dictum "common things occur commonly" applies to transplant recipients too. However, in evaluation of risk factors for infections various things should be kept in mind including specific infectious exposures within the community, geography, and socioeconomic status.

The duration, severity, and the frequency of multiple simultaneous processes are features that differentiate these patients from the normal host. Some of the infections may be latent, while others may be due to the result of unappreciated active infection in the donor at the time of transplantation. The efficiency of transmission is also enhanced in immunosuppressed parents. Living and deceased organ donors are both screened routinely to avoid transmission of certain infections to transplant recipients; however, still transmission of infections from donor to recipient may still occur. Donor-derived infections include bacterial, fungal (*Candida* spp.), viral (HIV, HBV, HCV, CMV), and parasitic infections (malaria). Transmission of resistant organisms such as MRSA, azole-resistant *Candida* spp. continues to occur with increasing frequency despite routine surgical prophylaxis. Carbapenem-resistant *Klebsiella pneumoniae* (CRKP) infections derived from the donor are associated with high morbidity and mortality and donation of organs from such donors should be avoided.

Hypogammaglobulinemia with immunoglobulin G (IgG) levels < 400 mg/dL during the 1st year post-transplantation is associated with a significant increase in the risk for fungal, respiratory infections, CMV infections, and higher all-cause mortality among recipients of SOT. IgG levels monitoring post-transplant and replacing intravenous immunoglobulin (IVIg) to keep IgG level > 700–800 mg/dL may help to bring down infection rates in these patients, although prospective controlled trials are lacking in this regard. Hence the identification and correction of modifiable risk factors are very essential for the prevention and treatment of infection.

Ref:
1. Fishman JA. Infection in solid-organ transplant recipients. N Engl J Med. 2007;357(25):2601-14.
2. Fishman JA. Infection in Organ Transplantation. Am J Transplant. 2017;17(4):856-79.
3. Florescu DF, Kalil AC, Qiu F, Schmidt CM, Sandkovsky U. What is the impact of hypogammaglobulinemia on the rate of infections and survival in solid organ transplantation? A meta-analysis. Am J Transplant. 2013;13(10):2601-10.
4. Varotti G, Dodi F, Marchese A, Terulla A, Bertocchi M, Fontana I. Fatal donor-derived carbapenem-resistant Klebsiella pneumoniae infection in a combined kidney-pancreas transplantation. Case Rep Transplant. 2016; 2016:7920951.

3. Ans. A

Urinary tract infection is the most common bacterial infection affecting renal transplant recipients. The incidence is higher than those found in general population and more in females. The incidence of UTI in renal transplant is more as compared to other SOT. UTI is the most common source of sepsis associated with high morbidity if left untreated.

Gram-negative bacilli are common causes of UTI in renal transplant recipient as in general population. *E. coli* is the most common organism. The other common organisms implicated include *Pseudomonas aeruginosa, Enterobacter cloacae,* coagulase negative *Staphylococci, Enterococcus, Klebsiella pnuemoniae,* and *Morganella morganii.* The spectrum of organisms causing cystitis and pyelonephritis vary slightly.

Organism causing cystitis	Organism causing pyelonephritis
Escherichia coli	Escherichia coli
Enterococcus faecalis	Pseudomonas aeruginosa
Klebsiella pneumoniae	Klebsiella pneumoniae
Enterococcus faecium	Morganella morganii
Proteus mirabilis	Enterococcus faecalis
Klebsiella oxytoca	
Morganella morganii	
Pseudomonas aeruginosa	

Pyelonephritis can develop in the transplanted kidney. Infection in the graft may result in graft failure. Graft infection warrants early diagnosis and treatment. Graft pyelonephritis presents as lower abdominal pain and fever. Differential diagnosis includes appendicitis and diverticulitis. In female ectopic pregnancy, pelvic inflammatory disease, ovarian cyst torsion should be considered. Graft rejection can produce fever and pain over the transplanted kidney. An abscess or other space-occupying lesion should be considered in the patient with UTI when fever persists beyond 48–72 hours despite appropriate antimicrobial therapy.

Cystitis should be treated with empiric antibiotic. The local antibiotic resistance pattern should be taken into consideration while making a choice of antibiotic. The drug of choice for treatment of UTI includes quinolone, oral cephalosporin, and fosfomycin. The recommended duration of therapy is 10–14 days.

Ref:
1. Pellé G, Vimont S, Levy PP, Hertig A, Ouali N, Chassin C, et al. Acute pyelonephritis represents a risk factor impairing long-term kidney graft function. Am J Transplant. 2007;7(4):899-907.
2. Senger SS, Arslan H, Azap OK, Timurkaynak F, Cağir U, Haberal M. Urinary tract infections in renal transplant recipients. Transplant Proc. 2007;39(4):1016-7.
3. López-Medrano F, García-Bravo M, Morales JM, Andrés A, San Juan R, Lizasoain M, et al. Urinary tract infection due to Corynebacterium urealyticum in kidney transplant recipients: An underdiagnosed etiology for obstructive uropathy and graft dysfunction-results of a prospective cohort study. Clin Infect Dis. 2008;46(6):825-30.

4. **Ans. C**

Urinary tract infection in kidney transplant recipients is associated with acute cellular rejection, impaired allograft function, allograft loss, and in a few cases even death. Ideally among all transplant recipients, screening urine cultures should be obtained at 2, 4, 8, and 12 weeks post-transplant. Regular screening for asymptomatic bacteriuria more than 3 months post-transplant is not recommended because the incidence is highest in this period and screening beyond this period is not recommended because of unnecessary administration of antibiotics. Untreated UTI is associated with increased incidences of graft dysfunction and rejection.

The administration of prophylactic antibiotics to prevent UTI is recommended for all kidney transplant recipients. Daily single-strength tablet of trimethoprim-sulfamethoxazole orally usually acts for UTI prevention in most cases and it is continued for at least 6 months to 1 year post-transplant. Few centers continue prophylaxis indefinitely. Cephalexin 500 mg orally twice daily for 3 months for the few who are unable to take trimethoprim-sulfamethoxazole or are allergic to it.

Renal transplant recipients with signs or symptoms of UTI should undergo thorough evaluation with a urine dipstick, urine microscopy, urine culture, and blood culture. In a few patients with complicated UTI imaging may be needed to exclude potentially correctable structural or functional abnormalities of the urinary tract. It is ideal to perform an ultrasound scan of both transplant kidney along with the native kidney and bladder in patients who present with UTI within 1 month of transplantation have past history of nephrolithiasis or three or more UTIs within the same year call (Recurrent UTI).

The optimal imaging modality is not defined but ultrasonography of the urinary system is usually the first investigation because of its ease to perform and lack of side effects including radiation exposure. Patients who have autosomal dominant polycystic disease (ADPKD) should be investigated using computed tomography (CT) or positron emission tomography (PET) scan. In patient with recurrent UTI, ideally a CT scan, urodynamic study or voiding cystourethrography should be done depending on the clinical scenario. Rarely cystoscopy may be done to detect abnormalities of the urethra.

Asymptomatic bacteriuria is the presence of >10^5 bacterial colony forming units per milliliter (CFU/mL) of urine on urine culture with no local or systemic symptoms of UTI. In patients with asymptomatic bacteriuria within the first 3 months of transplantation, treatment with an oral antibiotic is recommended while after 3 months it can be taken on case-to-case basis as per the treating clinician. An oral antibiotic based upon the susceptibility pattern of the microorganism is used for treatment and treatment should be given for at least 5 days.

Simple cystitis is the presence of >10^5 CFU/mL on urine culture with local urinary symptoms such as dysuria, frequency, or urgency, but no systemic symptoms or allograft pain. While in patients with simple cystitis empirical treatment with an oral antibiotic based on the antibiotic resistance patterns, patient's past causative organisms and antibiotic experience is usually recommended. The treatment should be tailored as per the causative organism and time since transplant.

Complicated UTI is the presence of $>10^5$ CFU/mL on urine culture with fever and one of the following—allograft pain, chills, malaise and/or positive blood culture with the same organism as is in urine, or biopsy with findings consistent with pyelonephritis. Recurrent UTI is three or more episodes of UTI in 1 year.

Renal transplant recipients with complicated UTI require therapy with intravenous (IV) antibiotics that cover both gram-negative and gram-positive bacteria (Grade 2C). And treatment should be modified once the causative organism and susceptibility pattern are known. Patients should be treated for at least 14–21 days, while longer duration treatments of greater than the usual 14- to 21-day course are required in cases of recurrent UTI.

Ref:
1. *Parasuraman R, Julian K; AST Infectious Diseases Community of Practice. Urinary tract infections in solid organ transplantation. Am J Transplant. 2013;13(Suppl 4):327-36.*
2. *Säemann M, Hörl WH. Urinary tract infection in renal transplant recipients. Eur J Clin Invest. 2008;38(Suppl 2):58-65.*
3. *Ariza-Heredia EJ, Beam EN, Lesnick TG, Kremers WK, Cosio FG, Razonable RR. Urinary tract infections in kidney transplant recipients: role of gender, urologic abnormalities, and antimicrobial prophylaxis. Ann Transplant. 2013;18:195-204.*
4. *Lee JR, Bang H, Dadhania D, Hartono C, Aull MJ, Satlin M, et al. Independent risk factors for urinary tract infection and for subsequent bacteremia or acute cellular rejection: a single-center report of 1166 kidney allograft recipients. Transplantation. 2013;96(8): 732-8.*

5. **Ans. D**

Nocardia is gram-positive branching bacilli, partially acid fast, commonly found in soil and water. Infection with *Nocardia* is common in immunosuppressed patients on steroid especially in SOT recipients. It has the ability to cause localized or systemic suppurative disease.

Inhalation of bacteria present in dust is the main mode of transmission and major organ affected is the lungs. Infection may present either as pneumonitis, nodular lesion or cavitation. It may also present as consolidation, interstitial infiltrates or rarely as pleural effusion. Chest X-ray and CT scan findings are diverse and may mimic TB, malignancy, or fungal infection. Definitive diagnosis can be made only by microbiological diagnosis that includes modified ZN stain and culture.

Trimethoprim-sulfamethoxazole is the drug of choice. If the patient is allergic then desensitization should be done if possible. It is given in the dose of 15 mg/kg orally in 3–4 divided doses for immunocompromised individuals whereas it is 5–10 mg/kg in immunocompetent individuals. In severe disease combination of TMP-SMX with amikacin or imipenem is recommended. Initially IV therapy is recommended for 6 weeks or till patient shows good signs of clinical improvement. No clear guideline exists on the duration of therapy; however, the treatment should be continued for a duration of 6–12 months in immunocompromised individual.

Other antibiotic found to be effective against *Nocardia* includes imipenem, meropenem, third generation cephalosporins, minocycline, and fluoroquinolones. They can be used either in clinically refractory disease to TMP-SMX or drug resistance.

Ref:
1. *Jorna T, Taylor J. Disseminated Nocardia infection in a renal transplant patient: the pitfalls of diagnosis and management. BMJ Case Rep. 2013;2013:pii: bcr2012007276.*
2. *Khadka P, Basnet RB, Khadka P, Shah DS, Pokhrel BM, Rijal BP, et al. Disseminated Nocardiosis in renal transplant recipient under therapy for pulmonary tuberculosis: a case report. BMC Res Notes. 2017;10(1):83.*
3. *Yaich S, Charfeddine K, Zaghdane S, El Aoud N, Masmoudi M, Kharrat M, et al. Pulmonary nocardiosis in a kidney transplant recipient: a case report and review of the literature. J Transplant Technol Res. 2011;1:101.*

6. **Ans. C**

Risk of development of TB is highest (50%) in the 1st year after transplant. Chronic liver disease, immunosuppression states, chronic malnutrition and patients on chemotherapy have a high risk of developing this disease. CMV infection can activate latent TB. Infection spread by inhalation of MTB bacilli that remains suspended in the air in form of aerosol. Prior exposure to MTB increases the chances of development of disease post-transplant. The disease occurs as a result of reactivation of previously acquired infection. Reinfection occurs in only a few and drug-resistant TB should be suspected in these cases.

Lung is the most common site of involvement and patients may present with cough, hemoptysis or shortness of breath. MTB infections in transplant recipient present in an unusual pattern with fever being the first presentation in contrast to general population and pyrexia of unknown origin (PUO) can be a presenting feature. It can also present in a disseminated form involving both lungs and the pleura. TB should be suspected in any patient who has pulmonary infiltrates on chest X-ray and cavitation is not a common feature seen in these patients. Approximately 30–50% of TB cases post-transplant are extra-pulmonary or disseminated and can involve liver, bone marrow, miliary disease, pericardial disease or meninges.

Detection of acid-fast bacilli (AFB) by microscopy is the most frequently employed method for diagnosis of TB. If the sputum production is scanty then bronchoscopy with BAL, gastric juice aspiration or sputum induction should be done. Culture and sensitivity should always be done to detect DR TB cases as the prevalence of DR-TB cases is increasing. Imaging methods like high-resolution CT scan or PET scan can also be used for diagnosis. Molecular techniques like polymerase chain reaction (PCR) can amplify the genetic material by using DNA probes and they have a specificity nearing 100% with variable sensitivity. Nucleic acid amplification test (NAAT) assays are available for rapid diagnosis of TB and can be done easily on direct tissue samples. The Centers for Disease Control and Prevention (CDC) recommends sending the first sputum sample for NAA testing. These assays can detect target specific MTB complex DNA sequences with nucleic acid probes in 24–48 hours. Xpert® MTB/RIF assay (Commonly called GeneXpert) an automated cartridge-based NAA test can detect presence of MTB complex along with the presence or absence of rifampicin resistance in approximately 2 hours and is now widely used for the diagnosis. Tissue biopsy for histopathological evaluation, AFB smear and culture should be obtained from the tissue or fluid. Purified protein derivative test (PPD) or interferon gamma detection is not useful for diagnosis of active TB infection. Treatment of TB consists of appropriate anti-TB therapy based on the sensitivity.

Ref:
1. Anand M, Nayyar E, Concepcion B, Salani M, Schaefer H. Tuberculosis in kidney transplant recipients: a case series. World J Transplant. 2017;7(3):213-21.
2. Sundaram M, Adhikary SD, John GT, Kekre NS. Tuberculosis in renal transplant recipients. Indian J Urol. 2008;24(3):396-400.

7. **Ans. B**

Multidrug regimen administered in adequate doses and for appropriate duration with drug compliance with minimal drug interactions forms the cornerstone of management in renal transplant patient with TB. INH, rifampicin, and pyrazinamide are the first-line essential drugs while ethambutol and one of the quinolones form the first-line supplemental agents as antituberculous treatment (ATT). They form the mainstay of treatment.

Ideally even in postrenal transplant patients, first-line is always preferred and the second-line agents [fluoroquinolones, aminoglycosides, peripheral anterior synechiae (PAS), thioacetazone, bedaquiline, etc.] are used under proper supervision only when there is resistance to first-line agents. They are associated with severe toxicity.

Isoniazid, ethambutol, and pyrazinamide are safe agents in renal transplant patients with ethambutol requiring dose adjustment as per the creatinine clearance. Rifampicin, one of the main drugs in the ATT regimen, is a strong inducer of the cytochrome-c P450 microsomal enzyme system responsible for metabolizing tacrolimus, sirolimus (mTor) inhibitors and prednisolone. Due to this reaction of enzyme induction nearly 30% patients can present with acute rejections while 20% can have allograft loss. Rifampicin, hence, is best avoided in SOT patients. If the clinician in some situations still wants to use rifampicin then the dose of immunosuppressive medications may have to be increased two- to fivefold to overcome this effect with regular drug level monitoring. Few of the drugs from the fluoroquinolone group (moxifloxacin or ofloxacin) have antimycobacterial property. They are added to make up the four-drug regimen in such situations. They can be as effective as ethambutol with fewer side effects. However, the use of fluoroquinolone is not approved in some countries for this indication.

Monitoring for side effects should be done in patients on ATT. Hepatic dysfunction, peripheral neuropathy, and rarely, psychoses are seen with INH. Hepatotoxicity is also seen with pyrazinamide along with hyperuricemia. Allopurinol should not be used to control hyperuricemia in patients on azathioprine because it potentiates the marrow toxicity of azathioprine. Ocular toxicity is seen with ethambutol and its use warrants periodic eye evaluation.

Different centers vary in their protocols with respect to dose and duration of ATT. These are based on individual and center experience. *Sundaram et al.* recommend the following four-drug regimen—pyrazinamide (3 months); ofloxacin (9 months); and INH and ethambutol (18 months). Dose adjustment should be done for INH and ethambutol adjusted for the degree of renal function.

To conclude the drug interactions between ATT drugs and immunosuppressive agents should be considered while prescribing. The duration of treatment should be prolonged. Drug-resistant (DR) TB and atypical mycobacterial infections are emerging problems. They should be suspected in cases of nonresponding patients.

Ref:
1. Sundaram M, Adhikary SD, John GT, Kekre NS. Tuberculosis in renal transplant recipients. Indian J Urol. 2008;24(3):396-400.

2. Singh N, Paterson DL. Mycobacterium tuberculosis infection in solid-organ transplantation recipients: impact and implications for management. Clin Infect Dis. 1998;27:1266-77.
3. John GT, Shankar V. Mycobacterial infections in organ transplant recipients. Semin Respir Infect. 2002;17(4):274-83.

8. Ans. D

Clostridioides difficile (*C. difficile*) infection (CDI), formerly called as *Clostridium difficile* infection, is the most common healthcare associated infection. It is associated with increasing morbidity and mortality amongst elderly hospitalized patients. It is common cause of antibiotic induced diarrhea. *C. difficile* colonizes the human intestinal tract after the normal gut flora has been disrupted after antibiotic therapy and is the causative organism of antibiotic-associated diarrhea and pseudomembranous colitis. The clinical presentation can range from asymptomatic carriage to fulminant diarrhea. It produces two types of toxins—type A is an enterotoxin while type B is a cytotoxin and they result in bloody diarrhea. Sigmoidoscopy reveals a characteristic pseudomembrane. Clinical features of CDI-associated infection are tabulated here.

Nonsevere diarrhea	Severe fulminant colitis	Recurrent disease
• Symptoms begin 2 weeks to 1 month after antibiotic therapy • Watery diarrhea • Lower quadrant abdominal pain • Nausea and vomitting • Leukocytosis	• Profuse diarrhea • Lower quadrant or diffuse abdominal pain, with abdominal distention • Fever • Hypovolemia • Lactic acidosis, hypoalbuminemia • Marked leukocytosis with deranged kidney functions	• Reappearance of Diarrhea after 2–8 weeks of completion of therapy • Can present as mild, severe or fulminant disease

Prolonged antibiotic use is the most common risk factor for development of *C. difficile* diarrhea. However, other risk factors include elderly population, history of hospitalization and immunosuppressed patients including patients of SOT and HIV. Antibiotics most commonly associated with *C. difficile* diarrhea are mentioned below in a tabulated form.

Antibiotic frequently associated with causing diarrhea	Antibiotic less frequently associated with diarrhea
Clindamycin	Aminoglycoside
Ampicillin	Metronidazole
Amoxicillin	Vancomycin
Cephalosporin	Teicoplanin
Chloramphenicol	Rifampicin
Erythromycin	
Quinolones	
Cotrimoxazole	

9. Ans. D

The laboratory diagnosis of CDI requires examination of freshly passed stool sample for detection of the presence of toxin A, toxin B and GDH by enzyme immunoassay. NAAT can also be performed to detect the toxigenic gene. Detection of toxin by enzyme immunoassay is highly specific and rapid for diagnosis of CDI. NAAT is highly specific and sensitive but is costly.

The other modalities available for diagnosis include culture, cytotoxicity testing from the sample, and cytotoxicity testing from culture. Although these techniques are quite sensitive, the cost, requirement of at least 48–72 hours for results and difficult availability are the major drawbacks.

Hence, in hospitalized patients who have more than three loose stools in 24 hours period and are not on laxative stool GDH plus toxin detection by enzyme-linked immunosorbent assay (ELISA) or GDH plus toxin detection arbitrated by NAAT should be performed. Repeat testing (within 7 days) during the same episode should not be performed.

10. Ans. A

Ideally patients should be stratified into three groups either nonsevere disease, severe disease or fulminant/complicated *C. difficile* diarrhea. Oral metronidazole (500 mg three times daily or 250 mg four times daily) and oral vancomycin (125 mg four times daily) have similar rates of efficacy, with response rates of 90–97% for 10–14 days, orally. Most *C. difficile* infections respond to either vancomycin or metronidazole, and the lack of a response should prompt an evaluation of compliance, a search for an alternative diagnosis, or an assessment for ileus or toxic megacolon should be sought for, since these conditions may prevent the drug from reaching the target site. For recurrent infection Pulsed doses of vancomycin (125 mg on alternate days) or fidaxomicin is given. Fidaxomicin is a poorly absorbed, orally administered macrolide antibiotic that is bactericidal toward *C. difficile* as compared to metronidazole and vancomycin, which are bacteriostatic.

There is reduction in the gut bacteroides and firmicutes in recurrent *C. difficile* infections. Fecal microbiota transplant causes re-inoculation of these gut microbiota from a healthy donor thus restoring the short-chain fatty acid (SCFA) production by gut microbiota. The cure rate estimated is 91–96%.

Nonsevere disease	Severe disease	Fulminant disease
White blood cell count ≤15,000 cells/mL and serum creatinine <1.5 mg/dL	White blood cell count >15,000 cells/mL and/or serum creatinine ≥1.5 mg/dL	Hypotension or shock, ileus, megacolon

Contd...

Contd...

Nonsevere disease	Severe disease	Fulminant disease
Initial episode Metronidazole 500 mg orally three times daily for 10 days Or Vancomycin 125 mg orally four times daily for 10 days	Vancomycin 125 mg orally four times daily for 10 days Or Fidaxomicin 200 mg orally twice daily for 10 days	Enteric vancomycin plus parenteral metronidazole Or Vancomycin 500 mg orally or via nasogastric tube four times daily And Metronidazole 500 mg intravenously every 8 hours

First recurrence
• If vancomycin was used for the initial episode:
  – Vancomycin pulsed-tapered regimen: 125 mg orally four times daily for 10–14 days, then 125 mg orally twice daily for 7 days, then 125 mg orally once daily for 7 days, then 125 mg orally every 2 or 3 days for 2–8 weeks
Or
  – Fidaxomicin 200 mg orally twice daily for 10 days
• If fidaxomicin or metronidazole was used for the initial episode:
  – Vancomycin 125 mg orally four times daily for 10 days
		Rectal vancomycin retention enema (500 mg in 100 mL normal saline per rectum; retained for as long as possible and readministered every 6 hours) in cases of ileus

Second or subsequent recurrence Vancomycin pulsed-tapered regimen (outlined above), Or Fidaxomicin 200 mg orally twice daily for 10 days		Rifaximin 400 mg three times daily for 20 days Or Fecal microbiota transplantation

11. Ans. D

Prevention and control of CDI requires judicious use of antibiotic, following contact precaution and adequate environmental cleaning. Judicious use of antibiotic should include written guidelines on correct antimicrobial use. The antibiotic susceptibility report should be discussed by the microbiologist and the treating physician or infectious disease specialist and the prescription of antibiotics should be controlled and monitored. Use of broad spectrum antibiotics should be avoided.

Contact precaution should be followed for symptomatic patients. Contact precautions include cohorting of patients in separate rooms, use of dedicated equipment and use of personal protecting equipment (PPE) by the healthcare workers. Frequent hand washing is the crux for preventing the spread of *C. difficile* infections. *C. difficile* spores are resistant to alcoholic disinfectants. Adequate cleaning of the room is required. Terminal cleaning of the room with approved disinfectants after the discharge of the patients is mandatory.

Ref:
1. Bouza E, Muñoz P, Alonso R. Clinical manifestations, treatment and control of infections caused by Clostridium difficile. Clin Microbiol Infect. 2005;11(Suppl 4):57-64.
2. McDonald LC, Gerding DN, Johnson S, Bakken JS, Carroll KC, Coffin SE, et al. Clinical Practice Guidelines for Clostridium difficile Infection in Adults and Children: 2017 Update by the Infectious Diseases Society of America (IDSA) and Society for Healthcare Epidemiology of America (SHEA). Clin Infect Dis. 2018;66(7):987-94.
3. Bagdasarian N, Rao K, Malani PN. Diagnosis and treatment of Clostridium difficile in adults: a systematic review. JAMA. 2015;313(4):398-408.
4. Kelly CP, LaMont JT. Clostridium difficile—more difficult than ever. N Engl J Med. 2008;359(18):1932-40.
5. Hopkins RJ, Wilson RB. Treatment of recurrent Clostridium difficile colitis: a narrative review. Gastroenterol Rep (Oxf). 2018;6(1):21-8.

12. Ans. C

This patient has CMV colitis. It can be as a consequence of immunosuppressive agents. It can present with fever and diarrhea ± blood. It can present as an exacerbation of inflammatory bowel disease (IBD) patients in those on immunosuppressive medications. Inclusion bodies are characteristic at biopsy. It will respond well to an antiviral agent ganciclovir.

Cytomegalovirus is one of the most common infections in a postrenal transplant recipient. It is associated with high morbidity and mortality. Invasive infection due to CMV has become less common in recent years due to available effective antiviral agents and widespread availability of monitoring and diagnostic assays. CMV latent infection or low-level replication can have a widespread implication on the graft and patient survival. Clinical manifestations of CMV are divided into two groups. Direct effects are also called viremic or cytopathic effects and include CMV syndrome which is viremia associated with fever, neutropenia, leukopenia, thrombocytopenia, or variable features of infectious mononucleosis including pharyngitis, lymphadenitis, and hepatitis. Other direct effects include pneumonitis, esophagitis, colitis, gastritis, bleeding or perforation, hepatitis, meningoencephalitis, pancreatitis, chorioretinitis, hemolytic uremic syndrome or thrombotic microangiopathy. These direct effects except chorioretinitis are usually observed within 1–6 months post-transplant in absence of prophylaxis, while chorioretinitis is usually observed later in the post-transplant course and at low levels of viral replication.

Indirect effects are called cellular or immunologic effects of CMV and are a result of the suppression of the host defence mechanism and predispose the host to variety of infections such as *Candida, Aspergillus* species, *P. jirovecii* and other fungal and bacterial pathogens. CMV also contributes to graft rejection, PTLD, acceleration of hepatitis C infection and also increases the risk of death.

Ref:
1. *Azevedo LS, Pierrotti LC, Abdala E, Costa SF, Strabelli TMV, Campos SV, et al. Cytomegalovirus infection in transplant recipients. Clinics (Sao Paulo). 2015;70(7):515-23.*
2. *Requião-Moura LR, de Matos AC, Pacheco-Silva A. Cytomegalovirus infection in renal transplantation: clinical aspects, management and the perspectives. Einstein (Sao Paulo). 2015;13(1):142-8.*

13. Ans. A

This lady has presented with the classical symptoms of CMV infection which is a cause of increased morbidity and mortality in renal transplant patients. The diagnosis should be suspected based on the clinical manifestations and CMV should always be one of the differential diagnoses in renal transplant patients who present with leukopenia, neutropenia, and graft dysfunction. CMV cultures from respiratory secretions are time consuming and insensitive and hence have little clinical utility. Serology is not useful in the post-transplant period as seroconversion is usually delayed and hence clinically useful in the pretransplant period. Identification of CMV inclusion bodies can be used for diagnosis but these techniques are labor intensive and less sensitive hence not preferred as the first choice investigations.

Newer techniques are qualitative detection of CMV-DNA, branched DNA assay, and the nucleic acid sequence-based amplification, which amplifies large quantities of RNA. Molecular assays (Direct DNA PCR) are highly sensitive and specific for detection of viremia. These have revolutionized the noninvasive diagnosis of CMV especially in central nervous system (CNS) and gastrointestinal tract (GIT) disease. Quantification of CMV in plasma, blood, or other body fluids helps in identifying patients who are at highest risk for developing disease, determine treatment duration and also prompt recognition of DR CMV strains. The total CMV burden expressed as copies/mL correlates with disease, severity, and response to therapy. PCR results vary significantly among various laboratories and hence require standardization.

Ref:
1. *Brennan DC. Cytomegalovirus in renal transplantation. J Am Soc Nephrol. 2001;12(4):848-55.*

14. Ans. B

Cytomegalovirus infection and disease is associated with increased mortality and graft loss. The CMV serostatus of the donor/recipient pair is the primary risk factor for CMV infection/disease. CMV donor-positive/recipient-negative (D+/R−) patients are at the highest risk for developing CMV disease through primary virus infection. CMV R+ patients have a similar risk of CMV infection as CMV D+/R− patients but are at lower risk of CMV disease. On the other hand CMV D−/R− patients are at lowest risk for CMV infection and disease. Other risk factors include use of lymphocyte-depleting agents (e.g., ATG) for induction immunosuppression use of mycophenolate or high-dose glucocorticoids, multiple organ transplantation, such as combined kidney-pancreas transplantation. Prophylaxis helps to reduce the risk of infection and disease.

Cytomegalovirus prevention can be pre-emptive or prophylactic. All patients with risk factors should be given prophylaxis and it is preferred over pre-emptive therapy due to prevention of low-level CMV replication, ease of administration, and the relatively minor and reversible side-effect profile of valganciclovir. Valganciclovir is started in the immediate post-transplant period once creatinine values become near normal. Oral ganciclovir is usually not recommended due to poor oral bioavailability whereas valacyclovir should be used with precaution due to risk of thrombotic microangiopathy.

Guidelines recommended valganciclovir 900 mg orally once daily for 6 months following transplantation, with the dose adjusted for renal function for CMV D+/R−patients. For CMV R+ patients valganciclovir 900 mg orally once daily for 3 months following transplantation, with the dose adjusted for renal function while in CMV D−/R− patients acyclovir 200 mg orally twice daily for 3 months following transplantation for HSV prophylaxis is usually recommended.

Overdosing is associated with the risk of drug toxicity, whereas underdosing increases the risk of treatment failure and antiviral resistance. In centers which adopt pre-emptive strategy, weekly monitoring for CMV replication using PCR for 3 months following transplantation is required. If active CMV infection is detected, valganciclovir or IV ganciclovir should be given at treatment doses until repeat CMV nucleic acid testing is negative and for a minimum of 21 days. If pre-emptive strategy is used HSV prophylaxis with acyclovir 200 mg orally twice daily for 3 months following transplantation needs to be given. Few minor noteworthy adverse effects of valganciclovir include leukopenia and diarrhea.

Ref:
1. *Kotton CN, Kumar D, Caliendo AM, Asberg A, Chou S, Danziger-Isakov L, et al. Updated international consensus guidelines on the management of cytomegalovirus in solid-organ transplantation. Transplantation. 2013;96(4):333-60.*

2. Brennan DC, Garlock KA, Singer GG, Schnitzler MA, Lippmann BJ, Buller RS, et al. Prophylactic oral ganciclovir compared with deferred therapy for control of cytomegalovirus in renal transplant recipients. Transplantation. 1997;64(12):1843-6.
3. Azevedo LS, Pierrotti LC, Abdala E, Costa SF, Strabelli TM, Campos SV, et al. Cytomegalovirus infection in transplant recipients. Clinics (Sao Paulo). 2015;70(7):515-23.

15. Ans. C

Timely diagnosis and treatment are required to optimize outcomes. A common approach is to group patients as either having a CMV infection or an active CMV disease.

Active CMV infection is defined as the presence of detectable CMV replication in blood regardless of whether signs or symptoms are present. Treating active CMV infection in the absence of signs and symptoms aims to reduce the progression to CMV syndrome and tissue-invasive organ disease. It is called pre-emptive therapy. Goal in these situations is to control virus progression and include decreasing dose of immunosuppression and adding antivirals. Lot of centers recommend stopping the antimetabolite immunosuppressant (i.e., azathioprine/mycophenolate) first, before adding the antiviral drug and repeat the PCR 1 week after stopping the antimetabolite to assess response and add an antiviral if there is continued evidence of viremia. Antiviral treatment is started even in the absence of symptoms if the viral load continues to increase. CMV PCR quantitative should be checked at least weekly.

Cytomegalovirus disease is defined as the presence of detectable CMV in a clinical specimen accompanied by other clinical manifestations. All transplant recipients with CMV disease should be managed by reducing the immunosuppression and by addition of antiviral therapy.

The severity of current CMV illness, viral load, ability to tolerate oral medication, and the ability to administer IV therapies are the factors that should be borne in mind while selecting the appropriate antiviral medication. However, IV ganciclovir is preferred in patients with GIT disease.

Antiviral therapy includes injectable ganciclovir, oral valganciclovir, injectable foscarnet and cidofovir. These drugs target the CMV DNA polymerase by interfering in the viral replication. Treatment in patient with life-threatening illness such as severe gastrointestinal disease, pneumonitis, and meningoencephalitis, high viral loads with full doses of ganciclovir, 5 mg/kg IV every 12 hours (adjusted for renal function) is recommended. Side effects of ganciclovir are milder and well tolerated and include leukopenia, thrombocytopenia, and diarrhea. If a patient on treatment for CMV disease develops leukopenia, it is not recommended to reduce the dose of antivirals. Other drugs like mycophenolate, azathioprine or cotrimoxazole should be sought for as a cause of leukopenia and their dose should be reduced. Also granulocyte colony stimulating factor (G-CSF) should be given, because reducing the doses of antivirals may give rise to drug resistance and hence is not recommended.

For patients with mild CMV disease with minimal signs and symptoms full treatment doses of valganciclovir, 900 mg orally twice daily (adjusted for renal function) is recommended. It has good oral bioavailability. In a study it was found to be noninferior to ganciclovir, with equivalent rates of viremia eradication and treatment success in less severe disease.

The duration of therapy depends on the clinical and virological response to treatment and the severity of disease. Ideally the typical duration of treatment is 21 days but can vary from 14 to 28 days or even longer like in patients with GIT disease.

Once symptoms and viremia are resolved, 1–3-month course of oral valganciclovir at 900 mg once daily (adjusted for renal function) to prevent relapse this is secondary prophylaxis.

Virological response monitoring to treatment with weekly PCR should be done in order to identify refractory disease and virological resistance. A decrease in the viral load generally correlates with a clinical response to treatment.

Ideally it is not recommended to restart antiproliferative immunosuppression till the conclusion of CMV treatment (i.e., when symptoms have resolved and PCR is negative), since viremia is a sign of excessive immunosuppression. However, if there is an increased risk of rejection, antimetabolites can be reintroduced at a lower dose. CMV replication by PCR should be monitored at weekly intervals for 4 weeks to ensure that CMV does not reactivate at the lower antimetabolite dose. If CMV recurs, the antimetabolite should be discontinued indefinitely and restart treatment with antivirals.

Ref:
1. Razonable RR, Humar A; AST Infectious Diseases Community of Practice. Cytomegalovirus in solid organ transplantation. Am J Transplant. 2013;13(Suppl 4):93-106.
2. Asberg A, Humar A, Rollag H, Jardine AG, Mouas H, Pescovitz MD, et al. Oral valganciclovir is noninferior to intravenous ganciclovir for the treatment of cytomegalovirus disease in solid organ transplant recipients. Am J Transplant. 2007;7(9):2106-13.
3. Gardiner BJ, Chow JK, Price LL, Nierenberg NE, Kent DM, Snydman DR. Role of secondary prophylaxis with valganciclovir in the prevention of recurrent

cytomegalovirus disease in solid organ transplant recipients. Clin Infect Dis. 2017;65(12):2000-7.
4. Kotton CN, Kumar D, Caliendo AM, Asberg A, Chou S, Danziger-Isakov L, et al. Updated international consensus guidelines on the management of cytomegalovirus in solid-organ transplantation. Transplantation. 2013;96(4):333-60.
5. Razonable RR, Åsberg A, Rollag H, Duncan J, Boisvert D, Yao JD, et al. Virologic suppression measured by a cytomegalovirus (CMV) DNA test calibrated to the World Health Organization international standard is predictive of CMV disease resolution in transplant recipients. Clin Infect Dis. 2013;56(11):1546-53.

16. Ans. B

A rising viral load or persistently elevated viral load or a rebounding viral load in the setting of CMV disease treated with adequate doses of antiviral therapy for 2 weeks should point toward the CMV disease. And when drug resistance is suspected a genotypic assay for drug resistance should be performed. Refractory CMV disease is mostly due to ganciclovir resistance. The incidence of drug resistance is around 1–2% of kidney transplant recipients with CMV infection or disease.

Drug resistance occurs in situations of chronic immunosuppression and inadequate exposure to ganciclovir either due to inadequate doses or therapy interruption causes emergence of virions that have DNA polymerase gene mutations.

Drug-resistant CMV disease is usually treated with foscarnet; however, sometimes an increased dose of ganciclovir may produce a clinical response. The preferred anti-CMV regimen depends on which mutation confers ganciclovir resistance. Common resistance mutations include the genes that encode UL97 phosphotransferase (80%), responsible for the initial phosphorylation of ganciclovir (required for its antiviral activity), and the viral DNA polymerase gene UL54. UL54 mutations usually confer dual ganciclovir-cidofovir resistance. In a significant number of patients with ganciclovir-refractory CMV disease no mutation is usually detected.

If genotypic testing identifies UL97 mutations injectable foscarnet at 60 mg/kg every 8 hours or 90 mg/kg every 12 hours (adjusted for renal function) is treatment of choice in patients with uncontrolled disease or high and increasing viral loads. Foscarnet being highly nephrotoxic warrants aggressive hydration and close laboratory monitoring. Cidofovir may be used in cases with ganciclovir and foscarnet resistance; however, it is relatively contraindicated in kidney transplant recipients due to its intense nephrotoxicity. An alternative approach can be to use letermovir, a CMV-specific antiviral compound. It inhibits the formation and release of infectious CMV virions.

It is US Food and Drug Administration (FDA) approved for CMV prevention in allogeneic hematopoietic cell transplant recipients. A phase III trial for letermovir prophylaxis in kidney transplant recipients is ongoing.

Cytomegalovirus immune globulin (CMV Ig) and IVIg should be considered in patients with life-threatening disease such as CMV pneumonitis that progresses despite appropriate antiviral agents and reduction of immunosuppression agents.

Two newer antiviral drugs, i.e., maribavir and brincidofovir are in various phases of clinical trials development for the management of CMV infection and may be useful in the treatment of multidrug-resistant CMV disease.

Ref:
1. Lurain NS, Chou S. Antiviral drug resistance of human Cytomegalovirus. Clin Microbiol Rev. 2010;23(4):689-712.
2. Fisher CE, Knudsen JL, Lease ED, Jerome KR, Rakita RM, Boeckh M, et al. Risk factors and outcomes of ganciclovir-resistant cytomegalovirus infection in solid organ transplant recipients. Clin Infect Dis. 2017;65(1):57-63.
3. Chou S, Waldemer RH, Senters AE, Michels KS, Kemble GW, Miner RC, et al. Cytomegalovirus UL97 phosphotransferase mutations that affect susceptibility to ganciclovir. J Infect Dis. 2002;185(2):162-9.
4. Razonable RR, Humar A; AST Infectious Diseases Community of Practice. Cytomegalovirus in solid organ transplantation. Am J Transplant. 2013;13(Suppl 4):93-106.
5. Chou S. Rapid in vitro evolution of human cytomegalovirus UL56 mutations that confer letermovir resistance. Antimicrob Agents Chemother. 2015;59(10):6588-93.
6. Papanicolaou GA, Silveira FP, Langston AA, Pereira MR, Avery RK, Uknis M, et al. Maribavir for refractory or resistant cytomegalovirus infections in hematopoietic-cell or solid-organ transplant recipients: a randomized, dose-ranging, double-blind, phase 2 study. Clin Infect Dis. 2019;68(8):1255-64.
7. Marty FM, Winston DJ, Rowley SD, Vance E, Papanicolaou GA, Mullane KM, et al. CMX001 to prevent cytomegalovirus disease in hematopoietic-cell transplantation. N Engl J Med. 2013;369(13):1227-36.

17. Ans. B

The common cause of AKI in post-transplant patient is prerenal, acute tubular injury, UTI and calcineurin toxicity. Since the condition did not improve after hydration prerenal cause is ruled out. Urine analysis does not show any significant findings and it further rules out acute tubular necrosis. To rule out calcineurin-induced toxicity renal biopsy is ideal and should be performed. The other probable cause of increased creatinine in this case could be CMV nephropathy or BK virus nephropathy.

BK virus is a small nonenveloped icosahedral double stranded DNA virus known to cause interstitial nephritis and allograft failure in renal transplant recipients. BK virus infection is acquired in childhood and with increasing age the seroprevalence stabilizes or wanes. Primary infection with BK virus is subclinical or may manifest as mild respiratory illness as the virus is ubiquitous in the environment. The seroprevalence rate is around 80% worldwide. The virus has a tendency to remain latent in the uroepithelial and tubular epithelial cells. In cases of intense immunosuppression the virus has a tendency to get reactivated. Replication of BK viremia (BKV) occurs during states of immune suppression and has been reported in cancer, HIV infection, pregnancy, diabetes, and transplantation.

The BK virus multiplies in the interstitium and crosses into the peritubular capillary resulting in viremia. It invades the allograft, leading to tubulointerstitial lesions and nephropathy. One-third of patients with viruria develop BKV and, without intervention, progress to BKV nephropathy (rates ranging from 1 to 10%).

Various risk factors have been implicated for BKV infection reactivation including high-dose immunosuppression, pulse steroid therapy, increased human leukocyte antigen (HLA) mismatches, and ischemia reperfusion injury.

Clinical spectrum of BKV infections includes BK viruria, BK viremia, BKV nephropathy or rarely ureteral stenosis or ulcerations. The highest prevalence of viruria or viremia is after 2–3 and 3–6 months, respectively. It commonly manifests as symptomatic rise in serum creatinine during the 1st year postrenal transplantation but has been reported to occur as early as 1 week to up to 6 years post-transplant. Clinical presentation is usually as sterile pyuria reflecting the shedding of infected tubular and ureteric epithelial cells. These cells contain sheets of virus and are detected in urine as decoy cells. Sometimes it can present as obstructive uropathy as ureteric stenosis.

Ref:
1. Drachenberg CB, Hirsch HH, Papadimitriou JC, Gosert R, Wali RK, Munivenkatappa R, et al. Polyomavirus BK versus JC replication and nephropathy in renal transplant recipients: a prospective evaluation. Transplantation. 2007;84(3):323-30.
2. Hirsch HH. Polyomavirus BK nephropathy: A (re-)emerging complication in renal transplantation. Am J Transplant. 2002;2(1):25-30.
3. Pahari A, Rees L. BK virus-associated renal problems—clinical implications. Pediatr Nephrol. 2003;18(8):743-8.
4. Shah KV. Human polyomavirus BKV and renal disease. Nephrol Dial Transplant. 2000;15(6):754-5.

18. **Ans. A**

BKV infections progress through well-characterized stages. Firstly, BKV DNA is detected in the urine, followed by detection in the plasma, and, finally, in the kidney, i.e., with BKV nephropathy (BKVN).

BKV nephropathy is preceded by a period of asymptomatic viruria followed by viremia and these can be detected weeks to months before there is a detectable increase in the serum creatinine; hence, routine screening and pre-emptive treatment is an effective strategy to prevent progression of asymptomatic BKV infection to clinically evident BKVN among transplant recipients. Screening should be pre-emptive as it is superior.

The data suggest that BK viruria which is the earliest clinical manifestation without viremia poses minimal risk; whereas minimization of immunosuppression upon detection of BK viremia is associated with excellent graft survival, low rejection rates, and preserved renal function at 5 years; hence such an approach may prevent clinically evident BKVN.

Guidelines recommend monthly screening for the first 6 months and then at 9, 12, 18, and 24 months post-transplant. This approach is based upon the observation that 85% of patients who develop BK viremia do so within the first 3–4 months after transplantation. Also screening should be performed whenever renal allograft dysfunction occurs or when an allograft biopsy is performed for allograft dysfunction.

There are no clear guidelines regarding the optimal method of screening. Urine cytology for decoy cells or PCR-based detection of urine BKV DNA or VP-1 mRNA is recommended. Decoy cells are tubular epithelial cells infected with BK virus are shed in the urine. They have large and basophilic nuclei with viral inclusions. Detection of decoy cells in the urine is a less sensitive marker as compared to urine PCR. Sensitivity is 25% and specificity is 80%. Haufen, icosahedral aggregates of polyomavirus particles and Tamm–Horsfall protein can be detected in the urine of kidney transplant patients with BKVN using negative-staining electron microscopy.

Once a positive test is obtained it should be confirmed within 4 weeks by one of the quantitative diagnostic adjunctive assays using quantitative real time PCR. Also, the threshold levels for presumptive disease being urine DNA load $> 10^7$ copies/mL, plasma DNA load $> 10^4$ copies/mL or urine VP-1 mRNA load $> 6.5 \times 10^5$ copies/ng total RNA. If either of these adjunctive test results is above threshold values, an allograft biopsy should be obtained to diagnose BKVN definitively.

Renal biopsy is the gold standard for the diagnosis of BK nephropathy.
Ref:
1. Hirsch HH, Brennan DC, Drachenberg CB, Ginevri F, Gordon J, Limaye AP, et al. Polyomavirus-associated nephropathy in renal transplantation: interdisciplinary analyses and recommendations. Transplantation. 2005;79(10):1277-86.
2. Bohl DL, Brennan DC, Ryschkewitsch C, Gaudreault-Keener M, Major EO, Storch GA. BK virus antibody titers and intensity of infections after renal transplantation. J Clin Virol. 2008;43(2):184-9.
3. Coleman DV, Gardner SD, Field AM. Human polyomavirus infection in renal allograft recipients. Br Med J. 1973;3(5876):371-5.
4. Randhawa P, Brennan DC. BK virus infection in transplant recipients: an overview and update. Am J Transplant. 2006;6(9):2000-5.

19. **Ans. E**

Renal biopsy is indicated when the viral load is more than log 4 copies/mL with rising serum creatinine. The leading lesion is interstitial nephritis. In the early stages of nephropathy, the tubules appear normal without any inflammation in the interstitium. In moderate nephropathy, the tubules are enlarged with large nuclei due to the presence of viral inclusions. The histology of BKVN is characterized by tubular atrophy and fibrosis with an inflammatory lymphocytic infiltrate that can be mistaken for acute cellular rejection. The BK virus infection is confirmed by the presence of SV 40 T antigen by immunohistochemistry. Positive SV 40 T antigen staining is 100% sensitive for BK virus nephropathy. Two core biopsies ideally from the medulla are required to confirm the diagnosis of BKVN.
Ref:
1. Sawinski D, Goral S. BK virus infection: an update on diagnosis and treatment. Nephrol Dial Transplant. 2015;30(2):209-17.

20. **Ans. A**

BK virus disease is caused by reactivation of latent infection. Since specific effective antiviral therapy does not exist, decreasing the immunosuppressive medications remains the cornerstone of therapy. The treatment regimen is usually center-specific. Reduction of the antimetabolite, dose reduction of the calcineurin inhibitor (CNI) by 25–50% targeting significantly lower levels (tacrolimus 3–4 ng/mL and cyclosporine 50–100 ng/mL, or even less) or switching from tacrolimus to cyclosporine is the treatment of choice. It is useful to monitor the response by doing regular 2 weekly plasma viral load measurements. During these treatment approaches it is ideal to monitor renal functions at least twice weekly along with drug levels and viral load, and sometimes a repeat biopsy may be needed for poor responses. Rapid reduction in the viral load is associated with improved glomerular filtration rate.

The use of specific antiviral medications remains controversial for the treatment of BKVN. Some centers recommend using cidofovir in doses of 0.25–1 mg/kg every 2 weeks. Leflunomide, an immunosuppressant used for treatment of rheumatoid arthritis and fluoroquinolones have been used with mixed results. Treatments with immunoglobulins have shown promising results in small studies. None of these treatment options have been approved by the FDA. Other treatment options include changing over to rapamycin [i.e., mechanistic target of rapamycin (mTOR inhibitors)] or brincidofovir or retinoic acids.

Retransplantation has been done successfully in patients with failed allografts due to BKVN. It should be deferred until BK viremia is resolved.
Ref:
1. Vasudev B, Hariharan S, Hussain SA, Zhu YR, Bresnahan BA, Cohen EP. BK virus nephritis: risk factors, timing, and outcome in renal transplant recipients. Kidney Int. 2005;68(4):1834-9.
2. The American Society of Transplantation Infectious Diseases Guidelines. Am J Transplant. 2009;9(Suppl 4):S92.
3. Celik B, Shapiro R, Vats A, Randhawa PS. Polyomavirus allograft nephropathy: sequential assessment of histologic viral load, tubulitis, and graft function following changes in immunosuppression. Am J Transplant. 2003;3(11):1378-82.
4. Humar A, Michaels M; AST ID Working Group on Infectious Disease Monitoring. American Society of Transplantation recommendations for screening, monitoring and reporting of infectious complications in immunosuppression trials in recipients of organ transplantation. Am J Transplant. 2006;6(2):262-74.

21. **Ans. C**

Progressive multifocal leukoencephalopathy is a demyelinating disease involving the white matter of the brain caused by JC virus belonging to *Polyomaviridae* family. It is commonly seen in patients with advanced HIV, patients with hematologic malignancies and in patients receiving certain lymphocyte-targeted agents, such as natalizumab. Infection with JC virus post-transplant is rarely observed but has been reported.

The disease presents as focal neurological deficit or sometimes seizures, however, it can gradually progress to death following extensive demyelination and associated increased neurological deficits. Hemiparesis, ataxia, cognitive impairment, aphasia, cranial nerve deficits, and visual field deficits are common presenting findings. PML needs to be differentiated from calcineurin neurotoxicity which may cause posterior reversible encephalopathy syndrome (PRES); both however respond to reduced immunosuppression. No proven therapies exist for PML in post-transplant recipients; however, reduction in immunosuppression is used commonly on similar lines to immune reconstitution in AIDS patients with PML where it is commonly observed.

Ref:
1. Fishman JA. Infection in kidney recepients. In: Morris PJ, Knechtle SJ (Eds): Kidney Transplantation - Principles and Practise, 7th edition. Edinburgh: Elsevier; 2014. p. 507.
2. Astrom KE, Mancall EL, Richardson EP Jr. Progressive multifocal leuko-encephalopathy; a hitherto unrecognized complication of chronic lymphatic leukaemia and Hodgkin's disease. Brain. 1958;81(1):93-111.
3. Tan CS, Koralnik IJ. Progressive multifocal leukoencephalopathy and other disorders caused by JC virus: clinical features and pathogenesis. Lancet Neurol. 2010;9(4):425-37.

22. Ans. D

Etiology of anemia in renal transplant recipients is multifactorial. Parvovirus B19 infection is not a frequent cause of anemia in post-transplant patients. Common causes include acute/chronic blood loss; immunosuppression/antiviral medications induced generalized bone marrow suppression, iron deficiency, hyperparathyroidism, use of angiotensin converting enzyme (ACE) inhibitors or angiotensin receptor blockers (ARBs), CMV infection, and allograft dysfunction.

The common clinical manifestations of Parvovirus B19 infection can be nonspecific including fever, rash, arthralgia, or only fatigue. Severe normochromic normocytic anemia with lack of reticulocyte response due to arrest of erythrocyte maturation and erythropoietin resistance clinches the diagnosis.

Diagnosis can be made by serology, direct viral detection by reverse transcriptase polymerase chain reaction (RT PCR) or bone marrow examination. Serologic testing for B19 virus-specific antibodies is most practical and is measured using enzyme immunoassays (EIA), which usually uses recombinant capsid proteins. IgM antibodies indicate acute infection, while previous infection detects IgG antibodies in the absence of IgM antibody. However, serology is not useful in immunosuppressed patients as they may not mount an antibody response. Also diagnosis can be confounded by administration of IV immunoglobulin or blood products which can produce false-positive IgG antibody tests. Thus, RT-PCR for identification of viral DNA is preferred for diagnosis. Bone marrow aspiration shows a hypocellular bone marrow with reduced erythrocytosis and maturation arrest with giant pronormoblast.

Presently no antiviral drugs are available for the treatment of Parvovirus B19 infection. However, IVIg in the dose of 400 mg/kg/day for 5 days is found to be beneficial in these patients. Additional courses of IVIg are used in patients with recurrence. Also immunosuppression dose reduction contributes in the resolution of infection. Development of recombinant human Parvovirus B19 vaccine composed capsid proteins is underway.

Ref:
1. Waldman M, Kopp JB. Parvovirus B19 and the kidney. Clin J Am Soc Nephrol. 2007;2(Suppl 1):S47-56.
2. Pakkyara A, Jha A, Al Salmi I, Siddiqi WA, Al Rahbi N, Kurkulasurya AP, et al. Persistent anemia in a kidney transplant recipient with Parvovirus B19 infection. Saudi J Kidney Dis Transpl. 2017;28(6):1447-50.

23. Ans. A

Multinucleated giant cells are seen in infections with Herpes group of virus. The clinical diagnosis in this case would be herpes zoster.

Herpes zoster is caused by VZV belonging to Herpesviridae family. Chicken pox is the primary manifestation of VZV. Postinfection, the virus remains latent in the ganglionic cells and gets reactivated in case of immunosuppression. After renal transplant, patients become prone to reactivation of the latent VZV virus resulting in clinical manifestation of herpes zoster infection, though not very common. Sometimes, patients may present with disseminated infection. Disseminated infection results in involvement of extra-dermatomal sites and typically occurs 7-14 days after zoster infection. The clinical presentation is typically same as that of chicken pox.

Risk factor for dissemination includes reduction in the CMI which can occur due to multiple reasons such as cancer chemotherapy, prolonged use of steroids, and SOT recipients. Use of mycophenolate mofetil has shown to be associated with development of herpes zoster infection in renal transplant recipients.

Herpes zoster in renal transplant recipient may be associated with increased risk of complication such as cutaneous scarring, postherpetic neuralgia, encephalitis, pneumonitis, hepatitis, disseminated intravascular coagulation, and graft rejection.

Diagnosis is made using Giemsa staining of the scraping from the base of vesicle (Tzanck smear) that shows typical multinucleated giant cells. Detection of varicella antigen using direct immunofluorescence (DFA) is another technique that can be employed. PCR and virus isolation on culture are techniques that are less commonly used.

Acyclovir is the treatment of choice for chickenpox as well as herpes zoster given in the dose of IV 10-15 mg/kg (or 500 mg/m^2) intravenously every 8 hours for ≥7 days. Mild-to-moderate localized infection can be treated with oral acyclovir in the dose of 800 mg five times daily × 7–10 days. Other drugs that can be used include valacyclovir, famciclovir. In case of acyclovir-resistant herpes zoster foscarnet in the dose of 60–90 mg/kg intravenously every 12 hours until healed (≥10 days) can be used. However, it is commonly associated with nephrotoxicity and electrolyte imbalance.

Ref:
1. Tarvade SM, Shahapurkar A, Dedhia NM, Bichu S. Herpes zoster in renal transplant recipient—case report and review of literature. Indian J Nephrol. 2005;15:245-7.
2. Gnann JW Jr. Antiviral therapy of varicella-zoster virus infections. In: Arvin A, Campadelli-Fiume G, Mocarski E (Eds). Human Herpesviruses: Biology, Therapy, and Immunoprophylaxis. Cambridge: Cambridge University Press; 2007. p. 65.

24. Ans. D

The yellow green fluorescence under Wood's lamp is the key factor here; none of the other answers fluoresce in this way. Hence vitiligo is not correct and the history of hypothyroidism is irrelevant. The description is not consistent with seborrheic dermatitis and the distribution of the rash is not consistent with either pityriasis alba or seborrheic dermatitis which typically affects the face.

Pityriasis versicolor also called Tinea versicolor is a superficial cutaneous fungal infection caused by *Malassezia furfur*. This fungus most commonly affects the trunk. It is one of the most common superficial fungal infections worldwide, particularly in tropical climates like India. PV is difficult to cure and the chances for relapse or recurrent infections are high due to the presence of *Malassezia* in the normal skin flora. Patches may be hypo-/hyperpigmented, pink or brown. Scaling is common with mild pruritus. Immunosuppression, malnutrition, Cushing's disease, poor transplant function, recent or multiple rejection episodes, hyperglycemia, leukopenia and older age can be the precipitating factors.

Management usually includes topical application of Ketoconazole shampoo as it is the most cost-effective if it involves larger areas. Other topical treatment includes zinc pyrithione and terbinafine. If extensive disease or failure to response to therapy occurs to topical treatment, treatment with oral itraconazole or fluconazole may be more appropriate and should be considered, with pramiconazole a possible future option. Maintenance or prophylactic therapy may be useful in preventing recurrent infection; however, at this time, there is limited research evaluating the efficacy of prophylactic antifungal treatment.

Ref:
1. Gupta AK, Foley KA. Antifungal treatment for pityriasis versicolor. J Fungi (Basel). 2015;1(1):13-29.
2. Gupta AK, Bluhm R, Summerbell R. Pityriasis versicolor. J Eur Acad Dermatol Venereol. 2002;16(1):19-33.

25. Ans. C

Infection caused by *Candida* species is the most common opportunistic infection in patients with supressed immunity. *Candida* infection arises from the endogenous flora that is present in human body. Colonization is followed by infection. Conditions that predispose colonization and overgrowth include diabetes mellitus, patients on long-term high-dose steroids, patients on cancer chemotherapy, prolonged hospitalization and SOT patients.

Mucocutaneous infections caused by *Candida* include infections of the oral cavity, esophagus, intertriginous sites and vagina. Incidence of mucocutaneous candidiasis is maximum within the 1st month of transplant, but can occur in later months also. *Candida* coats the superficial layer of the mucosa rarely it may cause erosive lesions. Oral candidiasis may be commonly associated with esophageal candidiasis. The other infections caused include UTI and intra-abdominal and disseminated candidiasis. Candiduria may be present but may be asymptomatic. The potential complication of *Candida* infection in the UTI may result in development of pyelonephritis and fungal ball formation. The diagnosis of oral candidiasis is clinical. Presence of creamy white patchy may hint toward *Candida* infection.

The treatment of oral candidiasis is clotrimazole oral application for 5 days. Alternative regimen includes nystatin and fluconazole. For esophageal candidiasis, oral fluconazole should be given for 14–21 days. In patients with prior fluconazole exposure or known fluconazole resistance, an echinocandin should be used. Posaconazole orally at 400 mg twice a day for 28 days appears to be promising in resistant patients. Special care must be taken for drug monitoring and dose reduction of CNI when fluconazole is used.

Ref:
1. Dongari-Bagtzoglou A, Dwivedi P, Ioannidou E, Shaqman M, Hull D, Burleson J. Oral Candida infection and colonization in solid organ transplant recipients. Oral Microbiol Immunol. 2009;24(3):249-54.
2. Pappas PG, Kauffman CA, Andes D, Benjamin DK Jr, Calandra TF, Edwards JE Jr, et al. Clinical practice guidelines for the management of candidiasis: 2009 update by the Infectious Diseases Society of America. Clin Infect Dis. 2009;48(5):503-35.

26. Ans. A

Urinary tract infection in post-transplant patients is a common entity. UTI can occur as early as 1 week to as late as 6 months. The most common source of UTI in the 1st month post-transplant is catheter-associated UTI (CAUTI).

The risk factor for development of *Candida* UTI remains the same as general population, i.e., use of immunosuppressive agents, previous exposure, prolonged antibiotic, and antibiotic prophylaxis. A single positive culture result for *Candida* species from a blood specimen necessitates the need for initiation of systemic antifungal therapy.

Elimination of source is the first step in management of lower UTI caused by *Candida* species. Once the source has been eliminated, fluconazole is the drug of choice in the treatment for most *Candida* species except for few species that are known to be inherently resistant to fluconazole, e.g., *Candida krusei* (*C. krusei*), *C. glabrata,* and few rare species. A dose of 200–400 mg orally, daily, for 2 weeks should be used as adequate concentration can be attained in the urine because of its highly water soluble nature. Other Azole do not attain adequate concentration in the urine, hence are not preferred for lower UTI. 5-flucytosine attains effective urine concentration, but is not preferred because of the associated toxicity. Liposomal amphotericin B does not attain adequate urinary concentration and hence is not a good drug for *Candida* cystitis. Bladder irrigation with amphotericin is known to produce good results in elimination of *Candida* from bladder.

Renal parenchymal infections can be effectively treated with fluconazole, posaconazole, and echinocandins. Echinocandins are effective in eliminating infections from the vascularized cortex and parenchyma. Their efficacy in eliminating infection from the collecting system is limited. Lipid formulation of amphotericin B should be used for elimination of renal candidiasis.

Upper UTI requires intense treatment with fluconazole 400 mg daily for 3–4 weeks. The concomitant presence of renal insufficiency affects the choice of antifungals and their dosing. Echinocandins are preferred in patients with prior exposure to azoles (caspofungin, 70-mg loading dose, then 50 mg daily; anidulafungin, 200-mg loading dose, then 100 mg daily; or micafungin, 100 mg daily) in cases of disseminated candidiasis but the lower UTI may not be eliminated and may result in relapse.

Ref:
1. Fisher JF, Sobel JD, Kauffman CA, Newman CA. Candida urinary tract infections—treatment. Clin Infect Dis. 2011;52(Suppl 6):S457-66.
2. Achkar JM, Fries BC. Candida infections of the genitourinary tract. Clin Microbiol Rev. 2010;23(2):253-73.
3. Sobel JD, Fisher JF, Kauffman CA, Newman CA. Candida urinary tract infections—epidemiology. Clin Infect Dis. 2011;52(Suppl 6):S433-6.
4. Kauffman CA. Diagnosis and management of fungal urinary tract infection. Infect Dis Clin North Am. 2014;28(1):61-74.

27. Ans. C

Pneumocystis jirovecii infections also called PCP (previously called *Pneumocystis carinii*) are common in the period of 3–6 months post-transplant. Overall incidence of PCP has reduced to 0.8 cases per 1,000 persons due to use of cotrimoxazole prophylaxis in transplant recipients. The incidence of PCP infection increases in those patients that require higher doses of immunosuppression or concomitant CMV infection.

This infection typically presents with cough, breathlessness, and hypoxemia. Radiological findings are nonspecific. X-ray may reveal perihilar and interstitial ground glass infiltrates. HRCT scan of the chest is more sensitive and may show diffuse and interstitial and nodular pattern. Hypoxemia caused by PCP has a broad gradient between the alveolar and arterial pressure. Other diagnostic feature includes raised serum LDH level > 300 IU/mL. Definitive diagnosis is established on the basis of identification of organism in induced sputum, BAL or transbronchial biopsy by immunofluorescence which demonstrates the trophic form.

The treatment includes high-dose trimethoprim sulfamethoxazole (TMP: 15–20 mg/kg—SMX: 75–100 mg/kg, IV or PO, divided into 3–4 doses daily). Alternatively in patients with sulfa allergy IV pentamidine (4 mg/kg/day for 14–21 days or atovaquone or clindamycin with primaquine can be used but all these are less effective. Treatment with adjuvant corticosteroids with rapid tapering is recommended. Low-dose trimethoprim-sulfamethoxazole is the most effective agent for prevention of infection.

Ref:
1. Fishman JA. Infection in kidney recepients. In: Morris PJ, Knechtle SJ (Eds). Kidney transplantation: Principles and Practise, 7th edition. Edinburgh: Elsevier; 2014. p. 507.
2. Iriart X, Bouar ML, Kamar N, Berry A. Pneumocystis pneumonia in solid-organ transplant recipients. J Fungi (Basel). 2015;1(3):293-331.
3. Goto N, Futamura K, Okada M, Yamamoto T, Tsujita M, Hiramitsu T, et al. Management of Pneumocystis jirovecii pneumonia in kidney transplantation to prevent further outbreak. Clin Med Insights Circ Respir Pulm Med. 2015;9(Suppl 1):81-90.

28. Ans. D

Mucormycosis is caused by fungus belonging to class Mucorales. Mucormycosis infections are common among diabetics, patients with hematological malignancies, HIV and immunosuppressed individuals including SOT recipients. The associated risk factors for mucormycosis include enhanced use of immunosuppressive therapy, prolonged prophylaxis with antifungals lacking activity against zygomycetes, the rising prevalence of diabetes mellitus, advances in diagnostic techniques, and increased awareness among the clinicians.

There has been an increasing incidence in infections caused by *Mucor* spp., ranging from 0.4 to 16%.

Mucormycosis can present as rhinocerebral, pulmonary, cutaneous, gastrointestinal, graft kidney or as disseminated infections. Rhinocerebral mucormycosis is the most common form, followed by pulmonary mucormycosis. The time frame for development of infection with *Mucor* postrenal transplant varies from as early as 1 month to as late as 4 years.

Diagnosis of mucormycosis is based on demonstration of fungal hyphae in the infected tissues. The morphologic features include broad, ribbon-like, thin-walled, nonseptate hyphae with wide-angle branching. Definitive diagnosis can be established by fungal culture, however, microbiological cultures are often negative with positive cultures on only one-third of the specimens. There are no available serological tests for routine diagnostics, and recently the use of PCR has been reported.

Treatment of mucormycosis involves a combination of surgical and medical management. Surgical management includes debridement of infected and necrotic tissues while medical management includes use of antifungal agents and decreasing the dose of immunosuppressive drugs. Only amphotericin B and posaconazole have activity against Mucorales. Liposomal amphotericin B in doses up to 10 mg/kg is the drug of choice for mucormycosis and is associated with least nephrotoxicity as compared to conventional amphotericin B. Posaconazole can be used as salvage therapy in resistant or refractory cases, or intolerance to side effects of amphotericin B. Combination therapy has been recommended to improve outcomes. Echinocandins have no role against the Mucorales while isavuconazole, a new broad-spectrum triazole antifungal agent is found to have good in vitro activity against various yeasts and molds including *Aspergillus* and *Mucorales*.

Ref:
1. Song Y, Qiao J, Giovanni G, Liu G, Yang H, Wu J, et al. Mucormycosis in renal transplant recipients: review of 174 reported cases. BMC Infect Dis. 2017;17:283.
2. Cornely OA, Arikan-Akdagli S, Dannaoui E, Groll AH, Lagrou K, Chakrabarti A, et al. ESCMID and ECMM joint clinical guidelines for the diagnosis and management of mucormycosis 2013. Clin Microbiol Infect. 2014;20(Suppl 3):5-26.

29. Ans. D

Cryptococcosis is caused by fungus *Cryptococcus neoformans* which is an opportunistic infection commonly seen in immunocompromised patients. *Cryptococcus*, an encapsulated yeast of 5–10 μ size is present in soil and bird droppings, and causes human disease.

Infection with *Cryptococcus* spp. occurs in late transplant period usually after 6 months posttransplant. Net state of immunosuppression is the main risk factor for development of infection in these patients. Infection caused by *Cryptococcus* ranges from asymptomatic pulmonary colonization to life-threatening meningitis and disseminated infection. CNS cryptococcosis is the common presentation of Cryptococcal infection in post-transplant patients; they can also present with pulmonary symptoms. Other presentation includes cutaneous involvement and disseminated infections.

A complete work-up to exclude the diagnosis should include India Ink Staining, cryptococcal polysaccharide antigen detection and culture. In immunocompromised patients with CNS disease, liposomal amphotericin B (3–4 mg/kg IV per day) or amphotericin B lipid complex (5 mg/kg IV per day) combined with flucytocine is strongly recommended for at least 2 weeks followed by oral Fluconazole 6 mg/kg/day for 8 weeks to 1 year. Treatment of nonmeningeal cryptococcosis is based on the symptoms. Pulmonary cryptococcosis associated with acute respiratory distress syndrome (ARDS) is treated like CNS cryptococcosis while in those with mild-to-moderate pulmonary involvement with no dissemination are treated with fluconazole 6 mg/kg/day for 6–12 months. If fluconazole is not available or is contraindicated, itraconazole (loading doses of 200 mg orally three times daily for 3 days, then 200 mg orally twice daily); voriconazole (loading doses of 6 mg/kg IV twice daily or 400 mg orally twice daily on the first day, then 200 mg orally twice daily); posaconazole or isavuconazole may be used.

Ref:
1. Dahdal S, Kalicki R, Von Steiger N, Sendi P. Disseminated cryptococcal infection in a patient who had kidney transplant: discrepancy between clinical symptoms and microbiological findings. BMJ Case Rep. 2017;2017: pii: bcr-2017-219234.
2. Perfect JR, Dismukes WE, Dromer F, Goldman DL, Graybill JR, Hamill RJ, et al. Clinical practice guidelines for the management of cryptococcal disease: 2010 update by the infectious diseases society of America. Clin Infect Dis. 2010;50(3):291-322.
3. Pappas PG, Perfect JR, Cloud GA, Larsen RA, Pankey GA, Lancaster DJ, et al. Cryptococcosis in human immunodeficiency virus-negative patients in the era of effective azole therapy. Clin Infect Dis. 2001;33(5):690-9.
4. Kerkering TM, Duma RJ, Shadomy S. The evolution of pulmonary cryptococcosis: clinical implications from a study of 41 patients with and without compromising host factors. Ann Intern Med. 1981;94(5):611-6.

30. **Ans. A**

This patient is likely to have had a prolonged period of immunosuppression post additional doses of high-dose immunosuppressive medications that have left him at risk of fungal infections. Fungal infections are the preserve of the immunosuppressed. They should be part of a differential diagnosis in patient undergoing chemotherapy, stem cell transplant or SOT, patient on immunosuppressive medications for autoimmune conditions and those that are HIV positive.

The patient above describes symptoms of active infection and also has the worrying symptoms of hemoptysis. Invasive aspergillosis is a medical emergency in transplant patients associated with high mortality rates. It is the third most common fungal infection in SOT patients after *Candida* and *Cryptococcus*. Lungs and sinuses are the most common sites of infection in more than 90% patients. Vascular invasion is the hallmark of invasive aspergillosis which accounts for infarction, hemorrhage, and systemic dissemination with metastatic invasion. Early in the course of transplantation CNS involvement due to *Aspergillus* is most common while after 1 year or later other fungi such as *Zygomycetes*, dematiaceous fungi become more prominent.

Presently, the conventional diagnostic methods like mycological examination (direct microscopic examination, histological examination, and culture), imaging, nonculture-based tests for the detection of galactomannan, β-(1,3)-glucan an extracellular glycoprotein, and molecular tests based on PCR used to detect this fungal infection. However, most of these methods do not detect the species *Aspergillus fumigatus* (*A. fumigatus*); they only allow the identification of genus *Aspergillus*. Fluorescent in situ hybridization (FISH)-based molecular methods can be a good alternative to achieve this purpose of identification of species.

Due to the high mortality associated with *Aspergillus* infection, it is important to identify and treat it quickly. Fluconazole is of no benefit. The first-line treatment is voriconazole which should be started intravenously before oral treatment in dose of primary therapy 6 mg/kg twice a day for 1 day, followed by 4 mg/kg IV twice a day; oral dosage is 200 mg twice a day. Duration of therapy for aspergillosis has not been optimally defined. Most experts recommend continuing treatment of infection until resolution or stabilization of all clinical and radiographic manifestations. Generally, treatment is continued for a minimum of 6–12 weeks.

Voriconazole has improved survival with better tolerability and less toxic side effects when compared to amphotericin B. Voriconazole is a strong cytochrome P450-3A4 inhibitor, hence tacrolimus dosage must often be adjusted accordingly. If tolerated better then liposomal amphotericin (3–5 mg/kg/day IV higher dosages are not more effective) should be used as oral voriconazole that may take at least 10 days to achieve the therapeutic levels. Combination antifungal therapy has been attempted to improve outcomes. Micafungin with voriconazole raises the minimal inhibitory concentration (MIC) and enhances maximal killing effects of voriconazole against *Aspergillus* hyphae, and may be considered. Other drugs such as caspofungin, posaconazole, micafungin, and itraconazole may be used in refractory cases.

Presently the high mortality rates and rising azole resistance necessitate a different approach to treatment of invasive fungal infections in immunocompromised hosts. IFN-γ therapy has shown promising results.

Ref:
1. Moura S, Cerqueira L, Almeida A. Invasive pulmonary aspergillosis: current diagnostic methodologies and a new molecular approach. Eur J Clin Microbiol Infect Dis. 2018;37(8):1393-403.
2. Estrada C, Desai AG, Chirch LM, Suh H, Seidman R, Darras F, et al. Invasive aspergillosis in a renal transplant recipient successfully treated with interferon-gamma. Case Rep Transplant. 2012;2012:493758.
3. Singh N, Husain S; AST Infectious Diseases Community of Practice. Aspergillosis in solid organ transplantation. Am J Transplant. 2013;13(Suppl 4):228-41.

CHAPTER 26

Infections in Liver Transplants

Parikshit S Prayag, Sujata Rege

1. A patient is admitted for a living donor liver transplant. The patient has end-stage liver disease from cirrhosis. 3 days prior to transplant, the nurse in the intensive care unit (ICU) sends a nasal swab for methicillin-resistant *Staphylococcus aureus* (MRSA) which is reported to be positive. The liver team calls the transplant infectious disease physician and asks him for an opinion in this situation. What should his response be?
   A. Cancel the transplant in view of the MRSA positive swab
   B. Screen the donor for MRSA
   C. Start teicoplanin or vancomycin today (3 days prior to transplant)
   D. Whole body imaging to look for active MRSA infection
   E. Go ahead with the transplant with or without nasal decolonization and note this information for future reference

2. Patient is referred to the infectious disease clinic for preliver transplant evaluation. The patient has alcoholic liver disease but has been sober for 8 months. While going through the chart the physician notes that the patient's rapid plasma reagin (RPR) test is positive. What should the approach be?
   A. Go ahead with the transplant with no further measures
   B. Repeat the RPR test
   C. Order a specific syphilis test
   D. Start therapy for primary syphilis
   E. None of the above

3. A patient comes to the infectious diseases outpatient department (OPD) prior to undergoing a living donor liver transplant. As a part of his pretransplant workup, several serologies are ordered. A week later, the patient comes back with his reports which indicate that the strongyloides immunoglobulin G (IgG) antibody is positive. He does not have any symptoms currently. What should the approach be in this setting?
   A. Ignore the result of the test
   B. Get donor serology
   C. Send a polymerase chain reaction (PCR) assay on stool
   D. Repeat the strongyloides test
   E. Give the patient ivermectin pretransplant

4. A patient undergoes a liver transplant from a living donor. The routine practice in the transplant center where this took place is to put patients on trimethoprim-sulfamethoxazole (TMP-SMX) prophylaxis for 6 months after transplant. Which of these statements is true about TMP-SMX used in this setting?
   A. It protects against only certain *Nocardia* in this setting
   B. It protects only against *Toxoplasma* in this setting
   C. It protects only against *Listeria* in this setting
   D. It protects against *Toxoplasma*, *Listeria*, and *Nocardia*

5. A patient undergoes a living donor liver transplant. Which of the following are indications for using anti-*Candida* prophylaxis in the posttransplant setting?
   A. Prolonged surgical time
   B. High transfusion requirement
   C. Patient being colonized with candida just before the transplant
   D. All of the above

6. A patient is sent to the transplant infectious diseases OPD for a pretransplant clearance. Which of the following is true about vaccines in the pretransplant setting?
   A. The pretransplant period is the time to ensure that the patient has received pneumococcal, influenza, diphtheria-tetanus-pertussis (DTP), and hepatitis B vaccines
   B. If the patient has received an measles, mumps, and rubella (MMR) vaccine, he can undergo a transplant in two weeks
   C. A live zoster vaccine can be given after transplant
   D. Following transplant, vaccines should be avoided for 3 years

7. A patient undergoes a deceased donor liver transplant. 3 weeks after the transplant the patient develops diarrhea. Stool testing is reported as

positive for the *Clostridium difficile* glutamate dehydrogenase (GDH) antigen as well as toxin production. He has three greenish bowel movements per day. White blood cell (WBC) count is 12,300 and creatinine and albumin are normal. What would be the best line of therapy?

A. Metronidazole alone
B. Intravenous (IV) vancomycin
C. Oral vancomycin
D. Oral vancomycin plus metronidazole
E. Tigecycline

8. A patient undergoes a deceased donor liver transplant. 7 months after his transplant the patient develops low grade fever. He is found to have a cytomegalovirus (CMV) viral load of 33,248. He is started on ganciclovir (induction dosing). 2 weeks into appropriately dosed therapy, the viral load is 89,382. The transplant physician sends a CMV resistance genotype panel. While awaiting the panel, what should he be switched to?

A. Higher dose of ganciclovir
B. Cidofovir
C. Foscarnet
D. Stop ganciclovir, give intravenous immunoglobulin (IVIG)

9. A patient undergoes a deceased donor liver transplant. 6 months after the transplant, he develops pancytopenia with transaminitis, low grade fevers, and diarrhea. A liver biopsy does not show any evidence of rejection. CMV PCR, toxoplasma PCR, and procalcitonin are negative. Blood adenovirus PCR shows 333,489 copies/mL. Herpes simplex virus (HSV) and varicella zoster virus (VZV) PCR in the blood are negative. Which of the following agents has the maximum activity against adenovirus in vitro?

A. Foscarnet   B. Ribavirin
C. Cidofovir   D. Oseltamivir
E. Ganciclovir

10. About 5 months after a living donor liver transplant, a patient develops fever. Immunosuppression regimen includes prednisone, mycophenolate, and tacrolimus. 3 days later, he develops difficulty in breathing, as well as icterus. A CT scan of the chest shows bilateral predominantly interstitial infiltrates. Echo reveals a reduced ejection fraction (EF) of 24% (baseline normal) at the time of transplant. Liver function tests show a bilirubin of 8 mg/dL, aspartate aminotransferase (AST) of 1,345 units per liter, alanine aminotransferase (ALT) of 190 units per liter. CMV viral load is undetectable. HSV and VZV PCRs in the blood are negative. The patient is on acyclovir prophylaxis. Blood cultures and procalcitonin are negative. A bronchoalveolar lavage (BAL) is done which is negative for adenovirus PCR, CMV PCR, atypical organisms (legionella PCR, mycoplasma PCR, chlamydia PCR, and Bordetella PCR). Which is the most likely diagnosis?

A. Disseminated histoplasmosis
B. Invasive aspergillosis (IA)
C. Disseminated strongyloidiasis
D. Severe CMV infection
E. Disseminated toxoplasmosis

11. A patient who has undergone deceased donor liver transplant 4 months back presents with progressive shortness of breath. He has also had subjective fevers and fatigue since a week. He is found to have hemoglobin of 4.3 g/dL. WBCs and platelets are within normal limits. Reticulocyte count is low. CMV PCR (blood) and adenovirus PCR (blood) are negative. He undergoes a bone marrow biopsy which reveals several giant erythroblasts with prominent intranuclear viral inclusions. What is the most effective therapy for this patient?

A. Ganciclovir
B. Foscarnet
C. Doxycycline or azithromycin
D. Intravenous immunoglobulin
E. Ribavirin

12. A patient undergoes right lobe living donor liver transplant. 14 months later, he comes to your clinic saying that his 1-year-old grandson has been confirmed to have chickenpox by his primary care physician. He lives with his grandson and cares for him, including feeding him lunch. You go through the records and find out that the patient is VZV IgG negative. He is no longer on acyclovir prophylaxis. What should be done?

A. Monitor clinically only
B. Either give varicella immunoglobulin or antiviral therapy
C. Send VZV PCR in the patient
D. Administer the zoster vaccine
E. Administer acyclovir to the infant

13. A patient develops fever 1 week after a right lobe living donor liver transplant. Clinically he does not have any focal symptoms. He has been on vancomycin and cefepime for the last 7 days. He has been started on fluconazole prophylaxis. Blood cultures are sent, which grow gram-positive cocci in 24 hours. A PCR-based assay identifies the presence of *VanA* gene, and the gram-positive cocci as *Enterococcus*. The treating physician changes the vancomycin to daptomycin. Patient remains febrile

over the next 48 hours. On the third day after the onset of fever, the blood culture report is available:

Antibiotic	Susceptibility
Vancomycin	R
Daptomycin	R
Linezolid	R
Aminoglycoside synergy	R
Teicoplanin	R
Tigecycline	R

The species is identified as *Enterococcus faecium*. Apart from ordering an echocardiogram and ensuring line removal, what would be the best agent for this infection?

A. Vancomycin alone in high dose
B. Vancomycin plus gentamicin
C. Daptomycin 10 mg/kg
D. Test for ceftaroline, if available use it with or without daptomycin
E. Linezolid plus vancomycin plus daptomycin

14. Which of the following solid organ transplants has been found to have the highest risk of developing posttransplant lymphoproliferative disorder (PTLD)?

A. Heart
B. Lung
C. Liver
D. Kidney
E. Intestine/multiorgan transplants

15. A patient with deceased donor liver transplant on steroids, tacrolimus, and mycophenolate presents with fever on day 7 of the transplant. He has been on meropenem. A blood culture sent from the central and peripheral line is growing *Klebsiella pneumoniae* which is resistant to meropenem, colistin, and ceftazidime-avibactam. What would be the best approach in this setting?

A. Use polymyxin B plus meropenem
B. Use polymyxin B plus fosfomycin
C. Use tigecycline
D. Test for the enzymes produced; if NDM and OXA-48 are both being produced use ceftazidime-avibactam plus aztreonam (also test for their synergy)
E. Continue meropenem

16. A patient develops a watery diarrhea three months after a living donor liver transplant. An assay for *C. difficile* is negative. Immunosuppression is reduced (mycophenolate is stopped), tacrolimus levels are low. A blood CMV and adenovirus PCR is negative. Stool examination does not show any parasites. Which of the following statements are true/actions would you take in this situation?

A. *Clostridium difficile* associated diarrhea is still possible
B. Start oral vancomycin
C. Start metronidazole
D. CMV colitis is still possible

17. A patient with fulminant liver failure undergoes a liver transplant. The organ that is available is from a donor who is hepatitis B core antibody positive. Which of the following recipient status denotes the highest risk of acquiring hepatitis B from the donor?

A. Hepatitis B core antibody positive
B. Hepatitis B surface antibody positive
C. Hepatitis B core and surface antibody positive
D. Hepatitis B core and surface antibody negative

18. What would be the best prophylactic agent for preventing hepatitis B in such patients?

A. Entecavir
B. Tenofovir plus lamivudine
C. Lamivudine
D. Hepatitis B immune globulin (HBIG)

19. Mr A, a living donor liver transplant recipient, on tacrolimus, mycophenolate mofetil, and steroids presents on postoperative day 42 with mild cough and fever. High-resolution computed tomography (HRCT) chest shows solid nodules with ground glass opacities. Serum galactomannan is 0.8, BAL galactomannan is 1.5. BAL; culture grows *Aspergillus* spp. diagnosed as probable invasive pulmonary aspergillosis (IPA). He is started on voriconazole with a trough level of 3 mg/L. He shows clinical and radiological worsening at week 3. Which of the following *Aspergillus* spp. could be the most likely pathogen causing IPA in this case?

A. *A. fumigatus*-wild type
B. *A. calidoustus*
C. *A. flavus*
D. *A. terreus*

20. A patient develops diarrhea 3 months after a deceased donor liver transplant. He reports five watery bowel movements daily. The stool *C. difficile* assay is negative. A stool multiplex PCR panel comes back positive for *Norovirus*. Which of the following actions/statements are true?

A. Give metronidazole
B. Nitazoxanide has proven benefit
C. IVIG has proven benefit
D. No proven therapy

21. A patient undergoes a deceased donor liver transplant. 3 weeks after the transplant he develops a fever. The blood cultures grow *Pseudomonas aeruginosa* which is resistant to all carbapenems, aminoglycosides, and cephalosporins. The meropenem minimum inhibitory concentration (MIC) is 8. Broth microdilution confirms colistin susceptibility. An Xpert Carba-R test shows production of New Delhi metallo-beta-lactamase (NDM). Which of the following is a good regimen for this patient?
    A. Aztreonam
    B. Ceftazidime-avibactam plus aztreonam
    C. Polymyxin plus rifampicin
    D. Polymyxin plus meropenem

22. A patient with alcoholic cirrhosis is planned for a living donor liver transplant. During his pretransplant visit, he is found to have a serum galactomannan of 1.4 (cutoff 0.5). He is afebrile and has no symptoms. What should be your approach in this situation?
    A. Go ahead with the transplant
    B. Cancel the transplant
    C. Thorough search for *Aspergillus* infection or colonization in the recipient
    D. Start voriconazole plus anidulafungin right now

23. A 68-year-old male postdeceased donor liver transplant recipient, undergoes reexploration for bowel perforation on day 21 posttransplant with concurrent reduction in immunosuppression. He goes on to develop mild acute cellular rejection for which he receives pulsed methylprednisolone. 2 weeks later, he presents with complaints of altered sensorium. MRI brain showed multiple cerebral abscesses, biopsy, and culture of which grow *Aspergillus fumigatus*. Antifungal susceptibility by Clinical and Laboratory Standards Institute (CLSI) protocol: amphotericin B (AmB) 1.0, voriconazole 0.25, and itraconazole 0.25. Which would be the preferred antifungal for treatment?
    A. Voriconazole
    B. Liposomal amphotericin B (LAmB)
    C. Echinocandin
    D. Posaconazole
    E. Combination of amphotericin plus anidulafungin

24. A 50-year-old male postdeceased donor liver transplant, on cyclosporine, mycophenolate mofetil, and steroids, presents 1 month posttransplant with complaints of fever and left flank pain. Ultrasonography (USG) abdomen shows a collection in left perinephric region which is aspirated. Smears of aspirated material showed broad aseptate hyphae and culture grows *Cunninghamella bertholletiae*. Which is the best management plan for this patient?
    A. LAmB + reduction in immunosuppression
    B. Posaconazole + reduction in immunosuppression
    C. Any AmB + surgery + deferasirox + reduction in immunosuppression
    D. Conventional AmB or posaconazole + surgery + reduction in immunosuppression

25. A patient who undergoes a liver transplant develops acute rejection 3 months after the transplant. He is treated with pulse steroids. 3 weeks later he presents with headache and fever. An MRI of the brain shows multiple abscesses. He undergoes a stereotactic brain biopsy, the cultures of which grow *Nocardia nova* complex. Which of the following therapies would be the optimum regimen in this patient?
    A. TMP-SMX monotherapy
    B. Ceftriaxone plus amikacin
    C. TMP-SMX plus imipenem
    D. Minocycline plus dapsone

26. A patient with chronic hepatitis B undergoes living donor liver transplant. 5 months later he develops a consolidation in the right upper lobe with fever and hemoptysis. He undergoes a BAL. The BAL GeneXpert ultra is positive. He is on tacrolimus, mycophenolate, and prednisone. No marker for rifampicin resistance is detected. Which of the following statements is true?
    A. This is likely to be a nontubercular mycobacterial infection
    B. Being a liver transplant, isoniazid (INH) is contraindicated
    C. Rifampicin may be avoided or if used then very careful monitoring of the tacrolimus levels should be done
    D. All of the above

27. A 54-year-old woman undergoes a living donor liver transplant for cryptogenic cirrhosis. On postoperative day 15, she develops a catheter-related bloodstream infection with *Candida auris*. Which of the following statements is false?
    A. *C. auris* requires strict infection control protocols like contact isolation, strict hand hygiene, and disinfection with quaternary ammonium compounds
    B. Sulfamethoxazole-voriconazole combination significantly enhances the survival of *Caenorhabditis elegans* infected with *C. auris*
    C. Micafungin and voriconazole exhibit synergistic activity against multidrug-resistant *C. auris* strains

D. *C. auris* can be misidentified when using traditional phenotypic methods for yeast identification such as VITEK 2 YST, BD Phoenix yeast identification system and MicroScan

28. A patient undergoes a living donor liver transplant. The CMV IgG serostatus is donor positive/recipient negative. He is planned for valganciclovir prophylaxis. Which of the following statements are true?
   A. Valganciclovir has a lower incidence of drug related cytopenias
   B. Ganciclovir is more effective than valganciclovir even in low level viremias without severe end organ involvement
   C. Patient also needs to be on HSV and VZV prophylaxis when on valganciclovir
   D. None of the above

29. A 40-year-old male status post-living donor liver transplant recipient presents a year after transplant with painful dark ulcerated nodules on his right leg with surrounding erythema. He had received linezolid at his local hospital with no improvement. Biopsy of the skin lesion shows dermal abscesses with septate hyphae on potassium hydroxide (KOH) mount. Culture of the tissue specimen grows *Fusarium* species. Which of the following statements is incorrect?
   A. Fusarial infections after solid organ transplantation tend to be localized and have better outcomes than in neutropenia
   B. Speciation and antifungal susceptibility testing of *Fusarium* species is not necessary
   C. Surgical resection alone may be effective for limited cutaneous or sinus disease
   D. Reversal of immunosuppression is recommended whenever possible

30. A patient with living donor liver transplant develops fever a month after transplant. He is found to have *C. auris* in the blood cultures. It is found to be resistant to fluconazole, but susceptible to all the three echinocandins—micafungin, anidulafungin, and caspofungin. The transplant hepatologist calls you and states "I want a drug that will have absolutely no interactions with the immunosuppressants that the patient is on". Which of the following drugs will fulfill the hepatologist's wish?
   A. Caspofungin
   B. Anidulafungin
   C. Micafungin
   D. Voriconazole

31. A 67-year-old female status postdeceased donor liver transplant, on tacrolimus, mycophenolate mofetil and prednisolone, receives antithymocyte globulin for antibody-mediated rejection 3 weeks post-transplant. She presents at 150 days posttransplant with complaints of low-grade fever, irritability, and headache. CSF cryptococcal antigen (CRAG) is positive and culture grows *C. neoformans*. Which of the following statements is true?
   A. Cerebral cryptococcomas are more common in patients with *C. neoformans* than with *C. gattii* infection
   B. Solid organ transplant recipients should receive primary prophylaxis against cryptococcosis in first 100 days post-transplant
   C. *C. gattii* has higher propensity for heteroresistance to fluconazole than *C. neoformans*
   D. Serum CRAG has high negative predictive value in isolated pulmonary cryptococcosis

ANSWERS WITH EXPLANATIONS

1. **Ans. E**
   Nasal swab being positive indicates colonization with MRSA. This is not a contraindication for a solid organ transplant. Pretransplant decolonization with intranasal application of mupirocin or chlorhexidine baths can be attempted, especially in units with high burden of MRSA, but the benefit is uncertain. Since this patient is not actively infected there is no benefit in starting MRSA therapy 3 days prior to transplant. This information can be used to identify high risk patients should they develop a post-transplant infection such as pneumonia and for infection control purposes.
   Ref:
   1. Avery RK, Snydman DR. Recipient screening prior to solid-organ transplantation. Clin Infect Dis. 2002;35(12):1513-9.

2. **Ans. C**
   It is important to screen for syphilis in the pretransplant period. The RPR test can be false positive in certain settings. Infections, autoimmune conditions, and recent immunization can affect the results of this test. Hence, it is important to confirm this by ordering a specific treponemal test. Following are the specific treponemal tests:
   - Fluorescent treponemal antibody absorption (FTA-ABS)
   - Microhemagglutination test for antibodies to *Treponema pallidum* (MHA-TP)
   - *T. pallidum* particle agglutination assay (TPPA)
   - *T. pallidum* enzyme immunoassay (TP-EIA)
   - Chemiluminescence immunoassay (CIA)

If the specific treponemal test is positive, then the patient needs to be treated after determining the likely stage of syphilis. It is ideal to complete therapy for syphilis before the transplant. However, in certain situations the need and urgency for the transplant can dictate this decision. This must be discussed with all the treating physicians involved.
Ref:
1. Larsen SA, Steiner BM, Rudolph AH. Laboratory diagnosis and interpretation of tests for syphilis. Clin Microbiol Rev. 1995;8(1):1-21.

3. **Ans. E**

Strongyloides is common in the tropical areas. In areas where it is endemic, it can persist in the intestines. After undergoing liver transplant when the patient receives immunosuppression, strongyloides can cause a hyperinfection syndrome which can involve the lungs. The radiograph usually reveals bilateral infiltrates. The larvae can penetrate the intestinal wall and enter the bloodstream; during this process bacteremias, especially with gram-negative bacteria can be seen. Hence, it is important to recognize the recipients who are at risk for this complication. Patients who show evidence of prior strongyloides infection can be given ivermectin in the pretransplant period. This is especially important in tropical settings with high prevalence of strongyloides infection. Ivermectin is more effective than albendazole for strongyloides infection. When the patient is asymptomatic in the pretransplant period, obtaining a PCR assay on the stool will not add anything to the management.
Ref:
1. Roxby AC, Gottlieb GS, Limaye AP. Strongyloidiasis in transplant patients. Clin Infect Dis. 2009;49(9):1411-23.

4. **Ans. D**

One single strength tablet taken daily or one double strength tablet taken three times every week are effective as prophylaxis for not only *Pneumocystis pneumonia* (PCP), but also *Toxoplasma* and *Listeria*. However, optimal dosing of TMP-SMX for the prevention of other pathogens is not very well established. Routine use of TMP-SMX prophylaxis has considerably reduced the incidence of PCP in the posttransplant period. Most centers administer 6-12 months of PCP prophylaxis; however, the incidence of PCP in a particular center, the cost of therapy, and other factors may affect this practice.

Parameter	TMP-SMX	Dapsone	Atovaquone
Effective as prophylaxis for PCP	+++	+	+
Toxoplasmosis protection	++	+ (with pyrimethamine)	+/−

Ref:
1. Martin SI, Fishman JA, AST Infectious Diseases Community of Practice. Pneumocystis pneumonia in solid organ transplantation. Am J Transplant. 2013;13:272-9.

5. **Ans. D**

Candida is the most common fungal infection in liver transplant recipients. It is useful to know the local epidemiology regarding the species of *Candida* and the susceptibility patterns. The 2013 American Transplantation Society guidelines recommend antifungal prophylaxis for *Candida* in the following situations in liver transplant recipients (if two or more risk factors present):
- Prolonged or repeat operation
- Retransplantation
- Renal failure
- High transfusion requirement (i.e., transfusion of ≥40 units of cellular blood products including platelets, packed red blood cells, and autotransfusion)
- Choledochojejunostomy
- *Candida* colonization during the perioperative period

Ref:
1. Silveira FP, Kusne S, AST Infectious Diseases Community of Practice. Candida infections in solid organ transplantation. Am J Transplant. 2013;13:220-7.

6. **Ans. A**

During the pretransplant visit, the infectious diseases physician must ensure that the patient has been adequately optimized as far as vaccines are concerned. He should receive vaccines like influenza, DTP, pneumococcal, and hepatitis B (if needed) during this period. Though serological response to vaccines can be reduced during this period, it is blunted further when the patient is started on immunosuppressive drugs after undergoing the transplant. Though the exact duration is unknown, the Infectious Disease Society of America (IDSA) recommends a gap of at least 4 weeks between getting a live vaccine and undergoing a solid organ transplant.

Live vaccines should be avoided after transplant when the patients are immunosuppressed. Again, the optimum time is unknown; however, it is safe to avoid all vaccines except influenza for about six months after transplant. Also, with respect to the hepatitis B vaccine, it is important to ensure that the patient has an adequate antibody titer (just having proof of administration may not suffice).

Ref:
1. Rubin LG, Levin MJ, Ljungman P, Davies EG, Avery R, Tomblyn M, et al. 2013 IDSA Clinical Practice Guideline for Vaccination of the Immunocompromised Host. Clin Infect Dis. 2014;58(3):e44-100.

7. **Ans. D**

   Clostridium difficile-associated diarrhea is one of the important causes of diarrhea in the solid organ transplant recipients. It is important to assess the disease severity. Severe *C. difficile* infection is suspected in the setting of leukocytosis (WBC > 15,000) and acute kidney injury. For nonsevere *C. difficile* oral vancomycin or fidaxomicin are the agents of choice. If these are unavailable only then should metronidazole monotherapy be used. For the first episode of severe *C. difficile*, a combination of metronidazole and oral vancomycin should be given. Tigecycline, though has anti-*C. difficile* activity, is not a first-line agent and can be considered only in *C. difficile* refractory to the usual therapy.
   Ref:
   1. McDonald LC, Gerding DN, Johnson S, Bakken JS, Carroll KC, Coffin SE, et al. Clinical Practice Guidelines for Clostridium Difficile Infection in Adults and Children: 2017 Update by the Infectious Diseases Society of America (IDSA) and Society for Healthcare Epidemiology of America (SHEA). Clin Infect Dis. 2018;66(7):e1-48.

8. **Ans. C**

   Cytomegalovirus is a significant problem in the solid organ transplant recipients. Drug resistance should be suspected when the viral loads fails to decrease despite 2 weeks of appropriate anti-CMV therapy. In this setting it is important to know the mechanism of resistance. UL97 mutations can confer resistance to ganciclovir and valganciclovir, whereas UL54 mutations can confer resistance to multiple antivirals. When the resistance for ganciclovir is due to a UL54 mutation there are high chances of cross resistance to cidofovir. Hence, in this setting foscarnet is used empirically.
   Ref:
   1. El Chaer F, Shah DP, Chemaly RF. How I treat resistant cytomegalovirus infection in hematopoietic cell transplantation recipients. Blood. 2016;128(23):2624-36.

9. **Ans. C**

   Cidofovir has activity against all the serotypes of adenovirus. Adenovirus can be an opportunistic infection in solid organ transplant recipients. When more than two organs are involved, it is defined as disseminated adenovirus infection. There is no consensus on management of adenovirus infection in solid organ transplant recipients. Reduction of immunosuppression if feasible is the cornerstone of management. In severe progressive or disseminated disease, most centers use cidofovir, though its dosage and duration in this setting remains unclear. Evidence is limited to case reports and nonrandomized studies. Nephrotoxicity remains the major dose limiting adverse effect, and whenever used, cidofovir should always be used with probenecid and adequate hydration. A lipid conjugate of cidofovir (brincidofovir) has potentially less nephrotoxicity and can be a future option. Ganciclovir and ribavirin have only limited activity and evidence for usage remains anecdotal.
   Ref:
   1. Hoffman JA. Adenovirus infections in solid organ transplant recipients. Curr Opin Organ Transplant. 2009;14:625-33.

10. **Ans. E**

    Toxoplasma can be an opportunistic infection in immunocompromised patients including transplant recipients. Unlike immunocompetent patients, the clinical manifestations in transplant recipients can be severe. This can be a de novo infection, reactivation or acquired through graft transmission. Graft transmission in more common in the heart transplant recipients. The clinical spectrum can include encephalitis, pneumonitis, chorioretinitis, meningitis, and disseminated toxoplasmosis with multiorgan involvement.

    The treatment regimen of choice is pyrimethamine 200 mg (oral) once, followed by 50–75 mg four times a day based plus sulfadiazine 4–6 g/day given in four divided doses plus folinic acid. Prophylactic Bactrim (used for preventions of pneumocystis) also protects against toxoplasmosis.
    Ref:
    1. Khurana S, Batra N. Toxoplasmosis in organ transplant recipients: evaluation, implication, and prevention. Trop Parasitol. 2016;6(2):123-8.

11. **Ans. D**

    This patient is likely to have pure red cell aplasia secondary to parvovirus infection. Parvovirus B19 infection can cause a refractory anemia in transplant recipients. Rarely it can disseminate and involve the lungs, liver, central nervous system (CNS) or heart. Several case reports have described the successful use of IVIG in the treatment of anemia caused by chronic Parvovirus B19. IVIG therapy has been shown to clear viremia and improve symptoms and cytokine dysregulation in Parvovirus B19-associated chronic fatigue. This viral infection is prevalent in the general population and IVIG contains a significant anti-Parvovirus B19 concentration. Screening for Parvovirus B19 in the pretransplant setting does not add much value to detection and outcomes in the posttransplant period.
    Ref:
    1. Eid AJ, Brown RA, Patel R, Razonable RR. Parvovirus B19 infection after transplantation: a review of 98 cases. Clin Infect Dis. 2006;43:40-8.

12. **Ans. B**

    Transplant recipients who are VZV IgG negative and have significant household exposures, should be either administered antiviral therapy or VZV immunoglobulin. In the outpatient settings, significant exposure is defined as exposure to a household contact

or nontransient face-to-face contact indoors. All transplant recipients should be monitored carefully after exposure regardless of therapy given.
Ref:
1. Pergam SA, Limaye AP, AST Infectious Diseases Community of Practice. Varicella zoster virus in solid organ transplantation. Am J Transplant. 2013;13 Suppl 4(Suppl 4):138-46.

13. Ans. C
Vancomycin-resistant enterococci (VRE) represent a formidable challenge in the liver transplant recipients. In this case the *Enterococcus* is resistant to almost all tested antimicrobials. Since it is *E. faecium*, quinupristin/dalfopristin, if available, can be tested.

The other option would be testing for ceftaroline and using it either alone (if susceptible) or in combination with daptomycin (if resistant to everything). It has been found that ceftaroline can enhance daptomycin surface binding with an associated increase in membrane fluidity and increase the net negative surface charge of the bacteria. Ceftaroline has been found to enhance killing of daptomycin-resistant VRE.

At the time of writing this chapter, ceftaroline is expected to be available in India within the next month.

Enforcing infection control measures including handwashing and contact precautions would be the other vital aspect of managing such patients.
Ref:
1. Sakoulas G, Rose W, Nonejuie P, Olson J, Pogliano J, Humphries R, et al. Ceftaroline restores daptomycin activity against daptomycin-nonsusceptible vancomycin-resistant Enterococcus faecium. Antimicrob Agents Chemother. 2014;58(3):1494-500.

14. Ans. E
The reported incidence of PTLD varies amongst different transplant centers, due to the differences in populations as well as immunosuppression regimens and practices. The greatest risk is in the first year. Amongst the various types of solid organ transplants, the highest incidence has been found in intestinal or multiorgan transplants. The cumulative incidence over 5 years ranges from 1 to 2% in hematopoietic cell transplantation (HCT) and liver transplants, 1 to 3% in renal transplants, 2 to 6% in heart transplants, 2 to 9% in lung transplants, and 11 to 33% in intestinal or multiorgan transplants.
Ref:
1. Cockfield SM. Identifying the patient at risk for post-transplant lymphoproliferative disorder. Transpl Infect Dis. 2001;3:70-8.

15. Ans. D
Gram-negative infections represent a serious problem in liver transplant recipients, especially in the immediate posttransplant period. In this case, the *Klebsiella* is resistant to meropenem. Testing for enzymes is useful—the common enzymes expected in this scenario in India would be NDM and OXA-48. Avibactam can inhibit OXA-48, whereas aztreonam can be stable in the face of NDM production and hence it is important to find the enzyme involved, test for synergy, and use this combination in the right scenarios.
Ref:
1. Marshall S, Hujer AM, Rojas LJ, Papp-Wallace KM, Humphries RM, Spellberg B, et al. Can ceftazidime-avibactam and aztreonam overcome β-Lactam resistance conferred by metallo-β-lactamases in Enterobacteriaceae? Antimicrob Agents Chemother. 2017;61(4):e02243-16.

16. Ans. D
Cytomegalovirus is a common viral pathogen that influences the outcome of liver transplantation. In addition to the direct effects of CMV syndrome and tissue-invasive diseases such as colitis, pneumonitis, hepatitis, and retinitis, CMV is associated with an increased predisposition to allograft rejection and other opportunistic infections. Risk factors for CMV disease include CMV donor positive/recipient negative serostatus, acute rejection, use of high-dose mycophenolate mofetil and prednisone, and the overall state of immunity.

The patient has a negative *C. difficile* assay, which would make *C. difficile* very unlikely. The sensitivity of the GDH antigen is high, and hence, a negative GDH antigen would be significant. Hence, there would be no utility in empirically treating for *C. difficile*-associated diarrhea. CMV colitis is still possible in this setting. The patient is in the window for opportunistic infections, and a negative blood PCR will not be able to rule out CMV colitis. The ideal way to diagnose or look for it would be to get a colonoscopic biopsy and look for evidence of CMV inclusion bodies.
Ref:
1. Razonable RR. Cytomegalovirus infection after liver transplantation: current concepts and challenges. World J Gastroenterol. 2008;14(31):4849-60.

17. Ans. D
Rejecting organs from hepatitis B core antibody positive donors can reduce the organ availability significantly. Recipients who have hepatitis B surface or core antibody at the time of transplantation are less likely to develop donor derived hepatitis B. The lowest risk of infection is in recipients who are positive for both the core and surface antibodies. Moderate risk is seen in recipients who have only one out of the two antibodies positive. The highest risk is seen in patients who are both anti-HBs and anti-HBc negative.
Ref:
1. Dickson RC, Everhart JE, Lake JR, Wei Y, Seaberg EC, Wiesner RH, et al. Transmission of hepatitis B by transplantation of livers from donors positive for antibody to hepatitis B core antigen. The National Institute of Diabetes and Digestive and Kidney Diseases Liver Transplantation Database. Gastroenterology. 1997;113(5):1668-74.

18. Ans. A

Such patients who receive a liver from a donor who is positive for hepatitis B core antibody often need lifelong prophylaxis. Hence, it is better to avoid lamivudine as it can be associated with higher rates of resistance. Entecavir and tenofovir are better options. Tenofovir can be associated with nephrotoxicity and the renal function should be carefully monitored. HBIG will not be effective as monotherapy as it cannot inhibit hepatitis B virus (HBV) replication in the liver.

Ref:
1. Bartholomew MM, Jansen RW, Jeffers LJ, Reddy KR, Johnson LC, Bunzendahl H, et al. Hepatitis-B-virus resistance to lamivudine given for recurrent infection after orthotopic liver transplantation. Lancet. 1997;349(9044):20-2.

19. Ans. B

Aspergillus is the most common invasive mold infection in solid organ transplant recipients, with shortest time to onset among heart and liver transplant recipients. The overall 12-week mortality of IA in solid organ transplant recipients exceeds 20%; prognosis is worse among those with CNS involvement or disseminated disease. Voriconazole is the drug of choice for treating IA and isavuconazole has also become a first-line targeted therapy as per recent European Society of Clinical Microbiology and Infectious Diseases (ESCMID) guidelines. However, concerns about changing epidemiology, including azole resistance or IA caused by cryptic *Aspergillus* spp. are rising.

Intrinsic resistance present among cryptic *Aspergillus* species.

	AmB	Azoles	Echinocandins
Aspergillus section fumigatin			
A. fumigatiaffinis	R	R	
A. lentulus	R	R	V
N. pseudofischeri	V	R	
A. viridinutans	R	R	
N. udagawae	R	R (vor)	
A. terreus (and A. alabamensis)	R		
A. flavus	R	R	
A. versicolor (and A. sydowi)	R	V	
A. calidoustus		R	V
A. allilaceus	V		V

(AmB: amphotericin B)

Ref:
1. Husain S, Camargo JF. Invasive Aspergillosis in solid-organ transplant recipients: Guidelines from the American Society of Transplantation Infectious Diseases Community of Practice. Clin Transplant. 2019;33(9):e13544.

20. Ans. D

Norovirus gastroenteritis is one of the common causes of diarrhea in transplant recipients. Unlike immunocompetent patients, these patients can have prolonged diarrhea and can shed the virus for months. Good infection control is important, as it can easily spread from person to person. It has a tropism for the small intestine. Treatment is primarily supportive, including reducing immunosuppression if feasible in severe cases. Immunoglobulins only have anecdotal evidence. The benefit with nitazoxanide needs further evaluation and current evidence is only anecdotal.

Ref:
1. Haessler S, Granowitz EV. Norovirus gastroenteritis in immunocompromised patients. N Engl J Med. 2013;368(10):971.

21. Ans. D

Gram-negative infections can complicate the early posttransplant period in transplant recipients. In this case, the *Pseudomonas* is producing a metallo-beta-lactamase enzyme. However, it can produce other enzymes such as AmpC or extended-spectrum beta-lactamases (ESBLs) such as PER and VEB which will not be detected by the test used in this scenario. Some of these will not be destroyed by avibactam and in turn will destroy aztreonam. Also, the polymyxin rifampicin combination in this situation will be tricky given the interactions between rifampicin and the immunosuppressive agents. The meropenem MIC in this case favors its use as an adjunctive agent.

Ref:
1. Livermore DM, Meunier D, Hopkins KL, Doumith M, Hill R, Pike R, et al. Activity of ceftazidime/avibactam against problem Enterobacteriaceae and Pseudomonas aeruginosa in the UK, 2015–16. J Antimicrob Chemother. 2018;73(3):648-57.

22. Ans. C

Aspergillus can be associated with a significant mortality in the post-transplant period. Earlier data suggested mortality rates as high as 100% with *Aspergillus* in liver transplant recipients, which led some centers across the globe to stop performing liver transplants in patients with active *Aspergillus* infection or those colonized with *Aspergillus*. More recent data indicates that these numbers may be improving. Nevertheless, it is important to thoroughly exclude the presence of *Aspergillus* in this patient with a positive galactomannan. Options include imaging, respiratory cultures and trending the galactomannan. Also this information can be used while deciding the need for mold active prophylaxis in the peritransplant period.

Ref:
1. Singh N, Avery RK, Munoz P, Pruett TL, Alexander B, Jacobs R, et al. Trends in risk profiles for and mortality associated with invasive aspergillosis among liver transplant recipients. Clin Infect Dis. 2003;36(1):46-52.

23. Ans. A

Central nervous system aspergillosis is a difficult condition to treat, associated with poor prognosis. The poor penetration of antifungal drugs into the CNS contributes to the mortality associated with it.

The CNS consists of multiple barriers which limit penetration of substances:
- The blood-cerebrospinal fluid (CSF) barrier consists of a fenestrated epithelial layer located at the choroid plexi through which drugs may penetrate more easily.
- Ependymal layer limits the penetration of drugs from CSF to brain tissue parenchyma.
- Voriconazole is the smallest triazole, which is moderately lipophilic and has excellent penetration into CSF and brain parenchyma.
- Itraconazole is another lipophilic large azole which has low CNS concentrations due to P-glycoprotein mediated efflux at the blood-brain barrier.
- Posaconazole resembles itraconazole structurally but is less lipophilic, also penetrates CSF poorly, but diffusion may be increased by meningeal inflammation.
- Amphotericin B is detectable at low concentrations in brain tissue and CSF, with no increase in levels with meningeal inflammation.
- Echinocandins are large amphipathic cyclic peptides which do not penetrate CSF and brain parenchyma.

The clinical efficacy of voriconazole in IA is due to its enhanced penetration into the CNS, including penetration into infected and non-infected brain tissue. Also it is the drug of choice for *A. fumigatus* species.

Combination antifungals have been used as salvage therapy in IA (voriconazole + echinocandin), especially in patients with suspected drug resistance, drug intolerance or refractory disease. There is however, no definitive data to support its benefit in all patients. Also the combination of azoles and amphotericin can be potentially antagonistic, while the combination containing echinocandins will not be effective due to limited penetration.

Ref:
1. Felton T, Troke PF, Hope WW. Tissue penetration of antifungal agents. Clin Microbiol Rev. 2014;27(1):68-88.

24. Ans. D

The teaching point here is to appreciate how *Cunninghamella* differs from other agents causing mucormycosis. In a fly model of infection, *C. bertholletiae* exhibited the highest degree of pathogenicity and relatively poorer prognosis compared with infection by *Rhizopus* and *Mucor* species. This is likely due to:
- Greater resistance of *Cunninghamella* spp. to human neutrophil-induced damage.
- *Cunninghamella bertholletiae* has been shown to suppress interleukin-8 (IL-8) release and increasing tumor necrosis factor (TNF)-alpha release from human neutrophils. Decreased IL-8 production diminishes chemotactic signals and reduces recruitment of satisfactory numbers of neutrophils to sufficiently damage hyphae. Enhanced TNF-alpha production by neutrophils exposed to *C. bertholletiae* compared with those exposed to *Rhizopus* spp. may generate a complex network of immunosuppressive mechanisms that give an advantage to the fungus for further tissue spread.
- *Cunninghamella bertholletiae* displays greater in vitro resistance to the iron chelator deferasirox than do *Rhizopus* spp. due to enhanced capacity for iron extraction from the environment or host, which may contribute to its enhanced pathogenesis in vivo.

Surgical resection is associated with favorable outcomes compared to antifungal therapy alone. High-dose conventional [amphotericin B deoxycholate (AmBd)] or LAmB has been traditionally used for therapy. The renal concentration of AmB in rat kidneys after AmBd administration is 10 times that in the serum, while the corresponding renal concentration after LAmB administration is one-third that of AmBd and only four times the serum concentration. However in recent studies in which a large set of clinical isolates of Mucorales was tested, *C. bertholletiae* demonstrated the highest resistance to AmB in vitro, with only 63% of the isolates tested showing MIC values under the working interpretative breakpoints described by the CLSI. Murine models have found high dose posaconazole to be efficacious in the treatment of *C. bertholletiae* infections, with reduced toxicity as compared to AmB.

Ref:
1. Pastor FJ, Ruíz-Cendoya M, Pujol I, Mayayo E, Sutton DA, Guarro J. In vitro and in vivo antifungal susceptibilities of the Mucoralean fungus Cunninghamella. Antimicrob Agents Chemother. 2010;54(11):4550-5.
2. Bellmann R, Smuszkiewicz P. Pharmacokinetics of antifungal drugs: practical implications for optimized treatment of patients. Infection. 2017;45(6):737-79.

25. Ans. C

Nocardia is a serious infection in immunocompromised hosts. Whenever *Nocardia* is isolated, it is important to get accurate antimicrobial susceptibilities. There are certain *Nocardia* species such as *N. farcinica* which can have unfavorable susceptibility patterns. For initial therapy for severe disease, TMP-SMX plus another IV agent is often preferred. The possibility of antimicrobial resistance among certain species of *Nocardia*, the demonstration of synergy with certain combinations of antibiotics in animal models, and the high mortality that may be associated with nocardiosis have all led to the recommendation that a combination of agents be used as initial therapy in persons who are seriously ill, those who have disseminated or CNS disease. For non-CNS nocardioisis, this second agent can be amikacin. However, for CNS involvement imipenem would be a better option. This should be tailored according to the susceptibility results. Meropenem, linezolid, and ceftriaxone are some of the other agents that can be considered in certain situations. *N. farcinica* is often resistant to ceftriaxone. The duration of therapy is usually very long.

Ref:
1. Clark NM, Reid GE, AST Infectious Diseases Community of Practice. Nocardia infections in solid organ transplantation. Am J Transplant. 2103;13:83-92.

26. Ans. C

Tuberculosis (TB) in transplant recipients represents a formidable challenge. In high burden countries, the utility of screening before transplants is uncertain, though these candidates should be thoroughly evaluated by an infectious diseases physician to decide the need for pretransplant treatment for latent TB. The question here is whether to use rifampicin or not.

The American Society of Transplantation states that a rifamycin-containing regimen is strongly preferred for both severe and localized nonsevere TB. The ESCMID recommends considering a regimen without rifampicin in cases of nonsevere TB provided there is no reason to suspect INH resistance.

Rifamycins are favored in patients with severe (e.g., cavitary or multilobar disease) or disseminated TB or when there is suspicion or documentation of INH resistance.

Rifampin should be used with caution due to significant interactions between this class of drug and the calcineurin inhibitors and rapamycin (sirolimus). The rifamycins reduce serum concentrations of tacrolimus, cyclosporine, rapamycin (sirolimus), and everolimus via induction of the cytochrome P450 isoenzyme CYP3A4.

Ref:
1. Subramanian AK, Morris MI, AST Infectious Diseases Community of Practice. Mycobacterium tuberculosis infections in solid organ transplantation. Am J Transplant. 2013;13:68-76.
2. Meije Y, Piersimoni C, Torre-Cisneros J, Dilektasli AG, Aguado JM, ESCMID Study Group of Infection in Compromised Hosts. Mycobacterial infections in solid organ transplant recipients. Clin Microbiol Infect. 2014;20:89-101.

27. Ans. A

Centers for Disease Control and Prevention (CDC) guidelines for infection control measures for *C. auris* include:

- Contact isolation
- Strict hand hygiene
- Use of an Environmental Protection Agency-registered hospital-grade disinfectant effective against *Clostridioides difficile* spores. Quaternary ammonium compounds may be inadequate for *C. auris*.

C. auris has been misidentified as *C. guilliermondii*, *C. famata*, *C. haemulonii*, *C. duobushaemulonii*, *C. catenulata*, *C. lusitaniae*, and *C. parapsilosis* when using traditional phenotypic methods for yeast identification.

There is some in vitro evidence that the combination of micafungin and voriconazole may be synergistic. Combinations of caspofungin with azole have exhibited indifferent interactions.

Another checkerboard assay identified sulfamethoxazole as the most effective sulfa drug that exhibited a synergistic activity with voriconazole against azole-resistant *C. auris* clinical isolates, and enhanced survival of nematodes infected with *C. auris*. The synergistic relationship between sulfamethoxazole and voriconazole depends on the overproduction or decreased affinity for the target of azole antifungals (Erg11p) as mechanism of azole resistance. On the other hand, efflux-activated mutant strains do not respond to the sulfamethoxazole-voriconazole combination, at the indicated concentrations.

Ref:
1. Centers for Disease Control and Prevention (CDC) (2019). Identification of Candida auris. [online] Available from: https://www.cdc.gov/fungal/candida-auris/recommendations.html [Last accessed February, 2020].

28. Ans. D

Valganciclovir is commonly used for prophylaxis in the transplant recipients. Although valganciclovir has been approved by the US Food and Drug Administration (FDA) for CMV prophylaxis in renal, lung, and pancreas transplant recipients, it has not been approved for liver transplant recipients because a clinical trial showed an increased incidence of CMV disease compared with those who received oral ganciclovir in patients who had undergone liver transplantation. Despite this data most centers use it for prophylaxis given the ease of administration.

The VICTOR trial did not show any perceivable difference in the incidence of cytopenias caused by ganciclovir and valganciclovir. Also clinical efficacy was similar (patients with severe end organ CMV involvement were excluded). Valganciclovir also has activity against HSV and VZV.

Ref:
1. Asberg A, Humar A, Rollag H, Jardine AG, Mouas H, Pescovitz MD, et al. Oral valganciclovir is noninferior to intravenous ganciclovir for the treatment of cytomegalovirus disease in solid organ transplant recipients. Am J Transplant. 2007;7:2106-13.

29. Ans. B

Culture identification is essential because *Fusarium* and other hyalohyphomycetes can have similar histopathological appearances. Although the genus *Fusarium* can be identified on culture by the production of hyaline, crescent or banana-shaped, multicellular macroconidia, species identification is difficult and may require molecular methods. Accurate species identification is important for optimal management. Molecular tests may be helpful but should be used only to supplement conventional laboratory tests.

The β-1,3-D-glucan test is usually positive in patients suffering from invasive *Fusarium* infections but cannot distinguish from *Candida* and *Aspergillus* infections. *Aspergillus* galactomannan may also be false positive in 50% cases of fusariosis. Antifungal susceptibility testing is important in order to optimize antifungal therapy. The most frequent etiological agents are *F. solani* and *F. oxysporum*, but other species such as *F. verticillioides*, *F. proliferate*, etc., have also been reported.

Optimal treatment for *Fusarium* spp. has not yet been established. Kontoyiannis et al. have analyzed that neutrophil recovery has the most impact in the outcome of fusariosis.

In vitro antifungal susceptibility profiles of *Fusarium* species demonstrate high MICs to most antifungal agents. *F. solani* species complex are usually resistant to azoles and show higher AmB MIC values than other species, whereas *F. oxysporum* may be susceptible to voriconazole and posaconazole. Hence it is important to know the species as well as the MICs. In severe disseminated cases, starting both voriconazole and amphotericin till the MICs are known may be a reasonable approach. Older azoles like itraconazole and fluconazole have high MICs to *Fusarium*. The echinocandins are not active against *Fusarium* spp.

Ref:
1. Tortorano AM, Richardson M, Roilides R, van Diepeningen A, Caira M, Munoz P, et al. ESCMID and ECMM joint guidelines on diagnosis and management of hyalohyphomycosis: Fusarium spp., Scedosporium spp. and others. Clin Microbiol Infect. 2014;20:27-46.

30. Ans. B

The mechanism by which caspofungin interacts with other drugs is unclear. It has been postulated that organic anion transporting polypeptides which mediate uptake of some drugs to hepatocytes may play a role in drug interactions of caspofungin. It can reduce the levels of tacrolimus by up to 20%. Also, drugs like rifampicin may induce caspofungin metabolism.

Micafungin may not affect tacrolimus but can reduce the clearance of sirolimus and cyclosporine.

Anidulafungin is the least likely to give rise to pharmacokinetic drug interactions because it is not a substrate, inhibitor, or inducer of cytochrome P450. These interactions are important to know while choosing an echinocandin in a transplant recipient.

Ref:
1. Sandhu P, Lee W, Xu X, Leake BF, Yamazaki M, Stone JA, et al. Hepatic uptake of the novel antifungal agent Caspofungi. Drug Metab Dispos. 2005;33(5):676-82.

31. Ans. C

Cryptococcosis is the third most commonly occurring invasive fungal infection in solid organ transplant recipients as per TRANSNET data. Approximately 8% of invasive fungal infections in solid organ transplant recipients are due to cryptococcosis with mortality of 5–20%.

Cryptococcosis is typically a late-occurring infection, usually occurring from 16 to 21 months posttransplant. The time to onset is earlier for liver and lung (<12 months) compared to kidney transplant recipients, which may be due to a higher intensity of immunosuppression in the former.

In pulmonary cryptococcosis without disseminated disease, serum CRAG can be negative, hence CT-guided biopsy with culture of pulmonary nodule is the ideal diagnostic method.

Studies from India have shown that *C. gattii* is significantly less susceptible than *C. neoformans* var. *grubii* to fluconazole, itraconazole, and voriconazole, with twofold higher MICs than *C. neoformans*.

Antifungal susceptibility testing is recommended for patients who:
- Fail primary therapy
- Have relapsed disease
- Develop cryptococcosis with prior fluconazole exposure
- Have *C. gattii* genotypes, since *C. gattii* isolates are associated with elevated fluconazole MICs.

Ref:
1. Setianingrum F, Rautemaa-Richardson R, Denning DW. Pulmonary cryptococcosis: a review of pathobiology and clinical aspects. Med Mycol. 2018;57(2):133-50.
2. Chowdhary A, Randhawa HS, Sundar G, Kathuria S, Prakash A, Khan Z, et al. In vitro antifungal susceptibility profiles and genotypes of 308 clinical and environmental isolates of Cryptococcus neoformans var. grubii and Cryptococcus gattii serotype B from north-western India. J Med Microbiol. 2011;60(7):961-7.
3. Baddley JW, Forrest GN, AST Infectious Diseases Community of Practice. Cryptococcosis in solid organ transplantation—Guidelines from the American Society of Transplantation Infectious Diseases Community of Practice. Am J Transplant. 2019;33:e13543.

CHAPTER 27

Infections in Bone Marrow Transplants

Samir Shah

1. **Severe combined immunodeficiency (SCID) can be treated with:**
   A. Intravenous immunoglobulin (IVIg)
   B. Hematopoietic stem-cell transplantation (HSCT)
   C. Thymic transplantation
   D. Immunotherapy

2. **Human immunodeficiency virus (HIV) is the major cause of secondary immunodeficiency (but not the only one). Which immune effector does it target?**
   A. B-cells and plasma cells
   B. Stem cells
   C. CD4 expressing T-cells
   D. CD8 expressing T-cells

3. **The transplantation of tissue from one part of the body to another is called an:**
   A. Autograft
   B. Isograft
   C. Allograft
   D. Xenograft

4. **Which type of rejection takes weeks to months following transplantation of a solid organ?**
   A. Ischemia/reperfusion injury
   B. Hyperacute rejection
   C. Acute rejection
   D. Chronic rejection

5. **Which of the following is not the indication for autologous stem cell transplant?**
   A. Hodgkin disease
   B. Non-Hodgkin lymphoma
   C. Multiple myeloma
   D. Thalassemia major
   E. Multiple sclerosis

6. **Which of the following is an indication for allogeneic stem cell transplant in first remission?**
   A. Multiple myeloma
   B. Hodgkin disease
   C. Non-Hodgkin lymphoma
   D. Acute promyelocytic leukemia
   E. Acute lymphoblastic leukemia in adults

7. **Which of the following is not the source of stem cells in stem cell transplant presently?**
   A. Autologous stem cells
   B. Human leukocyte antigen (HLA)-matched donor
   C. Cord blood
   D. Bone marrow
   E. Embryonic stem cells

8. **Principle of stem cell transplant consists of:**
   A. Conditioning chemoradiotherapy
   B. Immunosuppression to prevent graft-versus-host disease (GVHD)
   C. Stem cell infusion
   D. Blood product transfusions
   E. All of the above

9. **The risk of infections in transplant is due to:**
   A. Conditioning chemoradiotherapy
   B. Central line access devices
   C. Immunosuppression to prevent GVHD
   D. GVHD
   E. All of the above

10. **Which of the following are not infection risks in early transplant period?**
    A. Cytomegalovirus (CMV)
    B. Bacterial infections
    C. Herpes simplex
    D. Fungal infections
    E. Herpes zoster

11. **Which of the following is infection risk post-engraftment?**
    A. CMV
    B. Herpes zoster
    C. Bacterial infections
    D. *Pneumocystis*
    E. All of the above

12. **Which of the following are infection risks in the late post engraftment period?**
    A. Encapsulated bacteria
    B. *Nocardia*
    C. Herpes viruses
    D. Tuberculosis
    E. All of the above

13. Which of the following is not typical infection in the early transplant period?
    A. Pseudomonas
    B. Escherichia coli
    C. Klebsiella
    D. Enterococcus
    E. Neisseria meningitides

14. Which of the following is not typically associated with extended-spectrum beta-lactamase (ESBL) or carbapenem resistance?
    A. Staphylococcus
    B. Klebsiella pneumoniae
    C. Escherichia coli
    D. Acinetobacter baumannii
    E. Pseudomonas aeruginosa

15. The antibacterial prophylaxis for transplant patients is:
    A. Cephalosporins
    B. Penicillin
    C. Quinolones
    D. Macrolides
    E. Tetracycline

16. Which of the following is true for fluoroquinolone prophylaxis?
    A. Increases drug-resistant pathogens, but the benefits outweigh the risks
    B. Associated with Clostridium difficile diarrhea
    C. Reduces the rate of bloodstream infections but not the mortality
    D. Levofloxacin is more effective for broader coverage of Streptococcus viridans in the presence of mucositis
    E. All of the above

17. The overall risk is very high, except in which of the following?
    A. Allogeneic HSCT, especially in unrelated and mismatched donor
    B. Anticipated neutropenia >10 days
    C. GVHD with significant steroid treatment
    D. Autologous transplant
    E. Use of drugs such as tumor necrosis factor (TNF)-alpha inhibitors

18. In the event of fever in the setting of early transplant period, which of the following must be done?
    A. Blood cultures from central line and peripheral sample
    B. Identify the source of infection with imaging and additional cultures as needed
    C. Commence broad-spectrum antibiotics covering gram-positive and gram-negative bacteria
    D. Also excludes noninfectious causes of fever such as cytokine fever
    E. All of the above

19. Which of the following is not an early complication of conditioning regimen?
    A. Pancytopenia
    B. Alopecia
    C. Veno-occlusive disease of liver
    D. Cataract
    E. Convulsions

20. Which of the following is not a late complication of conditioning regimen?
    A. Sterility
    B. Endocrine abnormalities
    C. Secondary malignancies
    D. Veno-occlusive disease of liver
    E. Osteopenia

21. During empiric antimicrobial treatment for neutropenia, which of the following is true for de-escalation of therapy?
    A. High incidence of resistant pathogens
    B. High colonization rate of multiple drug-resistant pathogens
    C. Patient has history of infection with drug-resistant pathogen
    D. No randomized trial of therapeutic efficacy in HSCT of escalation versus de-escalation approach
    E. All of the above

22. Which of the following antifungal is not used as primary prophylaxis in stem cell transplant?
    A. Itraconazole
    B. Voriconazole
    C. Fluconazole
    D. Posaconazole
    E. Micafungin

23. Which of the following is the most common invasive fungal infection (IFI) in stem cell transplant?
    A. Aspergillosis
    B. Candida albicans
    C. Candida glabrata
    D. Mucormycosis
    E. Trichosporonosis

24. Risk factors for IFI are:
    A. Prolonged neutropenia
    B. CMV reactivation
    C. Secondary neutropenia
    D. GVHD
    E. All of the above

25. Which of the following statements is true?
    A. Invasive aspergillosis that develops during early neutropenic period is angioinvasive
    B. Post engraftment risk of Candida infection reduces with recovery of mucositis and neutrophils
    C. Candida albicans infections are markedly reduced by antifungal prophylaxis
    D. IFIs have a higher incidence in allogeneic than in autologous transplants
    E. All of the above

26. **For diagnosis of IFIs, one requires:**
    A. Chest X-ray and high-resolution chest CT scan
    B. Bronchoscopy, bronchoalveolar lavage (BAL), fluid samples, and lung biopsy
    C. Fungal cultures
    D. Galactomannan and beta-D-glucan
    E. All of the above

27. **For invasive aspergillosis (IA) treatment, which of the following is not true?**
    A. Itraconazole is the drug of choice
    B. Periodic galactomannan testing should be done during transplant period
    C. Voriconazole is the drug of choice
    D. Though CYP2C19 polymorphism affects voriconazole kinetics, clinical outcomes are not affected
    E. Treatment duration is at least 6–12 weeks

28. **The causes of breakthrough fungal infections during voriconazole treatment are:**
    A. Persistent immunodeficiency
    B. Neutropenia
    C. Low voriconazole concentration
    D. Poor vascular supply as with abscess or necrotic tissue
    E. All of the above

29. **In voriconazole refractory IA, which of the following must be considered?**
    A. Misdiagnosis or coinfection with another mold
    B. Inadequate voriconazole drug concentration
    C. Immune reconstitution syndrome
    D. Voriconazole-resistant aspergillosis
    E. All of the above

30. **Which of the following is found with *Pneumocystis jiroveci* infection?**
    A. Present with fever, breathing difficulty, and nonproductive cough
    B. Typical radiologic findings include bilateral diffuse infiltrate
    C. Usually occurs within 6 months of transplantation or later if there is ongoing immunosuppression for GVHD
    D. Can present with segmental consolidation or pneumothorax or ground-glass opacities
    E. All of the above

ANSWERS WITH EXPLANATIONS

1. **Ans. B**
   For patients with severe combined immunodeficiency (SCID), there are several treatment options amongst these hematopoietic stem-cell transplantation (HSCT) is potentially curative for all patients with SCID.
   Ref:
   1. Wahlstrom JT, Dvorak CC, Cowan MJ. Hematopoietic stem cell transplantation for severe combined immunodeficiency. Curr Pediatr Rep. 2015;3(1):1-10.

2. **Ans. C**
   HIV is a double-stranded, enveloped RNA retrovirus from the group lentiviruses, with a tropism for human CD4+ expressing cells, including T-cells and macrophages.
   Ref:
   1. Chinen J, Shearer WT. Secondary immunodeficiencies, including HIV infection. J Allergy Clin Immunol. 2010;125(2 Suppl 2):S195-S203.

3. **Ans. A**
   Bone or tissue transplanted from one part of a person's body to another part is called an autograft. Bone or tissue transplanted from the body of one person to another person is called an allograft.

4. **Ans. D**
   Acute rejection occurs days or weeks after transplantation and can be caused by specific lymphocytes in the recipient that recognize HLA antigens in the tissue or organ grafted. Finally, chronic rejection usually occurs months or years after organ or tissue transplantation.
   Ref:
   1. Justiz Vaillant AA, Waheed A, Mohseni M. Chronic Transplantation Rejection. [Updated 2019 Oct 18]. In: StatPearls [Internet]. Treasure Island (FL): StatPearls Publishing; 2020. Available from: https://www.ncbi.nlm.nih.gov/books/NBK535435/.

5. **Ans. D**
   Indications for hematopoietic cell transplantation in adults (generally age ≥18 years):

Indication and disease status	Allogeneic HCT	Autologous HCT
Acute myeloid leukemia		
CR1, low risk	N	C
CR1, intermediate risk	S	C
CR1, high risk	S	C
CR2	S	C

   Contd...

Contd...

Indication and disease status	Allogeneic HCT	Autologous HCT
CR3+	C	C
Not in remission	C	N
Acute promyelocyte leukemia		
CR1	N	N
CR2, molecular remission	C	S
CR2, not in molecular remission	S	N
CR3+	C	N
Not in remission	C	N
Relapse after autologous transplant	C	N
Acute lymphoblastic leukemia		
CR1, standard risk	S	C
CR1, high risk	S	N
CR2	S	C
CR3+	C	N
Not in remission	C	N
Chronic myeloid leukemia		
Chronic phase 1, TKI intolerant	C	N
Chronic phase 1, TKI refractory	C	N
Chronic phase 2+	S	N
Accelerated phase	S	N
Blast phase	S	N
Myelodysplastic syndromes		
Low/intermeditate-1 risk	C	N
Intermediate-2/high risk	S	N
Therapy related AML/MDS		
CR1	S	N
Myelofibrosis and myeloproliferative diseases		
Primary, low risk	C	N
Primary, intermediate/high risk	C	N
Secondary	C	N
Hypereosinophilic syndromes, refractory	R	N
Plasma cell disorders		
Myeloma, initial response	D	S
Myeloma, sensitive relapse	C	S
Myeloma, refractory	C	C
Plasma cell leukemia	C	C
Primary amyloidosis	N	C
POEMS syndrome	N	R
Relapse after autologous transplant	C	C

Contd...

Indication and disease status	Allogeneic HCT	Autologous HCT
Hodgkin lymphoma		
CR1 (PET negative)	N	N
CR1 (PET positive)	N	C
Primary refractory, sensitive	C	S
Primary refractory, resistant	C	N
First relapse, sensitive	S	S
First relapse, resistant	C	N
Second or greater relapse	C	S
Relapse after autologous transplant	C	N
Diffuse large B-cell lymphoma		
CR1 (PET negative)	N	N
CR1 (PET positive)	N	C
Primary refractory, sensitive	C	S
Primary refractory, resistant	C	N
First relapse, sensitive	C	S
First relapse, resistant	C	N
Second or greater relapse	C	S
Relapse after autologous transplant	C	N
Follicular lymphoma		
CR1	N	C
Primary refractory, sensitive	S	S
Primary refractory, resistant	S	N
First relapse, sensitive	S	S
First relapse, resistant	S	N
Second or greater relapse	S	S
Transformation to high grade lymphoma	C	S
Relapse after autologous transplant	C	N
Mantle cell lymphoma		
CR1/PR1	C	S
Primary refractory, sensitive	S	S
Primary refractory, resistant	C	N
First relapse, sensitive	S	S
First relapse, resistant	C	N
Second or greater relapse	C	S
Relapse after autologous transplant	C	N
T-cell lymphoma		
CR1	C	C
Primary refractory, sensitive	C	S
Primary refractory, resistant	C	N
First relapse, sensitive	C	S
First relapse, resistant	C	N
Second or greater relapse	C	C

Contd...

Contd...

Indication and disease status	Allogeneic HCT	Autologous HCT
Relapse after autologous transplant	C	N
Lymphoplasmacytic lymphoma		
CR1	N	N
Primary refractory, sensitive	N	C
Primary refractory, resistant	R	N
First or greater relapse, sensitive	R	C
First or greater relapse, resistant	R	N
Relapse after autologous transplant	C	N
Burkitt lymphoma		
First remission	C	C
First or greater relapse, sensitive	C	C
First or greater relapse, resistant	C	N
Relapse after autologous transplant	C	N
Cutaneous T-cell lymphoma		
Relapse	C	C
Relapse after autologous transplant	C	N
Plasmablastic lymphoma		
CR1	R	R
Relapse	R	R
Chronic lymphocytic leukemia		
High risk, first or greater remission	C	N
T-cell prolymphocytic leukemia	R	R
B-cell, prolymphocytic leukemia	R	R
Transformation to high grade lymphoma	C	C
Solid tumors		
Germ cell tumor, relapse	N	C
Germ cell tumor, refractory	N	C
Ewing's sarcoma, high risk	N	C
Breast cancer, adjuvant high risk	N	D
Breast cancer, metastatic	D	D
Renal cancer, metastatic	D	N
Non-malignant diseases		
Severe aplastic anemia, new diagnosis	S	N
Severe aplastic anemia, relapse/refractory	S	N
Fanconi's anemia	R	N

Contd...

Contd...

Indication and disease status	Allogeneic HCT	Autologous HCT
Dyskeratosis congenita	R	N
Sickle cell disease	C	N
Thalassemia	D	N
Hemophagocytic syndromes, refractory	R	N
Mast cell diseases	R	N
Common variable immunodeficiency	R	N
Wiskott–Aldrich syndrome	R	N
Chronic granulomatous disease	R	N
Multiple sclerosis	N	D
Systemic sclerosis	N	D
Rheumatoid arthritis	N	D
Systemic lupus erythematosus	N	D
Crohn's disease	N	D
Polymyositis-dermatomyositis	N	D

Recommendation categories: Standard of care (S); Standard of care, clinical evidence available (C); Standard of care, rare indication (R); Developmental (D); Not generally recommended (N).
Ref:
1. *Majhail NS, Farnia SH, Carpenter PA, et al. Indications for autologous and allogeneic hematopoietic cell transplantation: Guidelines from the American Society for Blood and Marrow Transplantation. Biol Blood Marrow Transplant. 2015;21(11):1863-9.*

6. **Ans. E**

Explanation discussed in previous question.
Ref:
1. *Majhail NS, Farnia SH, Carpenter PA, et al. Indications for autologous and allogeneic hematopoietic cell transplantation: Guidelines from the American Society for Blood and Marrow Transplantation. Biol Blood Marrow Transplant. 2015;21(11):1863-9.*

7. **Ans. E**

The source of stem cells are from bone marrow, blood, and umbilical cord blood.
Ref:
1. *InformedHealth.org [Internet]. Cologne, Germany: Institute for Quality and Efficiency in Health Care (IQWiG); 2006. Available from: https://www.ncbi.nlm.nih.gov/books/NBK65083/.*
2. *Harvesting blood stem cells for transplantation; 2013 [Updated December, 2016]. Available from: https://www.ncbi.nlm.nih.gov/books/NBK279428/.*

8. **Ans. E**

The first step involves administration of the conditioning regimen, which consists of either or both of chemotherapy and radiotherapy. The goal of the conditioning regimen is to ablate the recipient's own bone marrow and to induce sufficient immunosuppression to allow for the infused stem cells to engraft and to provide nonspecific immune therapy for ongoing disease control. Conditioning regimens can be myeloablative (full-dose) or non-myeloablative (reduced intensity), depending on recipient age and fitness.

Once the conditioning regimen is complete, the bone marrow or peripheral blood stem-cell graft is infused intravenously through a central catheter, and prophylaxis against a variety of infectious and noninfectious complications is instituted. Depending on the type of transplantation procedure, that prophylaxis might address bacterial infections, candidiasis, *Pneumocystis jirovecii*, herpes viruses, hepatic sinusoidal obstruction syndrome, and GVHD.

Ref:
1. Bazinet A, Popradi G. A general practitioner's guide to hematopoietic stem-cell transplantation. Curr Oncol. 2019;26(3):187-91.

9. **Ans. E**

The risks vary depending on the type of transplantation procedure, the conditioning regimen, the underlying disease, and the recipient's comorbidities. During the early post-engraftment period, patients remain at risk of infectious complications. The bone marrow or peripheral blood stem-cell graft is infused intravenously through a central catheter, and prophylaxis against a variety of infectious and noninfectious complications is instituted. The presence of GVHD and its treatment entail a greater degree of immunosuppression. Recipients with active GVHD are at higher risk of invasive fungal infections and viral reactivation.

Ref:
1. Bazinet A, Popradi G. A general practitioner's guide to hematopoietic stem-cell transplantation. Curr Oncol. 2019;26(3):187-91.

10. **Ans. A and E**

The infections commonly seen during this period are often related to neutropenia and consist of gram-positive and gram-negative bacteria, herpes simplex virus, candidiasis, and invasive aspergillosis.

Ref:
1. Bazinet A, Popradi G. A general practitioner's guide to hematopoietic stem-cell transplantation. Curr Oncol. 2019;26(3):187-91.

11. **Ans. E**

Pneumocystis jirovecii, encapsulated bacteria, fungi, varicella zoster virus, cytomegalovirus, respiratory syncytial virus, influenza virus, parainfluenza virus; infections are seen in post-engraftment patients

Ref:
1. Bazinet A, Popradi G. A general practitioner's guide to hematopoietic stem-cell transplantation. Curr Oncol. 2019;26(3):187-91.

12. **Ans. E**

The late infectious complications seen in transplantation patients includes *Pneumocystis jirovecii*, encapsulated bacteria, fungi, varicella zoster virus, cytomegalovirus, respiratory syncytial virus, influenza virus, parainfluenza virus.

Ref:
1. Bazinet A, Popradi G. A general practitioner's guide to hematopoietic stem-cell transplantation. Curr Oncol. 2019;26(3):187-91.

13. **Ans. E**

The infections commonly seen during this period are often related to neutropenia and consist of gram-positive and gram-negative bacteria, herpes simplex virus, candidiasis, and invasive aspergillosis.

Ref:
1. Bazinet A, Popradi G. A general practitioner's guide to hematopoietic stem-cell transplantation. Curr Oncol. 2019;26(3):187-91.

14. **Ans. A**

Extended-spectrum beta-lactamases (ESBL) are enzymes that confer resistance to most beta-lactam antibiotics, including penicillins, cephalosporins, and the monobactam aztreonam. Infections with ESBL-producing organisms have been associated with poor outcomes. Beta-lactamases are enzymes that open the beta-lactam ring, inactivating the antibiotic. The first plasmid-mediated beta-lactamase in gram-negative bacteria discovered was named TEM after the patient from whom it was isolated (Temoniera). Subsequently, a closely related enzyme was discovered and named TEM-2. It was identical in biochemical properties to the more common TEM-1 but differed by a single amino acid with a resulting change in the isoelectric point of the enzyme.

These two enzymes are the most common plasmid-mediated beta-lactamases in gram-negative bacteria, including *Enterobacteriaceae, Pseudomonas aeruginosa, Haemophilus influenzae,* and *Neisseria gonorrhoeae.*

Ref:
1. Munoz-Price LS. Extended-spectrum beta-lactamases. UpToDate; 2019. Available from: https://www.uptodate.com/contents/extended-spectrum-beta-lactamases.

15. **Ans. C**

Ref:
1. Horton LE, Haste NM, Taplitz RA. Rethinking antimicrobial prophylaxis in the transplant patient in the World of emerging resistant organisms—Where are we today?. Curr Hematol Malig Rep. 2018;13(1):59-67. doi: 10.1007/s11899-018-0435-0.

16. **Ans. E**

Ref:
1. Horton LE, Haste NM, Taplitz RA. Rethinking antimicrobial prophylaxis in the transplant patient in the World of emerging resistant organisms—Where are we today? Curr Hematol Malig Rep. 2018;13(1):59-67. doi: 10.1007/s11899-018-0435-0.

17. Ans. D

Overall infection risk and needs for antimicrobial prophylaxis after HSCT:

Risk	Examples of therapy	Antimicrobial prophylaxis
Intermediate	Autologus HSCT	**Bacteria**: Consider fluoroquinolone prophylaxis during neutropenia[a]
	Anticipated neutropenia less than 7–10 days	**Fungus**: Consider prophylaxis during neutropenia and for anticipated mucositis, consider PCP prophylaxis
		Virus: During neutropenia or longer depending on risks
High	Allogenenic HSCT including unrelated or family mismatched donor	**Bacteria**: Consider fluoroquinolone[a]
	Anticipated neutropenia more than 10 days	**Fungus**: Consider prophylaxis during neutropenia, consider PCP prophylaxis
	Prolonged neutropenia	**Virus**: During neutropenia or longer depending on risks
	Secondary neutropenia after engraftment	
	Status of malignancy not in remission	
	GHVD with significant steroids treatment (>20 mg/day of prednisolone equivalents)	
	Use of secondary immunosuppressive agents due to refractory GVHD (e.g., TNF-α inhibitor)	

[a]Recent data concern the correlation with fluoroquinolone prophylaxis and development of resistance or Clostridium difficile associated diarrhea.
(HSCT: hematopoietic stem-cell transplantation; PCP: *Pneumocystis jirovecii* pneumonia; GVHD: graft-versus-host disease; TNF-α: tumor necrosis factor-α).

Ref:
1. Cho SY, Lee HJ, Lee DG. Infectious complications after hematopoietic stem cell transplantation: current status and future perspectives in Korea. Korean J Intern Med. 2018;33(2):256-76.

18. Ans. E

Ref:
1. Heinz WJ, Buchheidt D, Christopeit M, et al. Diagnosis and empirical treatment of fever of unknown origin (FUO) in adult neutropenic patients: guidelines of the Infectious Diseases Working Party (AGIHO) of the German Society of Hematology and Medical Oncology (DGHO). Ann Hematol. 2017;96(11):1775-92.

19. Ans. D

Two of the most common early complications are oral complications/mucositis and sepsis. Some other relatively rare complications are also covered here: hemorrhagic cystitis (HC), endothelial damage (ED) syndromes including engraftment syndrome (ES), idiopathic pneumonia syndrome (IPS), diffuse alveolar hemorrhage (DAH), transplant-associated microangiopathy (TAM) and sinusoidal obstruction syndrome/veno-occlusive disease (SOS/VOD).

Ref:
1. Wallhult E, Quinn B. Chapter 9, Early and acute complications and the principles of HSCT nursing care. In: Kenyon M, Babic A (Eds). The European Blood and Marrow Transplantation Textbook for Nurses: Under the Auspices of EBMT. Springer, Cham; 2018. Available from: https://www.ncbi.nlm.nih.gov/books/NBK543661/. doi: 10.1007/978-3-319-50026-3.

20. Ans. D

Among the transplant community, it is common to define all events occurring beyond 3 months after allo-HSCT as late complications, and separate them into delayed (from 3 months to 2 years), late (2–10 years) and very late events (>10 years).

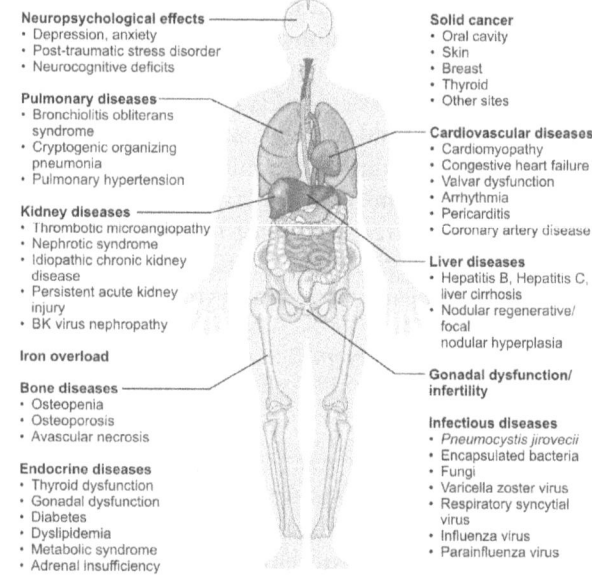

Source: Inamoto Y, Lee SJ. Late effects of blood and marrow transplantation. Haematologica. 2017;102(4):614-25. Available from: http://www.haematologica.org/content/102/4/614.

Ref:
1. Inamoto Y, Lee SJ. Late effects of blood and marrow transplantation. Haematologica. 2017;102(4):614-25. Available from: http://www.haematologica.org/content/102/4/614.

21. Ans. E

A "de-escalation" approach, with initial broad-spectrum antibiotics or combinations, should be used only in those patients with: (i) known prior colonization or infection with resistant pathogens; or (ii) complicated presentation; or (iii) in centers where resistant pathogens are prevalent at the onset of febrile neutropenia. In the latter case, infection control and antibiotic stewardship also need urgent review. Modification of the initial regimen at 72–96 hours should be based on the patient's clinical course and the microbiological results. Discontinuation of antibiotics after 72 hours or later should be considered in neutropenic patients with fever of unknown origin who are hemodynamically stable since presentation and afebrile for at least 48 hours, irrespective of neutrophil count and expected duration of neutropenia.

Ref:
1. Averbuch D, Orasch C, Cordonnier C, et al. European guidelines for empirical antibacterial therapy for febrile neutropenic patients in the era of growing resistance: summary of the 2011 4th European Conference on Infections in Leukemia [published correction appears in Haematologica. 2014;99(2):400]. Haematologica. 2013;98(12):1826-35.

22. **Ans. B**

Azoles represent the backbone of therapy for treating immunocompromised patients with invasive fungal infections (IFIs), isavuconazole; in addition, large studies support the use of mold-active azoles, posaconazole, as antifungal prophylaxis in HSCT recipients. The new mold-active agents, namely posaconazole and micafungin, have reduced the incidence of IFI compared to fluconazole and itraconazole; in addition, posaconazole have reduced transplant-related mortality significantly. Fluconazole remains the gold standard for primary prophylaxis in autologous HSCT recipients. For allogeneic HSCT recipients, the agent chosen for prophylaxis must be based on the patient's risk factors for IFIs.

Ref:
1. Busca A, Pagano L. Antifungal therapy in hematopoietic stem cell transplant recipients. Mediterr J Hematol Infect Dis. 2016;8(1):e2016039. doi: 10.4084/MJHID.2016.039.

23. **Ans. A**

Invasive fungal infections are major causes of morbidity and mortality after allogeneic HSCT. Invasive aspergillosis and candidiasis have traditionally been the predominant IFIs in this population.

Ref:
1. Corzo-León DE, Satlin MJ, Soave R, Shore TB, Schuetz AN, Jacobs SE, Walsh TJ. Epidemiology and outcomes of invasive fungal infections in allogeneic haematopoietic stem cell transplant recipients in the era of antifungal prophylaxis: a single-centre study with focus on emerging pathogens. Mycoses. 2015;58:325-36.

24. **Ans. E**

Variables associated with early phase include underlying pulmonary diseases, underlying nonmalignant stable or chronic disease at allo-HSCT, unrelated or family mismatched donor, and prolonged neutropenia. Variables associated with the late phase include high ferritin level at the time point of allo-HSCT, use of secondary immunosuppressive agents due to refractory GVHD, and cytomegalovirus reactivation.

Ref:
1. Choi JK, Cho SY, Yoon SS, Moon JH, Kim SH, Lee JH, et al. Epidemiology and risk factors for invasive fungal diseases among allogeneic hematopoietic stem cell transplant recipients in Korea: results of "RISK" study. Biology of Blood and Marrow Transplantation. 2017;23(10):1773-79.

25. **Ans. E**

Ref:
1. Vazquez JA, Miceli MH, Alangaden G. Invasive fungal infections in transplant recipients. Ther Adv Infect Dis. 2013;1(3):85-105.

26. **Ans. E**

Ref:
1. Ruhnke M, Behre G, Buchheidt D, Christopeit M, Hamprecht A, Heinz W, et al. Diagnosis of invasive fungal diseases in haematology and oncology: 2018 update of the recommendations of the infectious diseases working party of the German society for hematology and medical oncology (AGIHO). Mycoses. 2018;61(11):796-813.

27. **Ans. A**

Ref:
1. Park SY, Yoon JA, Kim SH. Voriconazole-refractory invasive aspergillosis. Korean J Intern Med. 2017;32(5): 805-12.

28. **Ans. E**

Possible causes of breakthrough invasive fungal diseases during voriconazole treatment.

Causes of antifungal therapy failure	N = 11 (%)
Host factor	
Severity of illness	
Stem cell transplantation (SCT), yes	7 (63.6%)
Persistence of immunodeficiency (e.g., neutropenia or use of corticosteroids)	
Prolonged neutropenia	6 (54.5%)
Graft-versus-host disease (GVHD)	4 (36.4%)
Receipt of corticosteroids (prednisolone ≥1 mg/kg/day)	9 (81.8%)
Mixed infection with other invasive fungal infection	1 (9.1%)
Low concentration of the drug at the site of infection	
Pharmacokinetic and pharmacodynamic (trough level <1 mg/L)	1 (9.1%)
Poor vascular supply (e.g., abscess and necrotic tissue)	1 (9.1%)

Ref:
1. Kim SB, Cho SY, Lee DG, et al. Breakthrough invasive fungal diseases during voriconazole treatment for aspergillosis: a 5-year retrospective cohort study. Med Mycol. 2017;55(3):237-45.

29. Ans. E

The severity of the illness and persistence of immunodeficiency, mixed infection, and low concentration of the treatment drug at the site of infection are identified as the causes of breakthrough invasive fungal diseases (bIFDs).

Ref:
1. Kim SB, Cho SY, Lee DG, et al. Breakthrough invasive fungal diseases during voriconazole treatment for aspergillosis: a 5-year retrospective cohort study. Med Mycol. 2017;55(3):237-45.

30. Ans. E

Ref:
1. Murray J, Agreiter I, Orlando L, Hutt D. Chapter 7, BMT settings, infection and infection control. In: Kenyon M, Babic A (Eds) The European Blood and Marrow Transplantation Textbook for Nurses: Under the Auspices of EBMT. Springer, Cham; 2018. Available from: https://www.ncbi.nlm.nih.gov/books/NBK543661/. doi: 10.1007/978-3-319-50026-3.

CHAPTER 28

Infections in the Eye

TP Lahane, Pooja D Chaturvedy

ORBIT AND LID

1. A 60-year-old recent retiree has been having uncontrolled diabetes. He has slowly developed orbital inflammation and proptosis. Invasion of blood vessels has caused "occlusive vasculitis" in him along with local black eschar formation in the sinus and orbit. His white blood cell (WBC) count is 2,800, chest X-ray is normal, and rapid plasma reagin (RPR) test is normal. A CT scan of the orbit and sinuses shows the following:

   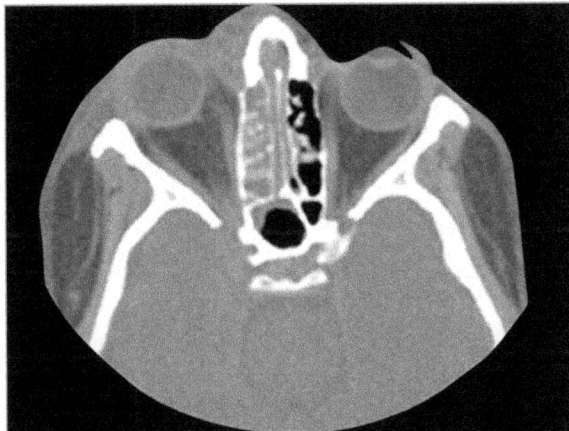
   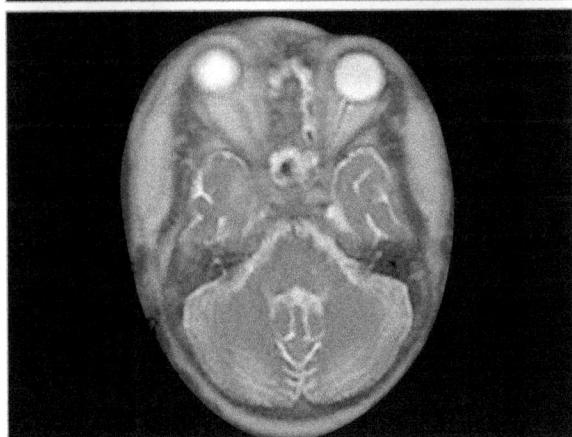

   Which of the following is the most likely diagnosis?
   A. Tuberculosis
   B. Mucormycosis
   C. Aspergillosis
   D. Syphilis

2. A 22-year-old law college student complains of red painful lid swelling of 8 mm since 3 days. She always has a habit of eye rubbing. On examination, the tarsal conjunctiva shows a bump, as seen in the picture below. In the next 20 days, only the pain and redness subside. She is still worried about her cosmesis.

   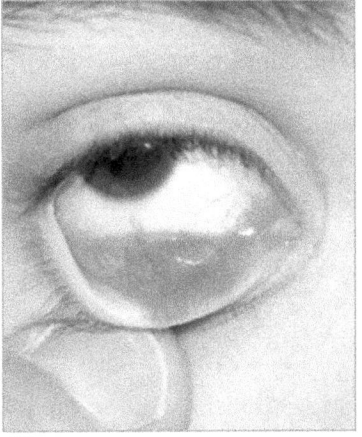

   The next step in management would be:
   A. Antifungals   B. Antiseptics
   C. Incision and curettage   D. Concretion removal

3. A 50-year-old woman presents with acute-onset painful swelling of 2 cm in between nose and left eye, as seen in the picture below. Watering of both eyes and yellowish discharge in the left eye are noted. She responds to oral medications very well within 5–7 days. Her WBC count is 10,000 and her chest X-ray is normal.

   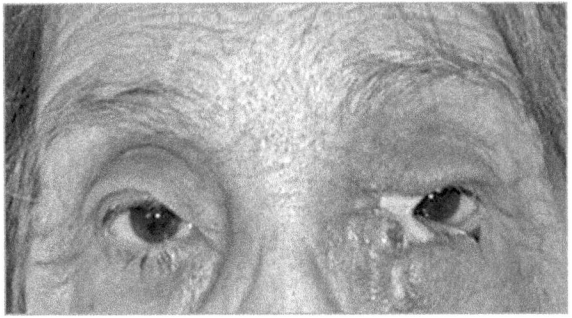

   The following is most likely the causative organism:
   A. *Acinetobacter*   B. *Chlamydia*
   C. *Klebsiella*   D. *Staphylococci*

4. A 10-year-old child, staying in poor hygienic conditions, complains of itching of both eyes with scruff noticed over both eyelids. On closer examination, it is found that the bases of lashes have brown opalescent pearly deposits with empty brown translucent shells too. His WBC count is 5,000 and his eosinophil count is high.
   The best step in management would be:
   A. Olopatadine eyedrops TDS
   B. Antibiotic drops QID
   C. Trimming of lashes with copious ointment
   D. Washing eyes with cold water

5. A 5-year-old known immunocompromised girl presents with three to four pale waxy umbilicated, raised spots on the lower eyelid. It does not transilluminate on examination. The ophthalmologist deals with this by cauterization. Her WBC count is 2,500 and her eosinophil count is normal.
   The most likely diagnosis is:
   A. Phthiriasis
   B. Molluscum contagiosum
   C. Rodent ulcer
   D. Cyst of Moll

CONJUNCTIVA

6. A young child, shown in in the picture below, is suffering from fever and sore throat and begins to complain of lacrimation and foreign body reaction. On examination, follicles were found in the lower palpebral conjunctiva with tender preauricular lymph nodes. Chest X-ray is normal and the WBC count is 2,000.

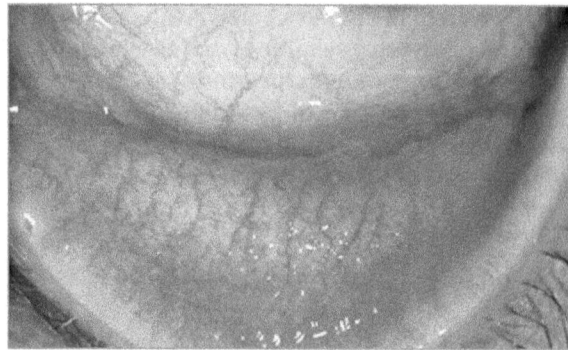

   The most probable diagnosis is:
   A. Trachoma
   B. Staphylococcal conjunctivitis
   C. Adenoviral conjunctivitis
   D. Phlyctenular conjunctivitis

7. A 19-year-old college student complains of watering and mild pain since 2 days with bilateral mild pink eye, which is more prominent only in the outer and inner canthi of eyes. The causative organism is seen in the picture below. The WBC count is 4,500, venereal disease research laboratory (VDRL) test is normal, and chest X-ray is normal.

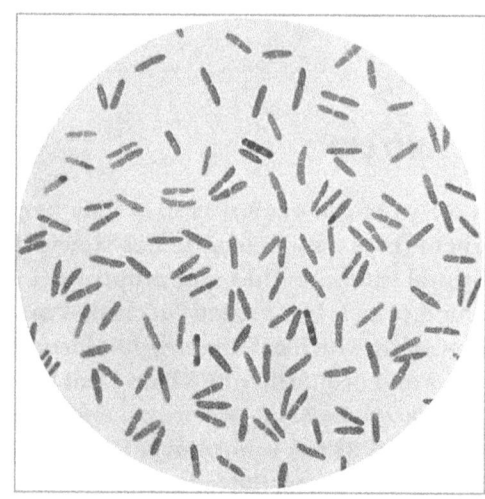

   Which is the causative organism?
   A. *Moraxella Axenfeld*
   B. Pneumococci
   C. Gonococci
   D. Adenovirus

8. A 30-year-old male, from a village of Punjab, presents with a subacute bilateral conjunctival infection, which is caused by a particular strain of chlamydia. The following is the picture of this patient who has superior pannus as well. The WBC count is 5,500.

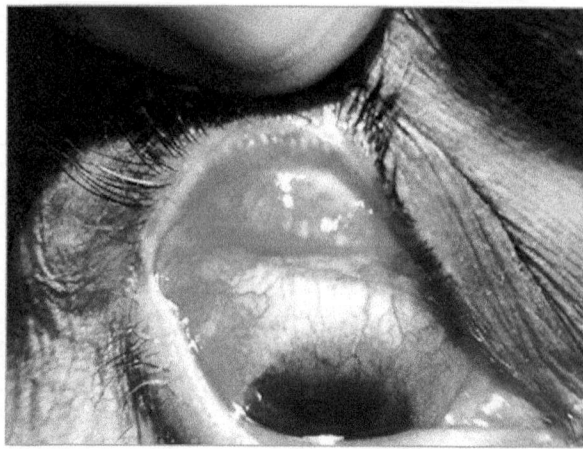

   At which stage of this peculiar infection is the patient most infectious to others?
   A. Arlt's line
   B. Herbert's pits
   C. Postinfective concretions
   D. Follicles in the palpebral conjunctiva

9. A 20-year-old medical student, as shown in the picture below, presents with acute-onset bilateral red eyes with pain and photophobia. The upper

tarsal conjunctiva shows beefy red velvety look. There is yellowish copious discharge in both eyes.

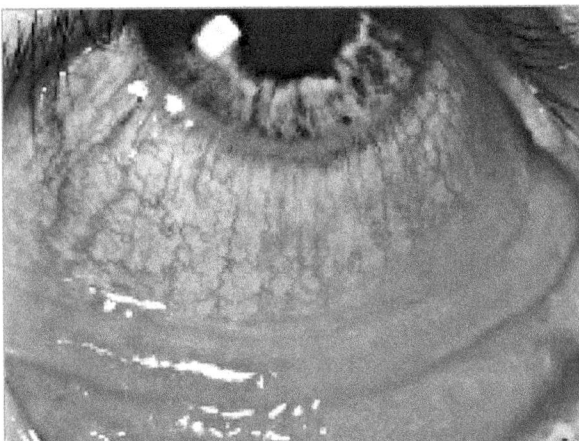

What is expected on the examination of lower tarsal conjunctiva?

A. Arlt's line
B. Papillary reaction
C. Follicular reaction
D. Concretion

10. A neonate, seen in the picture below, presented with bilateral swelling of eyes. He was unable to open both eyes, with copious white discharge. His mother was known to have a venereal disease.

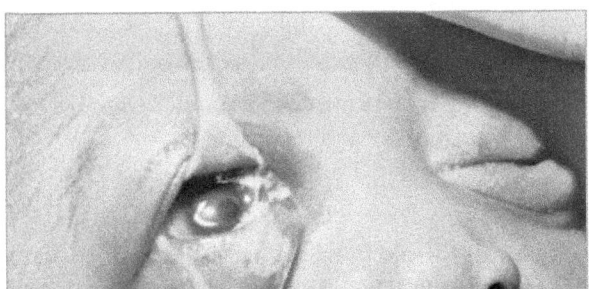

On microbiological examination, the most likely organism you would see is:

A. Gram-positive diplobacilli
B. Gram-positive diplococci
C. Gram-negative diplococci
D. Gram-negative diplobacilli

CORNEA

11. A 60-year-old diabetic comes to you with an acute bilateral eye condition. You have diagnosed the condition and written the prescription for all the relevant eye drops and ointments and are finally deciding whether to patch the patient's eye or not. Patching of the eye is contraindicated in:

A. Corneal abrasion
B. Allergic conjunctivitis
C. Mucopurulent conjunctivitis
D. After glaucoma surgery

12. A 30-year-old male truck driver complains of bilateral red eye and is found to have the following structures in eye on examination. This condition responded well to sulfacetamide eye drops.

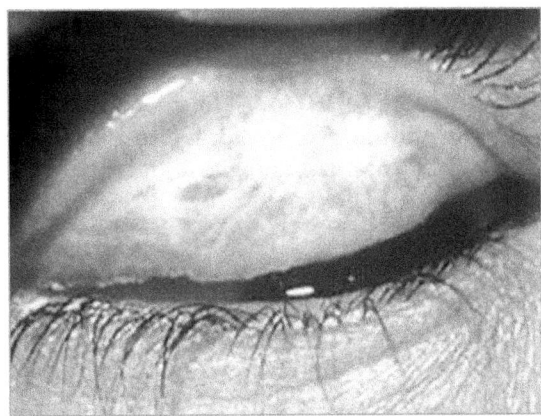

Corneal Herbert's rosettes are found in:

A. Mucopurulent conjunctivitis
B. Phlyctenular keratoconjunctivitis
C. Active trachoma
D. Spring catarrh

13. A 78-year-old man with severe cough comes to you with complaints of painful red eye. On examination, you see an acute keratoconjunctivitis with yellow discharge in fornix and a membrane.
The organism responsible is a gram-positive rod arranged beside each other in V or Y shapes. Which is this organism, which is known to also penetrate intact corneal epithelium?

A. *Moraxella Axenfeld*
B. *Staphylococcus aureus*
C. Meningococci
D. *Corynebacterium diphtheriae*

14. A 30-year-old gardener presents with a history of mild injury to the eye with a leaf 8 days ago and mild pain and photophobia of the left eye. On investigation, you find the following as in the picture:

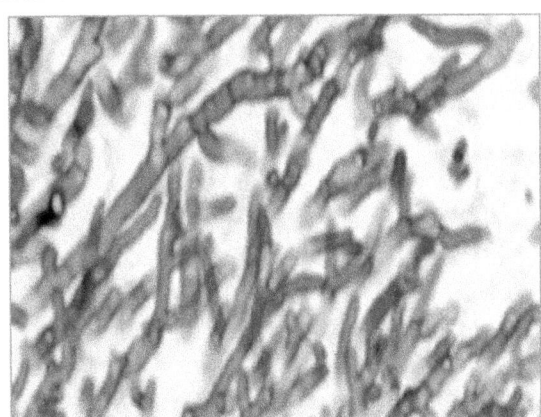

What would be the most likely pathology?

A. Tuberculous anterior uveitis
B. *Acanthamoeba* conjunctivitis
C. Fungal keratitis
D. Bacterial infection of corneal laceration

15. A 50-year-old villager goes to the local primary health care (PHC) for right eye pain, redness, and photophobia. He is referred to a higher center, where the ophthalmologist found this:

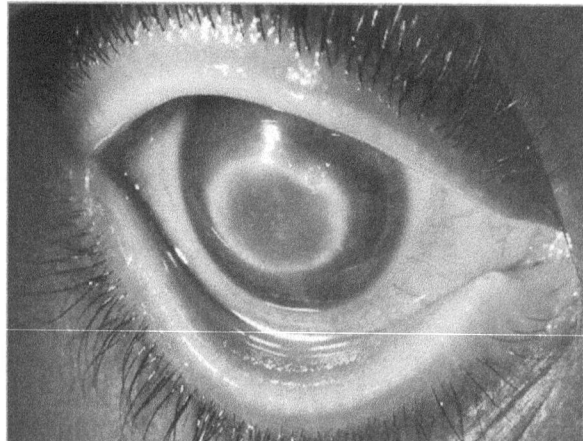

Which of the following statements is true regarding *Acanthamoeba* keratitis?

A. *Acanthamoeba* does not depend upon a human host for the completion of its life cycle
B. After isolation of the causative agent, it should be cultured on a nutrient agar plate
C. The causative agent *Acanthamoeba* is a tapeworm whose normal habitat is soil
D. Keratitis due to *Acanthamoeba* is not seen in the immunocompromised host

16. A 55-year-old female with a past history of common cold 15 days back presents with subepithelial keratitis and a painful eye. On examination, an anterior uveitis is present. The urine report is normal. The WBC count is 2,500.

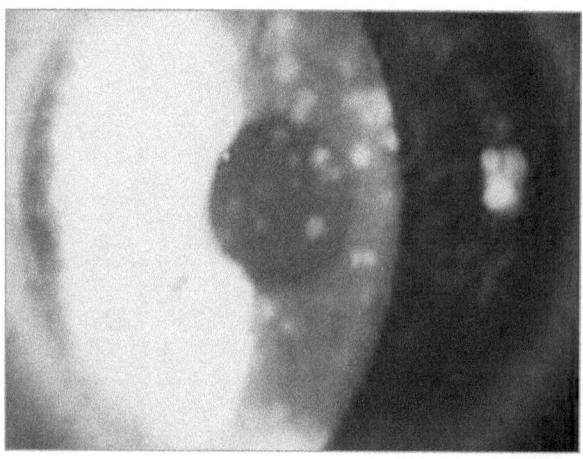

Which of the following would least likely be consistent with the underlying diagnosis of this infective uveitis?

A. Mutton fat keratic precipitates (KPs)
B. Raised IOP
C. Reduced corneal sensation
D. Sectoral iris transillumination

17. A 28-year-old female with the following staining pattern as seen in the picture below presents with painful red eye with circumcorneal congestion. The WBC count is 2,800 and chest X-ray is normal. Which of the following is characteristic feature to diagnose bacterial ulcer?

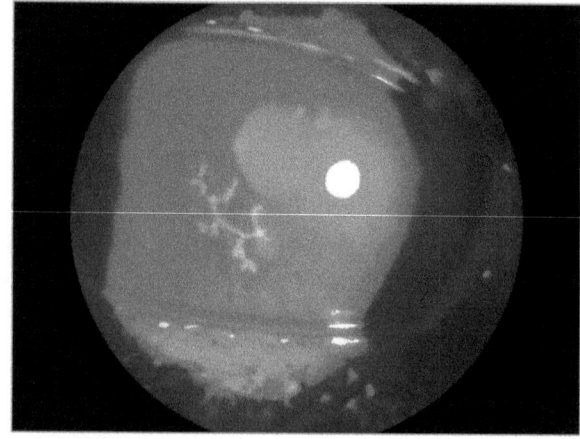

A. Presence of pus in the anterior chamber
B. No tendency to recurrence
C. Corneal hypesthesia
D. Tendency to perforate

18. A 35-year-old housewife presents with an acute red painful eye with lid edema and the following clinical picture. The WBC count is 8,500 and chest X-ray is normal.

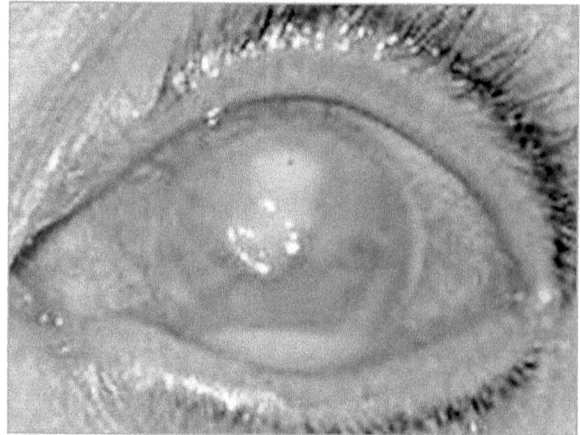

The most common cause of hypopyon corneal ulcer is:

A. *Moraxella* B. *Acinetobacter*
C. *Pneumococcus* D. *Acanthamoeba*

19. A 22-year-old medical intern complains of a sudden-onset painful small nodule near his right cornea with mild congestion. His WBC count is 5,500, erythrocyte sedimentation rate (ESR) is 35, urine examination is normal, and rheumatoid arthritis (RA) factor and antinuclear antibody (ANA) are normal. His liver function test (LFT) and kidney function test (KFT) are normal. The acid-fast bacillus in the picture is usually the causative factor.

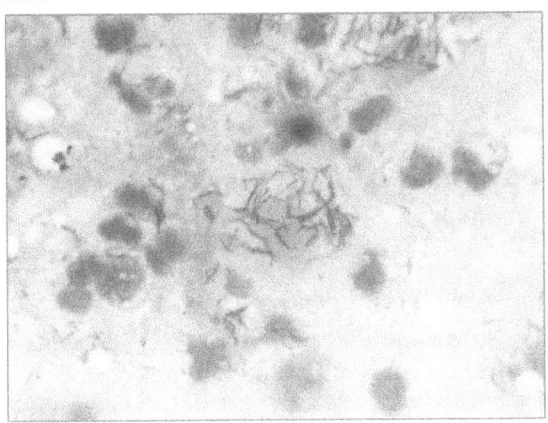

The diagnosis is:
A. Phlyctenular conjunctivitis
B. *Moraxella* conjunctivitis
C. Adenoviral conjunctivitis
D. Allergic conjunctivitis

20. A 19-year old presents to your eye infirmary with pain in the right eye. There is a history of blepharitis in the recent past. On examination, you see a 1.5 mm fluorescein-positive corneal ulcer at 6 o'clock position near limbus. It is associated with circumcorneal congestion. The WBC count is 4,500, X-ray is normal, and ESR is 15.
The causative organism is:
A. *Gonococcus*
B. *Staphylococcus*
C. *Chlamydia*
D. *Mycobacterium tuberculosis*

21. A 65-year-old male, who was vacationing in Goa since 10 days, comes with painful vesicles over his left eyelid and forehead, extending to the scalp on that side. This painful rash respects the midline. There is crusting of these lesions too. The Hutchinson sign is positive. He says he could not seek medical help earlier due to travel. His WBC count is 2,800 and his chest X-ray is clear. On slit-lamp examination, you find that his cornea is involved.
Which of the following corneal lesions is not a complication of this condition?
A. Epithelial keratitis   B. Nummular keratitis
C. Marginal keratitis   D. Disciform keratitis

22. A 22-year-old female came with history of epithelial viral keratitis 20 days back which settled after treatment. Now she complains of mild blurring of vision, and you find the signs as seen in the picture below—an intact corneal epithelium, a small 3 mm central patch of corneal edema with few KPs, and Descemet's folds.

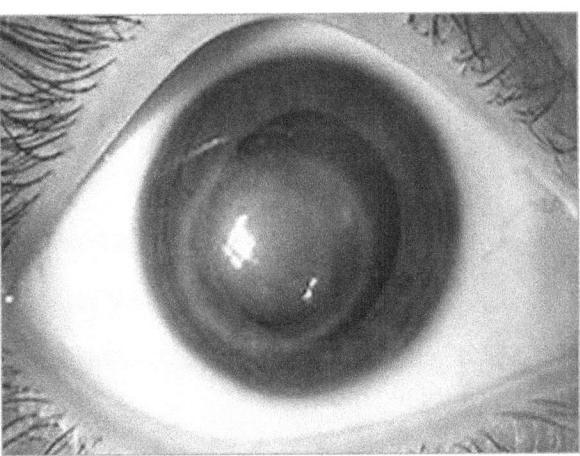

What will be your first option in treating this complication?
A. Tropicamide drops   B. Valacyclovir drops
C. Atropine ointment   D. Steroid drops

23. A 30-year-old banker with history of common cold 15 days back comes to your office with pain and photophobia of the right eye, with mild redness and no lid edema. When you start the patient on antibiotics, he does not improve at all. His WBC count is 2,800, urine examination is normal and chest X-ray is clear.
Which amongst the following is the most likely pattern of fluorescein staining you will find on slit-lamp examination?
A. Ulcus serpens   B. Satellite lesion
C. Dellen   D. Dendritic pattern

24. A 25-year-old lady with probable history of a sexually transmitted disease (STD) and complaints of blurring vision of both eyes comes to your office. On slit-lamp examination you find the epithelium intact, the endothelium not involved, stromal edema, "salmon patch," and stromal ghost vessels. VDRL was positive 2 months ago. The WBC count is 5,500.
What is the most likely diagnosis?
A. Epithelial keratitis   B. Interstitial keratitis
C. Marginal keratitis   D. Disciform keratitis

25. An 80-year-old man with an immunocompromised state comes to your office complaining of irritation, mild pain, mild blurring in vision, and mild redness in both eyes. On slit-lamp examination, you find a diffuse punctate epithelial keratitis, with mild

conjunctivitis. The patient responds poorly to steroid drops. The organism is seen below on a microscope with Brown and Hopps stain.

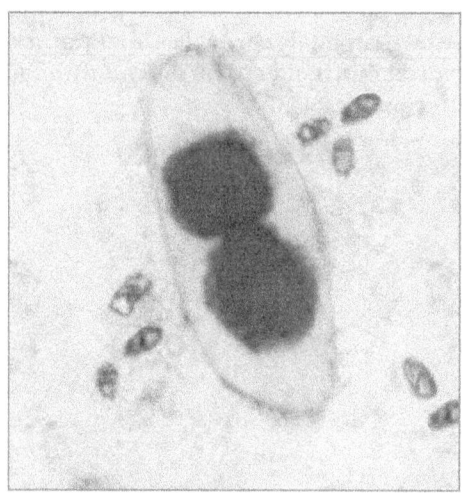

The most likely diagnosis is:
A. Adenoviral conjunctivitis
B. Staphylococcal keratitis
C. Fungal keratitis
D. Microsporidial keratitis

26. A 30-year-old actress who regularly uses contact lenses comes to your office quite anxious about mild blurring of vision and mild pain in the left eye since 4 days. You see pseudodendrites and radial keratoneuritis. Below is the picture of the organism. The WBC count is 4,500 and chest X-ray is normal.

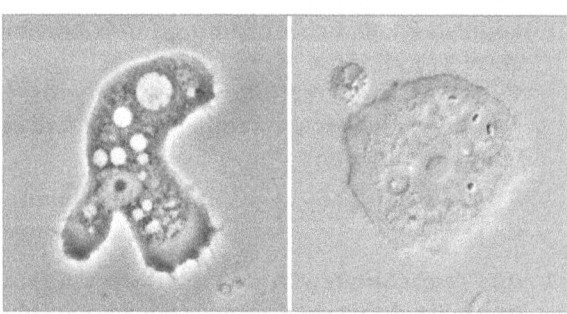

Which of the following is the most likely diagnosis?
A. Fungal keratitis
B. Bacterial keratitis
C. Viral keratitis
D. *Acanthamoeba* keratitis

UVEA

27. A 30-year-old female with night sweats and weight loss had complaints of floaters with blurring of vision. The anterior segment is clear. On indirect ophthalmoscopy, the patient had clear central fundus but there were inflammatory exudates in the very peripheral part. ESR is 40 and chest X-ray is as seen below.

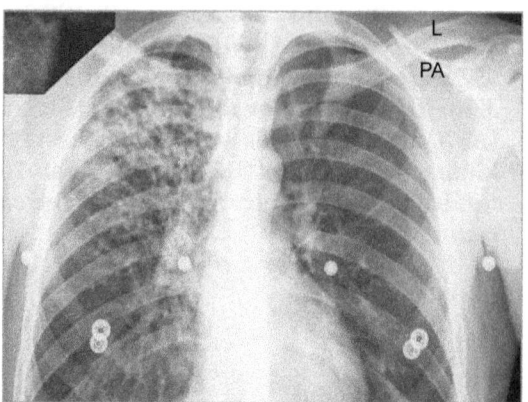

What is this finding on indirect ophthalmoscopy called?
A. Neovascularization B. Salmon patch
C. Snow-banking D. Candle wax dripping

28. An 18-year old complains of low vision in the right eye. On slit-lamp examination, you see few mutton fat KPs in the anterior segment. There is mild vitritis. He is fond of pets and has had them since childhood. The organism responsible for this is an obligate intracellular protozoan. The Sabin-Feldman dye test will be positive if done.
On indirect ophthalmoscopy, you will most likely see the following sign:
A. Salmon patch
B. Starburst pattern
C. "Headlight in fog" appearance
D. Tomato-catsup fundus

29. A homeless 65-year-old man seeks advice for his long-standing gradual visual loss. On slit-lamp examination, you find interstitial keratitis, mutton fat KPs few and old, iris pearls, miotic pupil, and madarosis. The organism looks as seen in the picture when stained with Ziehl-Neelsen (ZN) stain.

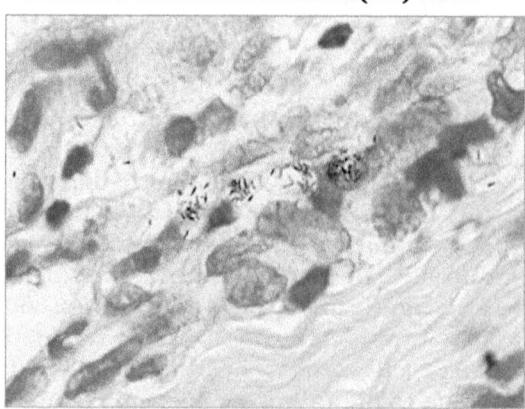

Which is the most likely systemic diagnosis?
A. Tuberculosis B. Syphilis
C. Toxoplasmosis D. Leprosy

30. A 45-year-old commercial sex worker presents with slowly progressing right eye blurring of vision. Pupillary reaction shows light-near dissociation. On slit-lamp examination, we see few dirty yellow KPs and iris roseolae. On indirect ophthalmoscopy, we find the following picture with neuroretinal involvement.

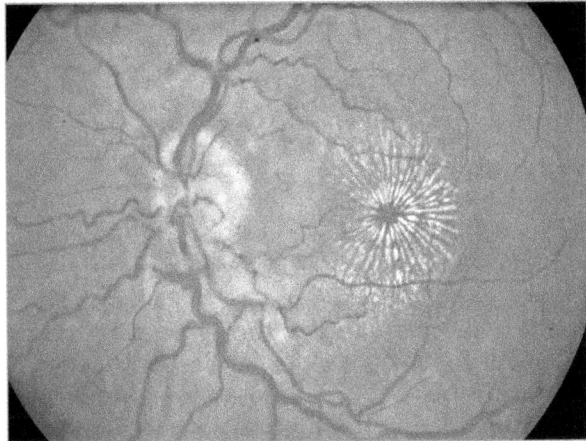

Which is the most likely organism involved?
A. Staphylococcus   B. Spirochete
C. Mycobacterium   D. Protozoan

31. A 65-year-old diabetic female with an in-dwelling catheter comes with a history of gradually progressing visual loss in both eyes since 1 month. The indirect ophthalmoscopy shows vitreous cotton balls as seen in the picture.

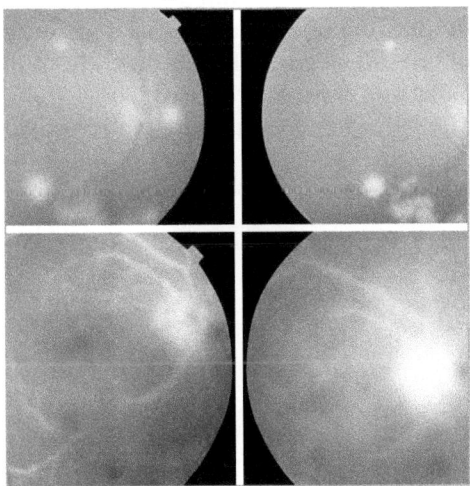

Which is the drug of choice for treatment?
A. Oral rifampicin   B. Oral flucytosine
C. Oral ciprofloxacin D. Oral acyclovir

32. A 45-year-old pilot by profession on HAART (highly active antiretroviral therapy) since few months is noted to have a falling CD-4 count. He comes with complaints of loss of vision of right eye since 15–20 days. On indirect ophthalmoscopy, it is noted to have a cheese and ketchup fundus with brushfire-like extension of exudates along blood vessels as seen in the picture below.

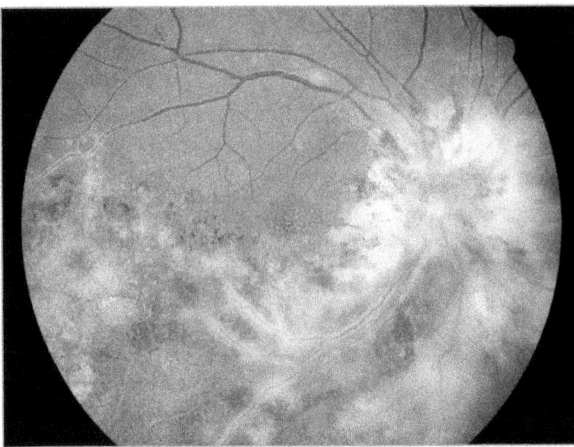

What is the definitive management step for his right eye?
A. Ganciclovir vitreous slow-release device
B. Vitreous depot steroid
C. Intravitreal vancomycin
D. Intravitreal amphotericin B

33. An infant was routinely examined by an ophthalmologist, as the mother was concerned regarding the smaller size of his eyes. The mother had not been properly vaccinated. He was found to have iris coloboma, pearly cataract, and salt and pepper retinopathy on fundus examination, as seen in the picture below.

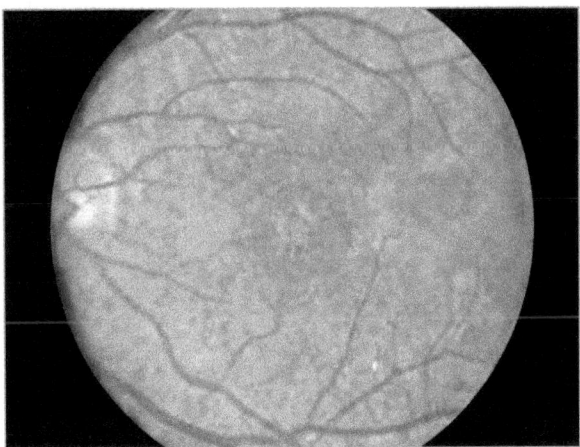

Salt and Pepper Retinopathy

One of the following tests will come positive for this baby:
A. Mantoux
B. Lepromin
C. TORCH (toxoplasmosis, rubella, cytomegalovirus, and HSV) titer
D. Triple H

34. A 40-year-old man who is a known case of AIDS has recently suffered from an opportunistic infection of herpes zoster ophthalmicus (HZO) 1 month back. He complains that he cannot see well, which was at a rapidly progressing speed. When optical coherence tomography (OCT) of retina was done, it was found that the outer layers have been necrosed. The diagnosis made is progressive outer retinal necrosis (PORN).

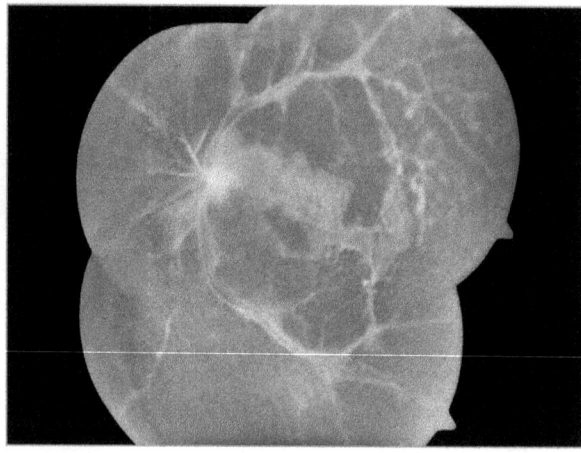

Which of the following is seen on fundus photography?
A. Tomato-catsup fundus
B. Cracked mud appearance
C. Bone spicule fundus
D. "Headlight in fog" appearance

35. A commercial sex worker comes to your clinic with complaints of mild blurring of vision. The patient is hesitant to give full medical/systemic history in a consistent manner. Following is the fundus picture seen on examination.

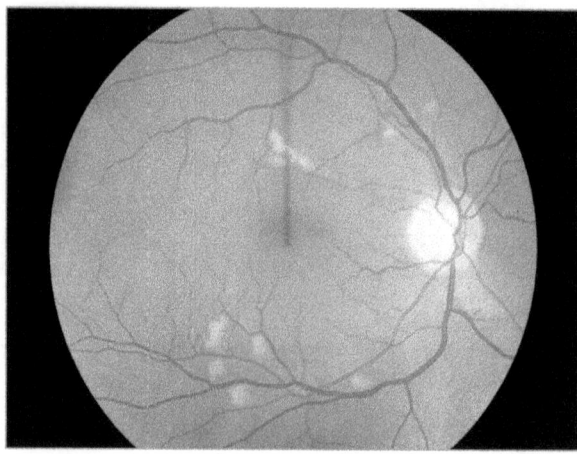

What is the most likely diagnosis?
A. TB
B. Endophthalmitis
C. Leprosy
D. HIV

36. A 32-year old returns from a mountain trekking trip with his friends. He complains to you of gradually developing low vision in the right eye with heaviness and discomfort in that eye. He says that he probably had an insect bite while he was trekking 3 weeks ago. You examine granulomatous iridocyclitis, pars planitis, and transient oculomotor nerve palsies. Chest X-ray is normal and ESR is 30.
Which of the following is the most likely diagnosis?
A. TB
B. Lyme disease
C. Candidiasis
D. Toxoplasmosis

ENDOPHTHALMITIS

37. A 45-year-old female with insulin-dependent diabetes mellitus and previous left corneal ulcer has an acutely irritable and painful left eye. The vision is reduced to bare hand movements and the cornea appears cloudy with loss of the fundus reflex. Pupils are normal.
Which of the following is the most likely diagnosis?
A. Conjunctivitis
B. Granulomatous anterior uveitis
C. Optic neuritis
D. Endophthalmitis

38. A 60-year-old female had a history of cataract surgery 1 year back. She has posterior capsule opacification (PCO) and got a yttrium-aluminum-garnet (YAG) laser capsulotomy done 3 weeks ago. She has complained of sudden-onset painful diminution of vision and was diagnosed as a case of late-onset endophthalmitis. The WBC count is 5,500 and chest X-ray is clear.
The following is the picture of the organism.

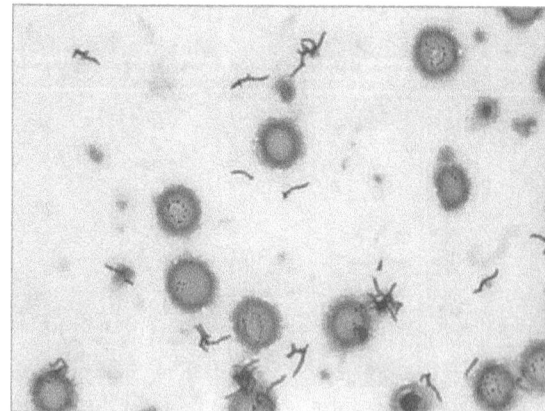

Which of the following organisms is most commonly implicated?
A. *Pneumococcus*
B. *Staphylococcus epidermidis*
C. *Candida albicans*
D. *Propionibacterium acnes*

39. A 50-year-old female had a history of cataract surgery 1 week back. She had complaints of sudden-onset painful diminution of vision, and redness and watering. On clinical examination she had hypopyon, anterior chamber cells, and flare with vitreous exudates on ultrasonography (USG). Which is the most common organism responsible for the condition?
    A. *Pseudomonas aeruginosa*
    B. *Staphylococcus epidermidis*
    C. *Candida albicans*
    D. *Propionibacterium acnes*

40. A 59-year-old diabetic banker goes for dialysis 3 days a week. He complains of severe eye pain and decreased vision in the left eye and is presented to the emergency room a few hours later. He underwent cataract surgery 2 days back. Pain is described as deep within the eye. Bright lights seem to make the pain worse and the vision seems very foggy with lots of floaters. The patient denies any fevers or chills. There is no witnessed trauma to that eye.
    What would be the best treatment for a patient presenting 2 days after cataract surgery with signs and symptoms of endophthalmitis and vision of 6/24?

    A. Arrange for the patient to go immediately to the operating room for a pars plana vitrectomy with vitreous cultures and placement of intravitreal broad-spectrum antibiotics
    B. Proceed with a "tap and inject" vitreous and/or aqueous for culture and inject intravitreal broad-spectrum antibiotics
    C. Close observation
    D. Give the patient a more broad-spectrum antibiotic topical drop to be used every 2 hours

41. Which of the following is the most important factor in the prevention of the endophthalmitis in cataract surgery?
    A. Preoperative preparation with povidone iodine
    B. One-week antibiotic therapy prior to surgery
    C. Trimming of eyelashes
    D. Use of intravitreal antibiotics

42. According to newer guidelines, which of the following drugs is the drug of choice in preventing postoperative endophthalmitis?
    A. Intracameral amphotericin B
    B. Intracameral amoxicillin
    C. Intracameral moxifloxacin
    D. Intracameral valacyclovir

ANSWERS WITH EXPLANATIONS

ORBIT AND LID

1. **Ans. B**

   Tuberculosis and syphilis of orbit is uncommon. In a diabetic, it is most commonly the mucormycosis fungal infection of the orbit, which causes black eschar and occlusive vasculitis. Mucor also crosses the blood-brain barrier. Aspergillosis, on the other hand, is seen more commonly in immunocompromised hosts; chest is usually always involved and black eschar is generally not a feature.
   Ref:
   1. Karadeniz Uğurlu Ş, Selim S, Kopar A, Songu M. Rhino-orbital mucormycosis: clinical findings and treatment outcomes of four cases. Turk J Ophthalmol. 2015;45(4):169-74.
   2. Mukherjee B, Raichura ND, Alam MS. Fungal infections of the orbit. Indian J Ophthalmol. 2016;64(5):337-45.

2. **Ans. C**

   Most of the internal hordeola settle with warm compresses and antibiotics; many do not completely resolve and can go cold painless and remain as a chalazion which eventually can grow at a slow pace. This could be cosmetically challenging if bigger than 4 mm. The definitive management of chalazion is incision and curettage.
   Ref:
   1. Lindsley K, Nichols JJ, Dickersin K. Interventions for acute internal hordeolum. Cochrane Database Syst Rev. 2013;4:CD007742.
   2. Kanski JJ. Clinical Ophthalmology: A Systematic Approach, 5th edition. Philadelphia: Butterworth-Heinemann; 2003. pp. 1-733.

3. **Ans. D**

   Dacryocystitis is characterized as an inflammatory state of the nasolacrimal sac. It is typically caused by an obstruction within the nasolacrimal duct and subsequent stagnation of tears in the lacrimal sac. When the lacrimal sac is inflamed and swells at the inferomedial canthus.

   An acute infectious state typically causes acute dacryocystitis. The most common organism is *Staphylococcus* and *Streptococcus* species, followed by *Haemophilus influenzae* and *Pseudomonas aeruginosa*.
   Ref:
   1. Taylor RS, Ashurst JV. Dacryocystitis. Treasure Island, FL: Stat Pearls Publishing; 2020.

2. Kanski JJ. Clinical Ophthalmology: A Systematic Approach, 5th edition. Philadelphia: Butterworth-Heinemann; 2003. pp. 1-733.

4. **Ans. C**

Phthiriasis palpebrarum is a rare condition which occurs due to infestation with pubic lice. It can be very easily misdiagnosed as a case of blepharitis. In neglected and misdiagnosed cases, it can lead to blepharoconjunctivitis.

Trimming lashes takes away its natural habitat, and application of an antibiotic ointment to smother the lice proved to be an easy and effective method.

Ref:
1. Ashraf M, Waris A, Kumar A, Akhtar N. A case of unilateral phthiriasis palpebrarum infestation involving the left eye. BMJ Case Rep. 2014;2014:pii: bcr2013203307.
2. Elder SD. Diseases of eye lids, system of ophthalmology. In: Ocular Adnexa. Vol XIII, Part-I. London: Henry Kimpton; 1974. pp. 195-9.

5. **Ans. B**

Molluscum is a pox viral infection of the skin and ocular adnexa affecting children and immunocompromised adults; lesions are seen as small pale waxy umbilicated papules on the lower lid.

Phthiriasis is infestation of eyelashes with brown shells and crablouse seen at roots of lashes. Cyst of Moll's sweat gland is not umbilicated, mostly transilluminates, and is also near the lid margin. Rodent ulcer, also known as basal cell cancer and usually seen in the elderly, is pearly, heaped margins indurated with a hard floor.

Ref:
1. Serin Ş, Bozkurt Oflaz A, Karabağlı P, Gedik Ş, Bozkurt B. Eyelid molluscum contagiosum lesions in two patients with unilateral chronic conjunctivitis. Turk J Ophthalmol. 2017;47(4):226-30.
2. Moyes AL, Verachtert AJ. Eyelid infections. In: Krachmer JH, Mannis MJ, Holland EJ (Eds). Cornea, 3rd edition. Philadelphia: Elsevier; 2011. pp. 415-24.
3. Wakeley C, Childs P. Basal-cell carcinoma (rodent ulcer) with special reference to lesions on neck, trunk, and limbs. Br Med J. 1949;1(4608):737-41.

CONJUNCTIVA

6. **Ans. C**

Trachoma would show follicular reaction initially, which becomes confluent and later scar into Arlt's line, with superior pannus, all of which is mostly seen in the upper lid. Phlyctenular reaction is bulbar and nodular. Bacterial conjunctivitis will have a papillary reaction. Adenoviral conjunctivitis will have foreign body sensation, follicular reaction, and whitish minimal discharge. Advanced cases can have pseudomembranes in the lower fornix.

Allergic conjunctivitis is the most common cause of a red itchy eye. Scant mucosal discharge and a papillary response on conjunctiva may also be found. Viral conjunctivitis presents with red eye and foreign body sensation. Tender preauricular lymph nodes may also be palpable on examination. Patients may express a history of upper respiratory tract infection.

Ref:
1. Bialasiewicz A. Adenoviral keratoconjunctivitis. Sultan Qaboos Univ Med J. 2007;7(1):15-23.
2. Mohammadpour M, Abrishami M, Masoumi A, Hashemi H. Trachoma: Past, present and future. J Curr Ophthalmol. 2016;28(4):165-9.

7. **Ans. A**

Moraxella Axenfeld are diplobacillary in structure with end-to-end alignment. They cause typical angular conjunctivitis. Pneumococci and Gonococci are not bacilli; also the conjunctival reaction in their infection is more generalized and all over bulbar and tarsal conjunctiva. The structures seen in the microscopic slide are not viruses. Adenoviral conjunctivitis would be a follicular reaction of the upper and lower tarsal and bulbar conjunctiva.

Ref:
1. Sathe SM. Angular conjunctivitis with associated dermatitis. Indian J Ophthalmol. 1955;3(1):1-9.
2. van Bijsterveld OP. New moraxella strain isolated from angular conjunctivitis. Appl Microbiol. 1970;20(3):405-8.

8. **Ans. D**

The World Health Organization (WHO) recommends a simplified grading system for trachoma.

Follicular trachoma (TF) is defined by the presence of at least five upper tarsal conjunctivas. It is believed that the presence of follicles is an indicator of active disease. It is now that the patient is in the most infective state, for others.

Involution of follicles in the limbal area may result in depressions that are called Herbert's pits. These lesions are pathognomonic of past active trachoma.

Trachomatous inflammation-intense (TI) is the pronounced inflammatory thickening and papillary hypertrophy of the upper tarsal conjunctiva.

Trachomatous scarring (TS) is the presence of white lines, bands, and sheets of fibrosis in the tarsal conjunctiva. TS is an indicator of a past inflammatory disease.

Trichiasis is the result of long-standing subconjunctival fibrosis over the tarsus.

Corneal opacity (CO) is the blindness stage of trachoma. Opacity includes pannus, epithelial vascularization, and infiltration.

Ref:
1. Mohammadpour M, Abrishami M, Masoumi A, Hashemi H. Trachoma: Past, present and future. J Curr Ophthalmol. 2016;28(4):165-9.

2. *Baneke A. Review: targeting trachoma—strategies to reduce the leading infectious cause of blindness. Travel Med Infect Dis. 2012;10(2):92-6.*

9. **Ans. B**

   Arlt's line is a sign of fibrosis scar seen in trachoma and that too in the very late stage of the disease, also mostly seen on the upper eyelid. The bacterial conjunctivitis has an angry red severe conjunctival congestion with the papillary reaction. The follicular reaction is seen in viral and allergic conjunctivitis.
   Ref:
   1. *Azari AA, Barney NP. Conjunctivitis: a systematic review of diagnosis and treatment. JAMA. 2013; 310(16):1721-9.*
   2. *Epling J. Bacterial conjunctivitis. BMJ Clin Evid. 2012;2012:pii: 0704.*

10. **Ans. C**

    Ophthalmia neonatorum caused by transfer of gonococcal infection from the mother's vaginal canal during normal delivery to the newborn is seen with copious whitish yellow discharge and swelling of both lids. *Neisseria gonorrhoeae* are gram-negative kidney-shaped diplococci.
    Ref:
    1. *Moore DL, MacDonald NE; Canadian Paediatric Society; Infectious Diseases and Immunization Committee. Preventing ophthalmia neonatorum. Paediatr Child Health. 2015;20(2):93-6.*
    2. *Costumbrado J, Ng DK, Ghassemzadeh S. Gonococcal conjunctivitis. Treasure Island, FL: Stat Pearls Publishing; 2020.*

CORNEA

11. **Ans. C**

    Mucopurulent bacterial conjunctivitis eye cannot be patched close as the heat generation can aggravate the bacterial infection and worsen the symptoms. Corneal abrasion is frequently patched to promote healing of abrasion. In a few cases of glaucoma surgery, patching is advised for managing postoperative low intraocular pressure (IOP).
    Ref:
    1. *Epling J. Bacterial conjunctivitis. BMJ Clin Evid. 2012;2012:0704.*
    2. *Kanski JJ. Clinical Ophthalmology: A Systematic Approach, 5th edition. Philadelphia: Butterworth-Heinemann; 2003. pp. 1-733.*

12. **Ans. C**

    Follicular trachoma—active trachoma—is defined by the presence of at least five follicles in upper tarsal conjunctivas. It is believed that the presence of follicles is an indicator of active disease. During which the patient is in the most infective state, for others. Involution of follicles in the limbal area may result in depressions that are called Herbert pits. These lesions are pathognomonic of past active trachoma.
    Ref:
    1. *Mohammadpour M, Abrishami M, Masoumi A, Hashemi H. Trachoma: Past, present and future. J Curr Ophthalmol. 2016;28(4):165-9.*
    2. *Baneke A. Review: targeting trachoma—strategies to reduce the leading infectious cause of blindness. Travel Med Infect Dis. 2012;10(2):92-6.*

13. **Ans. D**

    The answer is Corynebacterium. It is a gram-positive rod arranged beside each other in V or Y shapes. It is known to also penetrate intact corneal epithelium.
    Moraxella are gram-negative diplobacilli arranged end to end. *Staphylococcus* and meningococci are not bacilli.
    Ref:
    1. *Rubinfeld RS, Cohen EJ, Arentsen JJ, Laibson PR. Diphtheroids as ocular pathogens. Am J Ophthalmol. 1989;108(3):251-4.*
    2. *Eguchi H (2013). Ocular Infections caused by Corynebacterium species. [online] Available from https://www.intechopen.com [Last accessed February, 2020].*

14. **Ans. C**

    The organism in the picture is not an acid-fast Mycobacterium or a protozoan such as *Acanthamoeba*. It is not a gram-positive or gram-negative bacterium either. It is a picture of a Gram-stained branching fungal hyphae. Most commonly when history is of soil contamination, the keratitis is usually fungal. In *Acanthamoeba* infection, look for contact lens user or postswimming infection in the history.
    Ref:
    1. *Bharathi MJ, Ramakrishnan R, Vasu S, Meenakshi R, Puluniuppun R. Epidemiological characteristics and laboratory diagnosis of fungal keratitis. A three-year study. Indian J Ophthalmol. 2003;51(4): 315-21.*
    2. *Ansari Z, Miller D, Galor A. Current thoughts in fungal keratitis: diagnosis and treatment. Curr Fungal Infect Rep. 2013;7(3):209-18.*
    3. *Thebpatiphat N, Hammersmith KM, Rocha FN, Rapuano CJ, Ayres BD, Laibson PR, et al. Acanthamoeba keratitis: a parasite on the rise. Cornea. 2017;26(6):701-6.*

15. **Ans. A**

    The *Acanthamoeba* is a genus of free-living amoebae, which does not need a human host to complete its life cycle. It is not a tapeworm. It grows on non-nutrient agar. The keratitis it causes and infestation are definitely seen in a systemically and local immunocompromised state.

1. *Thebpatiphat N, Hammersmith KM, Rocha FN, Rapuano CJ, Ayres BD, Laibson PR, et al. Acanthamoeba keratitis: a parasite on the rise. Cornea. 2017;26(6):701-6.*
2. *Kilvington S, Gray T, Dart J, Morlet N, Beeching JR, Frazer DG, et al. Acanthamoeba keratitis: the role of domestic tap water contamination in the United Kingdom. Invest Ophthalmol Vis Sci. 2004;45(1):165-9.*

16. **Ans. A**

    Mutton fat KPs are seen in granulomatous uveitis, such as tuberculosis, syphilis, and sarcoidosis. In herpetic uveitis, as described in the clinical scenario, the raised IOP, reduced sensations, and sectoral transillumination are frequently seen in nongranulomatous uveitis such as herpetic infections.
    Ref:
    1. *Neumann R, Barequet D, Rosenblatt A, Amer R, Ben-Arie-Weintrob Y, Hareuveni-Blum T, et al. Herpetic anterior uveitis—analysis of presumed and PCR proven cases. Ocul Immunol Inflamm. 2019;27(2):211-8.*
    2. *Gaynor BD, Margolis TP, Cunningham ET Jr. Advances in diagnosis and management of herpetic uveitis. Int Ophthalmol Clin. 2000;40(2):85-109.*

17. **Ans. C**

    Bacterial ulcers would have a frank hypopyon or tendency to perforate. Here we see a dendritic viral/herpetic keratitis which is very well known to have associated corneal hypesthesia, no hypopyon, and tends to recur.
    Ref:
    1. *Neumann R, Barequet D, Rosenblatt A, Amer R, Ben-Arie-Weintrob Y, Hareuveni-Blum T, et al. Herpetic anterior uveitis—analysis of presumed and PCR proven cases. Ocul Immunol Inflamm. 2019;27(2):211-8.*
    2. *Gaynor BD, Margolis TP, Cunningham ET Jr. Advances in diagnosis and management of herpetic uveitis. Int Ophthalmol Clin. 2000;40(2):85-109.*

18. **Ans. C**

    Moraxella would cause an angular conjunctivitis. *Pneumococcus* is the most common bacteria to cause a fulminant bacterial keratitis and ulceration with a hypopyon. *Acanthamoeba* do not cause such florid response and a yellow hypopyon. *Acinetobacter* is known to cause pneumonitis, endocarditis, and meningitis. Keratitis is very rare.
    Ref:
    1. *Bourcier T, Thomas F, Borderie V, Chaumeil C, Laroche L. Bacterial keratitis: predisposing factors, clinical and microbiological review of 300 cases. Br J Ophthalmol. 2003;87(7):834-8.*
    2. *Al-Mujaini A, Al-Kharusi N, Thakral A, Wali UK. Bacterial keratitis: perspective on epidemiology, clinico-pathogenesis, diagnosis and treatment. Sultan Qaboos Univ Med J. 2009;9(2):184-95.*

19. **Ans. A**

    Phlyctenular keratoconjunctivitis is a known type IV reaction seen in tuberculosis patients. The acid-fast bacilli seen in the Ziehl-Neelsen-stained slide are *Mycobacterium tuberculosis*, not *Moraxella*. Viral and allergic conjunctivitis do not have the same clinical features as described above.
    Ref:
    1. *Gautam P, Shrestha GS, Sharma AK. Phlyctenular keratoconjunctivitis among children in the tertiary eye hospital of Kathmandu, Nepal. Oman J Ophthalmol. 2015;8(3):147-50.*
    2. *Bhandari A, Bhandari H, Shukla R, Giri P. Phlyctenular conjunctivitis: a rare association with spinal intramedullary tuberculoma. BMJ Case Rep. 2014;pii: bcr2013202010.*

20. **Ans. B**

    Marginal keratitis is known to afflict the lower peripheral cornea by *Staphylococcus* from the approximation of the lower lid to the inferior limbus, commonly after the patient has suffered from a Staphylococcal blepharitis.
    Ref:
    1. *Hoffman J, Hassan A. Severe staphylococcal marginal keratitis presenting with hypopyon. BMJ Case Rep. 2015;pii: bcr2015211979.*
    2. *Dai E, Couriel D, Kim SK. Bilateral marginal keratitis associated with engraftment syndrome after hematopoietic stem cell transplantation. Cornea. 2007;26(6):756-8.*

21. **Ans. C**

    Marginal keratitis is known to afflict the lower peripheral cornea by *Staphylococcus* from the approximation of the lower lid to the inferior limbus. The clinical features described in the question are consistent with a herpes zoster infection, in which the corneal findings can range from an early epithelial keratitis to a late nummular or disciform keratitis.
    Ref:
    1. *Catron T, Hern GH. Herpes zoster ophthalmicus. West J Emerg Med. 2008;9(3):174-6.*
    2. *Li JY. Herpes zoster ophthalmicus: acute keratitis. Curr Opin Ophthalmol. 2018;29(4):328-33.*

22. **Ans. D**

    The clinical vignette describes a disciform keratitis which is the affliction of corneal endothelium in a postherpetic scenario. A topical corticosteroid agent in conjunction with an oral antiviral agent is the preferred treatment for herpes simplex virus (HSV) endothelial keratitis.

    A topical corticosteroid agent in conjunction with an oral antiviral agent for at least 10 weeks is the preferred treatment for HSV stromal keratitis.

    Antiviral agents alone are the treatment of choice for HSV epithelial keratitis. Topical corticosteroids should be avoided.

Ref:
1. *White ML, Chodosh J (2014). Herpes Simplex virus keratitis: a treatment guideline - 2014. [online] Available from https://www.aao.org/clinical-statement/herpes-simplex-virus-keratitis-treatment-guideline [Last accessed February, 2020].*
2. *Collum LM, Logan P, Ravenscroft T. Acyclovir (Zovirax) in herpetic disciform keratitis. Br J Ophthalmol. 1983;67(2):115-8.*

23. Ans. D

Ulcus serpens is seen in aggressive bacterial pneumococcal bacterial ulcer, which creeps up the cornea in a serpiginous fashion, along with a hypopyon. Satellite lesions are the hallmark of fungal keratitis. Dellen is a noninfective thinning of corneal periphery. The viral keratitis usually follows a branching dendritic pattern as seen on fluorescein-stained cornea.

Ref:
1. *Cosar CB, Sridhar MS. Clinical signs in cornea and ocular surface. Indian J Ophthalmol. 2018;66(2):202-6.*
2. *Parmar P, Salman A, Kalavathy CM, Jesudasan CA, Thomas PA. Pneumococcal keratitis: a clinical profile. Clin Exp Ophthalmol. 2003;31(1):44-7.*

24. Ans. B

Interstitial keratitis (luetic) is seen as a long-term sequela of syphilitic infection of the eye with a bacterium *Treponema pallidum*. It is also seen in many granulomatous infections such as leprosy and Lyme disease. It is an immune-mediated response to particular antigens which flares inflammation in the corneal stroma with classical findings such as salmon patch, intrastromal bleeding, and ghost vessels. Epithelial keratitis is usually not a feature in syphilis. Marginal keratitis is seen in staphylococcal infection. Disciform keratitis is a sequela of viral keratitis which affects the endothelium.

Ref:
1. *Gauthier AS, Noureddine S, Delbosc B. Interstitial keratitis diagnosis and treatment. J Fr Ophthalmol. 2019;42(6):e229-37.*
2. *Schwartz GS, Harrison AR, Holland EJ. Etiology of immune stromal (interstitial) keratitis. Cornea. 1998;17(3):278-81.*

25. Ans. D

Microsporidial keratitis is always of the mild type. Microsporidia are eukaryotic and spore-forming obligate intracellular protozoa. Punctate epithelial keratitis stains irregularly with mild conjunctivitis. It worsens by steroid treatment unlike subepithelial viral keratitis. Fungal keratitis would have an ulcer with satellite lesions with or without a white hypopyon. The above organism is not an adenovirus.

Ref:
1. *Alkatan HM, Al-Zaaidi S, Athmanathan S. Microsporidial keratitis: literature review and report of 2 cases in a tertiary eye care center. Saudi J Ophthalmol. 2012;26(2):199-203.*
2. *Joseph J, Sridhar MS, Murthy S, Sharma S. Clinical and microbiological profile of microsporidial keratoconjunctivitis in southern India. Ophthalmology. 2006;113(4):531-7.*

26. Ans. D

The organism in the picture is the *Acanthamoeba*, a genus of free-living amoebae. The typical contact lens solution might get infected by them and cause a keratitis with mild signs like where radial corneal nerves are involved, with a pseudodendritic picture. Bacterial keratitis is very aggressive and viral keratitis would be epithelial but with loss of corneal sensations. The above picture is not of a virus. Fungi have hyphae which could be branching or nonbranching and would cause an ulcer with white hypopyon or satellite lesions.

Ref:
1. *Thebpatiphat N, Hammersmith KM, Rocha FN, Rapuano CJ, Ayres BD, Laibson PR, et al. Acanthamoeba keratitis: a parasite on the rise. Cornea. 2007;26(6):701-6.*
2. *Kilvington S, Gray T, Dart J, Morlet N, Beeching JR, Frazer DG. Acanthamoeba keratitis: the role of domestic tap water contamination in the United Kingdom. Invest Ophthalmol Vis Sci. 2004;45(1):165-9.*

UVEA

27. Ans. C

The tubercular uveitis is usually associated with a granulomatous anterior segment reaction with or without intermediate uveitis, of which snow-banking is a classical finding. Candle wax drippings are seen in the posterior uveitis of sarcoidosis. Neovascularization is nonspecific and seen in many different cases. Salmon patch is seen in sickle cell anemia-related retinopathy.

Ref:
1. *Shah JS, Shetty N, Shah SK, Shah NK. Tubercular uveitis with ocular manifestation as the first presentation of tuberculosis: a case series. J Clin Diagn Res. 2016;10(3):NR01-3.*
2. *El-Asrar AMA, Abouammoh M, Al-Mezaine HS. Tuberculous uveitis. Middle East Afr J Ophthalmol. 2009;16(4):188-201.*

28. Ans. C

Mutton fat KPs are seen in granulomatous uveitis. The clinical history here is consistent with toxoplasmosis infection. It is an obligate intracellular protozoan where the posterior uveitis caused by toxo has a usual "headlight in fog" appearance of the optic disk through the hazy vitritis. A starburst pattern is seen in hypertensive or syphilitic retinopathy. Tomato-catsup fundus is seen in vasculopathy of retina such as choroidal hemangioma, which is a noninfective condition.

Ref:
1. Park YH, Nam HW. Clinical features and treatment of ocular toxoplasmosis. *Korean J Parasitol.* 2013;51(4): 393-9.
2. Butler NJ, Furtado JM, Winthrop KL, Smith JR. Ocular toxoplasmosis II: clinical features, pathology and management. *Clin Exp Ophthalmol.* 2013;41(1):95-108.

29. Ans. D

The clinical vignette describes a typical leprosy patient with its associated ocular findings and the ZN stain shows *Mycobacterium leprae* clusters of bacilli. Tuberculosis bacilli on acid-fast stain also look similar but are not seen in clusters. The clinical findings of iris atrophy, iris pearls, and madarosis are not seen in TB but are typical of leprosy. Syphilis is caused by a spirochete; toxoplasma is an obligate intracellular protozoan.

Ref:
1. Kaushik J, Jain VK, Parihar JKS, Dhar S, Agarwal S. Leprosy presenting with iridocyclitis: a diagnostic dilemma. *J Ophthalmic Vis Res.* 2017;12(4):437-9.
2. Espiritu CG, Gelber R, Ostler HB. Chronic anterior uveitis in leprosy: an insidious cause of blindness. *Br J Ophthalmol.* 1991;75(5):273-5.

30. Ans. B

Syphilitic neuroretinitis seen here is caused by the spirochete *Treponema pallidum*. *Staphylococcus* would not cause a retinitis such as this. The clinical features are not consistent with a mycobacterial or protozoal (toxo) infection.

Ref:
1. Zhang T, Zhu Y, Xu G. Clinical features and treatments of syphilitic uveitis: a systematic review and meta-analysis. *J Ophthalmol.* 2017;2017:6594849.
2. Emmons WW 3rd, Church LW. Syphilitic uveitis. *West J Med.* 1994;161(2):168-71.

31. Ans. B

The cotton balls on fundus examination and history are consistent with ocular candida infection treated with an antifungal. Rifampicin would be treating leprosy. Ciprofloxacin is an antibiotic. Acyclovir is an antiviral.

Ref:
1. Lin P. Infectious uveitis. *Curr Ophthalmol Rep.* 2015;3(3):170-83.
2. Shah CP, McKey J, Spirn MJ, Maguire J. Ocular candidiasis: a review. *Br J Ophthalmol.* 2008;92(4): 466-8.

32. Ans. A

The clinical picture and description are classical of retinitis of cytomegalovirus (CMV) opportunistic infection, seen in AIDS (acquired immunodeficiency syndrome) patients. Ganciclovir ocusert is the treatment. Steroid would worsen the infection. Vancomycin is an antibiotic and would not help in CMV viral infection. Amphotericin B is used to treat fungal endophthalmitis.

Ref:
1. Chiotan C, Radu L, Serban R, Cornăcel C, Cioboata M, Anghel A. Cytomegalovirus retinitis in HIV/AIDS patients. *J Med Life.* 2014;7(2):237-40.
2. Stewart MW. Optimal management of cytomegalovirus retinitis in patients with AIDS. *Clin Ophthalmol.* 2010;4:285-99.

33. Ans. C

Microphthalmia, pearly cataracts, and salt and pepper retinopathy are typical of congenital rubella infection. TORCH titer is a diagnostic screen run on patients suspected to have congenital infections. Mantoux test is for delayed-type hypersensitivity-tubercular testing. Triple H encompasses hepatitis B, HIV, and hepatitis C. Lepromin test is an intradermal test for leprosy antigen.

Ref:
1. Bypareddy R, Chawla R, Azad SV, Khokhar S. Rubella cataract and retinopathy. *BMJ Case Rep.* 2016;pii: bcr2016216112.
2. Givens KT, Lee DA, Jones T, Ilstrup DM. Congenital rubella syndrome: ophthalmic manifestations and associated systemic disorders. *Br J Ophthalmol.* 1993;77(6):358-63.

34. Ans. B

Cracked mud appearance is typical look of the retina in PORN seen in varicella zoster infection in AIDS patients. Tomato-catsup fundus is seen in choroidal vasculopathies; bone spicule appearance is typical of retinitis pigmentosa. "Headlight in fog" appearance is seen in ocular toxoplasmosis.

Ref:
1. Lo PF, Lim R, Antonakis SN, Almeida GC. Progressive outer retinal necrosis: manifestation of human immunodeficiency virus infection. *BMJ Case Rep.* 2015;2015:pii: bcr2014207344.
2. Coisy S, Ebran JM, Milea D. Progressive outer retinal necrosis and immunosuppressive therapy in myasthenia gravis. *Case Rep Ophthalmol.* 2014;5(1): 132-7.

35. Ans. D

The HIV-related vasculopathy in the retina is typical; multiple soft exudates are noted near blood vessels. HIV retinal microvasculopathy being the most common HIV-related ocular manifestation, history and picture are not consistent with endophthalmitis. TB has more of choroiditis nodules or intermediate uveitis and leprosy has more anterior segment signs.

Ref:
1. Abu EK, Abokyi S, Obiri-Yeboah D, Ephraim RK, Afedo D, Agyeman LD, et al. Retinal microvasculopathy is common in HIV/AIDS patients: a cross-sectional study at the Cape Coast Teaching Hospital, Ghana. *J Ophthalmol.* 2016;2016:8614095.
2. Feroze KB, Gulick PG. HIV Retinopathy. Treasure Island, FL: Stat Pearls Publishing; 2020.

36. Ans. B

The history of the tick bite is consistent with Lyme disease where the organism *Borrelia*, a Spirochete, causes a granulomatous iridocyclitis and pars planitis. Toxoplasmosis would cause a "headlight in fog" appearance or choroidal exudates. TB would have a different history of an abnormal X-ray. Candidiasis would show off as cotton balls floating in vitreous.

Ref:
1. *Mikkilä HO, Seppälä IJ, Viljanen MK, Peltomaa MP, Karma A. The expanding clinical spectrum of ocular lyme borreliosis. Ophthalmology. 2000;107(3):581-7.*
2. *Kauffmann DJ, Wormser GP. Ocular Lyme disease: case report and review of the literature. Br J Ophthalmol. 1990;74(6):325-7.*

ENDOPHTHALMITIS

37. Ans. D

Both corneal ulcers and diabetes predispose to infection, so the question is steering you toward an infective cause. Normal pupils rule out optic neuritis. Hence, the potential list is narrowed to either conjunctivitis or endophthalmitis. Given the prominent visual loss (not that common in conjunctivitis) and cloudy cornea (also not a feature of conjunctivitis), the answer must be endophthalmitis.

Ref:
1. *Sheu SJ. Endophthalmitis. Korean J Ophthalmol. 2017;31(4):283-9.*
2. *Kanski JJ. Clinical Ophthalmology: A Systematic Approach, 5th edition. Philadelphia: Butterworth-Heinemann; 2003. pp. 1-733.*

38. Ans. D

Late-onset endophthalmitis is most commonly associated with *Propionibacterium acnes*; also, these low-virulence gram-positive nonspore-forming bacillus is a commensal in the lens capsule and are known to be released after neodymium-doped (Nd) YAG capsulotomy to cause this late-onset low-grade endophthalmitis.

Ref:
1. *Buggage RR, Callanan DG, Shen DF, Chan CC. Propionibacterium acnes endophthalmitis diagnosed by microdissection and PCR. Br J Ophthalmol. 2003;87(9):1190-1.*
2. *Institute of Medicine. Propionibacterium acnes and chronic diseases. In: Bhatia A, Maisonneuve JF, Persing HD (Eds). The Infectious Etiology of Chronic Diseases: Defining the Relationship, Enhancing the Research, and Mitigating the Effects: Workshop Summary. Washington, DC: The National Academies Press; 2004.*

39. Ans. B

Staphylococcus (coagulase negative) is the most commonly implicated gram-positive Cocci in clusters responsible for postoperative endophthalmitis. Pseudomonas is mostly associated with keratitis-related endophthalmitis.

Haemophilus influenzae is most commonly associated with bleb-related endophthalmitis.

Candida endophthalmitis is more so of endogenous origin, rather than the exogenous nature of postoperative endophthalmitis.

Propionibacterium is commonly implicated in late-onset endophthalmitis post cataract surgery.

Ref:
1. *Verma L, Chakravarti A. Prevention and management of postoperative endophthalmitis: a case-based approach. Indian J Ophthalmol. 2017;65(12):1396-402.*
2. *Clarke B, Williamson TH, Gini G, Gupta B. Management of bacterial postoperative endophthalmitis and the role of vitrectomy. Surv Ophthalmol. 2018;63(5):677-93.*

40. Ans. B

Proceed with a "tap and inject". Take a vitreous and/or aqueous sample for culture and inject intravitreal broad-spectrum antibiotics. Based on the visual acuity, one would follow the protocol of "tap and inject."

Ref:
1. *Clarke B, Williamson TH, Gini G, Gupta B. Management of bacterial postoperative endophthalmitis and the role of vitrectomy. Surv Ophthalmol. 2018;63(5):677-93.*
2. *Verma L, Chakravarti A. Prevention and management of postoperative endophthalmitis: a case-based approach. Indian J Ophthalmol. 2017;65(12):1396-402.*

41. Ans. A

The most important source of infection is the patient's own lid and conjunctival flora. Topical povidone iodine helps prevent this.

Ref:
1. *Schwartz SG, Flynn HW Jr. Update on the prevention and treatment of endophthalmitis. Expert Rev Ophthalmol. 2014;9(5):425-30.*
2. *Verma L, Chakravarti A. Prevention and management of postoperative endophthalmitis: a case-based approach. Indian J Ophthalmol. 2017;65(12):1396-402.*

42. Ans. C

Intracameral moxifloxacin is recommended for prevention of postoperative endophthalmitis, which is mostly of bacterial etiology. Amoxicillin is not used intraocularly. Valacyclovir is an antiviral. Amphotericin B is not preventive, not used intracamerally, and is mostly used as treatment intravitreally.

Ref:
1. *Schwartz SG, Flynn HW Jr. Update on the prevention and treatment of endophthalmitis. Expert Rev Ophthalmol. 2014;9(5):425-30.*
2. *Verma L, Chakravarti A. Prevention and management of postoperative endophthalmitis: a case-based approach. Indian J Ophthalmol. 2017;65(12): 1396-402.*

CHAPTER 29

Vector-borne Diseases

Mala V Kaneria

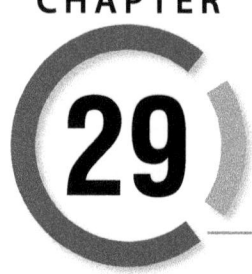

1. A 38-year-old male presented to the emergency room (ER) with fever and altered sensorium of 4 days duration. He was a chronic alcoholic and had been abstaining from alcohol for 2 years. On examination, he was febrile (temperature: 39.3°C), had tachycardia (Pulse rate: 108 beats/min, regular), was hypotensive (BP: 90 mm Hg, systolic), mildly pale and icteric. He was drowsy but arousable. There was no neck rigidity or focal neurological deficit and plantars were flexor. Besides a 3-cm palpable spleen, there were no other positive systemic findings. His hemoglobin level was 10.8 g%, total counts 6,800/mm³ and the platelet count was 40,000/mm³. The mean corpuscular volume (MCV) was 87, other red blood cell (RBC) indices being normal. *Plasmodium falciparum* trophozoites with schizonts were observed in the peripheral blood smear with a parasitemia of 4%. Total bilirubin was 7.8 mg% with the indirect fraction being 4.5 mg%, serum glutamic oxaloacetic transaminase (SGOT) 148 U/L, serum glutamic pyruvic transaminase (SGPT) 96 U/L, lactate dehydrogenase (LDH) 454. Renal function tests were within normal limits. The patient was treated with IV artesunate and his condition improved by day 4. He was subsequently shifted to artemether-lumefantrine combination to complete the course. On day 8, it was noted that his Hb dropped to 5.6 g%, bilirubin increased to 10.4 mg% (indirect 8.2 mg%) and LDH rose to 4,500. The patient continued to be afebrile and peripheral smear (PS) was negative for malarial parasites (the patient was probably hemolyzing). There was no glucose-6-phosphate dehydrogenase (G6PD) deficiency. What is the likely diagnosis?

   A. Megaloblastic anemia in an alcoholic patient
   B. Drug associated hemolysis
   C. Recrudescent malaria
   D. Autoimmune hemolytic anemia (AIHA)

2. A 29-year-old male presented with high-grade fever, severe bodyache, and yellowish discoloration of the sclera and oliguria for 4 days. He was a chronic alcoholic and the last bout of alcohol was 4 days ago. He had received treatment for these symptoms from a local general practitioner. He was toxic, conscious, oriented, highly febrile, deeply icteric, and tachypneic with a respiratory rate of 40 breaths/min. There was an evanescent macular rash on the trunk, subconjunctional hemorrhages in the eye, hepatosplenomegaly but no free fluid was detected clinically or abdominal tenderness. Chest examination revealed bilateral extensive crepitations. There were no flaps or focal neurological deficit. Hemoglobin was 6.0 g%, total counts 4,000/mm³, platelet count 38,000/mm³, MCV 106, total bilirubin 11.6 mg%, direct bilirubin 5.6 mg%, SGOT 148 U/L, SGPT 151 U/L, serum albumin 3.4 mg%, international normalized ratio (INR) 1.0, and serum creatinine 3.9 mg%. PS showed trophozoites of falciparum and vivax. Leptospira immunoglobulin M (IgM) enzyme-linked immunosorbent assay (ELISA) was positive. Arterial blood gas (ABG) revealed hypoxia (PO_2 60 mm Hg) and CO_2 washout (PCO_2 24 mm Hg) with the other parameters being normal. Chest radiograph showed bilateral interstitial shadows. Sonography of the abdomen revealed minimal free fluid and hepatosplenomegaly. The patient was treated with parenteral artesunate, ceftriaxone, oxygen, vitamin K, thiamine, and Bplex. Which would be the most appropriate immediate therapy in this situation?

   A. IV metronidazole B. Early dialysis
   C. IV methylprednisolone D. Anticoma treatment

3. A 24-year-old male presented with history of high-grade fever, severe bodyache and arthralgias of 5 days' duration. He was toxic, highly febrile, had bilateral conjunctival congestion, and a faint erythematous rash over the face, trunk and extremities. He gave a history of taking medicines from a general practitioner. Total count was 3,900/mm³, hemoglobin 17 g% and platelet count was 45,000/mm³. His fever profile, which included PS for malarial parasite, rapid malaria antigen test, dengue PCR, and IgM antibody capture enzyme-linked immunosorbent assay (MAC-ELISA) are negative. What is the likely diagnosis? Which investigations should be sent to confirm the diagnosis?

   A. Drug reaction
   B. Viral fever

C. Dengue fever
D. Chikungunya fever (CHIKF)

4. A 29-year-old female presented with high-grade fever, retro-orbital pain, arthralgias, and truncal rash which was mildly pruritic and of 3 days duration. Her NS1Ag for dengue tested positive. She visited a general practitioner for the above complaints and took some medications which relieved the symptoms. However, the rash worsened after 2 days, became intensely erythematous and pruritic and the fever recurred. What is the most likely diagnosis?
   A. Drug fever associated rash
   B. Saddleback fever of dengue
   C. Prodrome of viral hepatitis
   D. Infectious mononucleosis (IM) like illness

5. A 16-year-old female presented with clinical symptoms compatible with the diagnosis of dengue. Her IgM antibodies to dengue were positive on day 3, immunoglobulin G (IgG) was indeterminate, while her dengue PCR and NS1Ag test were negative. What is the most likely explanation for this?
   A. Primary dengue infection
   B. Recent probable dengue infection
   C. Secondary dengue infection
   D. False positive serological test

6. A 15-year-old female presented to the ER with fever, headache of 5 days' duration and acute onset altered sensorium in the form of not recognizing relatives, and muttering incoherently. There was no history of seizure. She was premorbid healthy and there was no preceding psychiatric history. She was febrile, altered, moving all four limbs, and had terminal neck rigidity. Tone was increased in all the four limbs with brisk tendon reflexes in upper and lower limbs and the plantars were bilaterally extensor. There was no pallor or icterus but a macular rash was visible on the chest wall. Rest of the systemic examination was unremarkable. PS for malarial parasite and rapid malaria antigen test (RMAT) were negative. Dengue NS1Ag, IgM antibody, and PCR were all positive. Total counts were 3,100/mm^3, hemoglobin 16.5 g%, platelet count 33,000/mm^3. Routine hematology and biochemistry results were normal apart from raised SGOT 350 IU/L and SGPT 250 IU/L. USG abdomen showed minimal ascites and the chest radiograph was within normal limits. MRI on T2 fluid attenuated inversion recovery demonstrated bilateral symmetrical hyperintense signals in thalamus, basal ganglia, and mid-brain. The areas of altered signal intensity in the bilateral thalami showed restriction of diffusion on diffusion weighted imaging (DWI) and loss of signal on GRE sequence. Cerebrospinal fluid (CSF) examination revealed—protein 130 mg%, cytology 70 cells/mm^3, and all the cells were lymphocytes. CSF herpes simplex virus (HSV) PCR was negative but JEV IgM antibody was positive. What is the most likely diagnosis?
   A. Dengue encephalitis
   B. Japanese encephalitis (JE)
   C. Viral encephalitis (HSV) in a patient with dengue
   D. Dual infection with dengue and JEV

7. A 43-year-old male presented with history of generalized weakness and lethargy for 10 days. He gave a history of fever with chills 10 days ago for which he received antimalarials from a local doctor. The fever resolved with the treatment but weakness persisted. He was afebrile and the general and systemic examination was unremarkable. His platelet count was 97,000/mm^3 and RMAT was positive for *Plasmodium falciparum*. All the other tests including PS were negative. What course of action would be most appropriate?
   A. Treat with a second-line antimalarial
   B. Treat with the same antimalarial
   C. Reassure the patient if no fever
   D. Repeat the RMAT from another laboratory

8. A 48-year-old male presented with history of fever, headache, bodyache, severe arthralgias, and rash for 2 days. There was no history of any respiratory complaints. He was febrile, toxic, and had bilateral conjunctival congestion but was hemodynamically stable. There was no pallor or icterus but there was minimal swelling and tenderness of the wrist and metacarpophalangeal joints. Chest examination revealed decreased air entry in the right infrascapular region, but no foreign sounds. He had no significant past history. Investigations showed total counts of 1,900/mm^3, hemoglobin 17.2 g%, PCV 51, platelet count 56,000/mm^3, SGOT 175 IU/L, SGPT 112 IU/L, NS1Ag positive by ELISA. Chest radiograph showed blunting of right costophrenic angle; abdominal sonography showed minimal ascites and gallbladder sludge. The patient was hydrated well and given paracetamol for the arthralgias. He subsequently developed pain in both knee joints and had difficulty in walking. What is the possible cause for this and which test should be sent?
   A. ESR and CRP
   B. Rheumatoid factor
   C. Anti-cyclic citrullinated peptide (anti-CCP)
   D. Chikungunya PCR

9. A 58-year-old male presented with fever and altered sensorium for 1 day. There was one episode of generalized tonic clonic seizures. On presentation, he was febrile, drowsy, mildly icteric, hemodynamically stable, with rest of the systemic examination being unremarkable. His PS showed trophozoites of *Plasmodium falciparum*. All the other biochemical parameters were normal except for an indirect hyperbilirubinemia (total bilirubin 3.8 mg% and indirect bilirubin 2.4 mg%). He was started on parenteral artesunate in a dose of 2.4 mg/kg, which was repeated 12 hours later and then 24 hours after the first dose. By day 3, the patient was afebrile, conscious, oriented, and taking orally. Which of the oral combinations is least preferred, while switching from parenteral to oral therapy?

    A. Artesunate plus mefloquine
    B. Artesunate plus lumefantrine
    C. Dihydroartemisinin plus piperaquine
    D. Artesunate plus amodiaquine

10. A 15-year-old female presented with fatigue, dyspnea and lethargy for 1 month. There was no history of fever, blood loss or any other symptoms. On examination, she was pale but had no icterus. There was no significant generalized lymphadenopathy. There was a 2-cm palpable spleen on per abdominal examination. Rest of the general and systemic examination was unremarkable. Hemoglobin was 8.4 g%, WBC count 5,200/mm^3, and platelet count 284,000/mm^3. RBC indices were normal. Scanty rings and trophozoites of *Plasmodium vivax* were seen on the PS. Renal and liver function tests were normal. Stool for occult blood was normal. Human immunodeficiency virus (HIV) and viral markers were negative. Chest radiograph and abdominal sonography were within normal limits. What would you do in this scenario?

    A. Request for an RMAT
    B. Treat the anemia only
    C. Treat the patient with antimalarials
    D. Repeat the PS from a good laboratory

11. A 24-year-old married female was recently treated for vivax malaria and had been started on primaquine for radical cure. She presented after 4 days with anemia (hemoglobin dropped from 9.5 to 6.0 g%) and high colored urine. Her G6PD which was sent earlier was reported as mildly deficient. What would be the further course of action?

    A. Stop primaquine
    B. Continue primaquine and monitor hemoglobin
    C. Decrease the dose of primaquine
    D. Continue primaquine presently but completely avoid it hereafter

12. A 21-year-old male presented in the monsoon with high-grade fever, severe bodyache, and retro-orbital pain of 3 days' duration. He was hemodynamically stable, tachypneic with a respiratory rate of 34 breaths/min, pulse rate of 120 beats/min. There was a maculopapular rash on the body, petechiae on the lower extremities and no icterus or pallor. He was conscious and oriented, and chest auscultation revealed crackles in both infrascapular regions. His total leukocyte count was 2,400/mm^3, Hb: 17 g%, platelet count: 33,000/mm^3, total bilirubin 1.2 mg%, SGOT: 45 IU/L, and SGPT: 40 IU/L. The PO$_2$ was 66 on room air. Chest radiograph showed bilateral fluffy shadows. Fever profile was awaited. Intravenous ceftriaxone and artesunate were started, along with other supportive measures. Considering the differentials, addition of which other antibiotic would be most appropriate at this stage?

    A. Doxycycline
    B. Levofloxacin
    C. Teicoplanin
    D. Amikacin

13. A 65-year-old Caucasian male and his wife make plans to visit India. They consult a travel physician regarding malaria chemoprophylaxis. They are both hypertensives and diabetics with chronic kidney disease and the travel is scheduled after 4 days. What is the most appropriate chemoprophylactic agent in this situation?

    A. Mefloquine
    B. Chloroquine
    C. Doxycycline
    D. Atovaquone-proguanil (malarone)

14. A 48-year-old female who was premorbid healthy, presented with acute onset fever, rash, and severe crippling joint pains. Her total count was 1,900/mm^3, hemoglobin 11.2 g%, and platelet count 105,000/mm^3. Liver and renal function tests were within normal limits. Tests for dengue and malaria were negative. Chikungunya PCR was positive. She was treated with NSAIDs, after which her joint pains significantly improved over 2–3 weeks. She had a relapse after that with severe polyarthralgias and morning stiffness. The affected joints were hands, knees, wrists, and shoulders, which were symmetrically involved. She was then started on steroids and subsequently on hydroxychloroquine (HCQ), with waxing and waning of her joint pains over a period of 2 years. Her ESR was 80, CRP 108, rheumatoid factor positive and anti-CCP antibody were negative. What is the possible reason for persistent arthralgias?

    A. Rheumatoid arthritis (RA)
    B. Undifferentiated polyarthritis

C. Chronic chikungunya arthritis (CCA)
D. Seronegative spondyloarthritis

15. A 63-year-old female presented with high-grade fever, rash, and bodyache. She was a known case of hypertension, diabetes mellitus type II, ischemic cardiomyopathy, and hypothyroidism. She was on regular medications for the above conditions. On the second day she developed severe pain in both ankle joints, which progressed rapidly to involve the knee, wrist, and shoulder joints. Movements became excruciating and she was immobilized. Routine blood biochemistry was normal and IgM and IgG antibodies against CHIKV were positive. She responded significantly to a combination of NSAIDs and steroids. 1 month later, she developed tingling and numbness of the right hand which was relieved with movement. Subsequently, she experienced weakness of the right thumb and index finger and difficulty in holding objects. X-ray of the cervical spine was normal. An ultrasound of the hand was suggestive of tenosynovitis. Electromyography and nerve conduction velocity were consistent with the diagnosis of carpal tunnel syndrome (CTS). Her free T3, free T4, and thyroid stimulating hormone (TSH) were within normal limits, on thyroxine tablets. What would be the most likely cause of CTS in this patient?

    A. Hypothyroidism
    B. Chikungunya fever
    C. Cervical spondylitis
    D. Menopause

16. An 18-year-old male presented with fever, headache, and vomiting of 3 days' duration. There was no history of seizures. On examination, he was highly febrile, toxic, and disoriented. Neck rigidity was present and plantars were bilaterally extensor. Pupils were sluggishly reacting to light and he moved all four limbs. There was no pallor or icterus and a faint macular rash was visible on the trunk. He was hemodynamically stable. All other systems were unremarkable on examination. There was a history of recurrent malaria and an episode of dengue in the preceding year. The total leukocyte count was 3,200/mm^3, hemoglobin 12.4 g%, platelet count 125,000/mm^3. Blood sugar, liver and renal function tests, and serum electrolytes were normal. There was no significant drug history. PS for malarial parasite done twice, RMAT, NS1Ag, dengue PCR, and blood culture were all negative. Chest radiograph and sonography of the abdomen were normal. Fundoscopy showed no papilledema and the brain imaging was normal. CSF examination was unremarkable. Electroencephalogram (EEG) was within normal limits. CHIK PCR in serum was positive, as was Zika IgM antibody. What is the possible cause of meningoencephalitis in this patient?

    A. Zika virus (ZIKV) infection
    B. Dengue virus infection
    C. Chikungunya virus infection
    D. Cerebral malaria

17. A 25-year-old male presented with high-grade fever, bodyache, rash, and joint pains of 5 days' duration. His total leukocyte count was 2,500/mm^3, hemoglobin 16 g%, platelet count 33,000/mm^3, SGOT 550 IU/L, SGPT 450 IU/L, and total bilirubin 1.2 mg%. Chest radiograph showed blunting of right costophrenic angle and abdominal sonography showed minimal free fluid. PS for malarial parasite and RMAT were negative and NS1Ag was negative. Which test would be most appropriate at this time?

    A. Dengue antibodies
    B. Blood culture
    C. Dengue PCR
    D. Viral markers

18. A 60-year-old postmenopausal woman presented with history of acute onset fever, rash, and debilitating joint pains of 2 days' duration. Her fever subsided but joint pains worsened over 4 weeks, with no response to NSAIDs. She was a known case of hypertension, diabetes mellitus type II, coronary artery disease, and RA (which was in remission). She was on irregular medications for her comorbidities and had poor glycemic control. She was initiated on tablet HCQ for her joint pains and asked to follow up. She returned after 2 months with complaints of decreased vision and pain in both eyes. Her joint pains persisted and she was on HCQ and NSAIDs. What is the most likely cause of her decreased vision?

    A. Ocular involvement in chikungunya
    B. Hypertensive and diabetic retinopathy
    C. Ocular toxicity of chloroquine
    D. Ocular involvement due to a flare up of RA

19. A 30-year-old unmarried male presented with history of difficulty in walking for the past 4 days. There was associated urinary and bowel retention and decreased sensations below T10. There was a history of fever with arthralgias preceding this. There was no history of vomiting, diarrhea, seizures, respiratory distress, trauma, lifting heavy weights, vaccination, or drug history. There was no history of weight loss or h/s/o any thyroid disorder. There was no history of visual disturbance or similar history in the past. There was no h/s/o cranial nerve involvement. The patient was conscious, oriented, power was 0/V in both lower extremities, knee and ankle jerks were absent, and plantars mute. There was no pallor, icterus, rash, or lymphadenopathy.

All other systems were unremarkable on examination. Hemoglobin was 14 g%, total counts 4,500/mm³, platelet count 86,000/mm³, SGOT 42 IU/L, SGPT 45 IU/L, sodium 138 mEq/L, potassium 3.5 mEq/L, blood sugar 84 mg%, creatine phosphokinase 110, and HIV and viral markers negative. Neuromyelitis optica (NMO) antibody against aquaporin 4 was negative. PS for malarial parasite and RMAT were negative, *Leptospira* IgM was negative, dengue IgM and IgG were negative, and chikungunya IgM was positive. Chikungunya PCR was negative and ZIKV antibody levels were not done. Chest radiograph and ECG were within normal limits. Ophthalmic examination for optic neuritis was negative. CSF studies were not performed. What is the most likely diagnosis?

A. Multiple sclerosis (first episode)
B. Acute transverse myelitis (ATM)
C. Hypokalemic periodic paralysis (HPP) (first episode)
D. Guillain–Barre syndrome (GBS)

20. A 33-year-old male has returned from a country endemic for ZIKV. There was an outbreak going on whilst he was there. He had suffered from respiratory symptoms a week earlier but did not get tested. He and his wife are trying to start a family. What advice would you offer him?

A. Abstinence or condom use for 3 months
B. Abstinence or condom use for 6 months
C. Abstinence or condom use for 9 months
D. Abstinence or condom use for 6 weeks

21. A 24-year-old healthy male was asked to donate blood for his sister who was critically ill. Before blood donation, he mentioned a history of hospitalization for dengue fever, a month ago. What is the policy regarding blood donation in dengue patients?

A. Cannot donate blood for 1 year
B. Cannot donate blood till dengue PCR positive
C. Cannot donate blood for 6 months
D. Cannot donate blood till dengue IgG positive

22. A 39-year-old male presented with history of fever and weight loss for 1 month, with chills, remittent, and without rigors. There was a history of listlessness and easy fatiguability for the past 2 weeks. There were no other complaints and he was premorbid healthy except for a history of hypertension. There was no history of addiction. On examination, he was conscious, oriented, and febrile, and there was severe pallor. There was generalized hyperpigmentation of the skin. There was no icterus, rash, clubbing, or significant lymphadenopathy. There was splenomegaly (6 cm below the left costal margin) and hepatomegaly (liver span 18 cm). All other systems were unremarkable on examination. Investigations revealed pancytopenia with hemoglobin 4.7 g%, leukocyte count 1,800/mm³ (neutrophils 41%, lymphocytes 42%, and monocytes 14%), platelet count 48,000/mm³, and corrected reticulocyte count 1.4%. RBC indices were normal. ESR was 40 mm/hour. PS for malaria parasite and RMAT were both negative. Dengue IgG antibody was positive. Blood Widal was negative. SGOT was 350 IU/L, SGPT 450 IU/L, total bilirubin 2.0 mg%, and serum LDH was 1029 U/L. Blood glucose and renal function were normal. Lipid profile was normal except for a high triglyceride level of 687 mg/dL. Blood and urine culture were sterile. Hepatitis B surface antigen, antihepatitis C virus, and HIV serology were negative. ANA was negative. INR was 1.4 with a normal activated partial thromboplastin time. Ultrasound of the abdomen showed hepatosplenomegaly but no lymphadenopathy or portal hypertension. Chest X-ray and 2D echo were normal. CT thorax and abdomen were normal except for hepatosplenomegaly. Esophagoduodenoscopy was normal. Bone marrow aspiration and biopsy were performed. What is the most likely diagnosis?

A. Chronic liver disease
B. Hyper-reactive malarial splenomegaly syndrome (HMSS)
C. Hemophagocytic lymphohistiocytosis (HLH) due to infection
D. Disseminated tuberculosis

23. If a mosquito bites an infected person, the chances of transmission of which viral infection to another human host, is the least?

A. Chikungunya virus
B. Dengue virus
C. Zika virus
D. Japanese encephalitis virus

24. A 59-year-old male residing in the United States of America is planning to travel to India (Agra) for a conference and leisure for a fortnight, in the monsoon season. He has received two doses of the JE vaccine 8 months earlier on a previous trip. Should he be advised to receive a booster dose now?

A. Not required
B. Should receive a month before travel
C. Should receive a week before travel
D. Should receive only if he goes to rural areas

25. A 33-year-old male, hailing from Jaunpur in Uttar Pradesh, presented with chronic intermittent fever with chills and swelling and redness over the left upper extremity, on and off for the past 5–6 months.

There were no other complaints. On enquiry there was no history of genital swelling or edema of the legs. He gave a history of occasional episode of blurring of vision. Physical examination was unremarkable. There were no palpable lymph nodes or edema of any extremity. Blood tests were normal except for eosinophils of 12% (total counts 8,400/mm^3). There were no microfilaria on PS. Antibody to filaria was positive. The patient was started on treatment with 6 mg/kg/day of diethylcarbamazine (DEC) in three divided doses for 15 days. On day 3 of treatment, the patient developed high-grade fever, pruritic rash, and worsening of visual disturbance.

A. Filarial infection of the eye
B. Central retinal artery occlusion
C. Drug reaction to DEC
D. Infective endocarditis

26. A 60-year-old patient presents with lymphedema and right leg elephantiasis. He also complains of scrotal swelling for the past 8 years. There is no history of fever on enquiry. What would be the best form of treatment?

A. Single dose of ivermectin combined with DEC
B. Single dose of ivermectin combined with albendazole
C. Single dose of DEC combined with albendazole
D. Leg elevation, exercises, and skin care

27. The best option for elimination of lymphatic filariasis (LF) is:

A. Single dose of DEC + albendazole + ivermectin
B. Single dose of DEC + albendazole
C. Single dose of DEC + albendazole + ivermectin repeated annually for 5 years
D. Single dose of DEC + albendazole+ ivermectin repeated annually for 3 years

28. Which of the following antibiotics has a role in the treatment of lymphatic filariasis (LF)?

A. Azithromycin   B. Ciprofloxacin
C. Doxycycline   D. Clindamycin

29. A 48-year-old farmer came with complaints of massive lower limb swelling for 4 years, which was bilateral and asymmetric, and was diagnosed as elephantiasis. The least likely cause in this patient would be:

A. Lymphatic filariasis
B. Podoconiosis
C. Leishmaniasis
D. Lymphogranuloma venereum (LGV)

30. A 30-year-old female presented with breathlessness and nocturnal dry cough, of 2 months' duration. She had been diagnosed as bronchial asthma based on these symptoms and was on metered dose inhalers. Her chest radiograph showed bilateral reticular shadows and since there was a doubtful history of fever and a raised ESR, she was started on four-drug weightwise antituberculous therapy for 15 days. After 2 months of therapy, there was neither symptomatic relief nor radiological improvement. General examination was unremarkable except for a respiratory rate of 24 breaths/min. Chest examination revealed bilateral rhonchi and scattered crackles. Rest of the systemic examination was normal. Her WBC count was 18,400/mm^3, DLC polymorphs 57%, lymphocytes 20%, eosinophils 19%, monocytes 04%, and absolute eosinophil count was 3,496/L. Liver and renal function tests, blood sugar, ECG, 2D echo were all normal. ABG showed a PO$_2$ of 118 and PCO$_2$ of 34. A repeat XRC showed the same findings, viz. bilateral reticulonodular shadows. Since her cough was dry, sputum examination could not be performed. Serum IgE was 1,800 IU/mL (NR 0–380 IU/mL). Considering the possibility of filarial tropical pulmonary eosinophilia (TPE), which is the least likely test to confirm the diagnosis?

A. Peripheral blood smear for microfilariae
B. Leukocytosis with peripheral eosinophilia >3,000/µm
C. Elevated serum IgE and filarial specific IgG and IgE
D. Clinical improvement with DEC

ANSWERS WITH EXPLANATIONS

1. **Ans. B**

   Patients with severe malaria treated with artesunate sometimes experience a delayed hemolytic episode. The rapid parasite clearing action of artesunate is based on pitting, a process whereby artemisinin-exposed rings are expelled from their host erythrocytes in the spleen. The erythrocytes then reseal rather than lyse. After being pitted, once-infected erythrocytes re-enter the circulation, now parasite free but with a reduced lifespan. Post-artemisinin delayed hemolysis (PADH) can occur 1–3 weeks after initiation of treatment with artemisinin-based antimalarials such as artesunate and is characterized by a decline in hemoglobin levels amid hemolysis. PADH occurs because of delayed clearance of once-infected erythrocytes, probably as a result of a pharmacologic effect of parenteral artesunate and not drug-related toxicity. Therefore, parenteral artesunate can still be considered a safe treatment for severe malaria and should remain an option for its treatment. Megaloblastic anemia in this patient is less likely in the absence of a normal MCV and no pancytopenia and the fact that the patient had been abstaining from alcohol for 2 years. Recrudescent malaria as the cause of hemolysis is unlikely as the patient had clinical and parasitological cure. AIHA is again unlikely in the absence of other relevant findings.

Ref:
1. Jauréguiberry S, Ndour PA, Roussel C, Ader F, Safeukui I, Nguyen M, et al. Postartesunate delayed hemolysis is a predictable event related to the lifesaving effect of artemisinins. Blood. 2014;124(2):167-75.
2. Paczkowski MM, Landman KL, Arguin PM; Centers for Disease Control and Prevention (CDC). Update on cases of delayed hemolysis after parenteral artesunate therapy for malaria - United States, 2008 and 2013. MMWR Morb Mortal Wkly Rep. 2014;63(34):753-5.
3. Angus BJ, Chotivanich K, Udomsangpetch R, White NJ. In vivo removal of malaria parasites from red blood cells without their destruction in acute falciparum malaria. Blood. 1997;90(5):2037-40.
4. White NJ. The assessment of antimalarial drug efficacy. Trends Parasitol. 2002;18(10):458-64.

2. **Ans. C**

The differentials in this patient would be severe mixed malaria (vivax + falciparum) with probable acute respiratory distress syndrome (ARDS) and leptospirosis with acute kidney injury (AKI); mixed malaria with leptospirosis with intrapulmonary hemorrhages secondary to leptospirosis, with AKI. Since the patient is a chronic alcoholic, the pancytopenia could be due to megaloblastic anemia (MCV 106) and/or hypersplenism secondary to portal hypertension, and spontaneous bacterial peritonitis with sepsis and AKI should also be considered. Fulminant viral hepatitis is a possibility, though less likely, where the liver enzymes may not be in thousands toward the end stage. In relevant situations, scrub typhus should also be considered and the presence of an eschar sought. Viral hemorrhagic fevers such as Hanta virus may present in a similar manner. The chest radiograph shows bilateral interstitial shadows, which is likely to represent intrapulmonary hemorrhages, i.e., severe pulmonary hemorrhage syndrome (SPHS) in the present scenario. Mixed infections with malaria and leptospirosis are common, especially in the monsoons. Thrombocytopenia, renal involvement, subconjunctival hemorrhages, hyperbilirubinemia, and ARDS are common to both these infections. In leptospirosis, the hyperbilirubinemia is much greater than the elevation in liver enzymes. IV methylprednisolone 1 g daily for 3 days followed by 1 mg/kg/day for 7 days is the preferred therapy for SPHS. Other therapies proposed are cyclophosphamide, vasopressin, and plasma exchange. Some recent studies have debated the role of corticosteroids, citing severe invasive fungal infections as a reason. Leptospira polymerase chain reaction (PCR) was reported as positive.

Ref:
1. Thunga G, John J, Sam KG, Khera K, Khan S, Pandey S, et al. Role of high-dose corticosteroid for the treatment of leptospirosis-induced pulmonary hemorrhage. J Clin Pharmacol. 2012;52(1):114-6.
2. Trivedi SV, Chavda RK, Wadia PZ, Sheth V, Bhagade PN, Trivedi SP, et al. The role of glucocorticoid pulse therapy in pulmonary involvement in leptospirosis. J Assoc Physicians India. 2001;49:901-3.
3. Hingorani RV, Kumar R, Hegde AV, Soman RN, Sirsat RA, Rodrigues C, et al. Is it time to rethink the use of steroids for pulmonary leptospirosis? J Assoc Physicians India. 2016;64(3):78-9.

3. **Ans. C**

The above clinical scenario along with the complete blood count is more likely to suggest dengue, in view of the hemoconcentration (hemoglobin 17) and platelet count of 45,000/mm^3. Viral fever and chikungunya do cause thrombocytopenia but usually not lower than 90,000/mm^3; fever in chikungunya is episodic and short-lasting. MAC-ELISA has a sensitivity and specificity of 90% and 98%, respectively but only when used 5 or more days after the onset of fever. Because antibodies are detected later, reverse transcription polymerase chain reaction (RT-PCR) has become a primary tool to detect virus early in the course of the illness, where it can be recovered for approximately the first 5 days of symptoms. Often times, both an acute and convalescent phase specimens are needed to make a diagnosis of dengue infection, especially when a day 5 or day 6 acute specimen is submitted initially. This is because the virus and IgM antibodies may be at undetectable levels around day 5. So, if a patient with suspected dengue infection submits a late acute phase specimen that is negative (i.e., by RT-PCR and MAC-ELISA) and does not submit a convalescent specimen, he is classified as a laboratory-indeterminate case. So, in this patient, dengue antibodies should be repeated. NS1Ag is another useful test which is positive in the first 5–7 days and helps in the early detection of dengue.

Ref:
1. Datta S, Wattal C. Dengue NS1 antigen detection: A useful tool in early diagnosis of dengue virus infection. Indian J Med Microbiol. 2010;28(2):107-10.

2. Peeling RW, Artsob H, Pelegrino JL, Buchy P, Cardosa MJ, Devi S, et al. Evaluation of diagnostic tests: Dengue. Nat Rev Microbiol. 2010;8(Suppl 12):S30-8.
3. Hunsperger EA, Yoksan S, Buchy P, Nguyen VC, Sekaran SD, Enria DA, et al. Evaluation of commercially available diagnostic tests for the detection of dengue NS1 antigen and anti-dengue virus IgM antibody. PLoS Negl Trop Dis. 2014;8(10):e3171.

4. **Ans. A**

Dengue initially causes a flushing erythema of the face, neck, and chest that typically occurs in the first 24–48 hours of the onset of symptoms and is thought to be the result of capillary dilatation. A second rash appears 3–5 days later in a large group of patients, which is a generalized morbilliform eruption with petechiae and islands of sparing (white islands in a sea of red) and is thought to be an immune response to the virus. A drug-induced rash is duskier, associated with severe pruritus and may be associated with eosinophilia. A patient with drug fever usually appears well in spite of the fever. Viral hepatitis is usually not associated with severe rash, and symptoms of nausea, vomiting, and fatigue are predominant. IM like illness is associated with oral lesions, pharyngitis, lymphadenopathy, and hepatosplenomegaly.

Ref:
1. Chadwick D, Arch B, Wilder-Smith A, Paton N. Distinguishing dengue fever from other infections on the basis of simple clinical and laboratory features: Application of logistic regression analysis. J Clin Virol. 2006;35(2):147-53.
2. Thomas EA, John M, Bhatia A. Cutaneous manifestations of dengue viral infection in Punjab (North India). Int J Dermatol. 2007;46(7):715-9.

5. **Ans. B**

Eighty percent of all dengue cases have detectable IgM antibody by day 5 of illness, and 93–99% of cases have detectable IgM by day 6 to day 10 of illness, which may remain elevated for 2–3 months after the illness. In a primary infection, IgM antibodies would not appear on day 3 and so this could be the result of an infection that occurred 2–3 months ago. In a secondary infection, high levels of IgG are detectable even in the acute phase, and since IgM levels are significantly low in a secondary infection, false negative IgM tests are very likely. In addition, there is cross reactivity with other flaviviruses including Japanese encephalitis virus (JEV), Yellow fever virus, West Nile virus, and St. Louis encephalitis virus, which could give rise to a false positive test. Hence, a past medical history, recent travel history, and vaccination record (especially yellow fever vaccination), should be recorded. So, this could be a recent probable dengue infection.

Ref:
1. Chanama S, Anantapreecha S, A-nuegoonpipat A, Sa-gnasang A, Kurane I, Sawanpanyalert P. Analysis of specific IgM responses in secondary dengue virus infections: Levels and positive rates in comparison with primary infections. J Clin Virol. 2004;31(3):185-9.
2. Shu PY, Chen LK, Chang SF, Yueh YY, Chow L, Chien LJ, et al. Comparison of capture immunoglobulin M (IgM) and IgG enzyme-linked immunosorbent assay (ELISA) and nonstructural protein NS1 serotype-specific IgG ELISA for differentiation of primary and secondary dengue virus infections. Clin Diagn Lab Immunol. 2003;10(4):622-30.
3. Blacksell SD, Doust JA, Newton PN, Peacock SJ, Day NP, Dondorp AM. A systematic review and meta-analysis of the diagnostic accuracy of rapid immunochromatographic assays for the detection of dengue virus IgM antibodies during acute infection. Trans R Soc Trop Med Hyg. 2006;100(8):775-84.

6. **Ans. A**

Dengue and JE are arboviral diseases that are common in the tropical countries. JEV is a classical neurotropic virus. The dengue virus (DENV), however, is usually not considered to be neurotropic, even though in recent years, reports of direct central nervous system (CNS) involvement in dengue have been described. Other causes of encephalopathy in dengue are due to metabolic disturbances, hepatic or renal involvement, or hypotension. This patient had magnetic resonance imaging evidence of bilateral thalamic and brainstem involvement with positive serologies for both dengue and JE. The clinical presentation and investigations in this patient point toward a dengue encephalitis. Both dengue and JEVs are flaviviruses and share some common antigens because of which serological cross-reactivity can occur with either infection. It is important to differentiate true JEV infections from false-positive JE results because of cross-reactive epitopes among flaviviruses. Since dengue PCR was positive, this patient certainly had dengue infection. Detection of virus genome or virus isolation in serum, plasma, or blood is very specific for JE diagnosis, which was not performed in this patient. So, it is difficult to say whether she had a single infection and cross-reactivity, or a true dual infection. However, JEV PCR is not sensitive, as virus levels are usually undetectable in clinically ill JE cases.

Ref:
1. Singh KP, Mishra G, Jain P, Pandey N, Nagar R, Gupta S, et al. Co-positivity of anti-dengue virus and anti-Japanese encephalitis virus IgM in endemic area: Co-infection or cross reactivity? Asian Pac J Trop Med. 2014;7(2):124-9.
2. Garg R, Malhotra HS, Gupta A, Kumar N, Jain A. Concurrent dengue virus and Japanese encephalitis virus infection of the brain: Is it co-infection or co-detection? Infection. 2012;40(5):589-93.

3. A-Nuegoonpipat A, Panthuyosri N, Anantapreecha S, Chanama S, Sa-Ngasang A, Sawanpanyalert P, et al. Cross-reactive IgM responses in patients with dengue or Japanese encephalitis. J Clin Virol. 2008;42(1):75-7.

7. Ans. C

Rapid malaria antigen test, especially one detecting PfHRP2 antigen for falciparum, may remain positive for 28 days after clinical cure. Hence, the RMAT may be false positive in this situation. Another scenario where PS is negative but RMAT is positive, may occur if the patient has received incomplete antimalarial treatment, especially a recent dose of artemisinin which has a very rapid fever clearance time (FCT) and parasite clearance time (PCT). Hence, eliciting a good history of recent treatment, completion of treatment and monitoring the patient for fever recurrence is important.

Ref:
1. WHO. Guidelines for the Treatment of Malaria, 3rd edition; 2015. p. 316.
2. Wongsrichanalai C, Chuanak N, Tulyayon S, Thanoosingha N, Laboonchai A, Thimasarn K, et al. Comparison of a rapid field immunochromatographic test to expert microscopy for the detection of Plasmodium falciparum asexual parasitemia in Thailand. Acta Trop. 1999;73(3):263-73.

8. Ans. D

Dengue and Chikungunya share many similarities. Both are arboviruses, share the same vector (*Aedes aegypti* and *Aedes albopictus*), have identical symptoms, and their geographical domain too is similar. Chikungunya is often misdiagnosed as the better known dengue fever. Misdiagnosis of dengue as chikungunya or missing a concurrent dengue infection in a patient of chikungunya risks delaying dengue-specific intensive supportive treatment. On the other hand, mistaking dengue for chikungunya leads to the inappropriate use of non-steroidal anti-inflammatory drugs (NSAIDs) to dengue patients which could lead to severe bleeding in patients with thrombocytopenia or dengue hemorrhagic fever. Also, concurrent with dengue and chikungunya occur in areas where these two viruses cocirculate. Studies have quoted the prevalence of coinfection to range from 0.9 to 19%. It is not known whether concurrent infections lead to more severe symptoms as compared to mono-infections, e.g., severe arthralgias in a patient of dengue or whether new symptoms are produced. The above patient has a clinical picture compatible with dengue hemorrhagic fever but has more severe arthralgias, with associated swelling of the joints, which is not commonly seen in dengue mono-infection. Chikungunya alone usually causes episodic, short-lasting fever; the platelet count not lower than a lakh and no capillary leakage.

Ref:
1. Singh J, Dinkar A, Singh RG, Siddiqui MS, Sinha N, Singh SK. Clinical profile of dengue fever and coinfection with chikungunya. Tzu Chi Med J. 2018;30:158-64.
2. Gandhi BS, Kulkarni K, Godbole M, Dole SS, Kapur S, Satpathy P, et al. Dengue and Chikungunya co-infection associated with more severe clinical disease than mono-infection. Int J Healthc Biomed Res. 2015;3(3):117-23.
3. Londhey V, Agrawal S, Vaidya N, Kini S, Shastri JS, Sunil S, et al. Dengue and Chikungunya virus co-infections: The inside story. J Assoc Physicians India. 2016;64(3):36-40.

9. Ans. A

Parenteral doses should be given for a minimum of 24 hours once started irrespective of the patient's ability to tolerate oral treatment earlier. Later on, a switch can be made to any of the WHO-recommended first-line oral artemisinin combination therapy (ACT). However, if the patient presents with neurological symptoms, as in cerebral malaria, mefloquine should be avoided in the combination due to its potent psychotropic potential. Severe psychiatric side effects due to mefloquine are well documented, including anxiety, panic attacks, paranoia, persecutory delusions, dissociative psychosis, and anterograde amnesia. Exposure to the drug has been associated with acts of violence and suicide. Due to the very long half-life of mefloquine, psychiatric symptoms can persist for weeks, necessitating an appropriate psychotropic treatment.

Ref:
1. WHO Malaria guidelines, 3rd edition; 2015. pp. 1-318.
2. FDA Drug Safety Communication (2013). FDA approves label changes for antimalarial drug mefloquine hydrochloride due to risk of serious psychiatric and nerve side effects. [online] Available from: https://www.fda.gov/drugs/drug-safety-and-availability/fda-drug-safety-communication-fda-approves-label-changes-antimalarial-drug-mefloquine-hydrochloride [Last accessed February, 2020].
3. Ritchie EC, Block J, Nevin RL. Psychiatric side effects of mefloquine: Applications to forensic psychiatry. J Am Acad Psychiatry Law. 2013;41(2):224-35.

10. Ans. C

In areas of stable transmission (endemic), with a high entomological inoculation rate (EIR), patients often develop immunity to the clinical symptoms of malaria and are asymptomatic in the presence of asexual blood stages. The WHO defines cure as not only the resolution of symptoms but also the documentation of parasitological clearance. Persistence of asexual blood stages is a common cause of anemia in endemic areas and should be treated.

Ref:
1. World Health Organization (2015). WHO Malaria Guidelines 2015. [online] Available from: https://www.who.int/docs/default-source/documents/publications/gmp/guidelines-for-the-treatment-of-malaria-eng.pdf?sfvrsn=a0138b77_2 [Last accessed February, 2020].

11. Ans. B

Primaquine, an 8-aminoquinoline is a time-tested medicine for treating relapses of *Plasmodium vivax* and *Plasmodium ovale* (*P. ovale*) malaria, due to its specific activity against malaria hypnozoites. It is the only currently available drug that actively clears mature *Plasmodium falciparum* (*P. falciparum*) gametocytes and prevents malaria transmission to mosquitoes. It induces dose-dependent acute hemolytic anemia in individuals with G6PD deficiency, a genetically X-linked disorder. It has a prevalence of 3–35% in tropical areas. The severity of hemolytic anemia depends on both the dose and the frequency of administration of primaquine and the variant of the G6PD enzyme. Most of the times, in mild and moderate deficiency, the hemolysis is self-limiting. A patient with mild G6PD deficiency can be given primaquine in the usual dose of 0.25 mg/kg body weight daily for 14 days. In moderate deficiency, the dose is 0.75 mg/kg weekly for 8 weeks (maximum dose 45 mg), whereas it should be avoided in severe deficiency. It should be avoided in pregnant and lactating women. A newer 8-aminoquinoline, tafenoquine (krintafel) is now approved for single dose radical cure. G6PD study should be done as far as possible, before prescribing oxidant drugs like primaquine.

Ref:
1. *White NJ. Primaquine to prevent transmission of falciparum malaria. Lancet Infect Dis. 2013; 13(2):175-81.*
2. *WHO (2016). Testing for G6PD deficiency for safe use of primaquine in radical cure of P. vivax and P. ovale malaria. [online] Available from: https://www.who.int/malaria/publications/atoz/g6pd-testing-pq-radical-cure-vivax/en/ [Last accessed February, 2020].*

12. Ans. A

The clinical presentation and investigations suggest dengue with ARDS. Leukopenia, thrombocytopenia and raised hemoglobin (due to capillary leak) go in favor of a diagnosis of dengue. There is no direct antiviral therapy available against the DENVs. Management is supportive primarily consisting of maintaining adequate intravascular volume. Doxycycline, an antibiotic derived from tetracycline with broad antimicrobial and anti-inflammatory activities has been shown to possess antiviral properties. It may prove helpful in providing clinical benefits in the treatment of DENV infection by modulating the cytokine cascade as well as by its ability to interact with the DENV E protein to inhibit a conformational change which is an essential step in the process by which the virus enters the susceptible cells. Doxycycline significantly inhibits viral entry and postinfection replication of the four dengue serotypes, with serotype-specific inhibition (high activity against DENV2 and DENV4 compared to DENV1 and DENV3). The antidengue activity and anti-inflammatory activity of doxycycline may prove to be helpful in reducing the severity of clinical symptoms such as dengue fever, severe dengue hemorrhagic fever, and dengue shock syndrome. Also, one of the differentials would be scrub typhus, even though an eschar was absent. Doxycycline would also work against this. Since this patient is unstable, ceftriaxone is appropriate for treating leptospirosis, even though doxycycline is effective.

Ref:
1. *Rothan HA, Mohamed Z, Paydar M, Rahman NA, Yusof R. Inhibitory effect of doxycycline against dengue virus replication in vitro. Arch Virol. 2014;159(4):711-8.*
2. *Fredeking TM, Zavala-Castro JE, González-Martínez P, Moguel-Rodríguez W, Sanchez EC, Foster MJ, et al. Dengue patients treated with doxycycline showed lower mortality associated to a reduction in IL-6 and TNF Levels. Recent Pat Antiinfect Drug Discov. 2015;10(1):51-8.*
3. *Garg P. Role of Doxycycline in the management of dengue fever. Indian Journal of Clinical Practice. 2018;29(2):132-5.*

13. Ans. C

Chemoprophylaxis in malaria can be causal (against exo-erythrocytic stage in the liver, i.e., tissue schizonticides) and suppressive (against asexual stages, i.e., blood schizonticides). Mefloquine, chloroquine, and doxycycline are blood schizonticides, whereas malarone is a blood and a tissue schizonticide. Chloroquine is not active against falciparum and hence would not be recommended for travel to India. Mefloquine and doxycycline are both active against falciparum, however, mefloquine has to be started 1–2 weeks prior to travel whereas this patient needs to travel within 4 days. Doxycycline can be started 1–2 days before travel and hence would be more appropriate in situations where a sudden trip is planned. The disadvantage of doxycycline is that it has to be taken daily whereas mefloquine is to be taken weekly. Malarone too has the advantage that it can be started 1–2 days before travel and be continued for just 7 days after return, as compared to other prophylactics which need to be continued for 4 weeks after return. However, it is contraindicated in severe renal failure and so may not be appropriate in this situation. No antimalarial drug is 100% protective and must be combined with the use of personal protective measures (i.e., insect repellent, long sleeves, long pants, sleeping in a mosquito-free setting or using an insecticide-treated bednet).

Ref:
1. *Castelli F, Odolini S, Autino B, Foca E, Russo R. Malaria prophylaxis: A comprehensive review. Pharmaceuticals (Basel). 2010;3(10):3212-39.*
2. *WHO. Guidelines for the Treatment of Malaria, 3rd edition. Geneva: World Health Organization; 2015.*

14. Ans. C

In several studies, 25–62% of patients had arthritic symptoms 18 months after the onset of CHIKF. Even at the 36-month follow-up, the prevalence of arthritis has been reported to be as high as 60%. The pathogenesis of CCA is not well understood. Proposed hypotheses include the persistence of a low level of replicating virus in the joints, the persistence of viral RNA in the synovium, and the induction of autoimmunity. Reports have also focused on CCA as an "RA mimic". A parallel to RA has been the finding of subchondral bone erosions, joint effusions, and joint thickening in patients with CCA. Among reports of CCA patients whose disease mimics RA, rheumatoid factor positivity has varied between 25 and 43%, and anti-CCP antibody positivity has been less frequent. Suggested risk factors for progression to long-term disease include female sex, age > 45 years, diabetes mellitus, hypertension, dyslipidemia, and previous rheumatic disease.

Ref:
1. *Amaral JK, Taylor PC, Teixeira MM, Morrison TET, Schoen RT. The clinical features, pathogenesis and methotrexate therapy of chronic chikungunya arthritis. Viruses. 2019;11(3). pii: E289.*
2. *Borgherini G, Poubeau P, Jossaume A, Gouix A, Cotte L, Michault A, et al. Persistent arthralgia associated with chikungunya virus: A study of 88 adult patients on reunion Island. Clin Infect Dis. 2008;47(4):469-75.*
3. *Schilte C, Staikowsky F, Couderc T, Madec Y, Carpentier F, Kassab S, et al. Chikungunya virus-associated long-term arthralgia: A 36-month prospective longitudinal study. PLoS Negl Trop Dis. 2013,7(3):e2137.*

15. Ans. B

Clinical conditions with a predilection for CTS are RA, obesity, diabetes mellitus, systemic lupus erythematosus, autoimmune disorders, hypothyroidism, etc. Musculoskeletal disorders, tumors, and normal aging, leading to wear and tear of the tissues in both the hand and wrist, have also been implicated. Tenosynovitis of the anterior wrist has been identified as the most important cause of CTS after virus infection. Thyroid function tests in this patient were within normal limits. Menopause has also been related to CTS. However, in this patient, CHIKV infection is the most likely cause and should be considered in the differential diagnosis of CTS in residents of endemic areas.

Ref:
1. *Puccioni-Sohler M, Salgado MC, Versiani I, Rosadas C, Ferry F, Tanuri A, et al. Carpal tunnel syndrome after chikungunya infection. Int J Infect Dis. 2016;53:21-2.*
2. *Chen YT, Williams L, Zak MJ, Fredericson M. Review of ultrasonography in the diagnosis of carpal tunnel syndrome and a proposed scanning protocol. J Ultrasound Med. 2016;35(11):2311-24.*
3. *Yurdakul OV, Mesci N, Cetinkaya Y, Geler Külcü D. Diagnostic significance of ultrasonographic measurements and median-ulnar ratio in carpal tunnel syndrome: Correlation with nerve conduction studies. J Clin Neurol. 2016;12(3):289-94.*

16. Ans. C

Dengue, Zika and chikungunya are all arboviruses and all three can cause an initial fever–arthralgia–rash syndrome and are associated with neurological complications. The strongest evidence of causality comes from demonstrating the virus in the CNS, which is most often shown by detecting viral RNA in the CSF by PCR. Cocirculation of chikungunya, Zika, and dengue viruses has been reported and is a potential problem in all areas of the world where *Aedes* mosquitoes are endemic. As is the case in other arboviral encephalitides, a CSF pleocytosis is not always seen in chikungunya encephalitis. Unlike encephalitis caused by other CNS pathogens such as HSV and cytomegalovirus, which have characteristic imaging abnormalities, chikungunya encephalitis in adults and children does not appear to show a distinct pattern and may be entirely normal. A positive Zika-IgM test can result from cross-reactivity of serum containing antibodies against DENV, as both are flaviviruses. Because chikungunya is an alphavirus, there is no serological cross-reactivity with the flaviviruses, making diagnosis more straightforward (in areas where other alphaviruses are not circulating). A positive blood test in a patient with neurological disease does not necessarily mean the virus caused the disease; infection may be coincidental, and care must be taken to exclude other possible causes. However, during an epidemic of chikungunya, neurological involvement may be attributed to it, after ruling out other causes.

Ref:
1. *Mehta R, Gerardin P, de Brito CAA, Soares CN, Ferreira MLB, Solomon T. The neurological complications of chikungunya virus: A systematic review. Rev Med Virol. 2018;28(3):e1978.*
2. *Smith DW, Mackenzie J. Zika virus and Guillain-Barré syndrome: Another viral cause to add to the list. Lancet. 2016;387(10027):1486-8.*
3. *Robin S, Ramful D, Le Seach' F, Jaffar-Bandjee MC, Rigou G, Alessandri JL. Neurologic manifestations of pediatric chikungunya infection. J Child Neurol. 2008;23(9):1028-35.*
4. *Chandak NH, Kashyap RS, Kabra D, Karandikar P, Saha SS, Morey SH, et al. Neurological complications of chikungunya virus infection. Neurol India. 2009; 57(2):177-80.*

17. Ans. C

The clinical picture is compatible with a diagnosis of dengue. Hepatic involvement is common in dengue, with SGOT being more than SGPT, unlike viral hepatitis where SGPT is more than SGOT. Liver enzymes can even increase to thousands in severe dengue. Dengue antibodies start rising only after 8–10 days, with the IgM being elevated for around 3 months and IgG for many years. NS1 levels peak around 4–5 days during primary infections and wane by day 7, but decline earlier in secondary infections. Also, in secondary infections, antibodies against DENV NS1 may be present in the patient's sample, forming antigen-antibody complexes, thereby reducing access to the target epitopes for the test articles. Another reason for false negative NS1Ag is the infecting DENV serotype, where DENV-4 sensitivity averaged only 50%. This could be due to the lower overall viremia and NS1 antigen levels in DENV-4 infections making it a less abundant target. Hence, whenever dengue is strongly suspected, dengue PCR should be sent even if NS1Ag is negative. Besides, resistance temperature detectors (RDTs) for NS1Ag are less sensitive as compared to ELISA tests.

Ref:
1. Sea VR, Cruz AC, Gurgel RQ, Nunes BT, Silva EV, Dolabella SS, et al. Underreporting of Dengue-4 in Brazil due to low sensitivity of the NS1 Ag test in routine control programs. PLoS One. 2013;8(5):e64056.
2. Sekaran SD, Ew CL, Subramaniam G, Kanthesh BM. Sensitivity of dengue virus NS-1 detection in primary and secondary infections. Afr J Microbiol Res. 2009;3(3):105-10.
3. Lima Mda R, Nogueira RM, Schatzmayr HG, dos Santos FB. Comparison of three commercially available dengue NS1 antigen capture assays for acute diagnosis of dengue in Brazil. PLoS Negl Trop Dis. 2010;4(7):e738.

18. Ans. B

Chikungunya virus infection is known to cause different ocular manifestations such as nongranulomatous anterior uveitis, episcleritis, panuveitis, granulomatous anterior uveitis, optic neuritis, 6th nerve palsy, retrobulbar neuritis, retinitis with vitritis, neuroretinitis, keratitis, central retinal artery occlusion, multifocal choroiditis, exudative retinal detachment, and secondary glaucoma. However, this patient developed visual symptoms after 2 months. Flare up of RA is less likely as her disease was in remission.

Retinal toxicity from HCQ is rare, but even if the medication is discontinued, vision loss may be irreversible and may continue to progress. And before treatment is initiated with HCQ, a complete ophthalmic examination should be performed to determine any baseline maculopathy. Previous reports indicate that toxicity is rare if dosing is <6.5 mg/kg/day. The risk factors for diabetic retinopathy are poor glycemic control, hypertension, duration of diabetes, hyperlipidemia, and proteinuria. Diabetic retinopathy is one of the important causes of visual disability in diabetic subjects during the period of active life. It is characterized by gradually progressive alterations in the retinal microvasculature, leading to increased vasopermeability, areas of retinal occlusion, and retinal neovascularization. Since this lady had poor glycemic control, diabetes and hypertension were the most likely causes of her visual defect.

Ref:
1. Muiesan ML, Grassi G. Assessment of retinal vascular changes in hypertension: New perspectives. J Hypertens. 2006;24(5):8134.
2. Marmor MF, Kellner U, Lai TY, Lyons JS, Mieler WF; American Academy of Ophthalmology. Revised recommendations on screening for chloroquine and hydroxychloroquine retinopathy. Ophthalmology. 2011;118(2):415-22.
3. Lalitha P, Rathinam S, Banushree K, Maheshkumar S, Vijayakumar R, Sathe P. Ocular involvement associated with an epidemic outbreak of Chikungunya virus infection. Am J Ophthalmol. 2007;144(4):552-6.

19. Ans. B

Multiple sclerosis is less likely as there was no earlier episode, NMO antibody was negative, and optic neuritis was ruled out. HPP is episodic; there may be preceding vomiting or diarrhea and the potassium is usually much lower than 3.5 mEq/L. Both ATM and GBS can occur after viral infections or vaccinations. It is often difficult to know whether direct viral infection or a postinfectious response to the infection causes the transverse myelitis. GBS has been associated with ZIKV too. Absent reflexes are a feature of GBS, though sensory involvement and bladder, bowel involvement are not common. ATM is sudden onset, with sensory involvement and bladder, bowel involvement. ATM is associated with exaggerated reflexes, but the stage of spinal shock may cause absent reflexes. Chikungunya is strongly believed to have neurotropism but has not been well studied like other neurotropic arboviruses. Encephalitis appears to represent the most common clinical manifestation and occurs either simultaneously or within few days of onset of systemic symptoms, during the period of viremia. A delay of >2 weeks has been reported with other complications like myelitis, GBS, and optic neuritis.

Ref:
1. Chandak NH, Kashyap RS, Kabra D, Karandikar P, Saha SS, Morey SH, et al. Neurological complications of Chikungunya virus infection. Neurol India. 2009;57(2):177-80.
2. Kumar R, Rajvanshi P, Khosla H, Arora S. Neuro-Chikungunya: Acute transverse myelopathy associated with Chikungunya virus infection. J Assoc Physicians India. 2019;67(7):84-5.

20. Ans. B

Zika virus can be transmitted between humans through sexual contact and this has important implications for public health, for people living in endemic regions, and for sexual partners of travelers returning to nonendemic regions from endemic regions because ZIKV infection during pregnancy can cause congenital infection of the fetus. ZIKV is more likely transmitted from men to women than from women to men. For other flaviviruses, evidence of sexual transmissibility is still absent. Very few men actually emit the whole virus, which is shed for a shorter duration and is potentially infectious. Fragments of viral RNA are shed for longer periods and are thought not to be infectious. Even in Ebola, the prolonged presence of viral RNA in the semen, was not associated with infectivity. However, both the Centers for Disease Control and Prevention (CDC) and the World Health Organization urge people who have been infected with Zika or have traveled to a place where Zika was spreading to put off trying to have a child for 6 months.

Ref:
1. Rasmussen SA, Jamieson DJ, Honein MA, Petersen LR. Zika virus and birth defects—reviewing the evidence for causality. N Engl J Med. 2016;374(20):1981-7.
2. Mead PS, Duggal NK, Hook SA, Delorey M, Fischer M, Olzenak McGuire D, et al. Zika Virus shedding in semen of symptomatic infected men. N Engl J Med. 2018;378(15):1377-85.

21. Ans. C

Dengue is known to be transfusion–transmitted since 2008. The testing to confirm dengue infection in patients is different from that of testing DENV in donated blood. There are currently no available licensed test kits to screen donated blood for DENV. Nucleic acid screening test (NAT) may be useful. Those infected with dengue must not donate blood for 6 months after recovery, according to the recent guidelines released by the National Blood Transfusion Council.

Ref:
1. Bianco C. Dengue and chikungunya viruses in blood donations: Risks to the blood supply? Transfusion. 2008;48(7):1279-81.
2. Petersen LR, Busch MP. Transfusion-transmitted arboviruses. Vox Sang. 2010;98(4):495-503.

22. Ans. C

Hemophagocytic lymphohistiocytosis is a rare clinicopathological condition, which causes inappropriate activation and proliferation of monocyte-macrophage-histiocytic lineage with uncontrolled hemophagocytosis, leading to fever, hepatosplenomegaly, cytopenia, liver dysfunction, hyperferritinemia, and hypertriglyceridemia. The primary form of the disease is genetic whereas another form occurs secondary to conditions like infections, malignancies, autoimmune diseases, or immunosuppression. Dengue, malaria, and visceral leishmaniasis (VL) can all lead to HLH. Diagnosing HLH is challenging as this may be easily confused with any systemic infection. In this patient, dengue IgG could be positive due to a past remote infection. The hyperpigmentation of the skin is likely to be because of kala azar (VL). Pancytopenia can be seen in VL too due to the massive splenomegaly. Tuberculosis is less likely as there is no e/o TB elsewhere in the body and the imagings show no lymphadenopathy. Bone marrow examination would confirm the diagnosis of HLH and also diagnose the infection responsible for the same.

Ref:
1. Henter JI, Horne A, Aricó M, Egeler RM, Filipovich AH, Imashuku S, et al. HLH-2004: Diagnostic and therapeutic guidelines for hemophagocytic lymphohistiocytosis. Pediatr Blood Cancer. 2007;48(2):124-31.
2. Ranjan P, Kumar V, Ganguly S, Sukumar M, Sharma S, Singh N, et al. Hemophagocytic lymphohistiocytosis associated with visceral leishmaniasis: Varied presentation. Indian J Hematol Blood Transfus. 2016;32(Suppl 1):351-4.

23. Ans. D

Humans become infected with JEV when bitten by an infected mosquito and are a dead-end host because of low viremia, preventing the virus from being transmitted further. In the other three infections, viral loads are very high during the viremia, thus increasing the chances of transmission, when the mosquito bites an infected person.

Ref:
1. WHO. Japanese encephalitis vaccines WHO position paper. Weekly Epidemiological Record. 2006; 81:325-40.
2. WHO (2015). Fact sheet N 386. [online] Available from: https://www.who.int/en/news-room/fact-sheets/detail/japanese-encephalitis [Last accessed February, 2020].

24. Ans. A

A booster dose (third dose) should be given if a person has received the two-dose primary vaccination series 1 year or more previously. JE is a very low-risk disease for most travelers to JE-endemic countries. However, some travelers will be at increased risk of infection based on factors including longer periods of travel, travel during the JEV transmission season, spending time in rural areas, participating in a lot of outdoor activities, and staying in accommodations without air conditioning, screens, or bednets.

Ref:
1. Centers for Disease Control and Prevention (CDC). In: Hamborsky J, Kroger A, Wolfe S (Eds). Epidemiology and Prevention of Vaccine-Preventable Diseases, 13th edition. Washington, DC: Public Health Foundation; 2015.
2. Vaccine Information Statement: Japanese Encephalitis Vaccine (What You Need to Know) Centers for Disease Control and Prevention (CDC) (2014). [online] Available from: http://www.cdc.gov/vaccines/hcp/vis/vis-statements/je-ixiaro.pdf [Last accessed February, 2020].

25. Ans. C

Search for coinfection is advisable when one form of microfilariasis is diagnosed. This is important especially if DEC is considered as a treatment option because of the severe reactions that may occur when DEC is administered to patients coinfected with O volvulus. The so-called "Mazzotti reaction" may be local (pruritus, skin rash, and visual disturbances) or systemic (fever, headache, joint pains, postural hypotension, collapse, and respiratory distress). DEC can aggravate existing eye lesions and precipitate new ones. For these reasons, DEC is either avoided or used after steroid administration to blunt inflammatory reactions. Often the treatment of choice is the combination of ivermectin and albendazole.

Ref:
1. Makunde WH, Kamugisha LM, Massaga JJ, Makunde RW, Savael ZX, Akida J, et al. Treatment of co-infection with Bancroftian filariasis and onchocerciasis: A safety and efficacy study of albendazole with ivermectin compared to treatment of single infection with bancroftian filariasis. Filaria J. 2003;2(1):15.
2. Hoerauf A. Control of filarial infections: Not the beginning of the end, but more research is needed. Curr Opin Infect Dis. 2003;16(5):403-10.

26. Ans. D

People with lymphedema and elephantiasis are unlikely to benefit from drug treatment because most people with lymphedema are not actively infected with the filarial parasite. To prevent lymphedema from getting worse, patients should ask their physician for a referral to a lymphedema therapist so they can be informed about some basic principles of care such as hygiene, elevation, exercises, skin and wound care, and wearing appropriate shoes. Surgery may be offered to patients with hydrocele.

Ref:
1. Centers for Disease Control and Prevention: CDC Guidelines (2018). Parasites—Lymphatic Filariasis. [online] Available from: https://www.cdc.gov/parasites/lymphaticfilariasis/index.html [Last accessed Feb., 2020].

27. Ans. D

A single dose of triple drug therapy is adequate to treat an episode of LF and is shown to be superior to dual drug therapy. However, single dose therapy regimens do not completely eradicate adult filarial worms or reduce the number of microfilariae in the community to sufficiently low levels; therefore, multiple rounds of treatment are required to interrupt transmission. In 2017, the WHO recommended the three-drug treatment to accelerate the global elimination of lymphatic filariasis.

Ref:
1. King CL, Suamani J, Sanuku N, Cheng Y1, Satofan S, Mancuso B, et al. A trial of triple-drug treatment for lymphatic filariasis. N Engl J Med. 2018; 379(19):1801-10.
2. WHO (2019). Fact Sheet on Lymphatic Filariasis. [online] Available from: https://www.who.int/news-room/fact-sheets/detail/lymphatic-filariasis [Last accessed February, 2020].

28. Ans. C

Endosymbiont rickettsiae found in onchocerciasis and LF parasites have an intimate relationship with the growth and reproduction of filarial parasites. Treatment of rickettsial infections with doxycycline has been shown to have profound effect on both microfilariae and adult worms in patients with onchocerciasis and LF. Studies have shown a reduction of 80–90% of adult worms in bancroftian filariasis with 200 mg/day doxycycline for 4 or 6 weeks and also showed reduction of lymph vessel dilation and of hydrocele. Lymphedema progression was halted and reversed in early stages. The other drugs used to treat LF such as albendazole, DEC, and ivermectin kill microfilariae but have no major effect on adult worms.

Ref:
1. Hoerauf A. Filariasis: New drugs and new opportunities for lymphatic filariasis and onchocerciasis. Curr Opin Infect Dis. 2008;21(6):673-81.
2. Sudomo M, Chayabejara S, Duong S, Hernandez L, Wu WP, Bergquist R, et al. Elimination of lymphatic filariasis in Southeast Asia. Adv Parasitol. 2010;72:205-33.
3. Hoerauf A, Mand S, Fischer K, Kruppa T, Marfo-Debrekyei Y, Debrah AY, et al. Doxycycline as a novel strategy against bancroftian filariasis-depletion of Wolbachia endosymbionts from Wuchereria bancrofti and stop of microfilaria production. Med Microbiol Immunol. 2003;192(4):211-6.

29. Ans. D

Elephantiasis, which is characterized by gross enlargement of an area of the body, especially the limbs, can be caused by a number of conditions such as LF, leishmaniasis, lymphogranuloma venereum, tuberculosis, repeated streptococcal infection, leprosy and environmental factors such as exposure to certain minerals like silica, red clay soil (podoconiosis), etc. However, LGV commonly causes genital elephantiasis and not limb elephantiasis.

Ref:
1. Palanisamy AP, Kanakaram KK, Vadivel S, Kothandapany S. Vulval elephantiasis. Indian Dermatol Online J. 2015;6(5):371.
2. Sethi A, Sethi D. Huge vulval elephantiasis of unknown aetiology. J Evol Med Dent Sci. 2014;3(13):3324-9.

30. Ans. A

Tropical pulmonary eosinophilia is caused by a hypersensitivity response to antigens from microfilariae of *Wuchereria bancrofti* and *Brugia malayi*. It is a syndrome of wheezing, fever, and eosinophilia seen predominantly in the Indian subcontinent and other tropical areas affecting <1% of patients with LF. The main radiological features include reticulonodular shadows more in the mid-to-lower zones and miliary mottling which make differentiation from miliary tuberculosis often difficult. While TPE due to hypersensitivity to filarial antigen is the most common, eosinophilia may also be due to roundworm, toxocara, strongyloides, and hookworm. Noninfectious causes mainly include bronchial asthma, allergic bronchopulmonary aspergillosis, acute and chronic eosinophilic pneumonia, Churg–Strauss syndrome, idiopathic hypereosinophilic syndrome, and drug reactions. In the absence of a specific and sensitive test, history suggestive of nocturnal symptoms mainly cough and dyspnea, pulmonary infiltrates on chest radiograph, leukocytosis with peripheral eosinophilia >3,000/µm, elevated serum IgE and filarial specific IgG and IgE, and clinical improvement with DEC may be used to diagnose TPE. Mature gravid human filarial parasites, living in the lymphatics periodically release microfilariae which are trapped within the pulmonary microcirculation. As a result, microfilaremia is rarely observed in TPE.

Ref:

1. *Mullerpattan JB, Udwadia ZF, Udwadia FE. Tropical pulmonary eosinophilia—A review. Indian J Med Res. 2013;138(3):295-302.*
2. *Udwadia FE. Tropical eosinophilia. In: Herzog H (Ed). Pulmonary Eosinophilia: Progress in Pulmonary Research. Basel: S Karger; 1975. pp. 35-155.*

CHAPTER 30

Pregnancy and Gynecological Infections

Duru Shah, Sabahat Rasool

1. **Which of the following statements is false about Zika virus infection in pregnant women?**
   A. Transmission occurs through Aedes mosquito bite
   B. It usually results in a mild viral illness lasting 2–7 days
   C. Breastfeeding with active Zika virus infection is contraindicated
   D. Congenital microcephaly, skull collapse, and vermian agenesis occur as a part of congenital Zika virus syndrome

2. **Which of the following statements is false about Zika virus?**
   A. *Aedes aegypti* is most active at night
   B. N,N-Diethyl-meta-toluamide (DEET)-based repellents are the most effective repellents and are safe in pregnant and breastfeeding mothers
   C. Couples considering pregnancy should use effective contraception for 3 months after returning from an area with risk for Zika virus transmission or last Zika virus exposure, if both partners have traveled
   D. Couples considering pregnancy should use effective contraception for 2 months after returning from an area with risk for Zika virus transmission or last Zika virus exposure, if only the female partner has traveled

3. **Which of the following statements is not true about hepatitis B virus (HBV) infection in pregnant women?**
   A. In unvaccinated populations, 2–10% infected individuals become long-term carriers
   B. 70–90% infants born to chronic carrier mothers will become chronic carriers
   C. The risk of a given individual in a sexually active age group becoming a chronic carrier is <5%
   D. None of the above

4. **Which of the following statements correctly represents pregnancy-induced immunological changes?**
   A. Increase in CD4-positive T-cells
   B. Increase in interleukins 4, 5, 10, 13
   C. Both A and B
   D. Increase in Th-1 type cytokines

5. **Regarding varicella-zoster virus (VZV) infection in pregnancy, which of the following statements is true?**
   A. Around 50% of adults have serological evidence of immunity
   B. The incubation period is 10–21 days
   C. Vaccinations reduced the incidence of adult varicella infections by 20%
   D. Mortality is predominantly due to encephalitis

6. **A pregnant woman tested positive for human immunodeficiency virus (HIV) infection during her first antenatal visit. Which of the following statements are correct regarding her infection?**
   A. In the absence of treatment, the risk of vertical transmission of HIV is 65–90%
   B. With antiretroviral medications, cesarean delivery prior to labor onset, and avoidance of breastfeeding, the vertical transmission risk drops to <2%
   C. Single-dose nevirapine (SD-NVP) decreases the transmission of HIV-1 by 10%
   D. With highly active antiretroviral therapy (HAART) in the antenatal period, the perinatal transmission reduces from 20 to 1–2%

7. **Which of the following statements is true about HIV in pregnancy?**
   A. Spermicides reduce HIV transmission
   B. PrEP decreases the transmission risk up to 20%
   C. Latex condoms are the only contraceptive that reduce HIV transmission by around 80%
   D. All of the above

8. **Which of the following statements is true about preconceptional care in HIV-positive patients?**
   A. Women with CD4 count <250/mL should be on ART before attempting conception
   B. Women should also be tested for other sexually transmitted infections

C. Dolutegravir can be continued in the first trimester of pregnancy but should be withheld thereafter
D. All of the above

9. A pregnant woman who is a cat lover presented with fever, malaise, and lymphadenopathy. She was prescribed TORCH (toxoplasmosis, rubella, cytomegalovirus, and herpes simplex virus) IgM screen for toxoplasmosis and she tested strongly positive for the same. Which of the following statements is true about her condition?
   A. Maternal–fetal transmission is highest in the first trimester
   B. The likelihood of transmission is highest in the first trimester
   C. A single blood test of IgM does not distinguish between acute and chronic infection
   D. Treatment with spiramycin reduces transmission and ocular sequelae

10. A pregnant lady presented with fever and painful genital ulcers at 36 weeks of gestation.
    Which of the following statements is true about her condition?
    A. 50–70% genital herpes simplex virus (HSV) infections are caused by HSV-1
    B. Seroconversion during pregnancy is 3.7% in women seronegative to both types
    C. Women with active lesions on buttocks, thighs, and anus should be delivered by cesarean section
    D. Transplacental transmission is higher with recurrent infection

11. Which of the following statements is not true about human papillomavirus (HPV) infection?
    A. It is the most common sexually transmitted virus worldwide
    B. It is the most common viral cause of cancer worldwide
    C. 80% sexually active adults acquire an HPV infection in their lifetime
    D. Vertical transmission during vaginal delivery can be as high as 90%

12. A pregnant lady presented with hyperpigmented pedunculated genital warts. What is the possible diagnosis?
    A. Condyloma acuminata
    B. Condyloma lata
    C. Acanthosis nigricans
    D. None of the above

13. A G2P1 36 weeks' gestation patient with diagnosed condyloma acuminata infection has presented to the antenatal clinic.
    Which of the following treatments is Centers for Disease Control and Prevention (CDC) recommended for her?
    A. Podofilox 0.5% gel
    B. Imiquimod 5% cream
    C. Sinecatechins 15% ointment
    D. 5-fluorouracil (5-FU)
    E. None of the above

14. Which of the following statements is true about syphilis in a pregnant woman?
    A. Transmission increases with gestational age
    B. Severity increases with gestational age
    C. Vertical transmission is lowest with primary syphilis
    D. Hutchinson's teeth, saddle nose, and CNS malformations are manifestations of early syphilis

15. Henderson–Patterson bodies are a classical histological feature of keratinocytes with cytoplasmic inclusion bodies. Which of the following conditions is it associated with?
    A. Molluscum contagiosum
    B. Chancroid
    C. Herpes simplex
    D. Syphilis

16. Which of the following treatments is recommended to chancroid?
    A. Azithromycin 1 g oral
    B. Ciprofloxacin 500 mg BD oral for 3 days
    C. Ceftriaxone 1 g IV BD for 7 days
    D. Amoxiclav 1.2 g IV BD for 2 weeks

17. Which of the following statements is true about urinary tract infections (UTIs) in pregnancy?
    A. Asymptomatic bacteriuria (ASB) increases the risk of pyelonephritis by 20–30 times
    B. Recurrent UTI is defined as three or more UTIs in 6 months
    C. Nitrofurantoin 100 mg three times daily can be used for suppressive therapy for recurrent UTIs
    D. Fosfomycin is the drug of choice for acute pyelonephritis in pregnancy

18. A pregnant woman presents at 34 weeks' gestation with leaking per vaginam for the last 34 hours. She is tachycardic, febrile, and dehydrated. The uterus is tender to touch, and fetal heart sounds are absent.

Which of the following statements is not true about her diagnosis?
A. Group B streptococcal (GBD) positivity is a risk factor
B. Neonatal pneumonia, meningitis, and hemorrhage are the sequelae if the fetus is alive
C. Both A and B
D. Cesarean section is the recommended mode of delivery

19. During the 2017–2018 H1N1 influenza epidemic, a pregnant lady at 29 weeks' gestation presented with fever, cough, and breathlessness.
Which of the following statements is correct about her illness?
A. There is no firm evidence that influenza A virus causes congenital malformations
B. ELISA (enzyme-linked immunosorbent assay) is the most sensitive and specific test to diagnose H1N1 infection
C. Tamiflu is an FDA category B drug
D. ACOG does not recommend influenza vaccination during pregnancy since it is a live attenuated vaccine

20. Which of the following statements about rubella in pregnancy is true?
A. Transmission occurs through nasopharyngeal secretions although the rate of transmission is 30–40%
B. All maternal infections are clinical
C. German measles virus belongs to the togavirus family
D. The virus can be isolated from blood and urine for up to 6 weeks after rash onset

21. A primigravida contacts German measles infection at 9 weeks' gestation. Which of the following statements would you like to counsel the patient with?
A. First-trimester infections have 90% congenitally infected fetuses
B. Congenital malformations in the second trimester infections reduce to 25%
C. Neonates born with congenital rubella syndrome (CRS) may infect other infants as well as susceptible adults
D. Extended rubella syndrome may develop clinically in the second and third decades of life in one-third neonates who are asymptomatic at birth
E. All of the above

22. A G2P1 mother reports to the OPD with fever and a bright red facial rash. Diagnosis of erythema infectiosum was made after serological testing. All of the following statements about the condition are incorrect, *except*:
A. It is the most frequent infectious cause of non-immune hydrops
B. The critical period of infection leading to fetal hydrops is 24–28 weeks
C. Most of the fetuses develop hydrops in the 1st week after infection
D. Hydropic fetuses have a mortality of 10% without transfusions

23. Which of the following is the route of fetal infection with maternal cytomegalovirus (CMV) infection?
A. Transplacental   B. During delivery
C. Breastfeeding   D. All of the above

24. Regarding maternal CMV infection, which of the following statements is correct?
A. Pregnancy does not increase the severity of maternal infection
B. There is no viral shedding in reactivation
C. Primary maternal CMV infection is transmitted to fetus in 2% cases
D. Recurrent maternal infection infects fetus in 10% cases

25. Which of the following statements is true about prenatal CMV infection?
A. Routine prenatal CMV screening is not recommended in all pregnant women
B. CMV IgM antibodies are always indicative of acute infection
C. Sonographic evidence and positive fetal blood or amniotic fluid cultures are predictive of a 25% risk of symptomatic congenital infection
D. CMV-NAAT of amniotic fluid has low specificity for diagnosing fetal infection

26. *Streptococcus agalactiae* colonizes the gastrointestinal and genitourinary tracts in 20–30% of pregnant women.
How does it affect the pregnancy outcome?
A. Preterm labor
B. Premature membrane rupture
C. Chorioamnionitis
D. All of the above

27. A neonate delivered to a GBS-positive mother developed apnea and hypotension 8 hours after birth. Which of the following statements is true about neonatal infections?
A. RDS is a differential diagnosis
B. Late-onset disease manifests as respiratory distress

C. Mortality rate for early onset sepsis is less compared to late-onset sepsis
D. Universal screening for GBS is recommended at 30 weeks' gestation

28. Which of the following women qualify for GBS prophylaxis intrapartum?
    A. GBS-positive rectovaginal cultures
    B. Previous child with GBS invasive disease
    C. Unknown GBS culture with ruptured membranes ≥18 hours
    D. All of the above

29. All of the following are recommended for GBS prophylaxis in labor in penicillin-allergic patients, *except*:
    A. Erythromycin   B. Vancomycin
    C. Clindamycin   D. Cefazolin

30. Methicillin-resistant *Staphylococcus aureus* (MRSA) is the most virulent *Staphylococcus* species. All of the following statements about MRSA are false, *except*:
    A. Community-acquired MRSA (CA-MRSA) is diagnosed when identified in an outpatient setting or within 48 hours of hospitalization
    B. MRSA colonizes 20% of population
    C. Most MRSA cases in pregnant women are hospital-acquired MRSA (HA-MRSA)
    D. All of the above

31. A pregnant woman returned after holidaying in Assam. She presented to the emergency department with high-grade fever, chills, and malaise. On blood smear examination, *Plasmodium falciparum* was detected.
    Which of the statements is correct about her condition?
    A. Thick and thin smears are the gold standard tests
    B. CDC recommends artemisinin-based regimens for uncomplicated falciparum malaria
    C. Chloroquine (CQ) and hydroxychloroquine (HCQ) are unsafe during pregnancy
    D. Primaquine is the prophylaxis of choice during pregnancy

32. What infection is most common in pregnant diabetic mothers?
    A. UTIs
    B. Candida vulvovaginitis
    C. Breast abscess
    D. Puerperal sepsis

33. What are the risk factors for bacterial vaginosis (BV) in pregnancy?
    A. Ethnicity   B. Chronic stress
    C. Douching   D. All of the above

34. Periodontal disease is known to increase preterm births. What are the odds that periodontitis will increase preterm birth?
    A. 6 times   B. 2.8 times
    C. 10.2 times   D. 21.6 times

35. What is the preferred first-line treatment for a pregnant woman with gonorrhea?
    A. Dual therapy with ceftriaxone and azithromycin
    B. Single-dose ceftriaxone
    C. 2 g azithromycin single dose
    D. All of the above

36. Which of the following is a risk factor for maternal sepsis?
    A. Black race   B. Nulliparity
    C. Multifetal gestation D. All of the above

37. Which of the following are the leading causes of sepsis in pregnant women?
    A. Septic abortion and UTI
    B. Chorioamnionitis and acute gastroenteritis
    C. Wound infection and pneumonia
    D. None of the above

38. What is the recommended empiric antibiotic for hospital-acquired pneumonia in pregnant women?
    A. Ceftriaxone
    B. Piperacillin-tazobactam
    C. Ampicillin plus gentamicin
    D. Cefotaxime and metronidazole

39. Which is the vasopressor of choice in maternal septicemic shock?
    A. Norepinephrine
    B. Dobutamine
    C. Dopamine
    D. None of the above

40. Which of the following is not a criterion used for Quick Sequential Organ Failure Assessment (qSOFA) score?
    A. Respiratory rate ≥ 22/min
    B. Change in mental status
    C. Systolic blood pressure ≤ 100 mm Hg
    D. Serum creatinine > 3.5 mg/dL

41. A 32-year-old woman at 34 weeks' gestation is admitted with fever, breathlessness, and cough. She is confused, has a temperature of 38°C, respiratory rate of 28/min, heart rate of 110/min, blood pressure of 80/49 mm Hg, and oxygen saturation of 80% on room air. Based on these observations, her qSOFA score is:
    A. 0   B. 1
    C. 2   D. 3

ANSWERS WITH EXPLANATIONS

1. Ans. C

Zika virus is transmitted by *Aedes* mosquito bite, blood transfusion, and sexually. The illness is a mild viral illness typically lasting 2–7 days, causing myalgias, fever, headache, rash, and conjunctivitis. Though viable virus is seen in breast milk, transmission is not confirmed. Therefore, benefits of breastfeeding outweigh the risks of Zika virus infant infection. Zika is a ribonucleic acid (RNA) virus and the first major mosquito-borne teratogen. The virus is detectable from blood at the time of symptoms and may persist for months. Immunoglobulin M (IgM) antibodies are detected within 2 weeks of infection and may persist for nearly 4 months. Regardless of maternal symptoms, the fetus can get infected in nearly 6% cases. Fetal mortality may reach 7%. Congenital Zika virus syndrome includes microcephaly, lissencephaly, intracranial calcifications, ventriculomegaly, ocular abnormalities, congenital contractures, and absent cavum septum pellucidum. Zika virus is isolated from maternal blood or urine by serological testing. Zika virus RNA detection by polymerase chain reaction (PCR) is the confirmation of diagnosis. No vaccines are available for Zika infection. Protective clothing, nets, and insecticides are used for vector control. Abstinence from a potentially infected partner is advised.

2. Ans. A

Aedes aegypti is most active during mid-morning and late afternoon. Travelers should cover up during daytime as much as possible. Clothing should be treated with an insecticide to kill mosquitoes. DEET-based repellents are most effective and safe in pregnant and breastfeeding women. Care should be taken to avoid ingestion and contact with mouth and eyes. If a couple is considering pregnancy, consistent use of effective contraception is advised to prevent pregnancy for 3 months after return from an area with risk for Zika virus transmission or the last possible Zika virus exposure, if both partners or only the male partner traveled, and for 2 months if only the female partner has traveled. The last possible Zika virus exposure is defined as either the date of leaving a high-risk area or the date on which the last unprotected sexual contact with a potentially infectious partner took place.

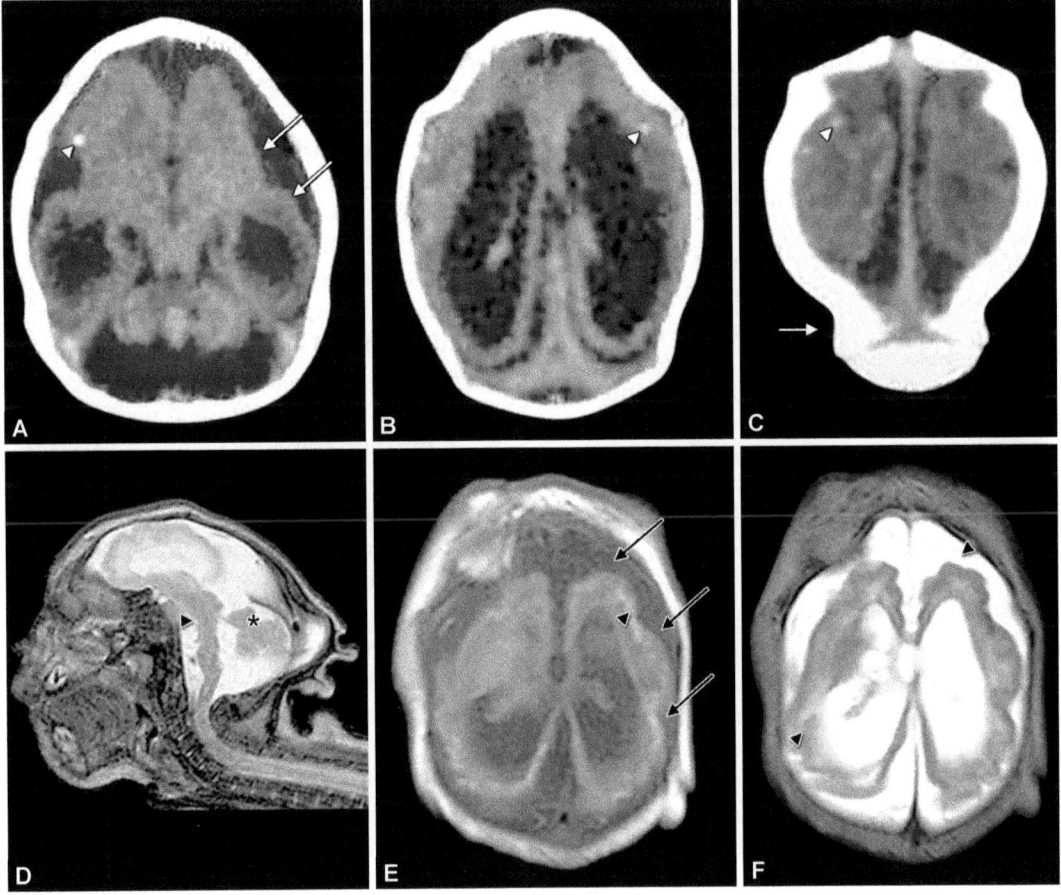

(A) Calcifications and shallow sulci; (B) Ventriculomegaly and punctate calcifications; (C) Small cranial vault and cerebellum; (D) Shallow sulci and calcifications.

3. Ans. D

Hepatitis B virus infection is often asymptomatic and detected during antenatal testing. There is some evidence linking maternal infection to preterm birth but not to pre-eclampsia and fetal growth restriction. Transplacental infection is uncommon. 10-20% of hepatitis B surface antigen (HBsAg) positive mothers infect their fetuses if no immunoprophylaxis is given. If the mother is both HBsAg and hepatitis B e antigen (HBeAg) positive, this rate increases to 90%. Immunoprophylaxis and hepatitis B vaccine prevents 90% of neonatal infections. Tenofovir is recommended as first-line drug in women with high HBV DNA levels. Maternal HBV infection is not a contraindication to breastfeeding. Seronegative women at risk can be given hepatitis B vaccine during pregnancy.

4. Ans. C

Pregnancy is associated with an increase in CD4-positive T-cells secreting cytokines such as interleukins 4, 5, 10, and 13 (Th-2 type cytokines). Interferon-gamma and interleukin 2 (Th-1 type cytokine) production is suppressed. This Th-2 bias affects the ability to contain certain intracellular pathogens. However, the Th-2 humoral immune response is maintained.

5. Ans. B

Varicella-zoster virus is a double-stranded deoxyribonucleic acid (DNA) virus acquired mostly during childhood, and 95% adults have serological evidence of immunity. The incidence of adult varicella infections is reduced by 74% after vaccine introduction. Primary infection is transmitted by direct contact and also by respiratory droplets. The incubation period is 10-21 days, and a nonimmune woman has 60-95% risk of infection after exposure and remains contagious from 1 day before the onset of rash until the lesions crust over. Primary varicella presents as flu-like prodrome and pruritic vesicular exanthems which crust in 3-7 days. Mortality is mostly due to varicella pneumonia, which is severe in pregnancy as well as adulthood. Nearly 5-20% of pregnant women with varicella infection develop pneumonitis. Fever, tachypnea, dyspnea, and dry cough are characteristics of VZV pneumonia. Fever and respiratory distress may persist for weeks. Risk factors for VZV pneumonia include smoking and >100 cutaneous lesions. Shingles is the reactivation of primary varicella and presents as dermatomal vesicular painful eruptions. Shingles or Zoster is not known to be more severe or frequent during pregnancy and very rarely lead to congenital varicella syndrome. Congenital varicella syndrome includes features such as chorioretinitis, microphthalmia, cerebral atrophy, hydronephrosis, limb hypoplasia, and cicatricial dermatological lesions. Active infection just before delivery puts the neonate at a significant risk of developing disseminated visceral and central nervous system (CNS) disease. Mortality rates approach 30%. Immunoglobulins should be given to neonates born to mothers with clinical evidence of varicella 5 days before and 2 days after delivery. Though maternal infection is diagnosed clinically, nucleic acid amplification testing (NAAT) can be used for confirmation in vesicular fluid and for fetal infection from amniotic fluid. Sonographic evidence of abnormalities due to VZV infection may be appreciated after 5 weeks of maternal infection. Exposed nonimmune pregnant mothers should be given VZ immunoglobulin (VZIg) ideally within 96 hours to 10 days of exposure. Once diagnosed with primary VZV infection, or herpes zoster, contact with pregnant women should be avoided. Seroconversion with varicella vaccine is 98%, but immunity may diminish over time. Vaccine is not recommended in pregnancy due to its live nature.

6. Ans. B and D

Human immunodeficiency virus is an RNA retrovirus and the causative agent of acquired immunodeficiency syndrome (AIDS). Most cases of AIDS are caused by HIV-1, which is more virulent than HIV-2. Sexual transmission is the most common mode, followed by infected blood and products, and mother-to-child transmission. Viral load is the primary determinant of vertical transmission. Primary infection causes mild viral illness with fever, headache, arthralgias, rash, lymphadenopathy, nausea, and diarrhea lasting up to 10 days. Host response lowers viremia to a set point, and the higher the viral burden at this time, the faster is the progression to AIDS. Pathogenicity of the viral strain, host response, size of inoculum, and route of infection—all affect the disease progression.

All women must be tested for HIV prenatally in an opt-out approach. Repeat testing is recommended in the third trimester before 36 weeks in all pregnant women. Viral burden is directly proportional to neonatal infection. Neonatal infection is <1% if the viral load is <400 copies/mL, and it reaches >23% if the viral load is 30,000 copies/mL. In the absence of treatment, the risk of vertical transmission of HIV is as high as 25-30%. Mother-to-child transmission of HIV is the most common source of pediatric HIV infection. SD-NVP decreases the risk of mother-to-child transmission of HIV-1 by 47% when compared with a short course of zidovudine. However, with the use of antenatal antiretroviral therapy (ART), the perinatal transmission reduced from 20% to 1.2%. The prevention of parent-to-child transmission of HIV in India was launched in 2002 with SD-NVP as the drug of choice. It reduced the risk of transmission to 12-15%. The National AIDS Control Organization (NACO) has initiated lifelong triple-drug ART for all pregnant and breastfeeding women living with HIV regardless of CD4 count and clinical stage of the disease. The NACO recommends a triple-drug regimen—tenofovir, lamivudine, and efavirenz. Infants should receive nevirapine for 6 weeks if the mother has been on ART for ≥4 weeks. For those infants whose mothers have been on ART for <4 weeks, nevirapine should be given for 12 weeks. Infants should be given 6-12 weeks of zidovudine if the mother has been previously exposed to nevirapine. Women on ART do not have a higher vertical transmission rate with amniocentesis or other invasive diagnostic procedures. Those who are not on ART have a twofold risk of transmission. Labor augmentation is used wherever necessary. Delayed cord clamping in preterm infants and labor analgesia are recommended. The use of ergot alkaloids should be discouraged since they cause severe peripheral vasospasm. The American College of Obstetricians and Gynecologists (ACOG) recommends cesarean delivery at 38 weeks for women with viral load >1,000 copies/mL. There is insufficient evidence to recommend cesarean delivery over vaginal delivery if viral load is ≤1,000 copies/mL and the patient is on ART. Such women may choose to deliver vaginally and if they opt for cesarean, it may be performed at 39 weeks. Breastfeeding increases vertical transmission and is not recommended in developed countries. However, the World Health Organization (WHO) recommends exclusive breastfeeding during the first 6-12 months in nutritionally deprived countries where diarrhea and malnutrition are the leading causes of infant deaths. ART regimens may be continued postpartum for viral suppression. All women planning conception should be on ART to optimally suppress viremia before pregnancy happens. For serodiscordant couples, the male infected partner should be on HAART and the uninfected female partner should receive pre-exposure prophylaxis (PrEP). Use of condoms is recommended with periovulatory condomless intercourse when conception is planned. Serodiscordant couples should consider intrauterine insemination and in vitro fertilization with washed semen to decrease transmission.

7. **Ans. C**
Latex condoms decrease HIV transmission by 80%. Spermicides do not reduce the transmission. HIV-positive patients should be on ART to decrease transmission to serodiscordant partners. PrEP has been shown to reduce the risk of transmission up to 83%. Such patients should receive pneumonia, influenza, and hepatitis B vaccines. Universal routine testing is recommended for all pregnant women at their maiden visit.

8. **Ans. B**
All women living with HIV who are contemplating pregnancy should be receiving ART irrespective of viral loads and CD4 counts and have a plasma viral load below the limit of detection prior to conception. When selecting or evaluating ART for women of childbearing age living with HIV, consider a regimen's effectiveness, a woman's hepatitis B status, teratogenic potential of the drugs in the ART regimen, and possible adverse outcomes for the mother and the fetus. HIV infection does not preclude the use of any contraceptive method; however, drug-drug interactions between hormonal contraceptives and ART should be considered. Partners living with HIV should attain maximum viral suppression before attempting conception to prevent HIV sexual transmission and, for women living with HIV, to minimize the risk of HIV transmission to the infant. For couples with differing HIV statuses, when the partner living with HIV is on ART and has achieved sustained viral suppression, sexual intercourse without a condom limited to the 2-3 days before and the day of ovulation (peak fertility) is an approach to conception with effectively no risk of sexual HIV transmission to the partner without HIV. For couples with differing HIV statuses who attempt conception via sexual intercourse without a condom (despite counseling) when the partner living with HIV has not been able to achieve viral suppression or when the viral suppression status is not known, administration of antiretroviral PrEP to the partner without HIV is recommended to reduce the risk of sexual transmission of HIV. Couples should still be counseled to limit sex (without condoms) to the period of peak fertility. When the woman is living with HIV, artificial insemination with semen from a partner without HIV during the periovulatory period is an option for conception that eliminates the risk of HIV transmission to the seronegative partner. When the man is living with HIV, the use of donor sperm from a seronegative man is an option for conception that eliminates the risk of HIV transmission to the seronegative partner. For couples with differing HIV statuses who attempt conception (condomless sexual intercourse limited to peak fertility) when the partner living with HIV has achieved viral suppression, it is unclear whether administering PrEP to a seronegative partner further reduces the risk of sexual transmission. Dolutegravir is a preferred integrase strand transfer inhibitor for use in pregnant women after the first trimester. When dolutegravir use is continued after delivery, clinicians should recommend the use of

postpartum contraception and discuss contraceptive options with patients. Dolutegravir is not recommended for use in nonpregnant women who are trying to conceive or during the first trimester of pregnancy due to concerns about a possible increased risk of neural tube defects (NTDs). A pregnancy test should be performed prior to the initiation of dolutegravir. Women who want to become pregnant or who cannot consistently use effective contraception should not initiate a dolutegravir-based regimen.

Plasma HIV RNA levels of pregnant women with HIV should be monitored at the initial antenatal visit, 2-4 weeks after initiating (or changing) ART, monthly until RNA levels are undetectable and then at least every 3 months during pregnancy. HIV RNA levels also should be assessed at approximately 34-36 weeks' gestation to decide about the mode of delivery. CD4 T lymphocyte (CD4) cell count should be monitored at the initial antenatal visit. For patients who have been on ART for ≥2 years and who have had consistent viral suppression and CD4 cell counts that are consistently >300 cells/mm^3, CD4 cell count should be monitored at the initial antenatal visit. CD4 cell counts do not have to be repeated for these patients during pregnancy. Women who have been on ART for <2 years, women with CD4 cell counts <300 cells/mm^3, and women with inconsistent adherence and/or detectable viremia should have CD4 cell counts monitored every 3-6 months during pregnancy. Women taking ART during pregnancy should undergo standard glucose screening at 24-28 weeks' gestation. Some experts suggest glucose screening early in pregnancy for women who are receiving protease inhibitor (PI)-based regimens initiated before pregnancy, in accordance with recommendations for women who are at risk for glucose intolerance. Amniocentesis, if clinically indicated, should be performed on women with HIV only after the initiation of an effective ART regimen and, ideally, when HIV RNA levels are undetectable. In women with detectable HIV RNA levels in whom amniocentesis is deemed necessary, consultation with an expert in the management of HIV in pregnancy should be considered.

9. **Ans. C**

   Toxoplasma gondii is an intracellular parasite whose life cycle has a feline stage and a nonfeline stage. Cat is a definitive host and toxoplasma oocytes are excreted in feline feces. Humans are intermediate hosts who ingest tissue cysts containing oocysts, which are digested by gastric juices to release bradyzoites, which infect small gut epithelium. They get converted into bradyzoites which infect all human cells. 38% women have toxoplasma immunity and incident infection in pregnancy is 0.2-1%. Maternal-fetal transmission occurs during the active phase of new infection. Maternal infections are subclinical mostly. Prepregnancy infection confers immunity and makes vertical transmission nearly impossible. Maternal infection increases preterm birth rates by fourfold. The transmission rate is around 30%. The severity and incidence of infection depend on the gestational age. The likelihood of transmission is 15% at 13 weeks, 44% at 26 weeks, and 71% at 36 weeks. A single blood test does not distinguish between acute and chronic infection nor does IgM versus IgG as both persist in chronic infection. Rising titers with four times or greater increase done at least 2 weeks apart indicate new infection. PCR of amniotic fluid and ultrasound surveillance of fetal anatomy and development are recommended if acute infection is documented. Clinically affected neonates have low birth weight, jaundice, hepatosplenomegaly, and anemia. Neurological disease with intracranial calcifications, convulsions, and micro- or hydrocephaly is seen in some. Later, children may develop learning disabilities and chorioretinitis. Treatment with spiramycin reduces serious neurological sequelae. However, it is unclear if it prevents transmission and ocular complications. Cooking meat to safe temperatures; proper cleaning of food items and utensils in contact with raw meat, seafood, poultry, fruits, and vegetables; and precautions while handling cat litter are some of the precautions needed to avoid contracting infection.

10. **Ans. B**

    About 50-70% genital herpes is caused by HSV-2. Genital HSV-1 increases in orogenital sex. Genital herpes affects 50 million adults and adolescents. The virus replicates at the entry site and then moves to cranial nerves and dorsal spinal ganglia. The incubation period is typically 6-8 days. Papular itching eruptions occur which become painful and vesicular and later ulcerate. Inguinal lymphadenopathy is severe and painful. Disseminated disease, hepatitis, encephalitis, and pneumonia are seen infrequently. Maternofetal transmission occurs peripartum in 85%, postnatal in 10%, and intrauterine in 5%. Transplacental transmission is rare. Primary maternal infection is associated with higher transmission rates at delivery than recurrent infections. Universal screening is not recommended. Diagnosis should be done by culture or PCR of the lesions. Serology can distinguish HSV type; IgM is indicative of active infection. Acyclovir and valacyclovir are the drugs of choice. Women with active lesions on vulva, vagina, or cervix should be delivered abdominally. Lesions elsewhere do not warrant a cesarean delivery.

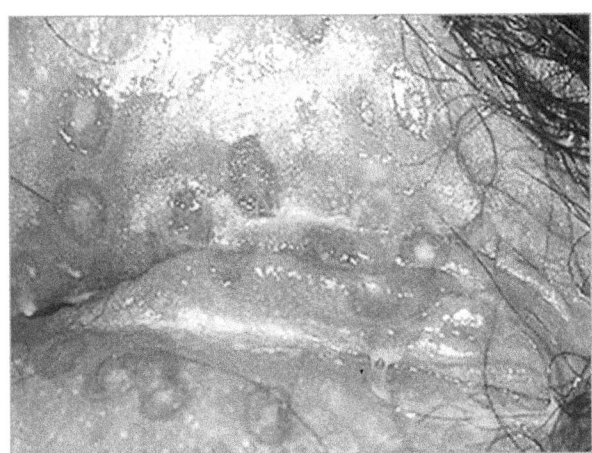

Herpes simplex 2 genital lesions.
Source: https://en.wikipedia.org/wiki/Genital_herpes.

11. **Ans. D**

Human papillomavirus (HPV) is the most common viral cause of cancer and sexually transmitted viral infection. It contributes to 5% of all cancers. The worldwide prevalence is around 10% although 80% sexually active adults acquire an infection in their lifetime. Young age, early sexual activity, polygamy, other sexual infections, and smoking are some of the risk factors. HPV's carcinogenic potential is related to E6 gene, which inactivates p53 tumor suppressor protein and *E7* gene associated with inactivation of the retinoblastoma apoptotic pathway.

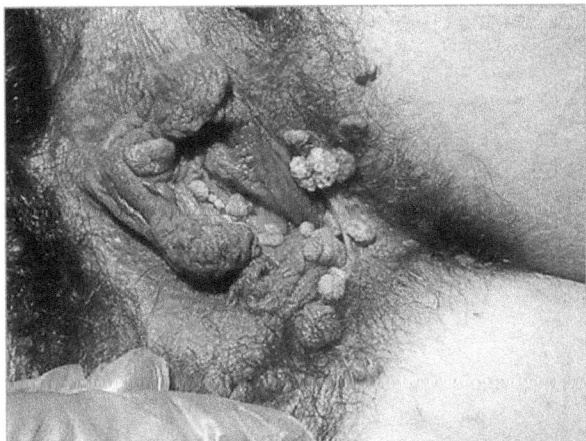

Condyloma acuminata genital lesions.
Source: https://en.wikipedia.org/wiki/Genital_wart#/media/File:SOA-Condylomata-acuminata-female.jpg.

12. **Ans. A**

Condyloma acuminata is caused by low-risk HPV 6 and 11 and presents as papillomatous growth around introitus. Warts vary in appearance—hyperpigmented, papilliform, flat, popular, or pedunculated in contrast to condyloma lata of syphilis which is flat and velvety. Genital warts increase in number and size during pregnancy. Some lesions may fill the vagina and cover the entire perineum, making vaginal delivery mechanically difficult. The prevalence of HPV infection is highest in younger women. Most infections are asymptomatic and transient. HPV 16 and 18 are the types with highest oncogenic potential.

13. **Ans. E**

Genital wart therapy in pregnancy is aimed at debulking the warts with minimum toxicity. Trichloroacetic acid 80-90% applied locally once a week is effective, so are cryotherapy and laser and surgical excision. Podophyllin, podofiox, imiquimod cream, 5-FU, and sinecatechins are not safe in pregnancy. Gardasil, a quadrivalent vaccine, and Cervarix, a bivalent vaccine, are available for long-term prevention. Newer vaccines such as Gardasil 9, a nonavalent vaccine, protect against HPV 6, 11, 16, 18, 31, 33, 45, 52, and 58. Vaccines are aimed at school girls aged between 9 and 14 years. Vaccines are not recommended during pregnancy, and if the woman is pregnant after starting the vaccination series, the remaining doses are delayed till after the delivery. Vertical transmission rates of HPV can lead to juvenile-onset recurrent respiratory papillomatosis which is a benign laryngeal neoplasm. Maternal genital HPV and prolonged labor increase the odds for infection. Abdominal delivery is not recommended for genital HPV.

14. **Ans. A**

Syphilis is caused by *Treponema pallidum* through vaginal abrasions. The bacterium replicates and spreads through lymphatics within days. The incubation period is a couple of weeks and depends on the inoculum size as well as the host response. The early stages of syphilis are primary, secondary, and early latent. Partner transmission rates during these stages are 30–60%. Primary syphilis is characterized by chancre, a painless solitary ulcer with a firm raised border without significant pus. Multiple chancres are found in immunocompromised hosts. Secondary syphilis has dermatological abnormalities such as rashes and target lesions, condyloma lata, in 90% patients. Constitutional symptoms such as fever, malaise, myalgias, and headaches develop in this stage. Latent syphilis develops when clinical manifestations resolve despite no treatment of primary and secondary syphilis. Syphilis during pregnancy is an uncommon condition nowadays. Pregnancy does not change the course of maternal disease. Transmission increases with gestational age, but severity decreases. Vertical transmission is highest with primary and secondary syphilis. Spirochetes cross the placenta and cause congenital infection. Treatment lowers the risk of transmission to 1–2%. Congenital syphilis is classified as early and late. Early syphilis prior to 2 years presents as rhinitis rash, hepatomegaly, and osteochondritis. Late syphilis after 2 years of birth presents as saddle nose, Hutchinson's teeth, keratitis, deafness, gumma, and skeletal and CNS malformations.

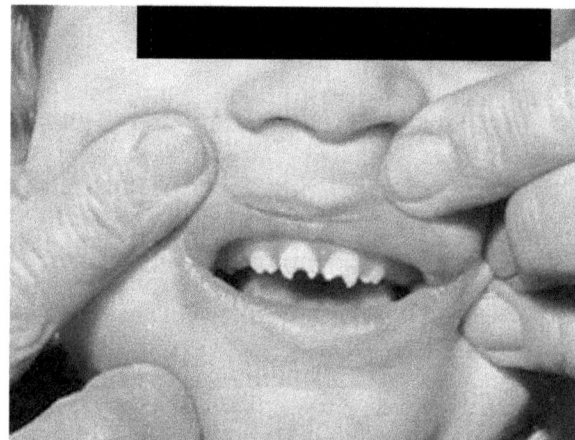

Source: https://commons.wikimedia.org/wiki/Category:Hutchinson%27s_teeth#/media/File:%ED%97%88%EC%B9%9C%EC%8A%A8_%EC%A0%88%EC%B9%98_%EC%9D%B4%EB%AF%B8%EC%A7%80.jpg

15. **Ans. A**

Molluscum contagiosum is caused by pox virus and spread through direct contact or through fomites. Diagnosis is clinical based on dome-shaped papules with central umbilication. Liquid nitrogen, cantharidin, and podophyllotoxins are some of the treatment options.

16. **Ans. A**

Chancroid is caused by *Haemophilus ducreyi* and causes painful nonindurated genital ulcers or soft chancres, which may be accompanied by suppurative inguinal lymphadenopathy. No Food and Drug Administration (FDA)-cleared PCR is available for testing as yet. Painful genital ulcers and negative syphilis and HSV testing lead to a diagnosis by exclusion. Azithromycin 1 g single oral dose, erythromycin 500 mg tds for 7 days, or 250 mg ceftriaxone single IV dose is recommended for therapy.

17. **Ans. A**

Urinary tract infection is the most frequent bacterial infection in pregnancy. ASB is the most common. Other types include cystitis and pyelonephritis. ASB is the persistent actively multiplying bacteria in the urinary tract in asymptomatic women. A positive urine culture irrespective of symptoms should prompt treatment. Left untreated, 25% women will develop symptomatic UTI. Screening for bacteriuria is recommended at the first antenatal visit in all patients. Recurrent UTI is defined as two UTIs in 6 months or three positive cultures. *Escherichia coli* is the pathogen in 75–90% cases. For treatment failures, nitrofurantoin 100 mg four times daily for 21 days may be used. For recurrent UTIs, nitrofurantoin 100 mg daily once can be used for suppressive therapy throughout pregnancy. Pyelonephritis is the leading cause of septic shock during pregnancy. It is unilateral and on the right side

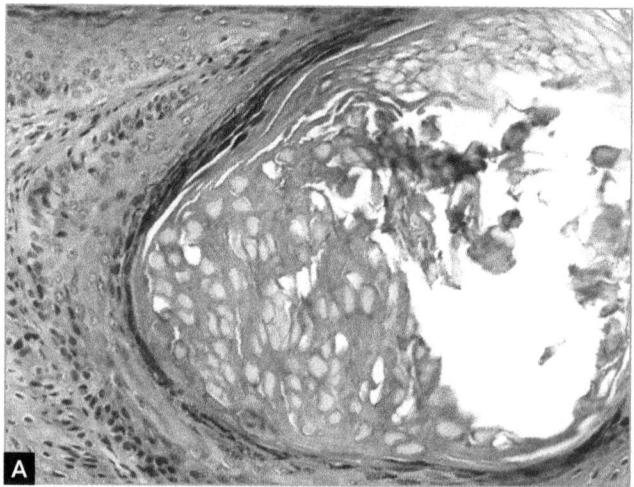
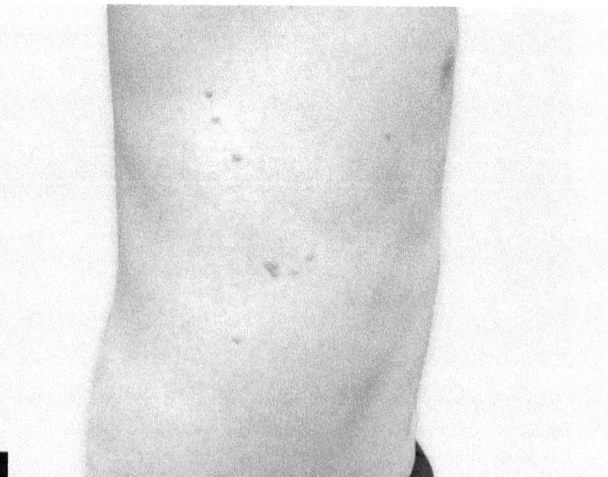

(A) Henderson–Patterson bodies in molluscum; (B) Molluscum lesions.

Sources: https://upload.wikimedia.org/wikipedia/commons/d/d9/Molluscum_conatgiosum%2C_vulva%2C_20X.jpg; https://commons.wikimedia.org/wiki/File:Molluscum_on_child.jpg.

in more than half of the cases. 20% of them develop acute renal injury. The drugs of choice for acute pyelonephritis are intravenous ceftriaxone, ampicillin, and gentamicin used in combination. Pyelonephritis increases the odds of preterm labor if not aggressively treated.

18. **Ans. D**

Intra-amniotic infections complicate nearly 5% of all births. Increased duration of membrane rupture, GBS positivity, prolonged labor, and multiple vaginal examinations are some of the risk factors. Chorioamnionitis is typically a polymicrobial infection. A positive amniotic fluid culture or Gram stain is an objective diagnosis, though majority are diagnosed clinically. Intravenous antibiotics are recommended. Cesarean delivery is restricted to obstetric indications.

19. **Ans. A**

Maternal influenza is characterized by dry cough, fever, malaise, and shortness of breath. Infections are uncomplicated in healthy individuals. Pregnant women are at risk of pulmonary complications. There is no firm evidence that influenza A virus causes congenital malformations. However, increased NTDs have been reported which are linked to hyperthermia. Transplacental passage of virus is rare. Influenza may be detected using antigen rapid detection assays from nasopharyngeal swabs. Reverse transcriptase-polymerase chain reaction (RT-PCR) is the most sensitive and specific test. Rapid diagnostic tests are most widely available but have a sensitivity of 40-70%. Antiviral medications should not be delayed pending tests results. Neuraminidase inhibitors are FDA category C drugs and their benefits outweigh the risks. Antibiotics should be added whenever secondary bacterial infection is suspected. Influenza vaccination is recommended during pregnancy by CDC and ACOG since it is an inactivated vaccine. A live attenuated influenza virus vaccine is available for intranasal use but contraindicated in pregnant women.

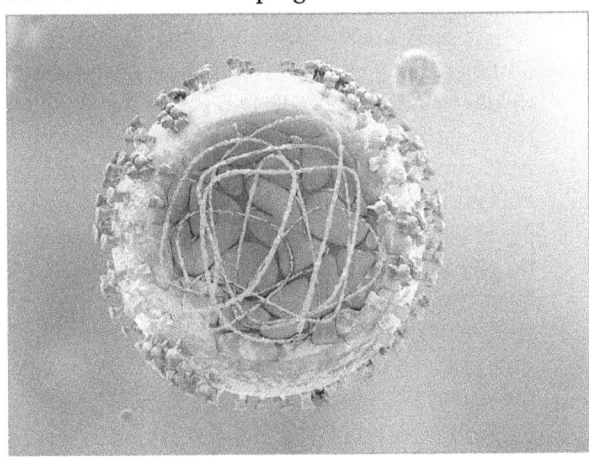

Swine flu virus

20. **Ans. C**

Rubella is an RNA togavirus which causes minor infections. Infection in the first trimester poses serious threat for severe congenital malformations and miscarriage. Women with rash during the first trimester have a congenitally infected fetus in 90% cases. At 13-14 weeks this incidence is 50%, and at the end of the second trimester it is 25%. The incubation period is 12-23 days. Up to half maternal infections are subclinical despite significant viremia. This may lead to severe congenital infections going undetected. Rubella virus is isolated from blood, urine, nasopharynx, and cerebrospinal fluid for up to 2 weeks from the onset of rash. 6% nonimmune women seroconvert during pregnancy. Rubella IgM can be detected for 4-5 days after the onset of rash but can persist for up to 6 weeks. Rubella virus reinfection can also transiently raise low levels of IgM. High IgG avidity indicates an infection at least 2 months prior. There is no specific treatment for rubella. Postexposure immunoprophylaxis may benefit if given within 5 days of exposure. The measles, mumps, and rubella (MMR) vaccine is recommended for all nonpregnant nonimmune women. Prenatal serological testing should be done in all women.

21. **Ans. E**

Fetuses have a 90% chance of rubella infection in the first trimester. The incidence decreases to 50% at 13 weeks and 25% at the end of the second trimester. Rubella vaccination should be offered to all nonimmune women of childbearing age and susceptible hospital personnel. Pregnancy should be avoided for 1 month after rubella vaccination, but vaccination is not an indication for termination of pregnancy.

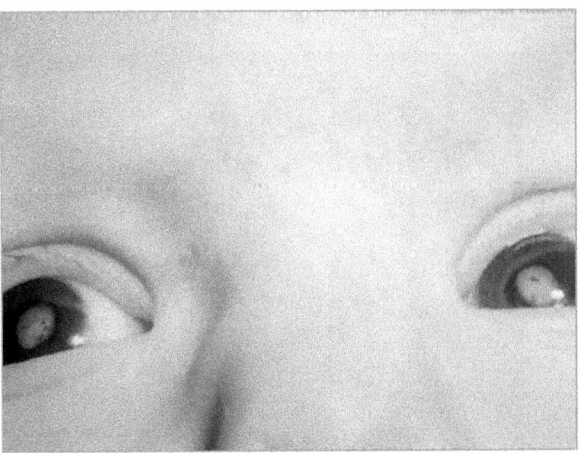

Congenital cataract in congenital rubella syndrome.

Source: https://upload.wikimedia.org/wikipedia/commons/0/07/Cataracts_due_to_Congenital_Rubella_Syndrome_%28CRS%29_PHIL_4284_lores.jpg.

22. Ans. A

Parvovirus B19 causes erythema infectiosum or fifth disease. This virus proliferates in erythroblast precursors, leading to anemia. Parvovirus is contracted from hand to mouth and respiratory contact. The maternal infection rate is highest in women with school-going children and in day-care workers but not in school teachers. Infection is asymptomatic in 30% adults. Flu-like symptoms are followed by a bright red malar rash giving slapped-cheek appearance. Vertical transmission happens in 30% cases. Fetal infection may lead to miscarriages, nonimmune hydrops, and stillbirths. 85% of cases of fetal hydrops develop within 10 weeks of maternal infection. The critical period for maternal infection leading to hydrops is between 13 and 16 weeks which coincides with gestation when fetal hepatic hemopoiesis is greatest. Serial sonography with middle cerebral artery Doppler should be performed every 2 weeks to predict fetal anemia. Fetal transfusion improves outcome depending on gestational age. Mortality rates in hydropic fetuses are as high as 30% without transfusion.

23. Ans. D

Cytomegalovirus is the most common perinatal infection in the developed countries. The virus is secreted into all body fluids and fetal infection occurs transplacentally, at the time of delivery or during breastfeeding. The virus becomes latent after primary infection. 25% of congenital CMV infection occurs from nonimmune mothers. Pregnancy does not alter the course of disease. Transmission rates for primary infection range from 30 to 36% in the first trimester, 34 to 40% in the second trimester, and 40–72% in the third trimester. Anti-CMV IgG antibodies do not prevent maternal recurrence, reactivation, or fetal infection.

24. Ans. A

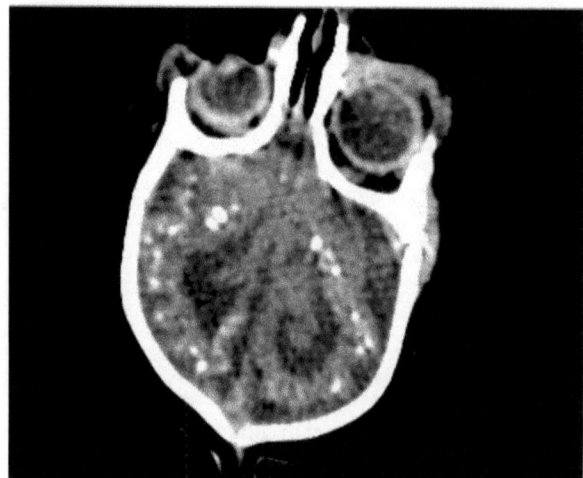

Microcephaly and intracranial calcification.

Source: https://radiopaedia.org/cases/congenital-zika-virus-infection-1?lang=us.

Cytomegalovirus reactivation disease is usually asymptomatic, but viral shedding is common. Primary maternal infection is transmitted to fetus in 40% cases compared to recurrent infection, which infects the fetus in 0.15–1%. Congenital CMV infection includes microcephaly, growth restriction, intracranial calcifications, chorioretinitis, hepatosplenomegaly, sensorineural deafness, and hemolytic anemia.

25. Ans. A

Pregnant women should be tested for CMV if they present with mononucleosis-like illness or if sonography is suggestive of fetal infection. CMV IgM may remain elevated for more than a year since primary infection. High IgG avidity indicates primary infection >6 months old. Sonographic evidence of microcephaly, growth restriction, intracranial calcifications, chorioretinitis, and hepatosplenomegaly or hydrops in combination with positive findings in amniotic fluid or fetal blood are predictive of 75% risk of symptomatic fetal infection. CMV-NAAT of amniotic fluid is the gold standard for diagnosis of fetal infection with a sensitivity ranging between 70% and 99%. No treatments or vaccines are proven to be of any help. Prevention of infection through good personal hygiene and hand washing is to be promoted.

26. Ans. D

Streptococcus agalactiae is a group B organism isolated in intermittent, transient, or chronic fashion throughout pregnancy. It may be an asymptomatic infection but can also lead to septicemia in both mother and fetus. GBS has been linked with preterm labor, premature rupture of membranes, chorioamnionitis, bacteriuria, pyelonephritis, osteomyelitis, mastitis, puerperal sepsis, and fetal infections. GBS septicemia is the leading infectious cause of infant mortality and morbidity in the United States. GBS neonatal septicemia is classified as early (infection <7 days after birth) and late (1 week to 3 months). Early onset sepsis presents as respiratory distress, hypotension, and apnea and must be differentiated from respiratory distress syndrome (RDS). Late-onset sepsis presents as meningitis, but the mortality rate is lesser compared to early-onset sepsis. Both CDC and ACOG recommend a culture-based approach (rectovaginal cultures taken at 35–37 weeks' gestation) to identify women who should be given intrapartum antibiotic prophylaxis. A risk-based approach is recommended for women in labor whose cultures are unknown but are delivering before 37 weeks, intrapartum fever ≥ 100.4°F, and ruptured membranes ≥ 18 hours.

Penicillin is the first-line agent for prophylaxis and ampicillin is a good alternative. Women with penicillin allergy should be given cefazolin as the first choice. Erythromycin is no longer used for such patients.

27. **Ans. A**

    Streptococcus agalactiae or group B *Streptococcus* colonizes genitourinary and gastrointestinal tracts in 10–25% women. The infection ranges from asymptomatic to septicemia and causes asymptomatic bacteriuria, pyelonephritis, mastitis, preterm births, prematurely ruptured membranes, chorioamniotis and neonatal infections. Early-onset neonatal sepsis occurs within <7 days of birth and causes respiratory distress, hypotension, and apnea. Late-onset sepsis manifests as meningitis. Mortality rate is higher with early-onset disease.

    Prophylaxis for GBS is either culture-based or risk-based. CDC and ACOG recommend screening pregnant women at 35–37 weeks and intrapartum prophylaxis to culture proven women. Antibiotics given 4 hours or more prior to delivery remains the antibiotic of choice, which may be replaced with ampicillin, cefazolin, clindamycin or vancomycin in penicillin-allergic women.

28. **Ans. D**

    Explanation same as in Ans 27.

29. **Ans. A**

    Explanation same as in Ans 27.

30. **Ans. A**

    Staphylococcus aureus colonizes nares, skin, genital tract, and oropharynx. MRSA colonizes only 2% population while as *S. aureus* is identified in 10–25% of obstetric patients. MRSA infections contribute significantly to mortality compared to methicillin-sensitive *Staphylococcus*. Skin and soft-tissue infections are the most common presentation. Most cases of MRSA in pregnant women are CA-MRSA, which is sensitive to trimethoprim-sulfamethoxazole. Linezolid is effective but should be avoided in pregnancy. Vancomycin remains the first line for MRSA infection. Prevention of infection is best achieved by hand hygiene and prevention of skin-to-skin contact or contact with infected wounds and linen. Decolonization is considered in women who develop recurrent infections. Nasal application of mupirocin, chlorhexidine-gluconate baths, and oral rifampicin are some of the decolonization measures. Women with CA-MRSA infection during pregnancy should be given single-dose vancomycin along with routine perioperative prophylaxis for cesarean deliveries and perineal tear repairs.

31. **Ans. A**

    Malaria is transmitted by a female *Anopheles* mosquito. Fever, chills, headaches, myalgias, and malaise are the presenting symptoms. Anemia and jaundice are a consequence of hemolysis. Falciparum malaria may lead to renal failure, convulsions, and death. Maternal malaria results in increased perinatal mortality and morbidity. Anemia, abortions, low birth weight, stillbirths, and preterm labor are common. Parasite identification by microscopic analysis of thick and thin blood smears is the gold standard for diagnosis. In women with low parasitemia, microscopy may not be diagnostic and malarial antigen testing may be used to arrive at a diagnosis. Most commonly used antimalarials are contraindicated in pregnancy. The CDC recommends using atovaquone–proguanil or artemether–lumefantrine only if other options are not available in pregnancy. All pregnant women with uncomplicated *vivax*, *ovale*, or *malariae* are CQ-sensitive *P. falciparum* must be treated with CQ and HCQ. For CQ-resistant falciparum malaria, mefloquine or quinine sulfate with clindamycin may be used. Mefloquine is the only chemoprophylaxis that can be used in pregnancy. Primaquine and doxycycline are contraindicated in pregnancy. Malaria control and prevention is based on vector control and prevention of mosquito bites.

    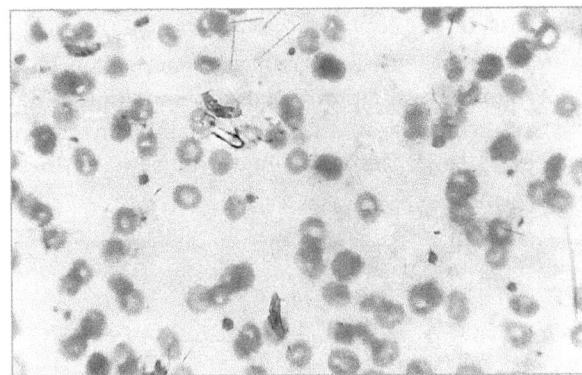

    Plasmodium falciparum gametocyte.
    Source: https://commons.wikimedia.org/wiki/File:Plasmodium_falciparum_gametocyte.jpg.

32. **Ans. B**

    At least 80% women with type 1 diabetes mellitus (DM) develop at least one infection during pregnancy compared with only 25% in those without diabetes.

33. **Ans. D**

    Normal hydrogen peroxide-producing *Lactobacilli* in vagina are replaced with anaerobes such as *Gardnerella vaginalis*, *Mobiluncus* species, and *Mycoplasma hominis* in BV. BV is associated with preterm labor, premature membrane rupture, chorioamnionitis, and amniotic fluid infection. Ethnicity, chronic stress, and vaginal douching are risk factors for developing BV.

34. **Ans. B**

    Periodontitis affects nearly 50% pregnant women and causes preterm birth. Treatment, however, does not prevent preterm birth but definitely improves gum inflammation.

35. **Ans. A**

Single marital status, poverty, low socioeconomic background, drug abuse, prostitution, and other sexually transmitted infections are some of the risk factors for developing gonorrhea in pregnancy. 40% cases have concomitant chlamydial infection. Infection is limited to the lower urogenital tract. Untreated *Gonococcus* may lead to septic abortions, preterm delivery, premature rupture of membranes, chorioamnionitis, and postpartum infections. These women should also be tested for HIV, syphilis, and chlamydia. NAAT is the diagnostic method of choice. For gonococcal infections, a dual therapy with ceftriaxone 250 mg single dose plus azithromycin 1 g single oral dose is recommended as first line. Neither doxycycline nor quinolones are used in pregnancy. Dual therapy should be given together on the same day, simultaneously and under direct supervision. Cefixime should be reserved for patients where ceftriaxone cannot be given, and a test of cure must be done 1 week after the treatment. Treatment of sexual partners is recommended.

36. **Ans. D**

Maternal sepsis is a significant cause of mortality and morbidity. Nulliparity, black race, multiple gestations, cesarean delivery, and assisted reproductive technology are all risk factors for maternal sepsis. More than 50% women dying of sepsis have a comorbidity like chronic renal, liver disease or congestive heart failure. Impaired immune system, invasive interventions, prolonged membrane rupture, and continued vaginal bleeding or discharge make the pregnant women more susceptible to sepsis. Sepsis should always be considered in otherwise-unexplained end-organ damage in the presence of an infection regardless of fever.

37. **Ans. A**

Sepsis is the leading cause for nearly 11% maternal deaths worldwide. The burden is greatest in Southern Asia and sub-Saharan Africa compared to high-income countries. The source of maternal sepsis can be either pelvic or nonpelvic. Antepartum sources most commonly are nonpelvic in origin, while intrapartum and postpartum causes have a leading pelvic source. 30% sepsis cases have no identifiable source. *Escherichia coli* and groups A and B *Streptococcus* are the most common pathogens in maternal sepsis. 15% cases are polymicrobial infections, the reason why broad-spectrum antibiotics are recommended. Blood, urine, respiratory, and other relevant cultures should be taken in addition to checking serum lactate levels in all women suspected of or diagnosed with sepsis.

Sequential Organ Failure Assessment (SOFA) score.					
System	Score 0	Score 1	Score 2	Score 3	Score 4
Respiration					
PaO_2/FiO_2 mm Hg (kPa)	≥400	<400	<300	<200 with respiratory support	<100 with respiratory support
Coagulation					
Platelets, × 10^3/μL	≥150	<150	<100	<50	<20
Liver					
Bilirubin (mg/dL)	<1.2	1.2–1.9	2.0–5.9	6.0–11.9	>12.0
Cardiovascular	MAP ≥ 70 mm Hg	MAP < 70 mm Hg	Dopamine < 5 or Dobutamine any dose[a]	Dopamine 5.1–15 or Epinephrine < 0.1 or Norepinephrine < 0.1[a]	Dopamine > 15 or Epinephrine > 0.1 or Norepinephrine > 0.1[a]
Nervous system					
Glasgow Coma Scale	15	13–14	10–12	6–9	<6
Renal					
Serum creatinine (mg/dL)	<1.2	1.2–1.9	2.0–3.4	3.5–4.9	>5.0
Urine output (mL/day)				<500	<200

[a]Catecholamines are given as μg/kg/min for at least 1 hour.
(FiO_2: fraction of inspired oxygen; MAP: mean arterial pressure; PaO_2: partial pressure of oxygen)
Source: Vincent JL, Moreno R, Takala J, et al. The SOFA (Sepsis-related Organ Failure Assessment) score to describe organ dysfunction/failure. Intensive Care Med. 1996;22:707-10.

38. Ans. B

Ceftriaxone, cefotaxime, ertapenem, or ampicillin plus azithromycin are the recommended antibiotics for community-acquired pneumonia. Low-risk patients with hospital-acquired pneumonia need piperacillin—tazobactam/meropenem/imipenem/cefepime. For high-risk patients, double coverage for pseudomonas (beta-lactam plus aminoglycoside or quinolone) and MRSA coverage with vancomycin or linezolid are recommended.

39. Ans. A

In hypotensive patients unresponsive to aggressive fluid management, vasopressors should be used to maintain blood pressure. They constrict the pathologically dilated systemic circulation. Norepinephrine is the drug of choice and mean arterial pressure (MAP) should be kept at <65 mm Hg. Dobutamine may be used where myocardial dysfunction is suspected.

40. Ans. D

SOFA score is used for assessing in-hospital mortality in septicemic patients. SOFA score includes assessment of respiratory PO_2, FiO_2, platelet count, bilirubin, serum creatinine, MAP, and Glasgow Coma Scale. The practical limitations and complexity of SOFA scoring led to a modified version of SOFA, also known as qSOFA. qSOFA includes 1 point each for a respiratory rate of >22/min, change in mental status, and systolic blood pressure < 100 mm Hg. A qSOFA ≥2 points indicates organ dysfunction.

41. Ans. D

Explanation same as in Ans 40.

SUGGESTED READING

1. Emedicine.com.
2. Medscape gynaecology/infectious diseases.
3. Uptodate.com.

CHAPTER 31

Imaging in Infectious Diseases

Shrinivas B Desai, Ritu K Kashikar, Shraddha Sinhasan, Chandresh Karnavat

INFECTIONS X-RAYS

1. A 56-year-old female with complaints of left sided chest pain and cough since 2 weeks and hemoptysis since 3 days.

   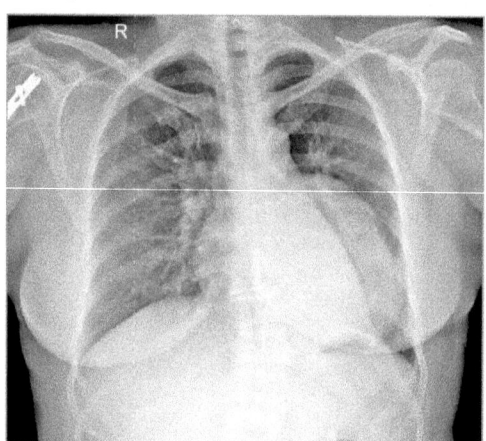

   The most likely diagnosis is:
   A. Lung malignancy
   B. Hydatid cyst
   C. Pneumonia
   D. Pleuropericardial cyst

2. Known c/o retroviral disease with CD4 count of 180 comes with complaints of cough and breathlessness.

   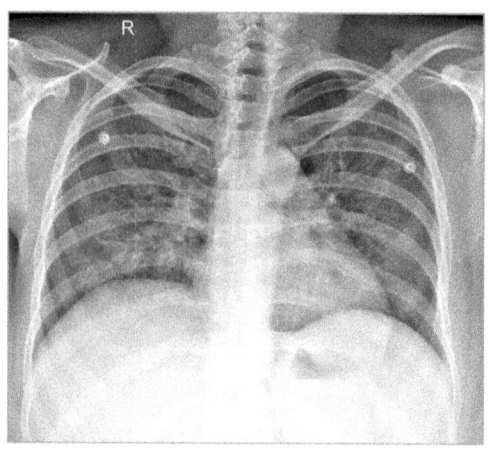

   The most likely diagnosis is:
   A. Cytomegalovirus (CMV) pneumonia
   B. Pulmonary edema
   C. *Pneumocystis carinii* pneumonia (PCP)
   D. Angioinvasive fungal infection

3. A 52-year-old female, known diabetes mellitus (DM) type II, on long-term steroids for systemic lupus erythematosus (SLE) came with history of fever and cough for 2 weeks. Routine antibiotic course did not lead to resolution of X-ray changes. The patient presently complains of breathlessness and decreased right lower lung air sounds.

   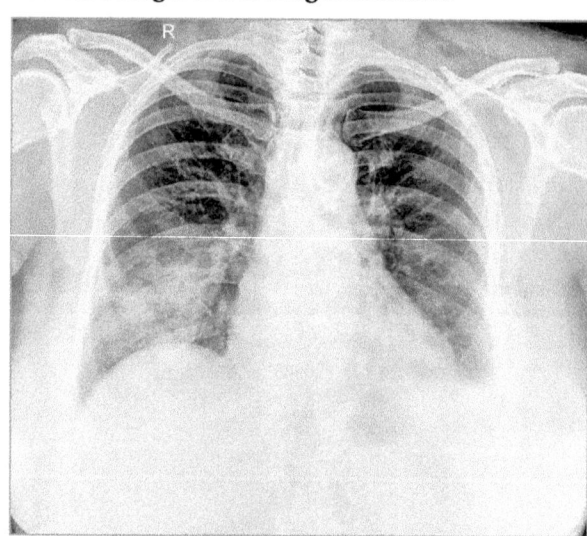

   The most likely diagnosis is:
   A. Pulmonary tuberculosis
   B. PCP
   C. Invasive fungal or fungal-like pneumonia
   D. SLE-related lung interstitial disease

4. A 13-year-old boy with lower lumbar pain for 2 weeks. The patient's blood tests reveal raised CRP and markedly raised ESR of 72. He also complains of low-grade fever and fatigue.

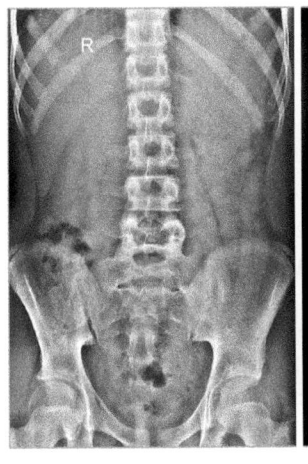
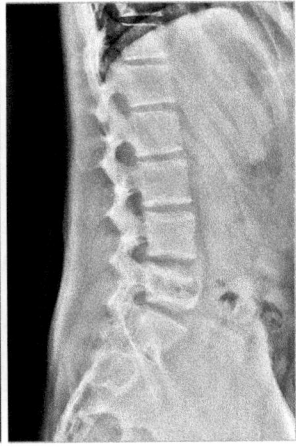

The most likely diagnosis is:

A. Eosinophilic granuloma
B. Tuberculous spondylitis
C. Sickle cell anemia
D. Metastasis from unknown primary

5. A 4-year-old child with high-grade fever, cough, and tachypnea. Routine blood test reveals WBC–18,000; ESR–30; platelets–1.9 lakh.

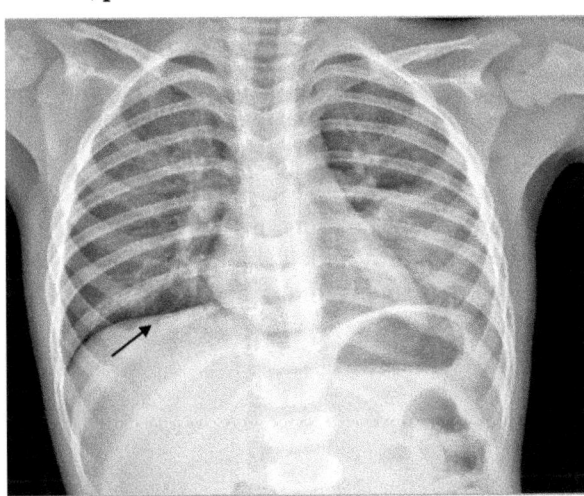

The most likely diagnosis is:

A. Pleuropericardial cyst
B. Round pneumonia
C. Primary lung neoplasm
D. Hydatid cyst

6. A 45-year-old male with fever and cough for 1 month. He also complains of weight loss of 8 kg in last 2 months. He had two episodes of hemoptysis in last 10 days.

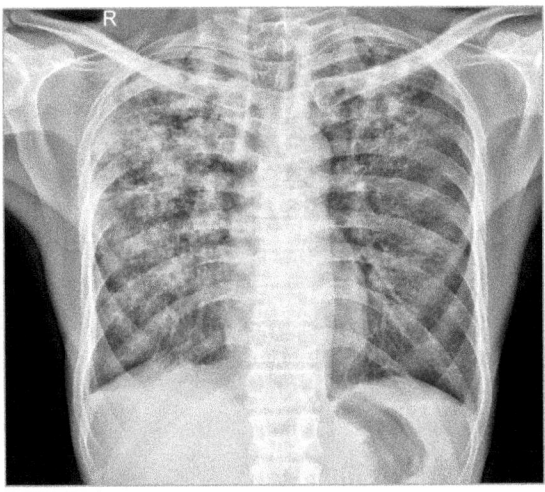

The most likely diagnosis is:

A. *Pneumocystis carinii* pneumonia
B. Community-acquired pneumonia
C. Aspergillosis
D. Pulmonary tuberculosis

7. A 35-year-old male with marked weight loss in the last 3 months with loss of appetite and fever. He is known c/o type I DM and was on immunosuppressants for ankylosing spondylitis.

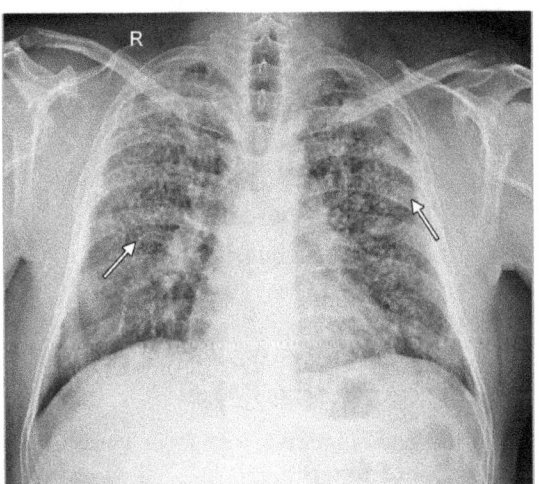

The most likely diagnosis is:

A. Miliary tuberculosis
B. Sarcoidosis
C. CMV
D. Carcinomatosis

8. A c/o 32-year-old male with sudden onset left sided chest pain and breathlessness.

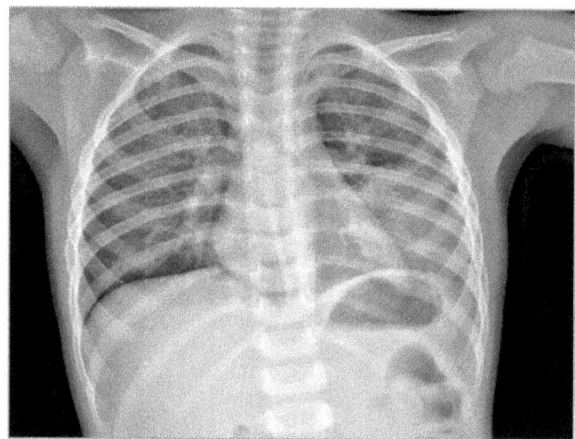

The most likely diagnosis is:
A. Left-sided hydropneumothorax
B. Ruptured pulmonary hydatid
C. Rising sun sign
D. All of the above

9. A 55-year-old male with neck pain for 1 month. He also complains of bilateral upper limb numbness and weakness (left > right).

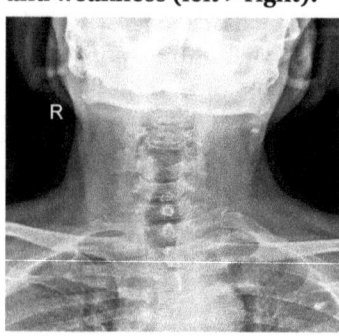 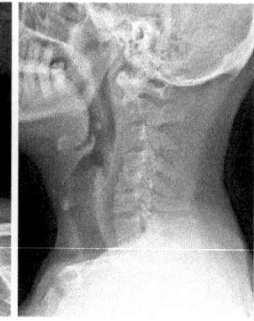

The most likely diagnosis is:
A. Block vertebra
B. Fracture of C4 and C5 vertebral bodies
C. C4/C5 cervical spondylodiscitis
D. Degenerative spondylosis

10. An 18-year-old female with fever, cough, weight loss and loss of appetite.

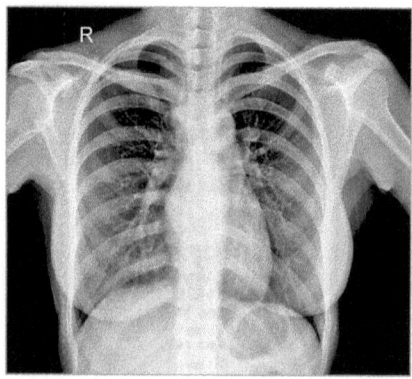

The most likely diagnosis is:
A. Normal X-ray
B. Mediastinal mass
C. Potts spine
D. Atrial septal defect (ASD)

11. A 40-year-old male with severe left hip pain for 10 days. Currently he is unable to walk. He is febrile with raised WBC counts in routine blood test.

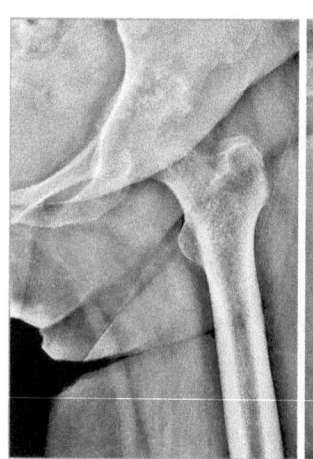 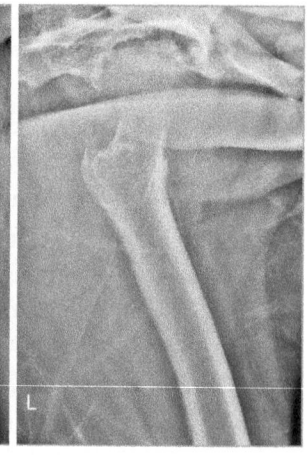

The most likely diagnosis is:
A. Septic arthritis
B. Avascular necrosis of head of femur
C. Lytic bone tumor of left acetabulum
D. Reactive arthritis

12. A 40-year-old female patient with lower back pain. The patient has severe pain during walking, predominantly on left side. There is left lower back tenderness also noted.

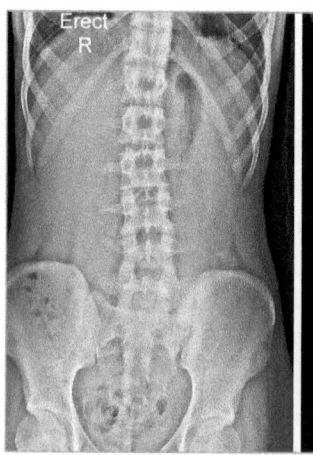 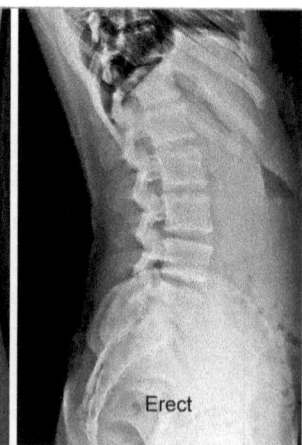

The most likely diagnosis is:
A. Lumbar spondylodiscitis
B. Osteitis condensans ilii
C. Ankylosing spondylitis
D. Tuberculous sacroiliitis

13. A 35-year-old male patient with bilateral osteonecrosis of head of femur, posted for hip replacement. This is the preoperative X-ray for fitness.

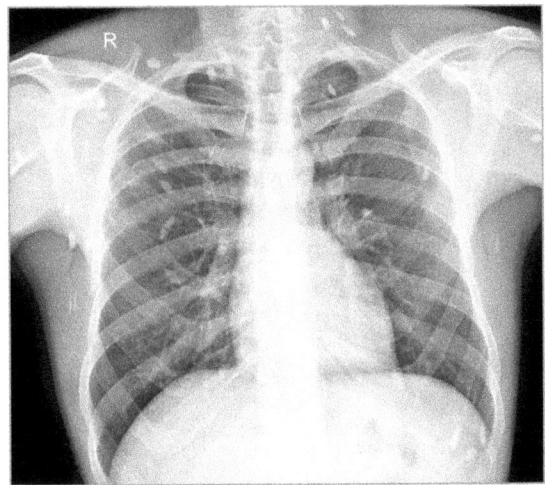

The most likely diagnosis is:
A. Dermatomyositis
B. Systemic lupus erythematosus
C. Guinea worm disease
D. Cysticercosis

14. A 55-year-old female with breathlessness and dropping SPO$_2$. She had high-grade fever for 7 days, headache, malaise, PSMP+ for vivax strain.

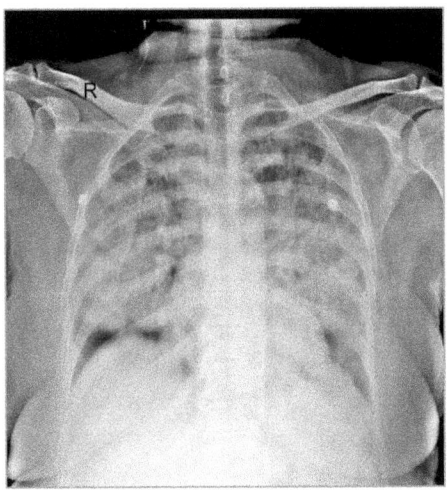

A. Pulmonary edema due to fluid overload
B. Acute respiratory distress syndrome (ARDS)
C. Bilateral lung infiltrates of bacterial etiology
D. Extensive fungal infection

CHEST

CASE 1

A 55-year-old with history of recent renal transplant presented with fever, cough with expectoration, dyspnea.

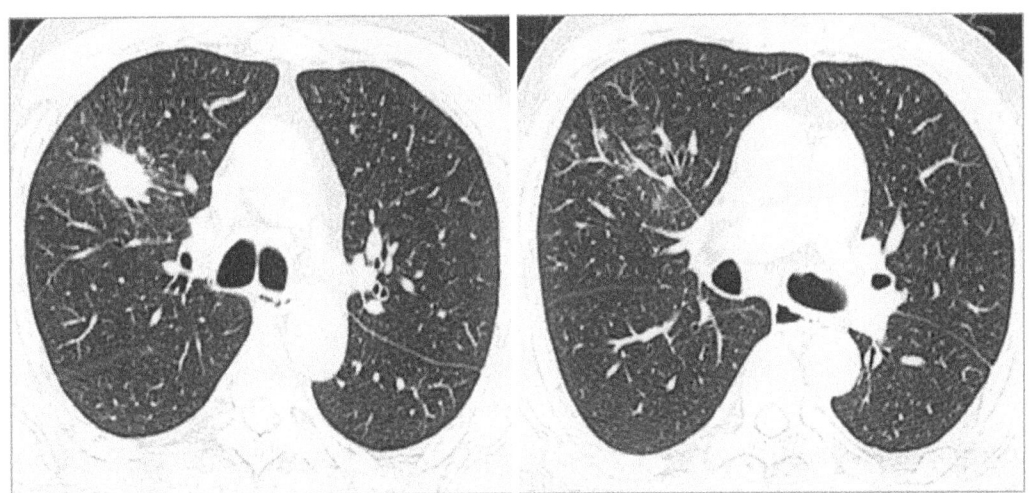

22/2/16
Rounded patch of consolidation in right upper lobe was seen.

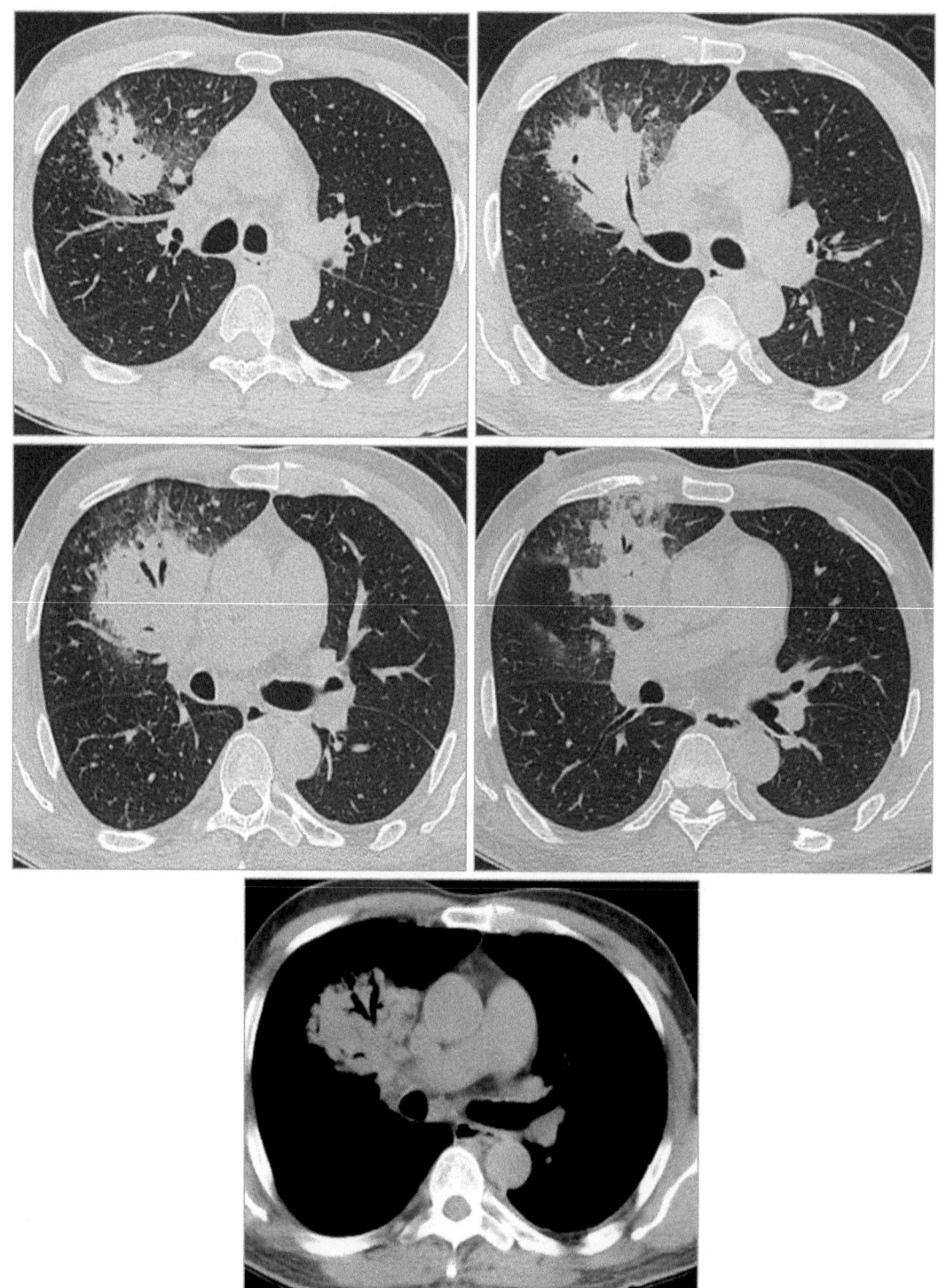

Follow-up scan showing rapid increase in size with small central cavitation.

15. **What is the differential diagnosis?**

   A. *Pneumocystis carinii* pneumonia
   B. Nocardiosis
   C. Tuberculosis
   D. Aspergillosis

CASE 2

A 35-year old female k/c/o chronic glomerulonephritis, renal transplant done in 2008 presented with fever, cough for 17 days, and breathlessness for 10 days duration.
- BiPAP continuously—did not improve.
- Diffuse ground-glass opacity: Symmetrically bilateral with peri-bronchial thickening.
- Diffuse ground-glass opacity: Bilaterally symmetrical.
- Bilateral pleural effusion.

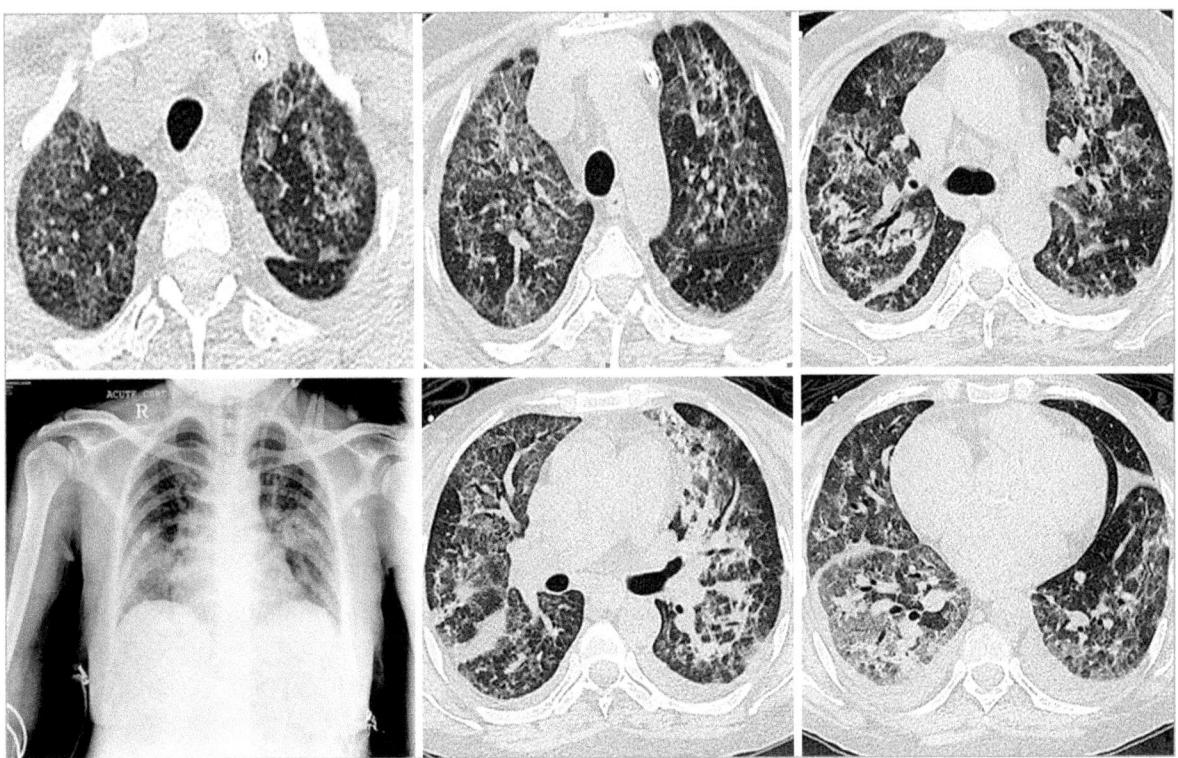

16. **What is the differential diagnosis?**
    A. *Pneumocystis carinii* pneumonia
    B. H1N1 pneumonia
    C. CMV pneumonia
    D. Tuberculosis

CASE 3

A 45-year-old male with history of allogeneic bone marrow transplant presented with fever and cough.
- Diffuse small nodules
- Mild interstitial septal thickening
- Bilateral, symmetric distribution
- No lymphadenopathy.

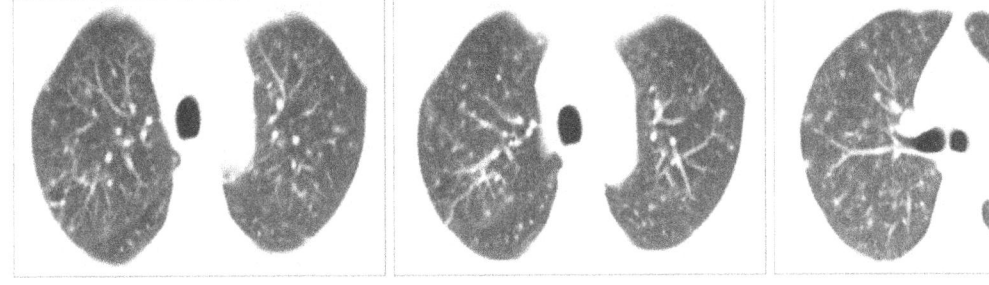

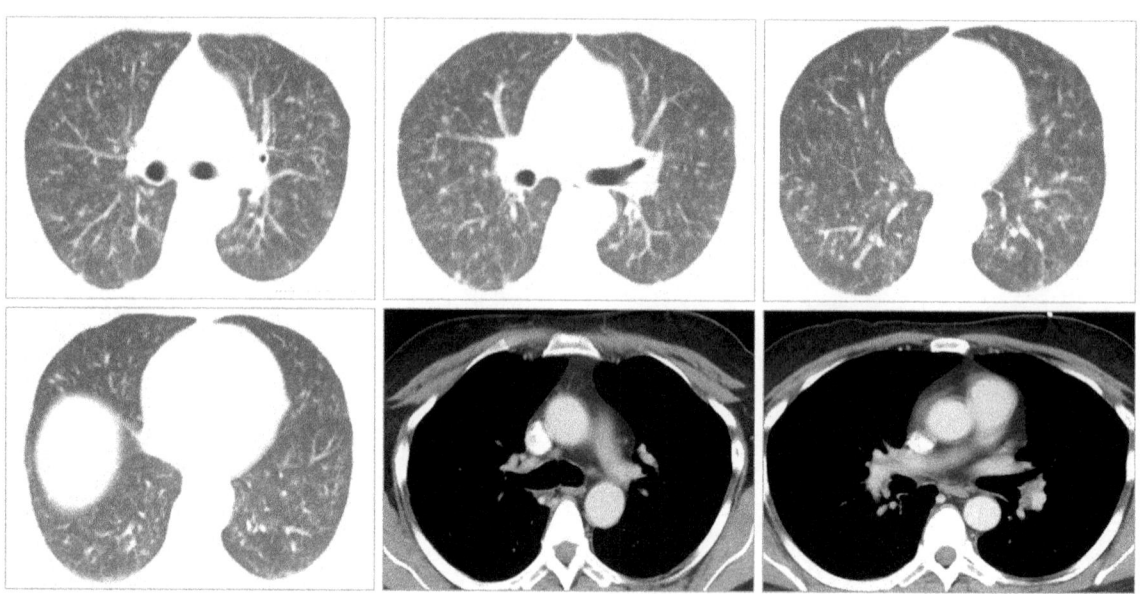

17. What is the differential diagnosis?

   A. CMV Pneumonia   B. PCP   C. Miliary TB   D. H1N1 pneumonia

CASE 4

A 44-year-old male, postrenal transplant presented with fever, severe cough, reduced oxygen saturation requiring ventilatory support.

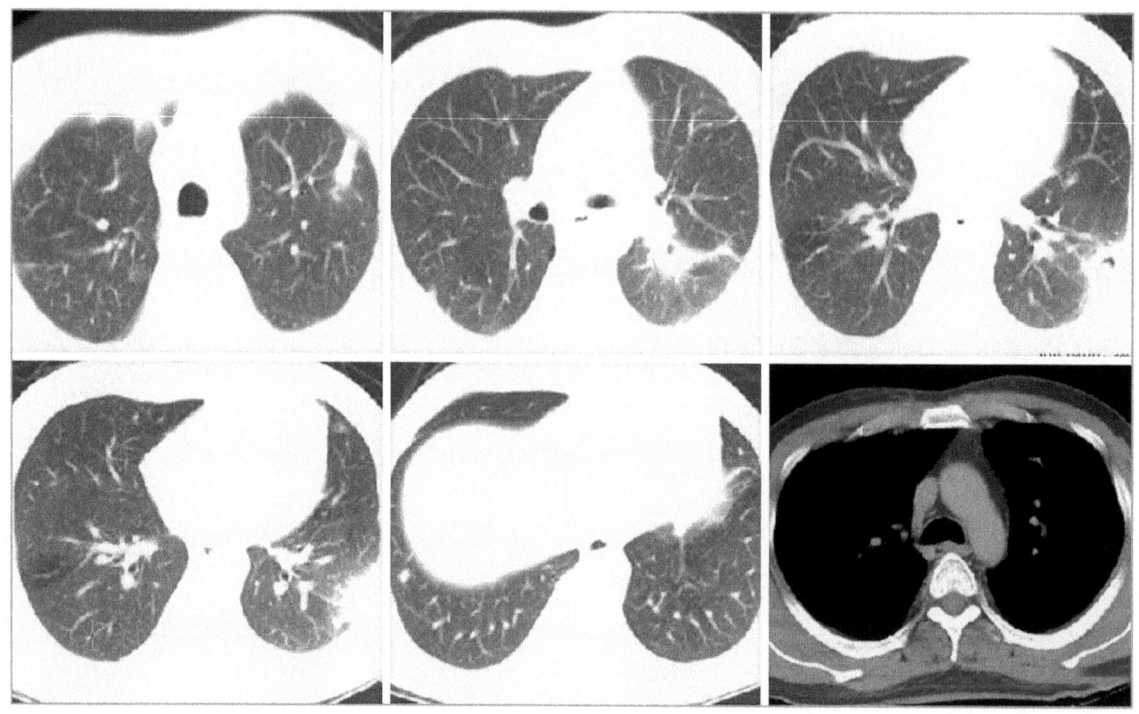

Cavitary nodules with surrounding ground-glass attenuation.

18. What is the differential diagnosis?

   A. Angioinvasive aspergillosis   B. Nocardiosis
   C. CMV pneumonia   D. Tuberculosis

CASE 5

A 25-year-old male with fever, cough with expectoration for 2 months, gradual loss of weight and appetite, no known comorbidities.

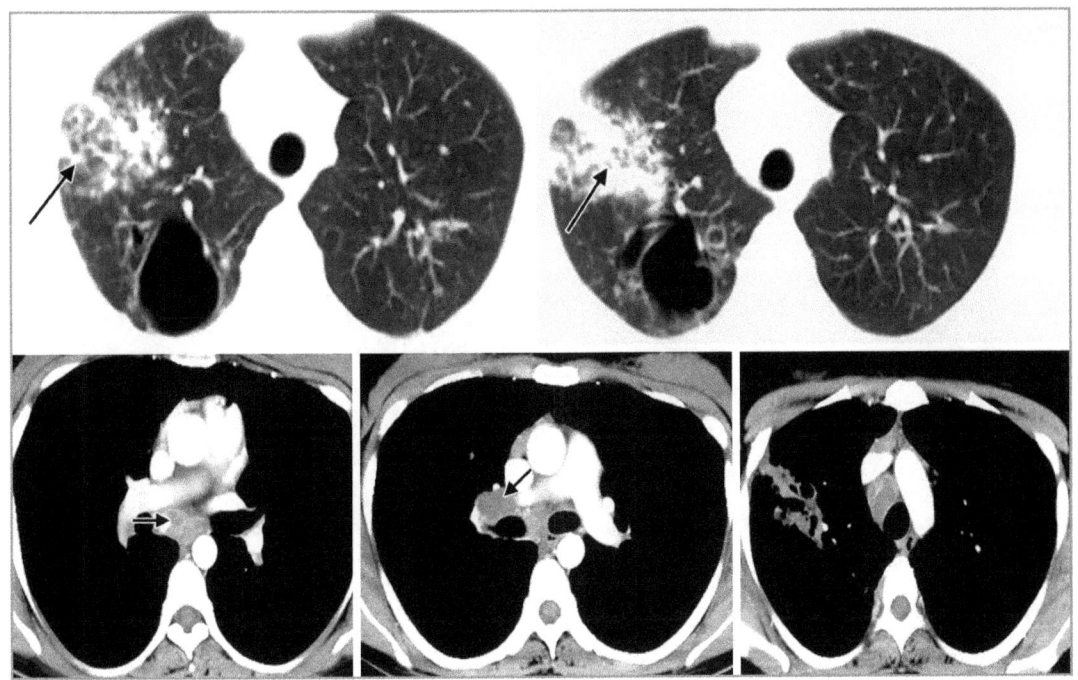

Centrilobular nodules, small consolidations in right upper lobe (arrows) with necrotic mediastinal and hilar adenopathy (small arrows).

19. What is the differential diagnosis?

    A. Tuberculosis   B. CMV   C. Aspergillosis   D. Nocardiosis

CASE 6

A 35-year-old seropositive male presented with fever, cough.

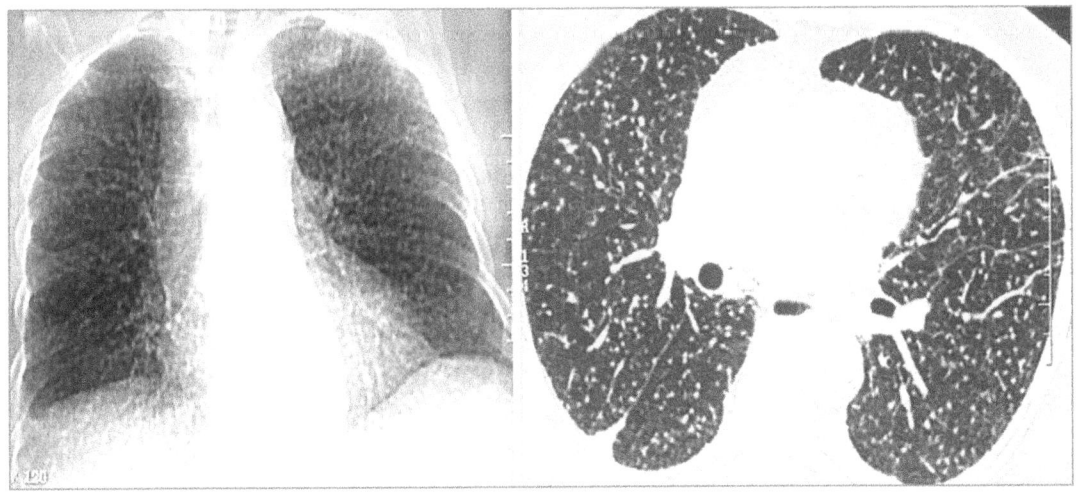

Multiple tiny randomly distributed nodules throughout both lungs.

20. What is the differential diagnosis?

    A. Miliary TB   B. CMV   C. PCP   D. Aspergillosis

CASE 7

A 42-year-old female, incidentally detected lesion in chest X-ray.

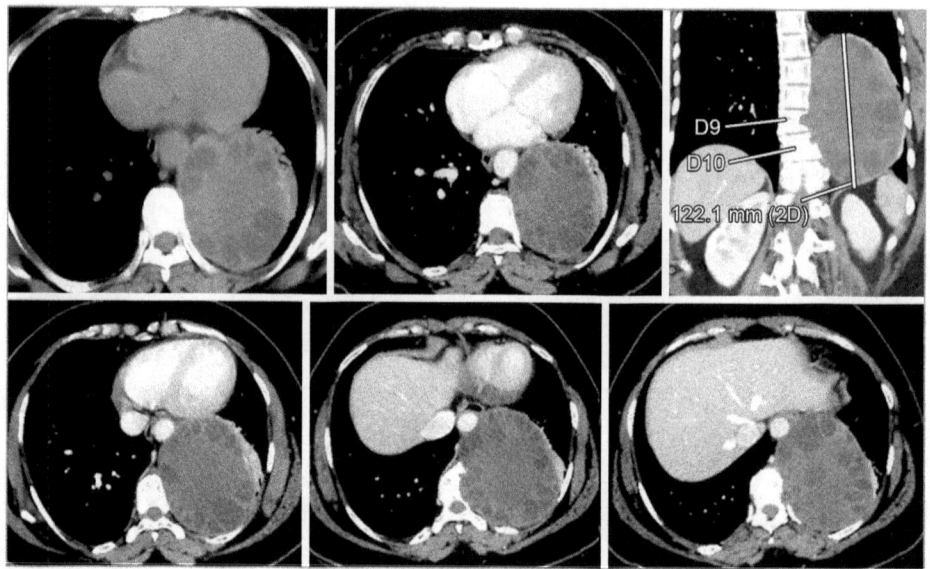

Well-defined rounded hypodense lesion in left lower lobe with peripherally arranged cysts eroding into vertebra.

21. **What is the differential diagnosis?**

    A. Tuberculoma B. Pulmonary carcinoma C. Hydatid cyst D. Fungal ball

CASE 8

A 45-year-old male k/c/o B-cell lymphoma on chemotherapy presented with high fever, cough. O/E—bilateral lower lobar crepts.

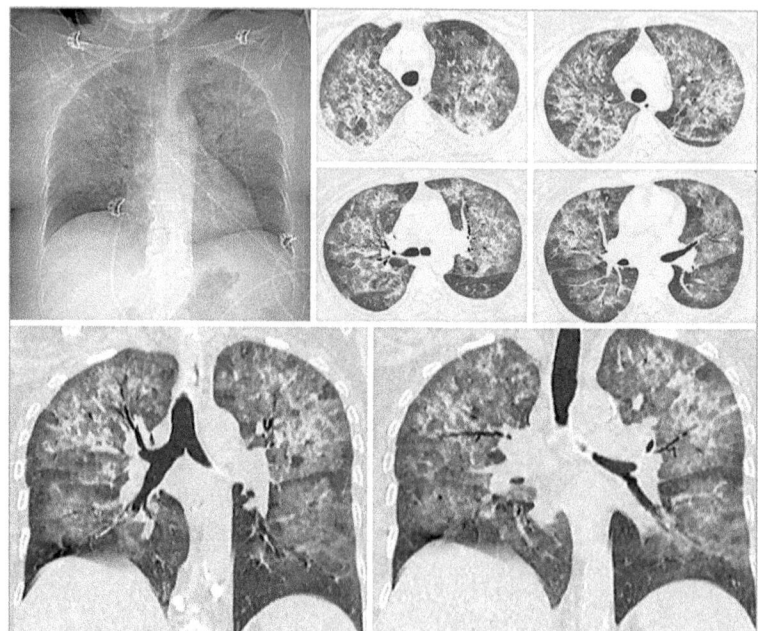

Diffuse ground-glass attenuation with septal thickening in both lungs predominantly in central perihilar regions.

22. **What is the differential diagnosis?**

    A. PCP B. Aspergillosis C. Viral pneumonitis D. Pulmonary edema

ABDOMINAL INFECTIONS

CASE 1

A 45-year-old alcoholic male presented with fever, pain in right upper quadrant. O/E—tenderness in right upper quadrant and palpable lump.

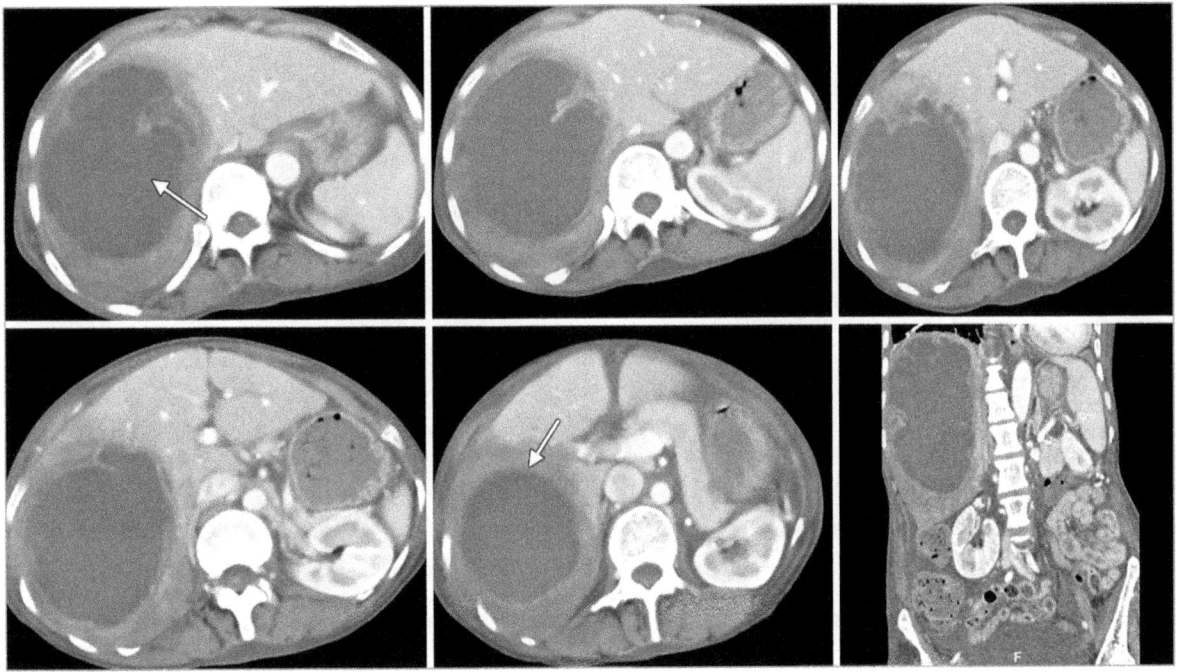

Well-defined hypodense wall enhancing lesion with internal septa in the right lobe of liver with surrounding edema in adjacent liver parenchyma.

23. **What is the differential diagnosis?**

    A. Tuberculoma B. Pyogenic abscess C. Hydatid cyst D. Amebic liver abscess

CASE 2

A 72-year-old female with fever, altered sensorium. Blood culture—gram negative sepsis (*E. coli*).

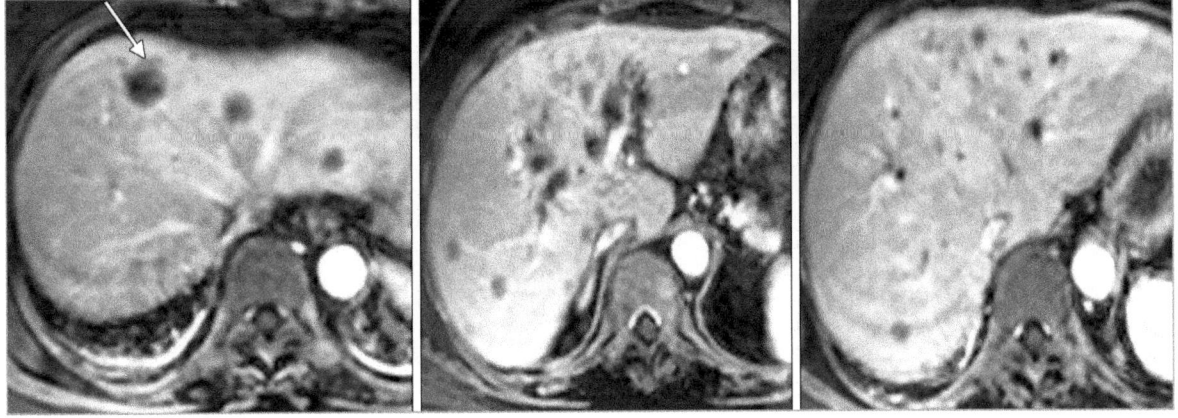

Postcontrast MR images reveals multiple peripherally enhancing lesions in both lobes of liver with dilated biliary radicals (arrow).

24. **What is the differential diagnosis?**

    A. Cholangitic abscess B. Amebic liver abscess C. Tubercular abscess D. Metastasis

CASE 3

A 45-year-old male with history of dull pain in right upper quadrant for 2–3 months. US s/o hypoechoic lesions in segment 8. Patient advised CT for further evaluation.

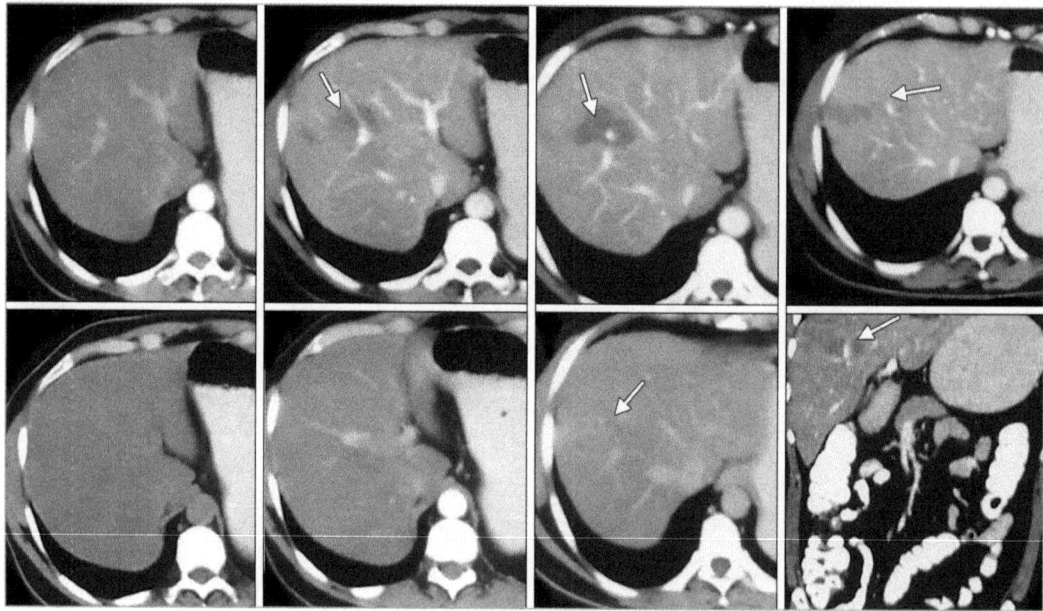

CT showing multiple hypodense conglomerate lesions in segment 8 (arrows).

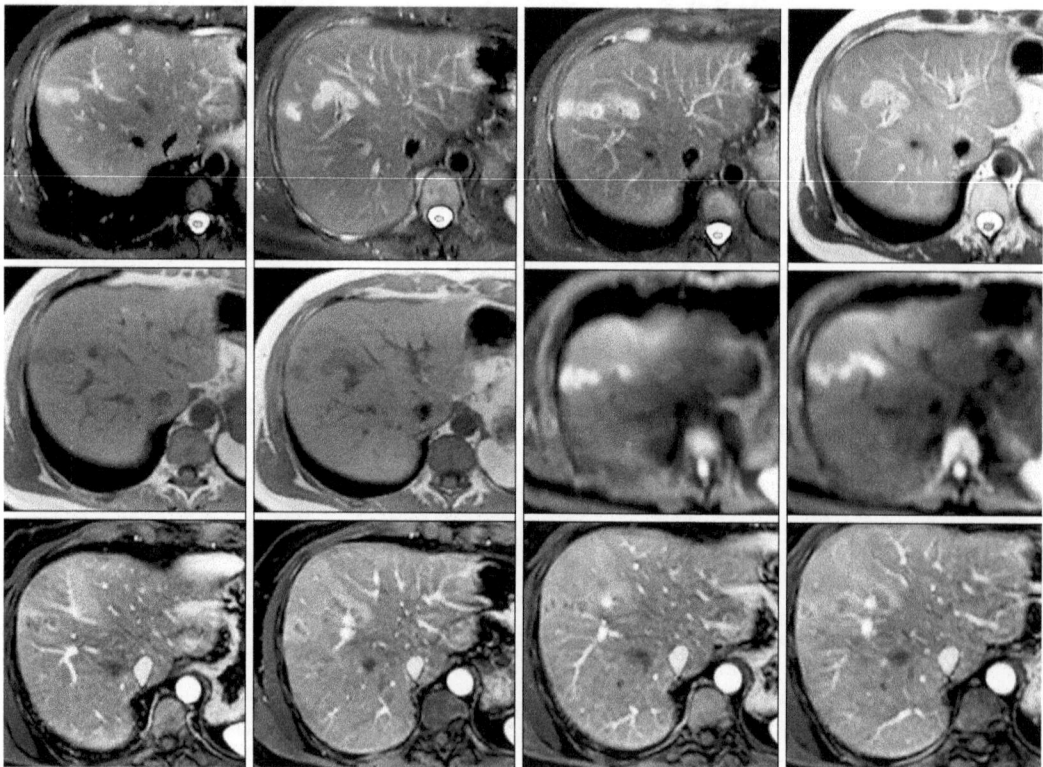

MRI showing lesions are hyperintense on T2 and show peripheral enhancement.

25. **What is the differential diagnosis?**
    A. Metastasis
    B. Abscess
    C. Tuberculous granulomas
    D. HCC

CASE 4

A 51-year-old male with pain and lump in right upper quadrant. O/E—hepatomegaly with lobulated lump. No comorbidities.

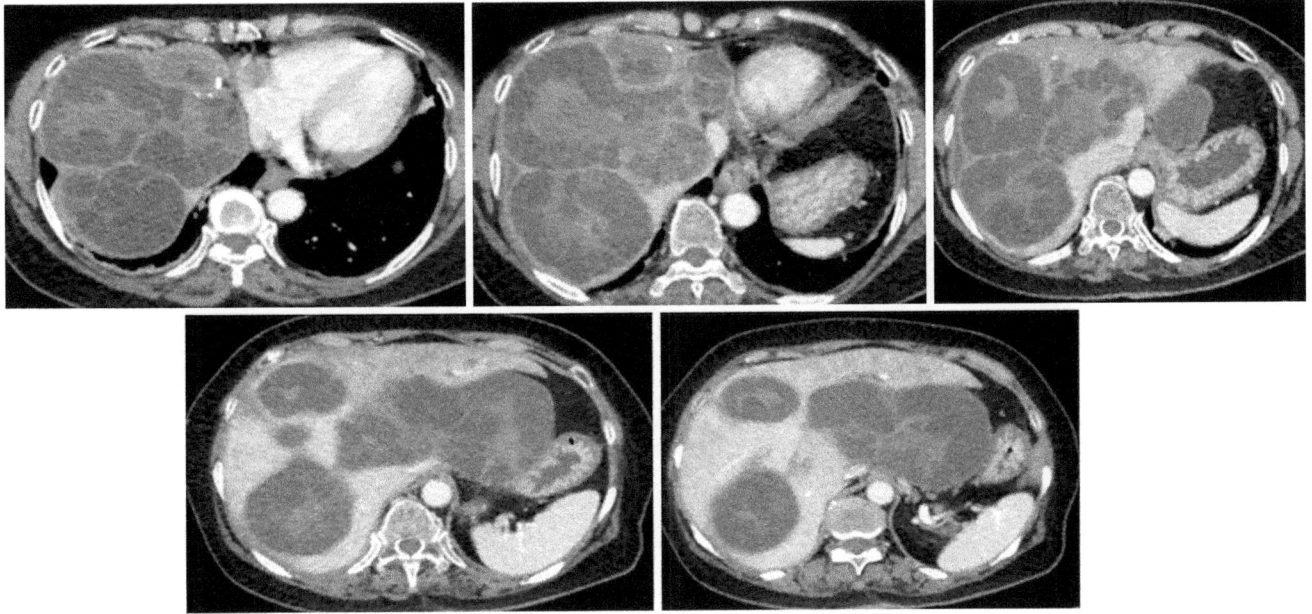

Multiple cystic lesions in both lobes with peripherally located daughter cysts.

26. **What is the differential diagnosis?**
    A. Amebic abscess
    B. Pyogenic abscess
    C. Hydatid cysts
    D. Tuberculomas

CASE 5

A k/c/o ALL, postallogenic BMT, presented with fever, deranged liver function tests.

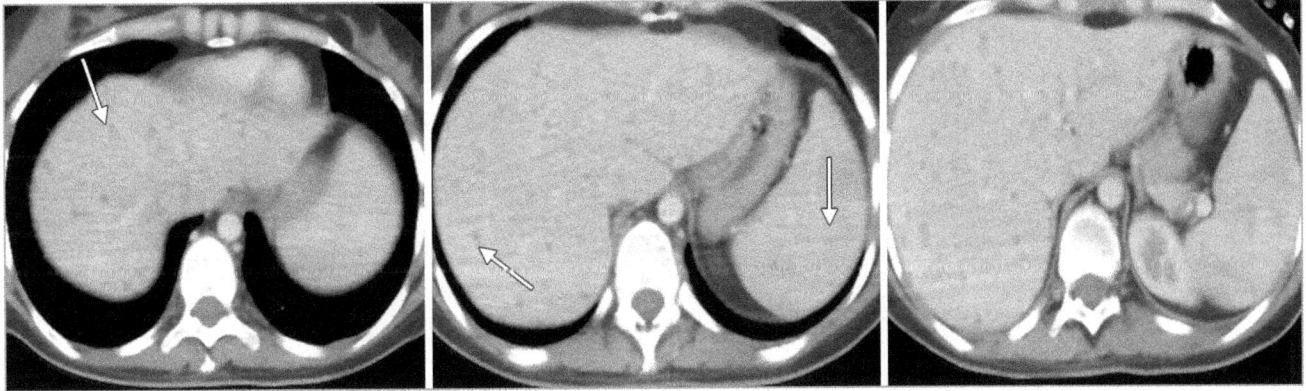

Multiple small minimally enhancing lesions in both lobes (arrows) and spleen.

27. **What is the differential diagnosis?**
    A. Fungal abscess
    B. Pyogenic abscess
    C. Tuberculomas
    D. Amebic liver abscess

CASE 6

A 32-year-old male with fever, weight loss, abdominal distension, c/o colicky abdominal pain for 2 months.

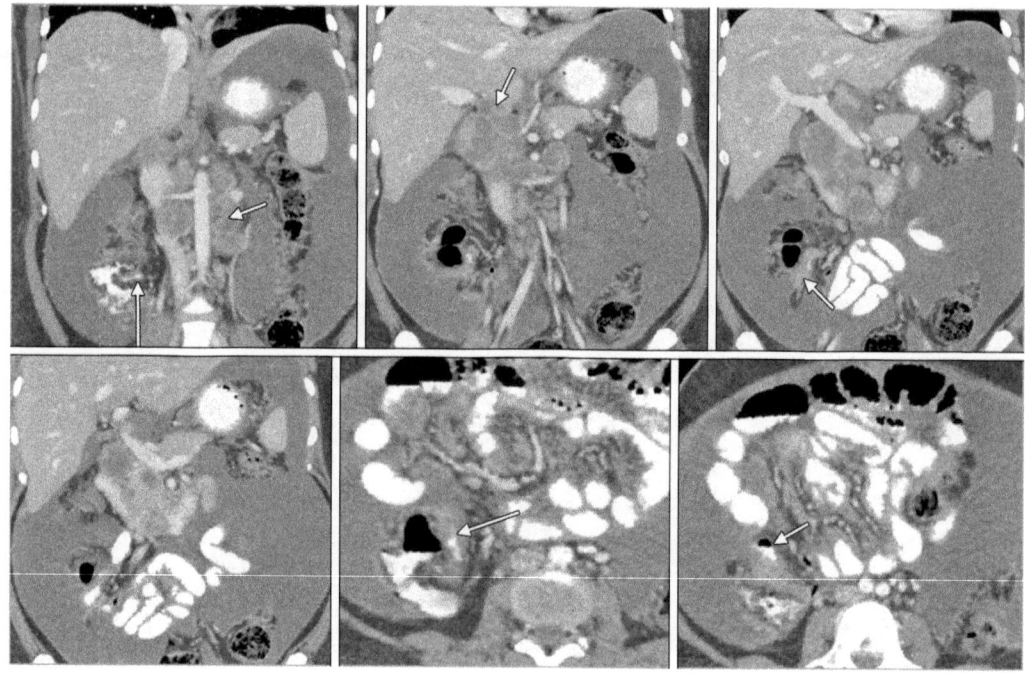

Thickening of ileocecal junction (long arrow) with gross ascites with extensive necrotic lymphadenopathy (small arrows)

28. **What is the differential diagnosis?**
    A. Abdominal tuberculosis
    B. Metastatic carcinoma
    C. Lymphoma
    D. Bacterial peritonitis

CASE 7

A 30-year-old seropositive male presented with diarrhea, fever and weight loss, abdominal pain, and hematochezia.

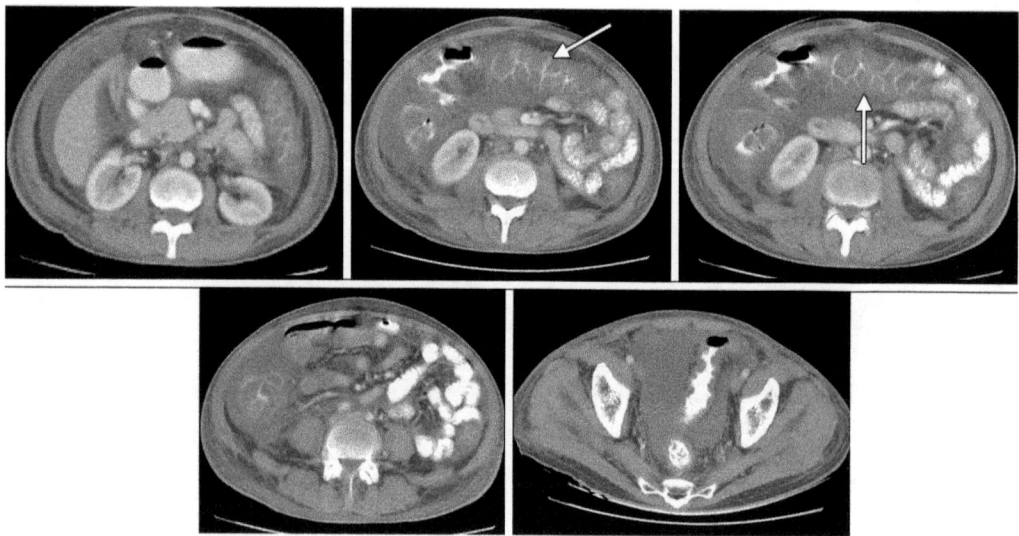

Long segment thickening of large bowel with marked mucosal edema (arrows) and ascites.

29. **What is the differential diagnosis?**
    A. Tuberculous colitis
    B. CMV colitis
    C. Pseudomembranous colitis
    D. Fungal colitis

CASE 8

A 45-year-old male presented with diarrhea, fever, raised white cell count, and abdominal pain with distension. History of 4 weeks of antibiotic therapy prior to symptom onset.

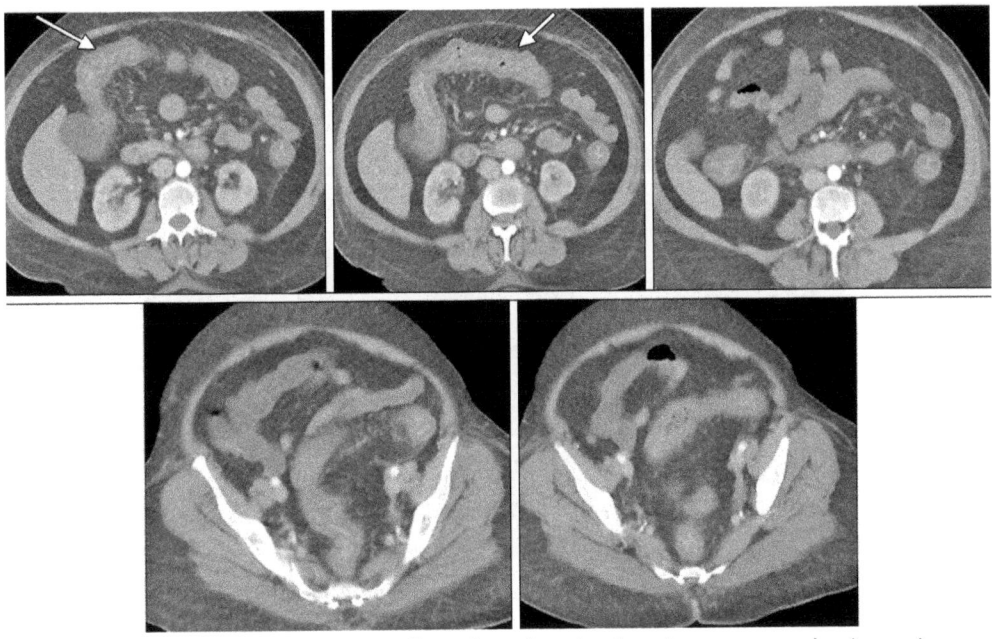

Diffuse long segment thickening of large bowel predominantly transverse colon (arrows).

30. **What is the differential diagnosis?**
    A. Tuberculous colitis
    B. CMV colitis
    C. Pseudomembranous colitis
    D. Fungal colitis

CASE 9

A 55-year old male, k/c/o CRF presented with fever, pain in abdomen, vomiting. Clinical signs—intestinal obstruction. Patient sent for plain CT abdomen in view of high creatinine.

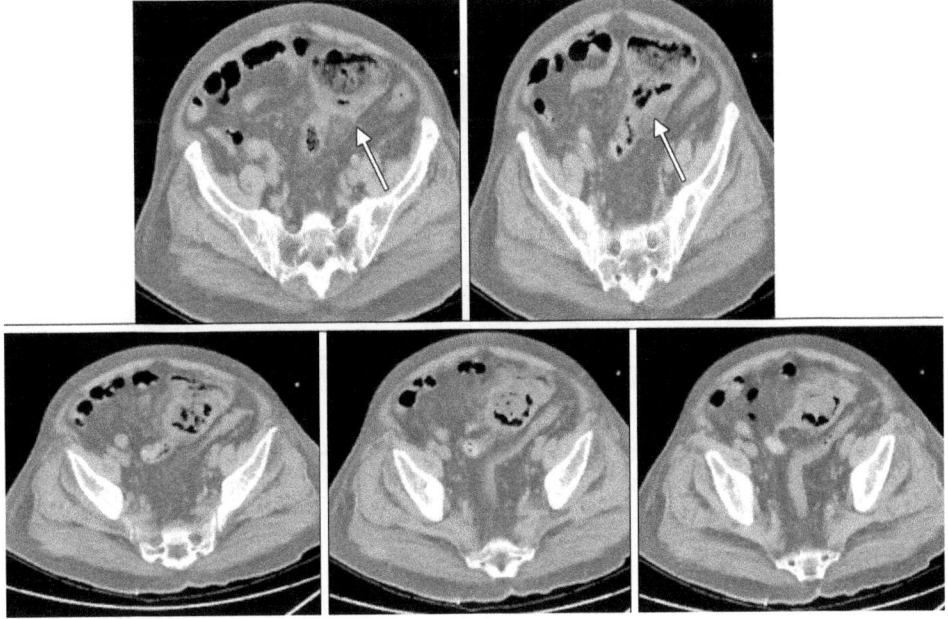

Inflammation in the colon (arrows) with wall thickening.

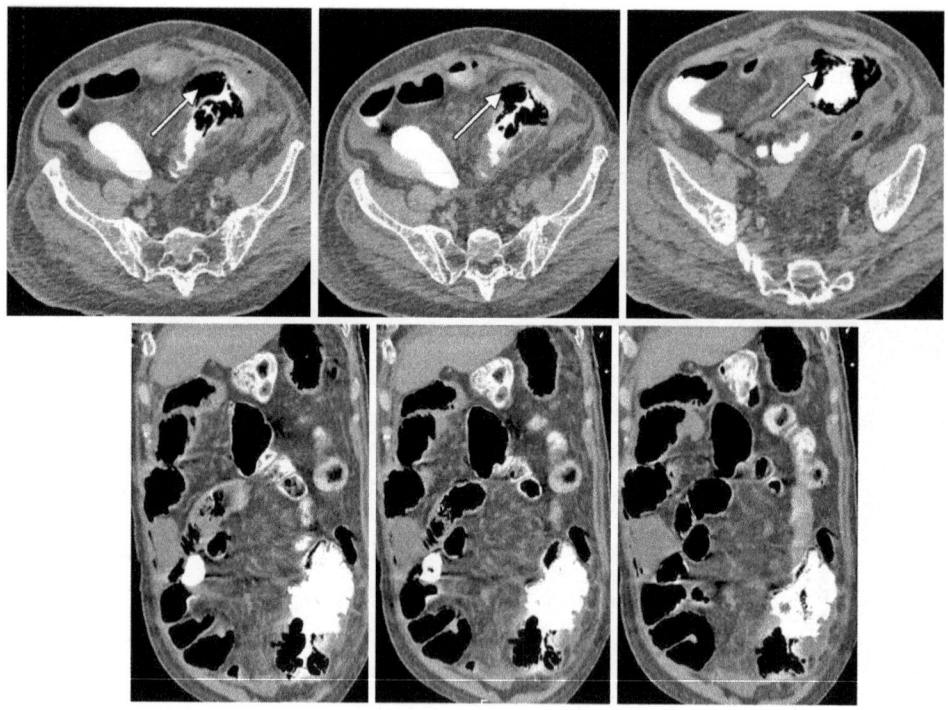

Patient started on IV antibiotics–continued to deteriorate.

31. **What is the differential diagnosis?**
    A. Ischemic bowel
    B. Amebic colitis with perforation
    C. Fungal colitis with perforation
    D. Neutropenic typhlitis

CASE 10

A 60-year-old male presented with low grade, intermittent fever, loss of weight, and appetite for duration of 4 months. He had lost about 7 kg in the past 6 months.
- General examination of the patient was normal.
- Routine blood examination, urine examination, renal function test, and chest X-ray were normal. Blood culture was sterile. The tests for malaria, tuberculosis, and HIV were negative. Ultrasonography of the abdomen revealed hepatosplenomegaly without any focal lesion. Both adrenal gland were enlarged and hypoechoic.

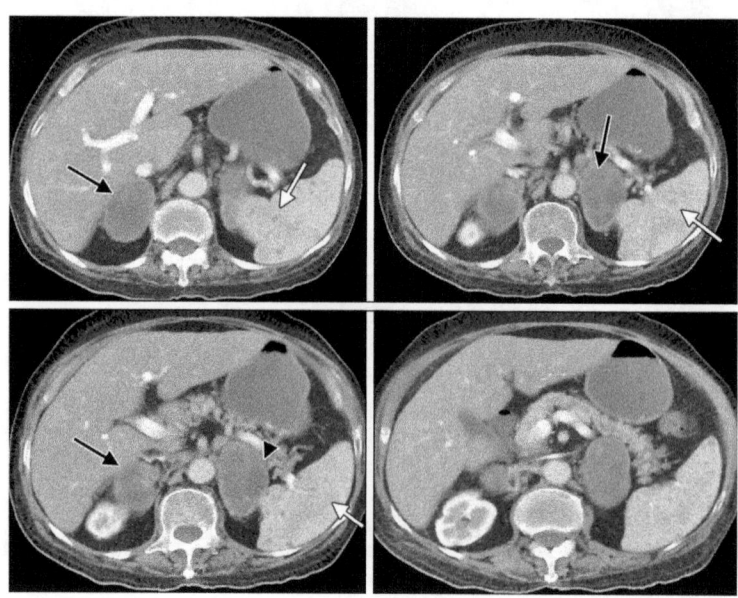

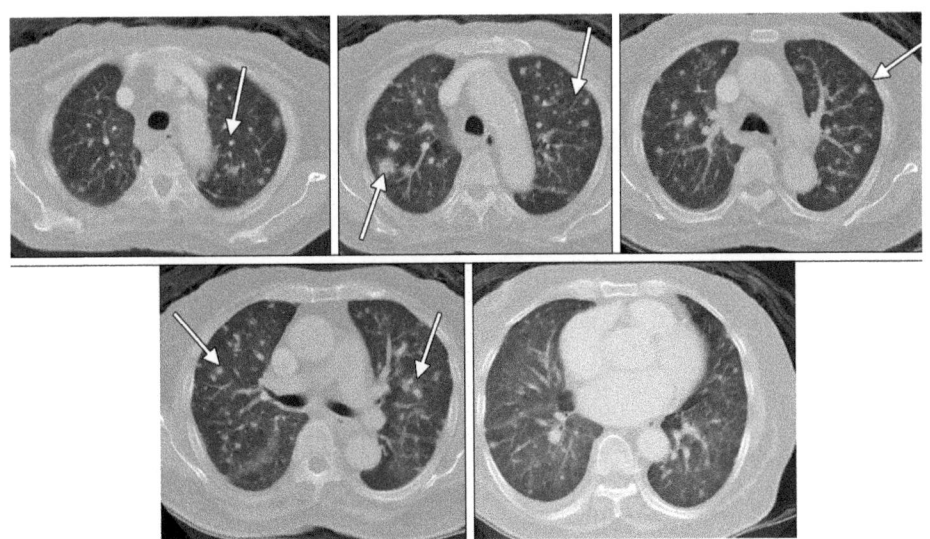

Bilateral adrenal masses with central low attenuation.
Hepatosplenomegaly with multiple hypodense lesions in spleen.
Multiple various sized pulmonary nodules.

32. **What is the differential diagnosis?**
    A. Pheochromocytoma with metastasis
    B. Primary adrenal carcinoma with metastasis
    C. Primary lung carcinoma with adrenal metastasis
    D. Granulomatous condition involving lungs/adrenals

MUSCULOSKELETAL

CASE 1

A 40-year-old with backache, fever, and tenderness over the dorsal spine.

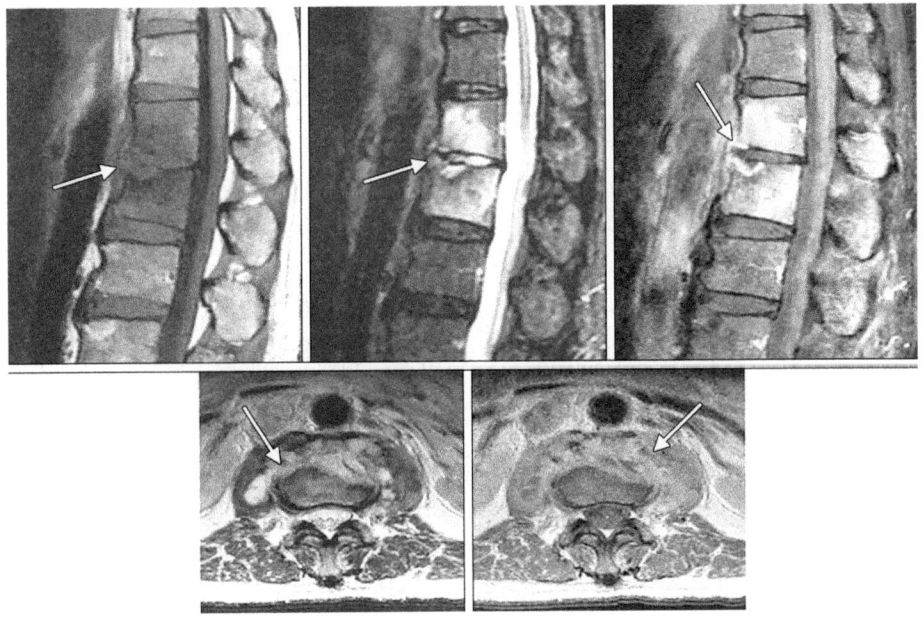

Hyperintense signal in disc with involvement of end plates, bone erosion.

33. **What is the differential diagnosis?**
    A. Pyogenic spondylitis
    B. Tuberculous infection
    C. Fungal infection
    D. Neoplastic

CASE 2

A 25-year-old female with low backache, fever.

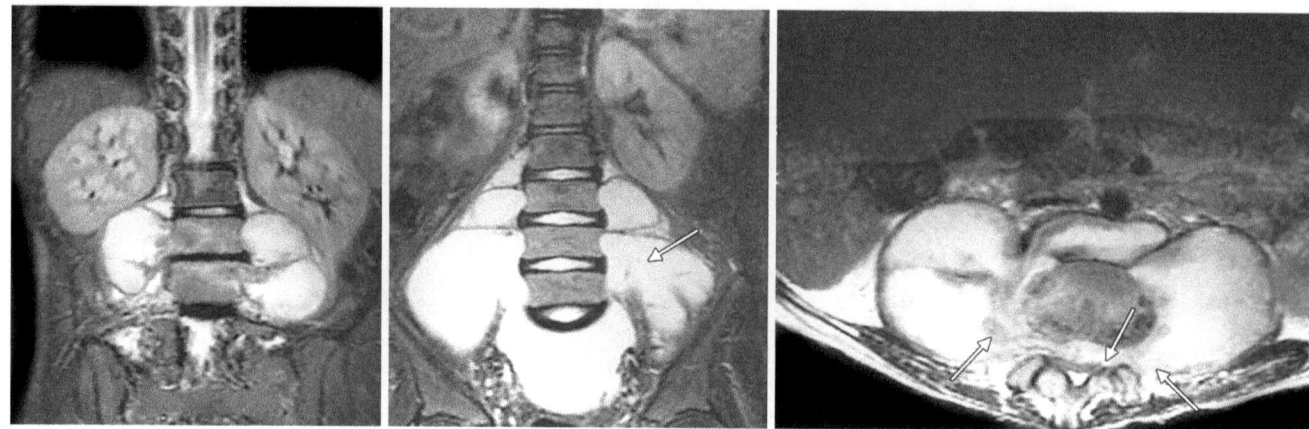

Large bilateral paravertebral abscesses with epidural extension (arrows) and associated vertebral destruction.

34. **What is the differential diagnosis?**
    A. Pyogenic spondylitis
    B. Tuberculous spondylitis with paravertebral abscess
    C. Fungal infection
    D. Neoplastic

CASE 3

A 45-year-old with backache, fever, pain with weakness in lower limbs.

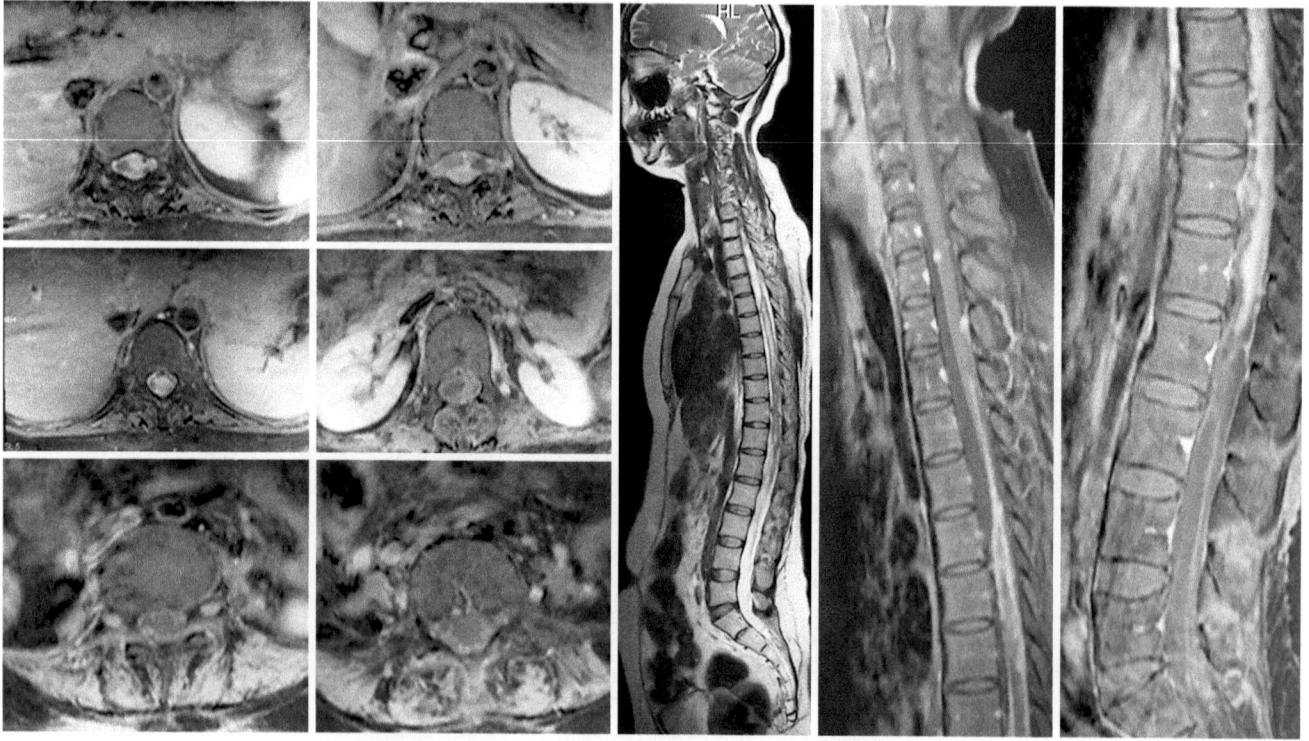

Loculated epidural collections with extensive arachnoiditis with multiple granulomas.

35. **What is the differential diagnosis?**
    A. Tuberculous arachnoiditis
    B. Metastasis
    C. Pyogenic
    D. Fungal infection

CASE 4

A 12-year-old male with history of chronic left hip and proximal thigh pain, nonradiating. No history of fever, elevated ESR or C-reactive protein. Hematologic parameters always had been within normal limits.
- *On examination*: No evidence of limb shortening, no wasting of muscles
- Difficult to flex or abduct the left leg
- No focal swelling in the left hip joint.

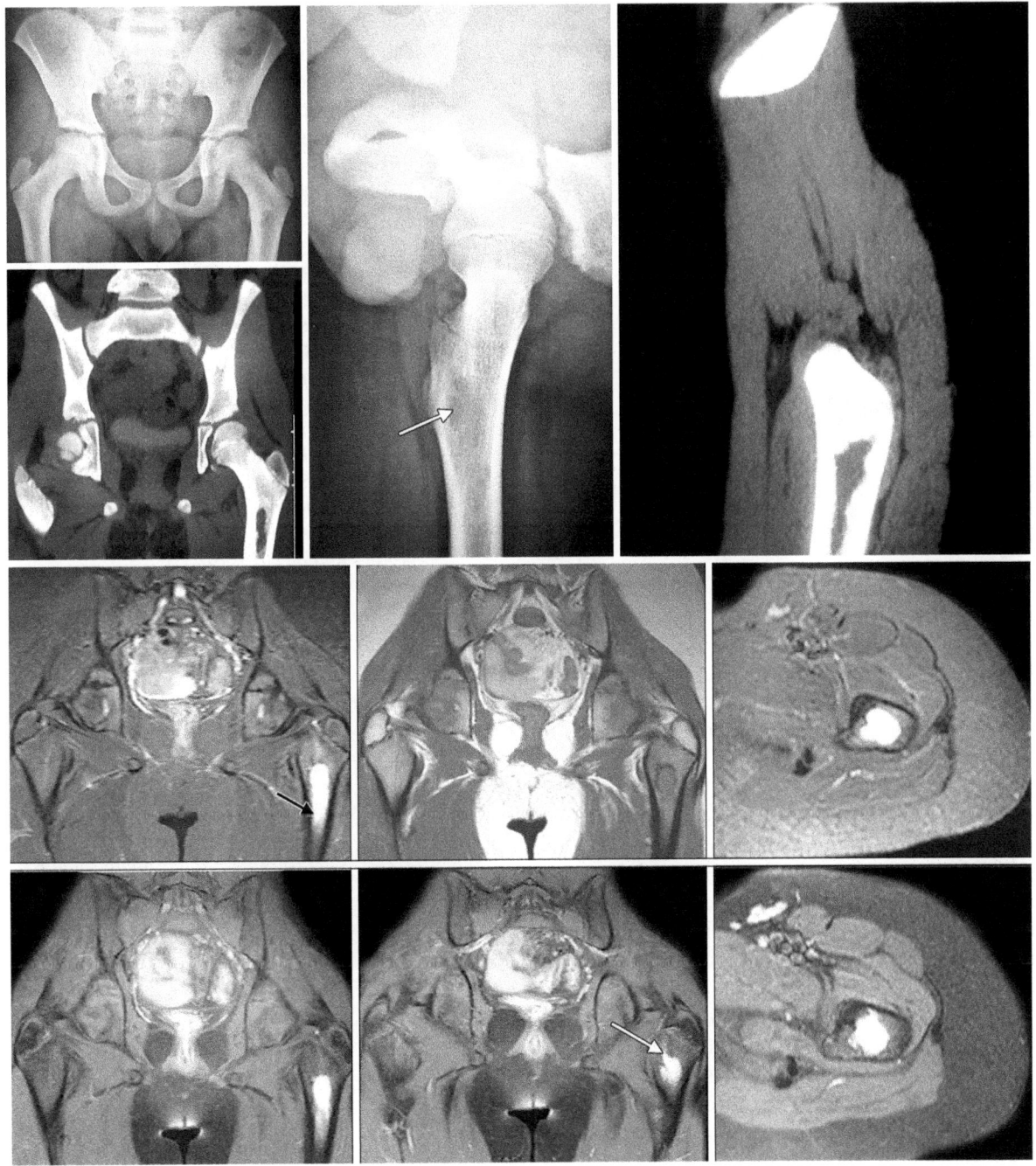

T2 hyperintense enhancing lesion in meta-diaphyseal region of left femur (black arrow) with tunneling toward the growth plate (white arrow). Lucency seen on X-ray and hypodensity on CT.

36. **What is the differential diagnosis?**

    A. Brodies abscess   B. Tuberculosis   C. Osteoid osteoma   D. Sclerosing osteomyelitis

ANSWERS WITH EXPLANATIONS

1. Ans. C

The above X-ray reveals a well-defined oval to round opacity in left lung with minimal wall calcification. The medial aspect of left hemidiaphragm is obscured; however, the left cardiac margin is well visualized through the opacity, thereby confirming the location of left lower lobe of lung. This is likely to represent a hydatid cyst.

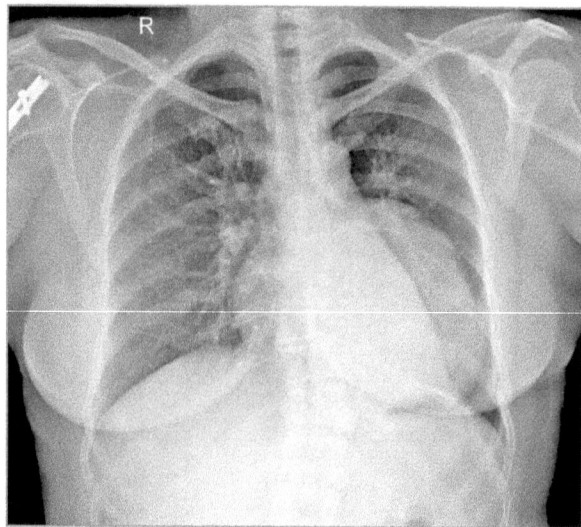

Hydatid disease is a zoonosis that can involve almost any organ in the human body by *Echinococcus* tapeworm in the larval stage.

Pulmonary hydatid infection by echinococcosis granulosus is the most common organ of involvement in children and second most common organ of involvement in adults, followed by liver.

Lungs are the second most frequent site of hematogenous spread in adults and have been reported as the most common site in children (15–25% of cases). Concurrent involvement of the liver and lungs is seen in approximately 6% of all patients. Cysts are more commonly located in lower lobes (60% cases) and can be multiple (30% cases), and bilateral (20% cases).

Uncomplicated smaller hydatid cysts of the lungs are usually asymptomatic, while larger cysts present with nonspecific clinical features such as coughing, chest pain, and hemoptysis, caused by larger cysts. Acute-onset chest pain, coughing, hemoptysis, and anaphylactic reactions may suggest cyst rupture.

X-ray features

An uncomplicated hydatid cyst appears as a well-defined homogeneous radio-opacity on a chest X-ray. Adjacent atelectasis of lung may be seen.

Cysts can assume polycyclic configuration due to pressure from adjacent structures. Notching can also occur in cysts, giving them a bilobed appearance. Calcification is very rare, but is known to occur. Multiple signs of rupture have also seen described on X-ray.

CT scan is the most standard modality for diagnosing hydatid. The early signs of rupture as well as complicated ruptured hydatid can be well evaluated on CT scan. The role of MRI for evaluation of hydatid remains minimal in adults; however, it may be used in pediatric population where radiation dose is a major concern.

Ref:
1. Gottstein B, Reichen J. Hydatid lung disease (echinococcosis/hydatidosis). Clin Chest Med. 2002;23(2):397-408.
2. Pomelov VS, Karimov SH, Nishanov KH. Surgical tactics in associated echinococcosis of the liver and lung. Khirurgiia (Mosk). 1991;11:69-74.
3. Aytac A, Yurdakul Y, Ikizler C, Olga R, Saylam A. Pulmonary hydatid disease: Report of 100 patients. Ann Thorac Surg. 1977;23:145-51.
4. Garg MK, Sharma M, Gulati A, Gorsi U, Aggarwal AN, Agarwal R, et al. Imaging in pulmonary hydit cysts. World J Radiol. 2016;8(6):581-7.
5. Balikian JP, Mudarris FF. Hydatid disease of the lungs. A roentgenologic study of 50 cases. Am J Roentgenol Radium Ther Nucl Med. 1974;122:692-707.

2. Ans. C

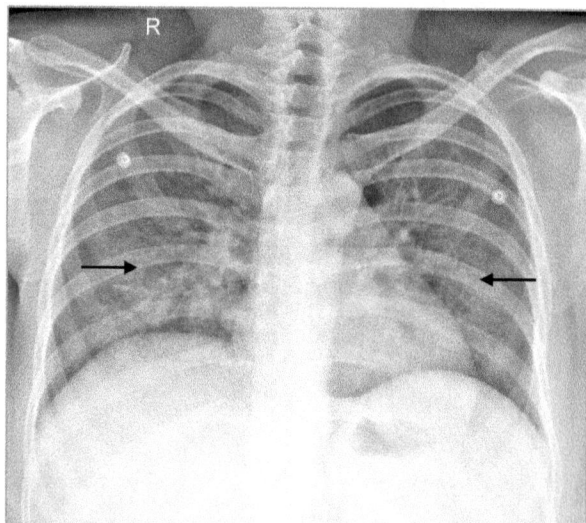

The above X-ray reveals diffuse ground-glass opacities predominantly in bilateral midzones (arrows), relatively sparing the periphery of lungs. Few small radiolucent cysts are seen in the left parahilar region. This is likely to represent PCP pneumonia.

The formation of cysts is very unlikely in the case of CMV pneumonia.

Pneumocystis jirovecii is an atypical yeast-like fungus of the genus *Pneumocystis*. Pulmonary *Pneumocystis jirovecii* infection, also referred to as *Pneumocystis jirovecii* pneumonia (PJP) and previously Pneumocystis pneumonia (PCP), is an atypical pulmonary infection and the most common opportunistic infection in immunocompromised patients, commonly seen in AIDS.

It typically occurs at CD4 counts < 200 cells/mm^3.

Features which are highly suggestive of PCP in patients with CD4 counts below 200/mm^3 include small pneumatoceles, subpleural blebs, fine reticular interstitial changes, and predominantly perihilar in distribution.

Pleural effusions are normally not a feature of PCP, seen in less than 5% of cases.

Ref:
1. Kanne JP, Yandow DR, Meyer CA. Pneumocystis jiroveci pneumonia: High-resolution CT findings in patients with and without HIV Infection. Am J Roentgenol. 2012;198:W555-61.
2. Dr Pir Abdul Ahad Aziz, Assoc Prof Frank Gaillard, et al. Hydatid disease. Radiopaedia; 2020.
3. Hidalgo A, Falcó V, Mauleón S, Andreu J, Crespo M, Ribera E, et-al. Accuracy of high-resolution CT in distinguishing between Pneumocystis carinii pneumonia and non-pneumocystis carinii pneumonia in AIDS patients. Eur Radiol. 2003;13(5):1179-84.

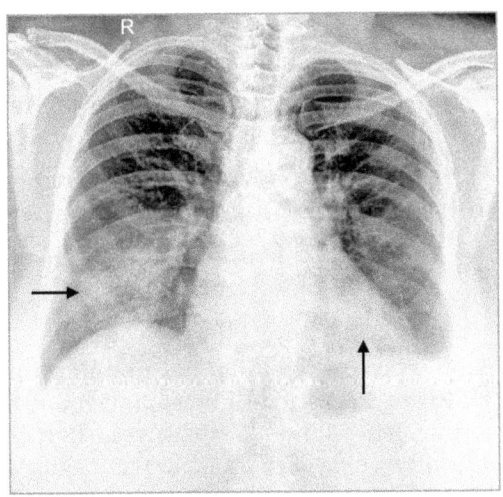

3. Ans. C

The X-ray reveals inhomogeneous patchy consolidations in right mid and lower zones with diffuse ground glass opacities in these regions (horizontal arrow). There is opacity also seen in retrocardiac region of left lung (vertical arrow) with left mild pleural effusion. Findings are likely to represent invasive fungal or fungal-like infection.

Invasive fungal and fungal-like infections contribute to substantial morbidity and mortality in immunocompromised individuals. The incidence of these infections is increasing—largely because of rising numbers of immunocompromised patients including those with neutropenia, human immunodeficiency virus, chronic immunosuppression, indwelling prostheses, burns, and diabetes mellitus, and those taking broad-spectrum antibiotics.

Invasive fungal pathogens include primary mycotic organisms such as *Histoplasma capsulatum*, *Coccidioides immitis*, *Blastomyces dermatitidis*, and *Paracoccidioides brasiliensis*, which are true pathogens and inherently virulent. Secondary mycotic organisms such as *Candida* and *Aspergillus* species, *Cryptococcus neoformans*, *Pneumocystis jirovecii*, and Mucorales fungi are opportunistic, less virulent pathogens. *Nocardia* and *Actinomyces* species are gram-positive bacteria that behave like fungi in terms of their growth pattern and cause fungal-like invasive indolent infections.

Invasive fungal and fungal-like pulmonary infections are most frequently diagnosed or suggested on the basis of chest radiographic findings and CT findings in particular. These infections have a wide spectrum of phenotypic characteristics, which range from nodules to lobar consolidations to chest wall invasion. There may be features of airway-centered bronchopneumonia with associated tree-in-bud nodules.

Ref:
1. Orlowski HLP, McWilliams S, Mellnick VM, Bhalla S, Lubner MG, Pickhardt PJ, et al. Imaging spectrum of invasive fungal and fungal-like infections. Radio Graphics. 2017;37:1119-34.
2. Connolly JE Jr, McAdams HP, Erasmus JJ, Rosado-de-Christenson ML. Opportunistic fungal pneumonia. J Thorac Imaging. 1999;14(1):51-62.

4. Ans. B

The X-ray reveals lytic lesion in L5 vertebral body (arrow). There is in addition, prevertebral soft tissue swelling seen (small arrow) with bilateral bulky psoas shadows. There are erosions seen along superior endplate of the vertebral body (arrowhead). These findings are consistent with tuberculous spondylitis.

Tuberculous spondylitis is one of the more common infections of spine in countries where TB is prevalent. It is the most common cause of vertebral body infection, with the majority of cases seen in patients under the age of 20. It is commonly associated with reduction in disk space with endplate erosions. TB can also affect the meninges of the spine, causing an intense pachymeningitis.

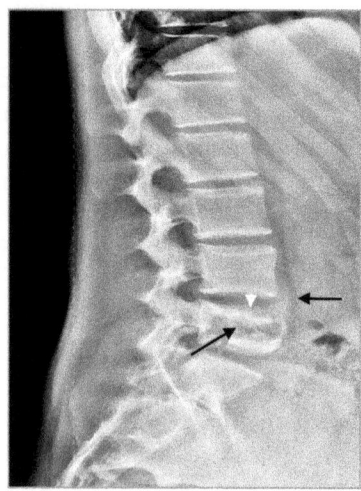

In 1779, Percivall Pott, for whom the disease is named, presented the classic description of spinal tuberculosis.

Discitis/osteomyelitis represents approximately 50% of all musculoskeletal tuberculosis, and usually affects the lower thoracic and upper lumbar levels of the spine.

MRI is the modality of choice for this, with CT with contrast being a distant second.

MRI reveals T1 hypointense and T2 and STIR hyperintense signal seen with contrast enhancement. The paraspinal collections are typically well circumscribed, with fluid centers and well-defined enhancing margins.

Ref:
1. Dr Pir Abdul Ahad Aziz, Dr Hani Makky ALSALAM, et al. Tuberculous spondylitis. Radiopaedia; 2020.
2. Burrill J, Williams CJ, Bain G, Conder G, Hine AL, Misra RR. Tuberculosis: a radiologic review. Radiographics. 2007;27(5):1255-73.
3. Hidalgo JA. Pott Disease (Tuberculous [TB] Spondylitis). Medscape; 2019.

5. **Ans. B**

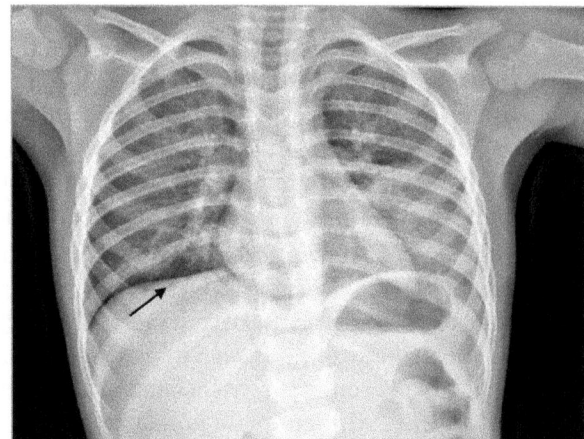

The X-ray reveals well-defined large rounded opacity in left mid and lower zones, extending into the left retrocardiac region. There is no significant air bronchogram seen within it. It does not reveal any calcification or cavitation within. It reveals irregular margins (arrow), unlike hydatids and pleuropericardial cysts which reveal well-defined smooth margins.

Round pneumonia is a type of pneumonia usually only seen in pediatric patients. They are well-defined, rounded opacities that represent regions of infected consolidation.

The mean age of patients with round pneumonia is 5 years. Round pneumonia is uncommon after the age of eight because collateral airways tend to be well developed by this age.

They are well-circumscribed with irregular margins. 98% times they are solitary.

Air bronchograms are often seen, however, rarely seen when it occurs in adults.

Ref:
1. Wagner AL, Szabunio M, Hazlett KS, Wagner SG. Radiologic manifestations of round pneumonia in adults. Am J Roentgenol. 1998;170(3):723-6.
2. Kim YW, Donnelly LF. Round pneumonia: imaging findings in a large series of children. Pediatr Radiol. 2007;37(12):1235-40.

6. **Ans. D**

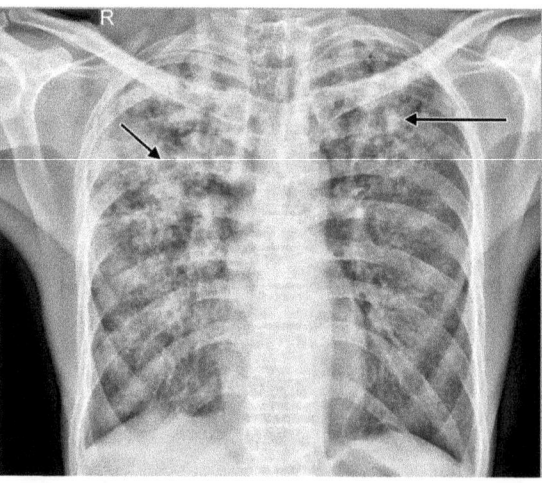

The X-ray reveals bilateral nodular and patchy infiltrates (long arrow) in apical, upper, and mid zones (right > left) with *cavitary* changes (short arrow) and few intervening fibrobronchiectatic changes. There is blunting of bilateral costophrenic angles suggestive of mild pleural effusion.

Tuberculosis (TB) is caused by mycobacterial species in the *Mycobacterium tuberculosis* complex. The lungs are the most common site of primary infection by TB and are a major source of spread of the disease.

Active disease can occur as primary tuberculosis, developing shortly after infection or postprimary tuberculosis, developing after a long period of latent infection.

Primary TB demonstrates radiologic findings that include lymphadenopathy, consolidation, pleural effusion, and miliary nodules. Postprimary TB demonstrates consolidations that are predominant in the apical and upper lung zones, nodules, and cavitation. Primary tuberculosis demonstrates radiologic findings that include lymphadenopathy, consolidation, pleural effusion, and miliary nodules. Postprimary TB demonstrates consolidations that are predominant in the apical and upper lung zones, nodules, and cavitation. Chest CT may be useful in identifying active TB even if the chest radiograph is negative, although chest CT is not the standard of practice.

In postprimary tuberculosis, cavitation is a common finding, seen in 20–45% of patients on chest radiographs. These have thick and irregular walls. Cavitary lesions are often seen within areas of consolidation and may be multifocal. Residual cavities may persist after treatment, findings that predispose to bacterial superinfection, mycetoma formation, or erosion of adjacent vasculature resulting in hemoptysis. The presence of an air-fluid level within a cavity may be related to the TB itself or to bacterial superinfection.

Ref:
1. Centers for Disease Control and Prevention. Self-study modules on tuberculosis. [online] Available from: http://www.cdc.gov/tb/education/ssmodules/. [Last accessed February, 2020]
2. Burrill J, Williams CJ, Bain G, Conder G, Hine AL, Misra RR. Tuberculosis: a radiologic review. Radiographics. 2007;27(5):1255-73.
3. Nachiappan AC, Rahbar K, Shi X, Guy ES, Barbosa EJM Jr, Shroff GS, et al. Pulmonary tuberculosis: Role of radiology in diagnosis and management. Radiographics. 2017;37(1):52-72.
4. Lee SW, Jang YS, Park CM, Kang HY, Koh WJ, Yim JJ, et al. The role of chest CT scanning in TB outbreak investigation. Chest. 2010;137(5):1057-64.

7. **Ans. A**

    The X-ray reveals diffusely scattered tiny noncalcified lung parenchymal nodules, approximately 1–3 mm in size (arrows). This is called "miliary mottling" and in the given clinical scenario consistent with miliary tuberculosis. The other differential diagnosis (DDs) of fungal etiology and miliary metastasis may be made in the light of clinical history. The other causes include pulmonary microlithiasis, miliary sarcoidosis, etc.

    The term miliary opacities refer to innumerable, small 1–4 mm pulmonary nodules scattered throughout the lungs. It is useful to divide these patients into those who are febrile and those who are not. It also helps to minimize the differentials on the basis of calcified and noncalcified nodules.

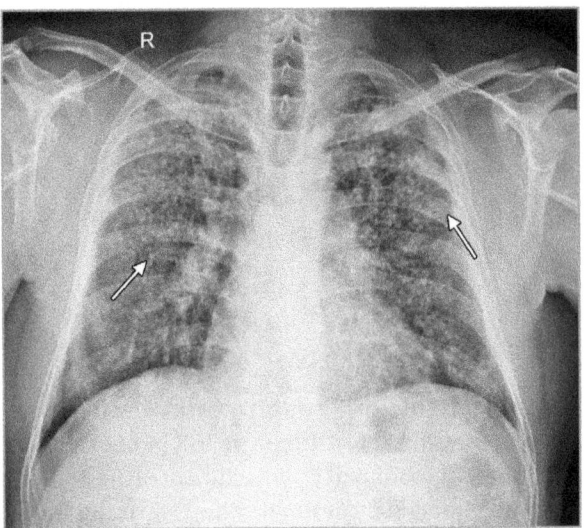

    Hematogenous dissemination results in miliary tuberculosis, especially in immunocompromised and pediatric patients. Miliary disease may occur in primary or postprimary tuberculosis. In primary tuberculosis, miliary disease often manifests as an acute, severe illness with high mortality.

    On the chest radiograph or CT image, miliary disease manifests as diffuse 1–3 mm nodules in a random distribution. Miliary TB is spread by hematogenous seeding, as demonstrated by the finding of a miliary nodule centered on a small blood vessel.

    Ref:
    1. Dr Daniel J Bell, Assoc Prof Frank Gaillard et al. Miliary opacities (lungs). Radiopaedia; 2019.
    2. Marchiori E, Souza AS, Franquet T, Müller NL. Diffuse high-attenuation pulmonary abnormalities: A pattern-oriented diagnostic approach on high-resolution CT. Am J Roentgenol. 2005;184(1):273-82.
    3. Rahbar K, Shi X, Guy ES, Barbosa EJM Jr, Shroff GS, Ocazionez D, et al. Pulmonary tuberculosis: Role of radiology in diagnosis and management. Radiographics. 2017;37(1):52-72.

8. **Ans. D**

    The given X-ray reveals a large left-sided hydropneumothorax due to ruptured pulmonary hydatid with left-sided chest drain in situ. There are two ovoid cysts seen in the collapsed left lung (white arrows) and one floating in the left pleural fluid (rising sun sign—black arrow).

    There is hydatid disease, which is a worldwide parasitic infection caused by the larval stage of *Echinococcus* tapeworm.

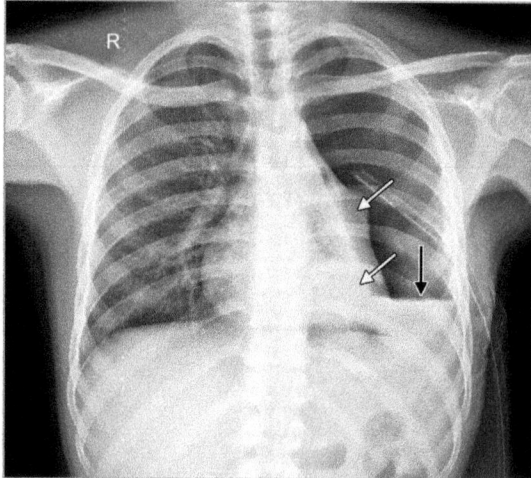

A hydatid cyst rupture is the most common complication occurring in up to 49% of cases. Ruptures may be contained (by detachment of the pericyst from the endocyst), communicating (with the bronchus), and direct (rupture of all membranes with spillage of contents).

The risk of rupture increases with the size and number of cysts.

Antihelminthic therapy and percutaneous aspiration are also known to cause cyst rupture and fatal complications. Cyst rupture can occur into bronchus (manifesting as coughing with sputum containing hydatid sand and membrane fragments) or the pleural cavity (manifesting as pneumothorax, effusion, and emphysema). Infection is the most common complication of cyst rupture, clinically presenting with features of lung abscess.

Uncomplicated hydatid cyst	Complicated hydatid cyst
Well circumscribed round radio-opacity (resembling canon ball on AP and rugby ball on lateral projection)	Crescent sign
Polycyclic and bilobed appearance	Cumbo or double arch sign
Slot sign (impending rupture)	Water lily or camelotte sign
	Rising sun sign
	Dry cyst sign

Ref:
1. Mehta P, Prakash M, Khandelwal N. Radiological manifestations of hydatid disease and its complications. Trop Parasitol. 2016;6(2):103-12.
2. Garg MK, Sharma M, Gulati A, Gorsi U, Aggarwal An, Agarwal R, et al. Imaging in pulmonary hydatid cysts. World J Radiol. 2016;8(6):581-7.
3. Moreno González E, Rico Selas P, Martínez B, García García I, Palma Carazo F, Hidalgo Pascual M. Results of surgical treatment of hepatic hydatidosis: current therapeutic modifications. World J Surg. 1991;15:254-63.

9. **Ans. C**

There is reduction in C4/C5 disc space (long arrow) with erosions and sclerosis along endplates. There is prevertebral soft tissue swelling seen (small arrows). There is addition in grade 1 retrolisthesis of C4 over C5 vertebral body with loss of cervical lordosis.

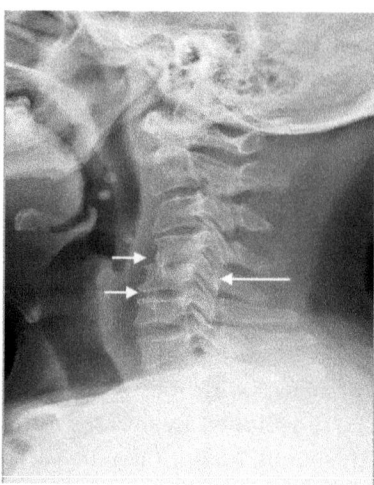

It is characterized by infection involving the intervertebral disk and adjacent vertebrae.

Spondylodiscitis has a bimodal age distribution, which many authors consider essentially as separate entities: (1) pediatric and (2) older population ~50 years

Discitis/osteomyelitis represents approximately 50% of all musculoskeletal tuberculosis, and usually affects the lower thoracic and upper lumbar levels of the spine.

Plain radiography is insensitive to the early changes of discitis/osteomyelitis, with normal appearances being maintained for up to 2-4 weeks. Thereafter, disc space narrowing and irregularity or ill definition of the vertebral endplates can be seen. In untreated cases, bony sclerosis may begin to appear in 10-12 weeks.

The earliest findings are radiolucencies and the loss of definition of the plate margins. The most common appearance consists of vertebral body destruction (predominantly anterior), loss of disc height, erosion of end plates, vertebral geodes, bone sequestration, sclerosis, and paravertebral masses. Calcification in paraspinal masses is highly suggestive of TB. However, the height of disc space can be preserved until the later stages of the infection.

Advanced stages of the disease are characterized by: Sclerosis from reparative processes, bony ankylosis, vertebral collapse and anterior wedging leading to progressive kyphosis and gibbus deformity.

Ref:
1. Dr Bahman Rasuli, Assoc Prof Frank Gaillard, et al. Spondylodiskitis. Radiopaedia; 2020.

2. Burrill J, Williams CJ, Bain G, Conder G, Hine AL, Misra RR. Tuberculosis: a radiologic review. Radiographics. 2007;27(5):1255-73.
3. Rivas-Garcia A, Sarria-Estrada S, Torrents-Odin C, Casas-Gomila L, Franquet E. Imaging findings of Pott's disease. Eur Spine J. 2013;22(Suppl 4):567-78.

10. Ans. C

There is reduction in D7/D8 and D8/D9 disc spaces (long arrows) with paravertebral shadows (small arrows), suggestive of Potts spine. Thickening of right paratracheal stripe (dotted arrow) is due to enlarged paratracheal lymph node, also tuberculous in etiology.

Tuberculosis continues to be an important public health problem in developed countries especially in deprived socioeconomic groups, older people, immunocompromised patients, drug-therapy resistant cases, and the immigrant population.

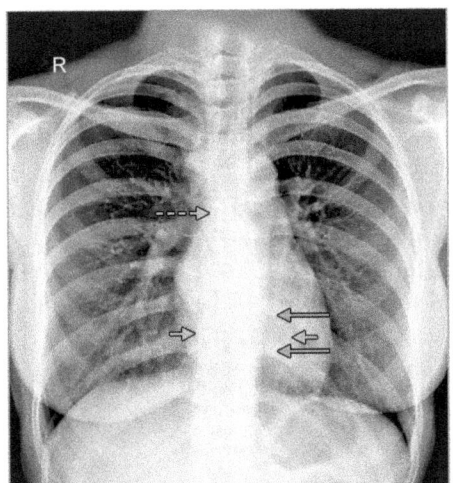

Diagnosis of TB cannot be established solely on the basis of clinical tests or imaging findings and biopsy may be required. Differential diagnosis between tuberculous and pyogenic spondylitis is of clinical importance, but may be difficult on the basis of radiological findings alone. Findings not pathognomonic but favoring tuberculous etiology include slow progression of lesions with late preservation of disc space, involvement of several contiguous segments, large intraosseous and paraspinal abscesses containing calcifications, and body collapse with kyphotic deformity.

The thoracic segments are the preferred sites in which infection spreads, followed by the lumbar levels.

The earliest findings are radiolucencies and the loss of definition of the plate margins. The most common appearance consists of vertebral body destruction (predominantly anterior), loss of disc height, erosion of end plates, vertebral geodes, bone sequestration, sclerosis, and paravertebral masses.

Advanced stages of the disease are characterized by: sclerosis from reparative processes, bony ankylosis, vertebral collapse, and anterior wedging leading to progressive kyphosis and gibbus deformity.

Ref:
1. Rivas-Garcia A, Sarria-Estrada S, Torrents-Odin C, Casas-Gomila L, Franquet E. Imaging findings at pott's disease. Eur Spine J. 2013;22(Suppl 4):567-78.
2. Cormican L, Hammal R, Messenger J, Milburn HJ. Current difficulties in the diagnosis and management of spinal tuberculosis. Postgrad Med J. 2006;82:46-51.
3. Jain R, Sawhney S, Berry M. Computed tomography of vertebral tuberculosis: patterns of bone destruction. Clin Radiol. 1993;47:196-9.
4. Lindahl S, Nyman RS, Brismar J, Hugosson C, Lundstedt C. Imaging of tuberculosis. IV. Spinal manifestations in 63 patients. Acta Radiol. 1996;37:506-11.
5. Moore SL, Rafii M. Imaging of musculoskeletal and spinal tuberculosis. Radiol Clin North Am. 2001;39(2):329-42.
6. Jevtic V. Vertebral infection. Eur Radiol. 2004;14:E43-52.

11. Ans. A

There is widening of left hip joint space with articular erosions. There are osteopenic areas seen in head of femur and acetabulum (arrows) with mild sclerosis. There is swelling surrounding the left hip joint.

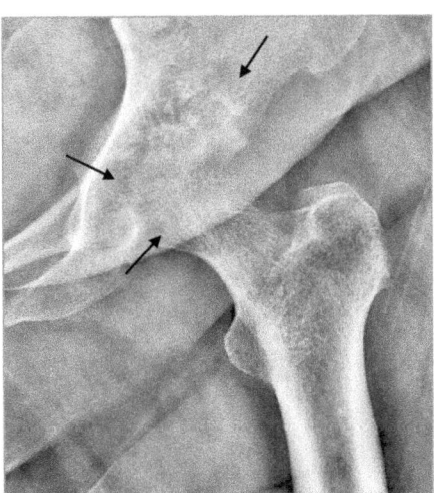

The diagnosis of joint sepsis is often considered straightforward. Patients often present with a painful joint, fever, and purulent synovial fluid.

In general, infectious arthritis is classified as pyogenic (septic) or nonpyogenic. Pyogenic septic arthritis is caused by *Staphylococcus aureus* in up to 80% of cases followed by other pathogens such as staphylococci, streptococci, *Gonococcus* species, *Escherichia coli*, *Haemophilus*, *Klebsiella*, *Pseudomonas*, and *Candida*.

X-rays may be normal in the very early stage of the disease.

Radiological features include joint effusion, juxta-articular osteoporosis due to hyperemia, narrowing of the joint space due cartilage destruction in the acute phase, destruction of the subchondral bone on both sides of a joint if left untreated, reactive juxta-articular sclerosis, and in severe cases, ankylosis develops.

If the patient is hemodynamically stable then attempts should be made to obtain a sample of joint fluid for microscopy and culture prior to starting treatment with antibiotics. This will allow focused treatment of the infection.

Ref:
1. *Bickle I, Radswiki, et al. Septic arthritis. Radiopaedia; 2020.*
2. *Nunez-Atahualpa L. Septic arthritis imaging. [online] Available from: https://emedicine.medscape.com/article/395381-overview [Last accessed February, 2020].*
3. *Goldenberg DL, Brandt KD, Cohen AS, Cathcart ES. Treatment of septic arthritis. Arthritis Rheum. 1975;18(1):83.*

12. **Ans. D**

There is widening of left sacroiliac joint space with subarticular sclerosis and articular erosions suggestive of infective sacroiliitis, proved to be tuberculous in etiology on biopsy.

Of all TB, approximately 10% occurs at the sacroiliac joint.

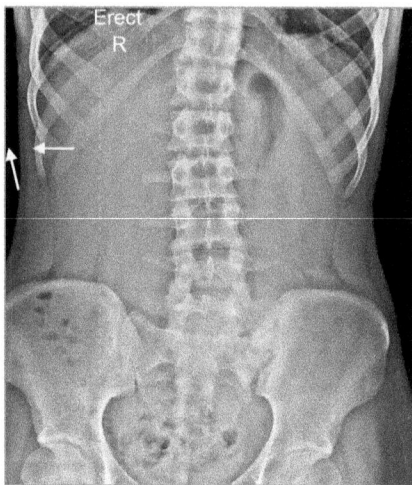

The joint is a synchondrosis and the hyaline cartilage is thinner on the ilial surface when compared to the sacral side. The presenting symptoms of sacroiliitis are vague and the distribution of pain varies due to close relationship between the joint, the lumbosacral plexus, and the ability of the abscess to track in any direction. Pain is worsened by walking, sitting, and physical activity.

X-rays reveal haziness initially, but this is replaced by joint widening, sclerosis of the margins, and possible sequestrae in the joint in the more advanced stages.

CT scans demonstrate the joint space widening, sequestrate, and calcification more clearly than X-rays. Earliest signs of capsular distension, bone edema, and destruction can be picked up on MRI.

In the early stages of the infection, aspiration using a closed needle biopsy is recommended. An open biopsy is essential when the aspirate yields no growth and in patients who present late with severe joint destruction as in our group of patients. Following the diagnosis and commencement of chemotherapy, bony ankylosis is to be expected.

Ref:
1. *Davies PD, Humphries MJ, Byfield SP, Nunn AJ, Darbyshire JH, Citron KM, et al. Bone and joint tuberculosis. A survey of notifications in England and Wales. J Bone Joint Surg Br. 1984;66(3):326-30.*
2. *Ramlakan RJS, Govender S. Sacroiliac joint tuberculosis. Int Orthop. 2007;31(1):121-4.*
3. *Kim NH, Lee HM, Yoo JD, Suh JS. Sacroiliac joint tuberculosis—classification and treatment. Clin Orthop Relat Res. 1999;358:215-22.*
4. *Attarian DE. Septic sacroiliitis: the overlooked diagnosis. J South Orthop Assoc. 2001;10(1):57-60.*

13. **Ans. D**

There are multiple small calcific opacities seen overlying the chest, neck, axillae and bilateral proximal arms resembling rice grain. This is pathognomonic of cysticercus infection in soft tissues.

Cysticercosis is a parasitic tissue infection caused by ingestion of tapeworm eggs through a fecal oral transmission or autoinfection. Humans act as a definitive host in this disease. The etiological agent is the tapeworm taenia solium.

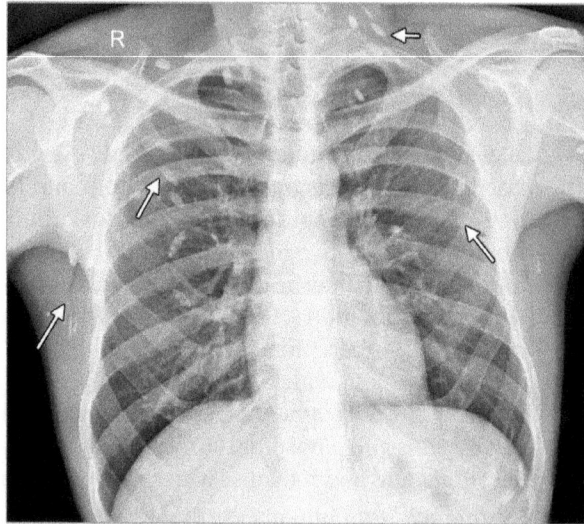

If the eggs contaminate food sources, upon ingestion they develop into larvae and result in cysticercosis. Hence, even people who do not consume pork, including vegetarians, can develop cysticercosis.

In skeletal muscles, cysticerci appear as oblong calcific specks in the skeletal muscles parallel to the muscle fibers, giving a characteristic appearance which has been termed rice-grain calcification owing to its resemblance to rice grains.

USG is an inexpensive, readily available, and radiation-free modality for the diagnosis of soft tissue cysticercosis. The most common USG appearance of soft tissue cysticercosis that we encountered in this study was that of an intramuscular abscess with an eccentrically situated typical cyst with a scolex within.

Ref:
1. Bell DJ, Firke V, et al. Cysticercosis. Radiopaedia; 2020.
2. Mittal A, Das D, Aiyer N, Nagaraj J, Gupta M. Masseter cysticercosis—a rare case diagnosed in ultrasound. Dentomaxillofac Radiol. 2008;37:113-6.
3. Naik D, Srinath MG, Kumar A. Soft tissue cysticercosis-Ultrasonographic spectrum of the disease. Indian J Radiol. 2011;21(1):60-2.

14. Ans. B

There are extensive patchy opacities seen in both lungs (arrows). There is relative sparing of the periphery and costophrenic angles. This is likely to represent ARDS in the given clinical setting.

Acute respiratory distress syndrome is a form of acute lung injury (ALI) and occurs as a result of a severe pulmonary injury that causes alveolar damage heterogeneously throughout the lung. It can either result from a direct pulmonary source or as a response to systemic injury.

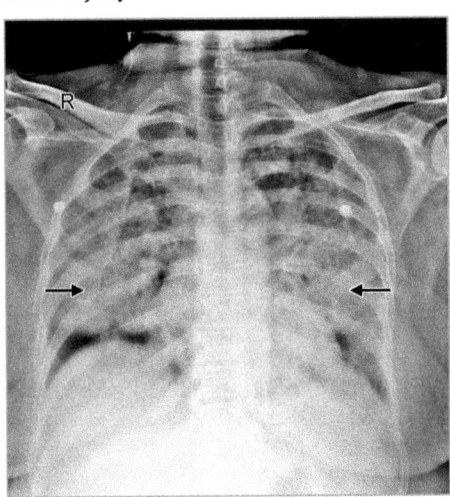

Chest radiographic findings of acute respiratory distress syndrome are nonspecific and resemble those of typical pulmonary edema or pulmonary hemorrhage. There are diffused bilateral coalescent opacities (the only radiological criterion defined by the Consensus Conference). The time course of ARDS may help in differentiating it from typical pulmonary edema.

Chest X-ray features usually develop 12-24 hours after initial lung insult as a result of proteinaceous interstitial edema. Within 1 week, alveolar pulmonary edema (hyaline membrane) occurs due to type 1 pneumocyte damage.

In contrast to cardiogenic pulmonary edema, which clears in response to diuretic therapy, ARDS persists for days to weeks. Also, as the initial radiographic findings of ARDS clear, the underlying lung appears to have a reticular pattern secondary to type 2 pneumocyte proliferation and fibrosis.

The role of chest radiography has been recognized since the first definition of ARDS. Lung opacities are bilateral, diffuse, patchy or homogeneous, involving at least three quadrants and cannot be fully explained by pleural effusion, atelectasis, or nodules.

In malaria, increased alveolar capillary permeability leading to intravascular fluid loss into the lungs is the main pathophysiologic mechanism. This defines malaria as another cause of ALI and ARDS. Pulmonary edema has been described most often in nonimmune individuals with *Plasmodium falciparum* infections as part of a severe systemic illness or as the main feature of acute malaria. *P. vivax* and *P. ovale* have also rarely caused pulmonary edema.

Ref:
1. Bell DJ, Amini B. Acute respiratory distress syndrome. [online] Available from: https://radiopaedia.org/articles/acute-respiratory-distress-syndrome-1 [Last accessed February, 2020].
2. Zompatori M, Ciccarese F, Fasano L. Overview of current lung imaging in acute respiratory distress syndrome. Eur Respir Rev. 2014;23:519-30.
3. Taylor WR1, Cañon V, White NJ. Pulmonary manifestations of malaria: recognition and management. Treat Respir Med. 2006;5(6):419-28.

CHEST

15. Ans. B

- Lobar consolidation with small cavity in right upper lobe showing rapid increase in size should raise possibility nocardiosis in setting of immunocompromised host.
- Sputum–Nocardia.
- IV Meropenem started.

Nocardiosis
- *Pulmonary nocardiosis* is an infrequent but severe opportunistic infection typified by necrotic or cavitary consolidation in an immunocompromised patient
- Most commonly caused by *Nocardia asteroides*
- Lobar or multilobar consolidation
    - Probably the predominant feature
    - Focal areas of decreased attenuation may reflect abscess formation
    - Cavitation in 30%
- Solitary lung masses and/or nodules.

Ref:
1. Kanne JP, Yandow DR, Mohammed TL, Meyer CA. CT findings of pulmonary nocardiosis. Am J Roentgenol. 2011;197(2):W266-72.
2. Buckley JA, Padhani AR, Kuhlman JE. CT features of pulmonary nocardiosis. J Comput Assist Tomogr. 1995;19(5):726-32.

16. Ans. B

- Throat swab sent for *H1N1*—positive
- *Oseltamivir*—improved

  H1N1—Caused by a type of influenza A virus of swine origin.

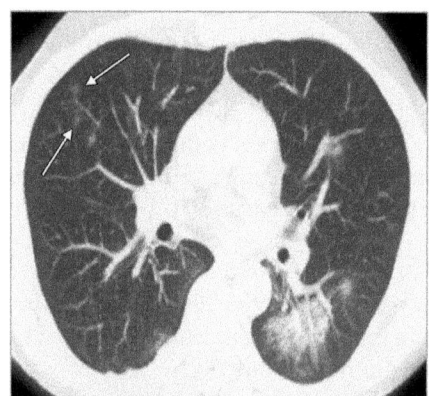

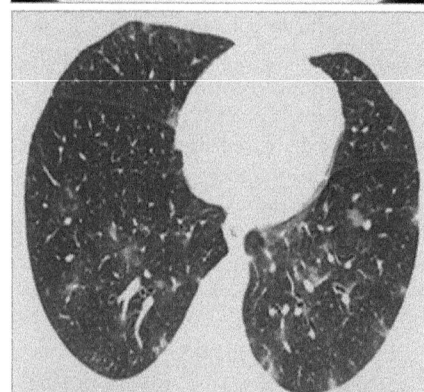

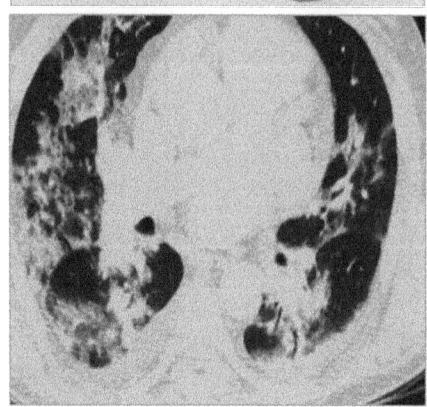

The predominant CT findings:

- Ground-glass opacities, areas of consolidation, or a mixed pattern of ground-glass opacities and areas of consolidation.
- Frequently bilateral; peripheral subpleural, peribronchovascular, lobular or random distribution.
- May be diffuse without zonal predominance.
- More rarely, unilateral.

  The main patterns of disease that are most suggestive of H1N1 are scattered lung consolidations, ground-glass opacities, or both in a peribronchovascular or subpleural distribution.

Opravil scoring in H1N1

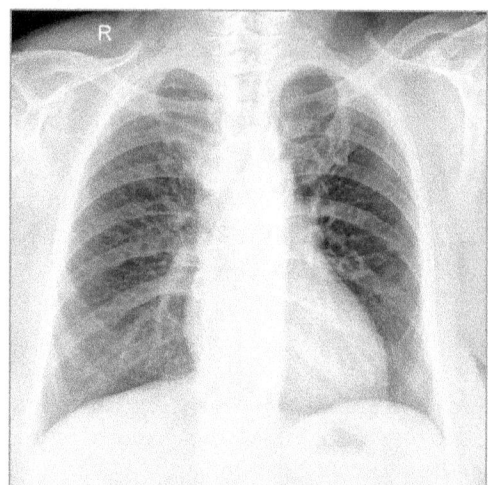

- In chest radiograph, each lung was divided into four regions with a total of eight regions in both lungs
- The radiological appearances were scored as follows:
  - 0—Normal
  - 1—Interstitial pattern
  - 2—Ground-glass pattern
  - 3—Consolidation
- This system allows a maximum score of 24 for both lungs.
- A higher score (>12) has been found to correlate well with a longer duration of hospital stay, the need for mechanical ventilation, and overall patient morbidity.
- Scoring allows a triage of H1N1 patients and predicting the need for invasive mechanical ventilation.

  Ref:
  1. *Agarwal PP, Cinti S, Kazerooni EA. Chest radiographic and CT findings in novel swine-origin influenza A (H1N1) virus (S-OIV) infection. Am J Roentgenol. 2009;193(6):1488-93.*
  2. *Aviram G, Bar-Shai A, Sosna J, Rogowski O, Rosen G, Weinstein I, et-al. H1N1 influenza: initial chest radiographic findings in helping predict patient outcome. Radiology. 2010;255(1):252-9.*
  3. *Elicker BM, Schwartz BS, Liu C, Chen EC, Miller SA, Chiu CY, et-al. Thoracic CT findings of novel influenza A (H1N1) infection in immunocompromised patients. Emerg Radiol. 2010;17(4):299-307.*

17. Ans. A

Likely CMV pneumonia, other possibility of miliary TB should be considered.

- Sputum was sent for AFB and C/S—Negative
- CMV PCR—Positive.

CMV pneumonia

- Frequent in immunosuppressed patients

- Characteristically presents with fever, pulmonary infiltrates, and hypoxia resulting in acute respiratory distress syndrome (ARDS)
- Patchy B/L foci of GGO or consolidation

- Scattered poorly defined nodules, masses
- Small nodules, diffuse
- Abnormalities tend to be B/L and symmetric
- Reticulation and septal thickening (resolving disease).

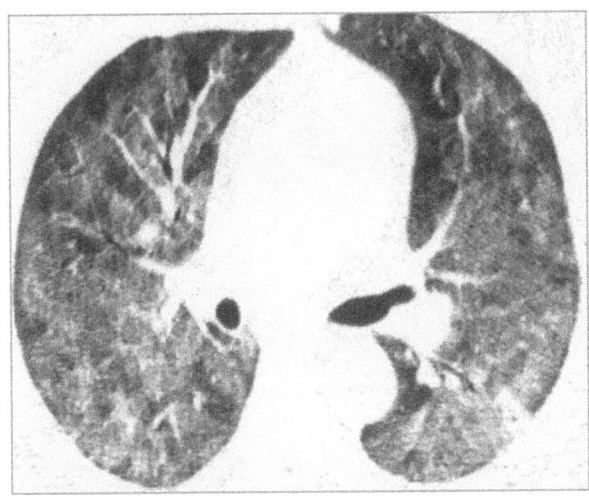
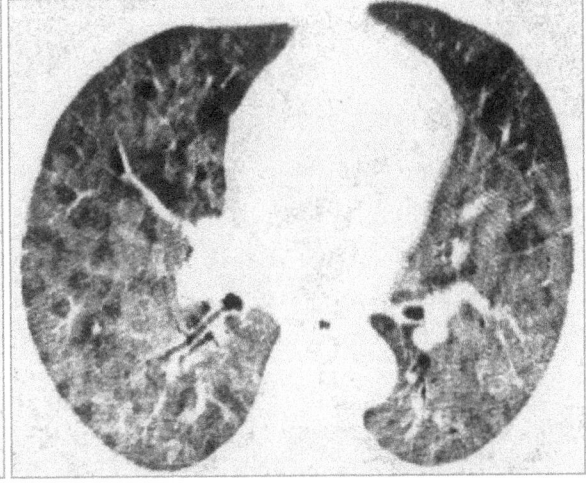

Ref:
1. Moon JH, Kim EA, Lee KS, Kim TS, Jung KJ, Song JH. Cytomegalovirus pneumonia: High-resolution CT findings in ten non-AIDS immunocompromised patients. Korean J Radiol. 2002;1(2):73-8.
2. Horger MS, Pfannenberg C, Einsele H, Beck R, Hebart H, Lengerke C, et al. Cytomegalovirus pneumonia after stem cell transplantation: Correlation of CT findings with clinical outcome in 30 patients. Am J Roentgenol. 2006;187(6):W636-43.

18. **Ans. A**

Aspergillosis
- Infection with a fungus of the *Aspergillus* species (usually *Aspergillus fumigatus*)
- Pulmonary Involvement
- Aspergilloma (saprophytic/noninvasive aspergillosis): The most common form seen radiographically

- Allergic bronchopulmonary aspergillosis (ABPA)
- Invasive aspergillosis:
  - Subacute invasive pulmonary aspergillosis [previously termed—chronic necrotizing aspergillosis (CNA) or semi-invasive aspergillosis]
  - Airway invasive aspergillosis (or bronchopneumonic aspergillosis)
  - Angioinvasive aspergillosis
- Obstructive bronchopulmonary aspergillosis.

Angioinvasive aspergillosis: Seen in immunocompromised hosts
- Nodules or focal consolidation with surrounding ground-glass attenuation (halo sign)
- Wedge-shaped pleural-based areas of consolidation.

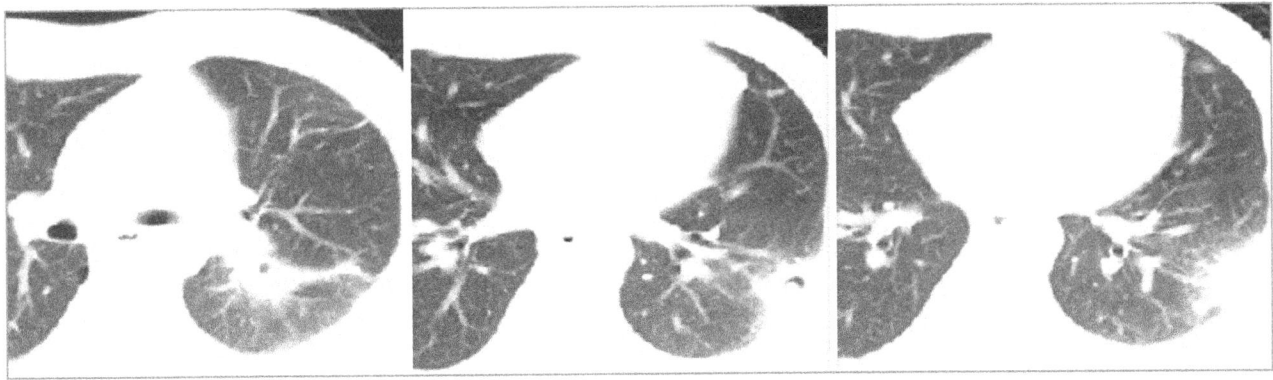

Aspergillus bronchiolitis and bronchopneumonia (airway invasive aspergillosis):
- Patchy peribronchial or lobular consolidation
- Small centrilobular nodules.

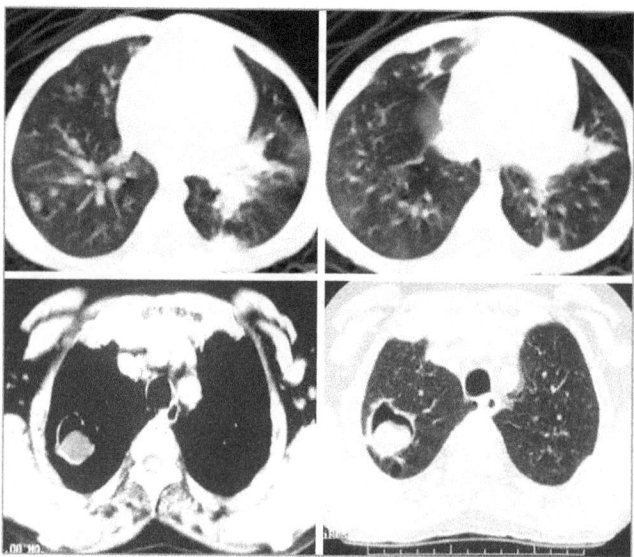

Aspergilloma

Cavitary lesion in right lobe fungal ball.
- Aspergillomas are mass-like fungus balls that are typically composed of *Aspergillus fumigatus* and are a noninvasive form of pulmonary aspergillosis.
- Aspergilloma can be seen on both plain film and CT as an intracavitary mass surrounded by a crescent of air.
- Correct term to describe the crescent of air is the Monod sign in the setting of aspergilloma developing in a pre-existing cavity.

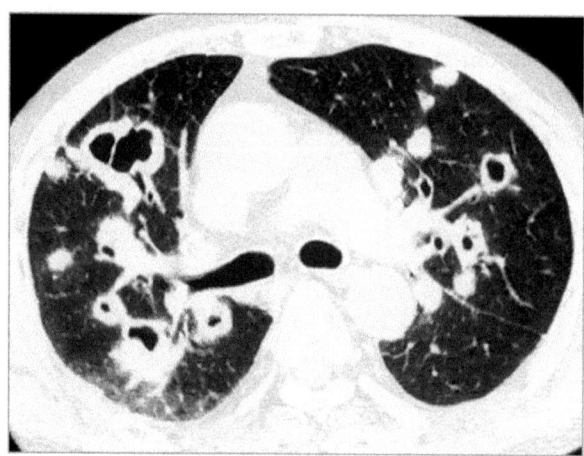

Allergic bronchopulmonary aspergillosis:
- Mild form of aspergillosis.
- Central, upper lobe saccular bronchiectasis involving segmental and subsegmental bronchi is characteristic mucoid impaction, results in a *bronchocele*.

Ref:
1. Franquet T, Müller NL, Giménez A, Guembe P, de La Torre J, Bagué S. Spectrum of pulmonary aspergillosis: histologic, clinical, and radiologic findings. Radiographics. 2001;21(4):825-37.
2. Kosmidis C, Denning DW. The clinical spectrum of pulmonary aspergillosis. Thorax. 2015;70(3):270-7.

19. Ans. A

Pulmonary tuberculosis
- Pulmonary manifestations of TB are varied and depend in part whether the infection is primary or postprimary
- The location of infection within the lung varies with both the stage of infection and age of the patient
- Primary infection can be anywhere in the lung in children whereas there is a predilection for the upper or lower zone in adults
- Postprimary infections have a strong predilection for the upper zones
- Miliary tuberculosis is evenly distributed throughout both lungs.

Primary pulmonary tuberculosis
- Patchy areas of consolidation or even lobar consolidation
- Ipsilateral hilar and contiguous mediastinal (paratracheal) lymphadenopathy, usually right-sided, usually necrotic
- May heal with calcification.

Postprimary tuberculosis
- Reactivation TB or secondary TB

- Most common in posterior segments of the upper lobes, superior segments of the lower lobes
- Patchy consolidation or poorly defined linear and nodular opacities
- Hilar nodal enlargement is seen in only approximately a third of cases.

Ref:
1. Jeong YJ, Lee KS. Pulmonary tuberculosis: up-to-date imaging and management. Am J Roentgenol. 2008;191(3):834-44.
2. Im JG, Itoh H, Shim YS, Lee JH, Ahn J, Han MC, Noma S. Pulmonary tuberculosis: CT findings-early active disease and sequential change with antituberculous therapy. Radiology. 1993;186(3):653-60.

20. **Ans. A**

Miliary tuberculosis
- Hematogenous dissemination of an uncontrolled tuberculous infection.
- It is seen both in primary and postprimary tuberculosis.
- 1-3 mm diameter nodules, which are uniform in size and uniformly distributed.

21. **Ans. C**

Pulmonary hydatid disease
- Lung is the second most common site of involvement with *Echinococcosis granulosus* in adults after the liver (10-30% of cases), and the most common site in children.
- Thoracic involvement may occur via trans-diaphragmatic route or hematogenous spread multiple or solitary cystic lesion, predominantly in the lower lobes.
- Rounded well-defined lesions with daughter cysts.

Complicated cysts may show:
- Meniscus sign or air crescent sign.
- *Cumbo sign or onion peel sign*: Gas lining between the endocyst and pericyst has the appearance of an onion peel. It is pathognomonic for a ruptured hydatid cyst.
- *Water-lily sign*: Detachment of the endocyst membrane which results in floating membranes within the pericyst that mimic the appearance of a water lily.
- Consolidation adjacent to the cyst.

Ref:
1. Polat P, Kantarci M, Alper F, Suma S, Koruyucu MB, Okur A. Hydatid disease from head to toe. Radiographics. 2003;23(2):475-94.
2. Pedrosa I, Saíz A, Arrazola J, Ferreirós J, Pedrosa CS. Hydatid disease: radiologic and pathologic features and complications. Radiographics. 2000;20(3):795-817.

22. **Ans. A**

Pneumocystis pneumonia
- Pulmonary *Pneumocystis jirovecii* infection, also referred to as *Pneumocystis jirovecii* pneumonia (PJP), and previously Pneumocystis pneumonia (PCP), is an atypical pulmonary infection and the most common opportunistic infection in patients with acquired immunodeficiency syndrome (AIDS)
- Common symptoms—dyspnea and/or non-productive cough
- Imaging—ground glass typically bilateral in perihilar distribution
- Reticular opacities or septal thickening
- Pneumatocele

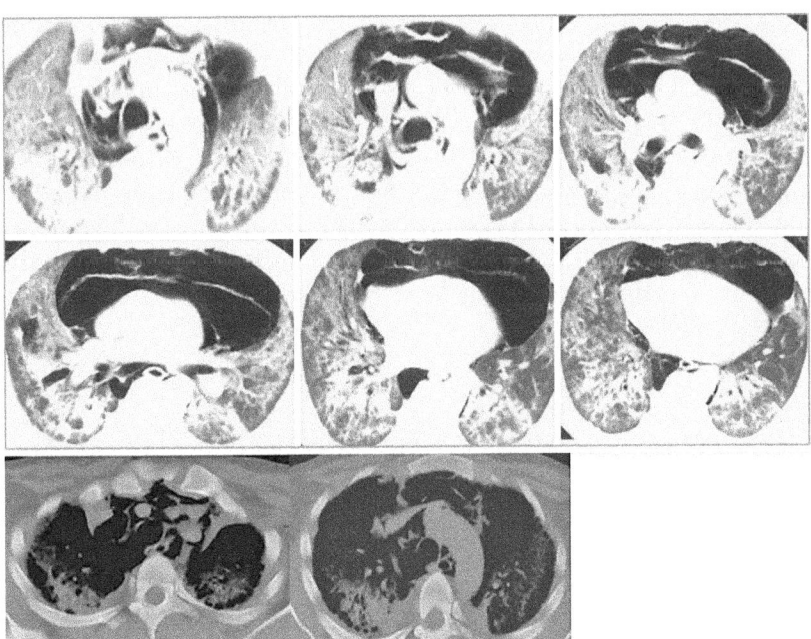

Pneumocystis pneumonia with pneumomediastinum.

Ref:
1. Hidalgo A, Falcó V, Mauleón S, Andreu J, Crespo M, Ribera E, et al. Accuracy of high-resolution CT in distinguishing between Pneumocystis carinii pneumonia and non- Pneumocystis carinii pneumonia in AIDS patients. Eur Radiol. 2003;13(5):1179-84.
2. Boiselle PM, Crans CA, Kaplan MA. The changing face of Pneumocystis carinii pneumonia in AIDS patients. Am J Roentgenol. 1999;172(5):1301-9.

ABDOMINAL INFECTIONS

23. Ans. D

Amebic liver abscess
- Amebic *hepatic abscesses* are a form of hepatic abscess resulting from *Entamoeba histolytica* infection.
- Incidence higher in alcoholic males.
- Rounded, well-defined lesions with attenuation values that indicate the presence of complex fluid (e.g., 10–20 HU).
- Enhancing wall and a peripheral zone of edema may be seen with wall thickness around 3–15 mm.
- The central abscess cavity can show septations and/or fluid-debris levels.
- May cause thrombosis of adjacent veins (portal > hepatic).
- Associated changes of amebic colitis can be seen.

Ref:
1. Mortelé KJ, Segatto E, Ros PR. The infected liver: radiologic-pathologic correlation. Radiographics. 2004;24(4):937-55.
2. Lodhi S, Sarwari AR, Muzammil M, Salam A, Smego RA. Features distinguishing amoebic from pyogenic liver abscess: a review of 577 adult cases. Trop Med Int Health. 2004;9(6):718-23.

24. Ans. A

Pyogenic abscess
- The mechanism of infection resulting in these lesions is through the portal system due to portal phlebitis from gastrointestinal infection, through the biliary tree from ascending cholangitis or hematogenous spread of infection.
- Most of the abscesses are polymicrobial and they are commonly caused by *Clostridium* species and gram-negative bacteria such as *Escherichia coli* and *Bacteroides* species.
- The clinical symptomatology associated is fever and severe right-sided abdominal pain.

Imaging
- Cluster of small low-attenuation or high-signal-intensity lesions.
- Some lesions may show heterogeneous central signal due to internal septae and content. The MRI signal of these lesions may vary depending on the protein content.
- The periphery of the abscess shows thick-walled smooth or irregular enhancement on contrast-enhanced CT and MR.

Ref:
1. Mortelé KJ, Segatto E, Ros PR. The infected liver: radiologic-pathologic correlation. Radiographics. 2004;24(4):937-55.
2. Radin DR, Ralls PW, Colletti PM, Halls JM. CT of amebic liver abscess. Am J Roentgenol. 1988;150(6):1297-301.

25. Ans. C

Patient underwent liver biopsy – Granulomas with AFB culture positive

Isolated hepatic tuberculosis
- Isolated hepatic TB now well-recognized and occurs usually in setting of immunocompetent host.
- Focal nodular lesions appearing as small solitary or conglomerate hypodense minimally enhancing lesions >2 mm in size.
- On MRI, these lesions are hypo or hyperintense on T2WI depending on the presence of caseous necrosis, showing nodular or ring-like enhancement.
- Focal abscess can be seen as a large hypodense lesion on CT showing thick, irregular peripherally enhancing walls.
- Conglomerate hypodense enhancing lesions seen around dilated biliary radicles mimicking cholangitic abscesses can be seen in biliary form.

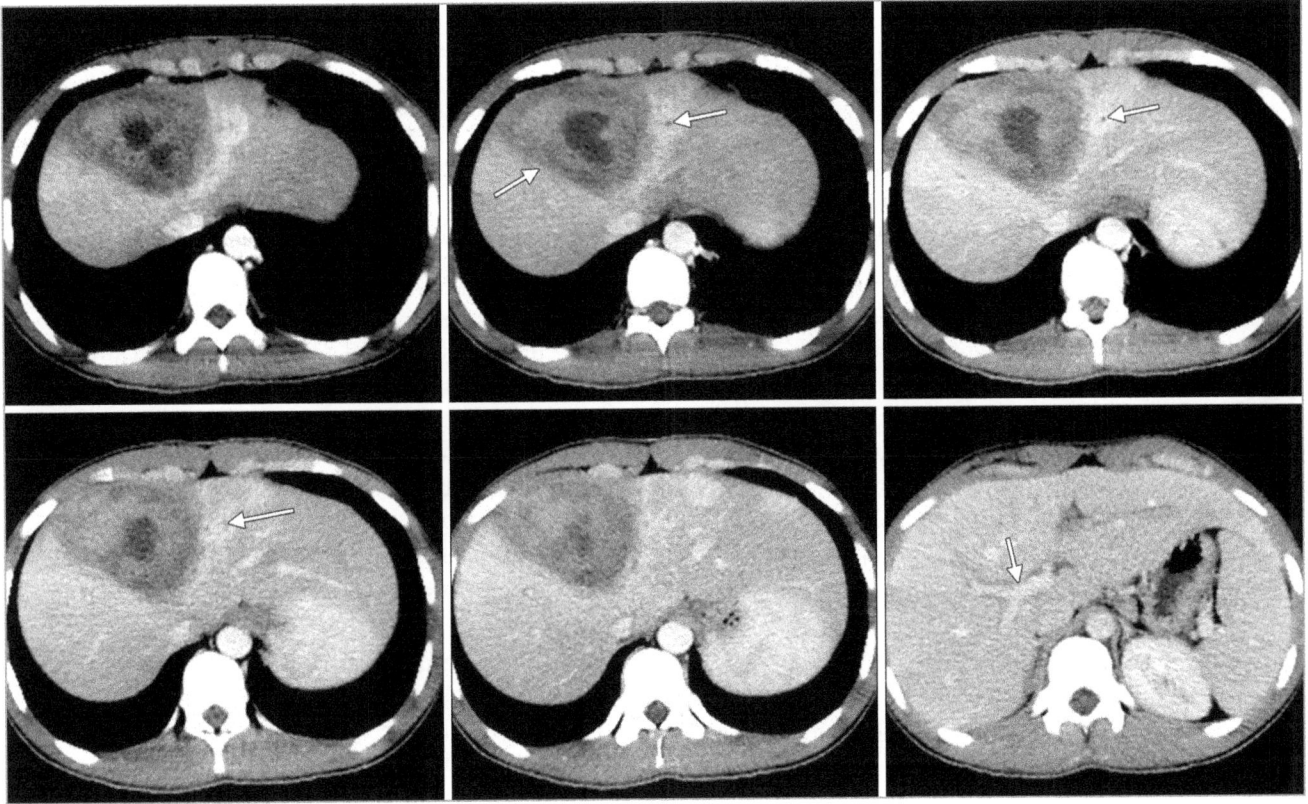

Tuberculous abscess

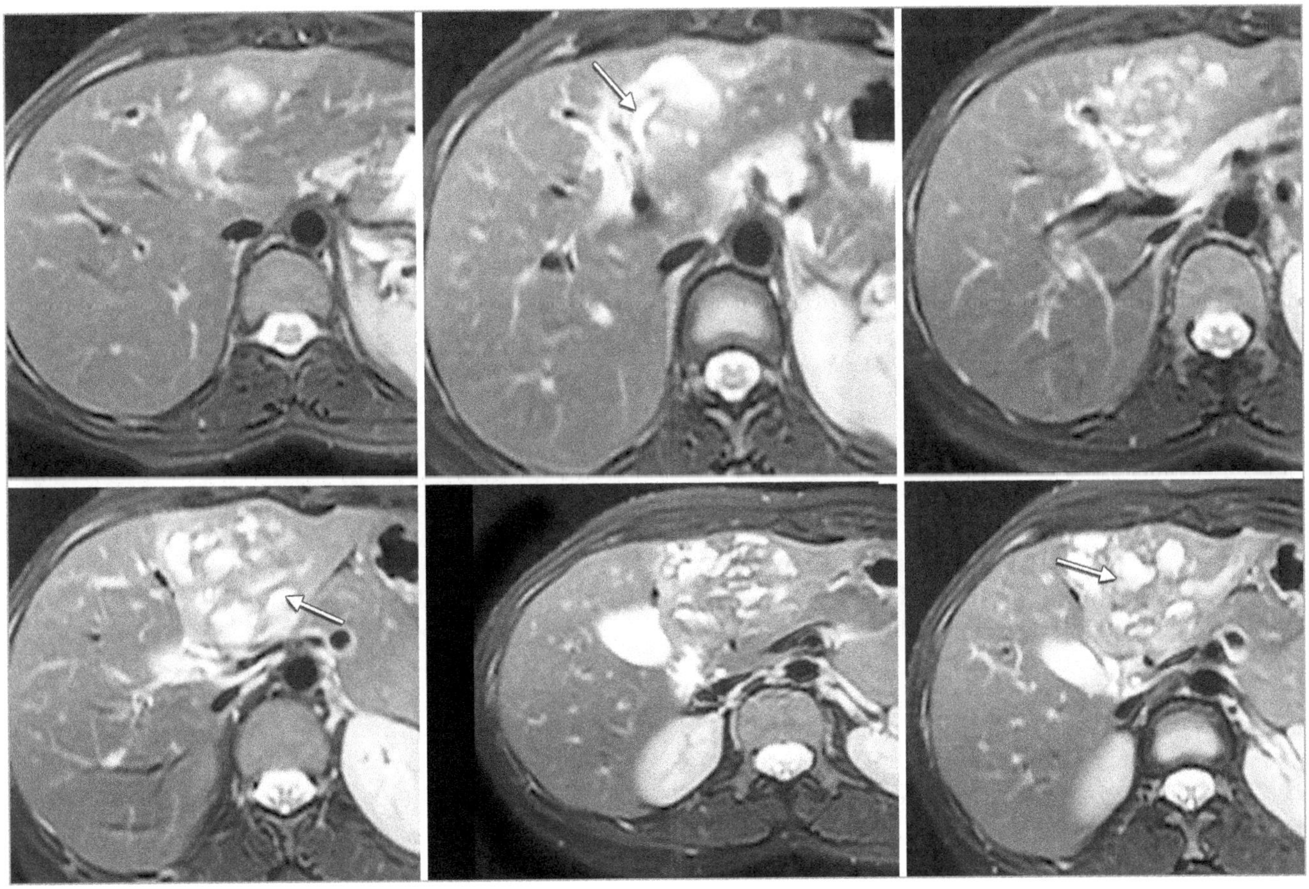

- Biliary form of isolated hepatic tuberculosis.
- Multiple conglomerate lesions in left lobe around biliary radicals (white arrows), which are mildly dilated.

Ref:
1. Kakkar C, Polnaya AM, Koteshwara P, Smiti S, Rajagopal KV, Arora A. Hepatic tuberculosis: a multimodality imaging review. Insights Imaging. 2015;6(6):647-58.
2. Harisinghani MG, McLoud TC, Shepard JA, Ko JP, Shroff MM, Mueller PR. Tuberculosis from head to toe. Radiographics. 2000;20(2):449-70.

26. Ans. C

Hepatic hydatid disease
- Humans become infected by ingestion of eggs of the tapeworm *Echinococcus granulosus*.
- Biochemical evaluation shows eosinophilia and positive serologic test in 25% of patients.
- Large unilocular or multilocular liver cysts with well-defined walls.
- Crescentic mural calcifications.
- Daughter cysts are seen as round peripheral structures that may have lower attenuation than fluid within the mother cyst.

MRI
- Fluid is typically low on T1-weighted and high on T2-weighted images.
- The pericyst appears as a hypointense rim on both T1-weighted and T2-weighted imaging.
- The hydatid matrix ("hydatid sand") is hypointense on T1-weighted imaging and hyperintense on T2-weighted imaging.
- Daughter cysts at the periphery are more hypointense than the matrix on both T1-weighted and T2-weighted imaging.

Ref:
1. Pedrosa I, Saíz A, Arrazola J, Ferreirós J, Pedrosa CS. Hydatid disease: radiologic and pathologic features and complications. Radiographics. 2000;20(3):795-817.
2. Malik A, Chandra R. Imaging appearances of atypical hydatid Cyst. 2016;26(1):33-9.

27. Ans. A

Fungal abscess
- These are usually seen in patients who are immunocompromised or have hematological malignancies especially leukemia with resultant disseminated fungal disease.
- There can be concomitant involvement of the spleen and occasionally the kidney.
- These are most often caused by *Candida albicans*.
- Typically fungal infection leads to the formation of micro abscesses.

- Multiple round small (2-20 mm), discrete hypodense foci showing central enhancement.

Ref:
1. Bächler P, Baladron MJ, Menias C. Multimodality imaging of liver infections: differential diagnosis and potential pitfalls. Radiographics. 2016;36(4):1001-23.

28. Ans. A

Tuberculosis
- *Tuberculous peritonitis* is a result of peritoneal involvement in tuberculosis.
- It is frequently seen in association with other forms of gastrointestinal tuberculosis.
- The abdomen is the most common site of extrapulmonary tuberculosis, with peritoneal disease being the commonest form within the abdomen.
- Peritoneal involvement is usually due to hematogenous spread.

Imaging
- CT imaging features seen with tuberculous peritonitis include:
  - Nodular or symmetrical thickening of the peritoneum and mesentery
  - Abnormal peritoneal or mesenteric enhancement
  - Ascites
  - Enlarged hypodense lymph nodes: low attenuation lymphadenopathy
- Ileocecal junction is a common site for intestinal involvement and is seen on imaging as bowel wall thickening with or without luminal narrowing.
- Retraction or deformity of ileocecal junction can be seen.

Ref:
1. Suri S, Gupta S, Suri R. Computed tomography in abdominal tuberculosis. Br J Radiol. 1999;72(853):92-8.
2. Gulati MS, Sarma D, Paul SB. CT appearances in abdominal tuberculosis. A pictorial essay. Clin Imaging. 1999;23(1):51-9.

29. Ans. B

Likely CMV colitis in the given setting.

CMV colitis
- Cytomegalovirus (CMV) infection of the gastrointestinal tract is usually seen in patients who are severely immunocompromised, such as solid organ transplantation and is common in HIV/AIDS
- Colon and rectum are more frequently involved in abdomen
- Mural thickening and surrounding stranding
- Can be diffuse or segmental.

Ref:
1. Murray JG, Evans SJ, Jeffrey PB, Halvorsen RA Jr. Cytomegalovirus colitis in AIDS: CT features. Am J Roentgenol. 1995;165 (1):67-71.
2. Reeders JW, Goodman PC. Radiology of Aids: A Practical Approach. Heidelberg: Springer Verlag; 2001.

30. **Ans. C**

Likely pseudomembranous colitis in the given setting.

Pseudomembranous colitis

- *Clostridium difficile* colitis, also known as *pseudomembranous colitis*, is a common cause of antibiotic-associated diarrhea, and increasingly encountered in sick hospitalized patients.
- CT findings include bowel wall thickening, thumb printing normal haustra become thickened at regular intervals appearing like thumbprints projecting into the aerated lumen, shaggy mucosal outline.
- Although typically the whole colon is involved, the right colon and transverse colon may be affected in isolation in up to 5% of cases.

Ref:
1. Kirkpatrick ID, Greenberg HM. Evaluating the CT diagnosis of Clostridium difficile colitis: should CT guide therapy? Am J Roentgenol. 2001;176(3): 635-9.
2. Roland GW, Lee MJ, Cats AM, Gaa JA, Saini S, Mueller PR. Antibiotic-induced diarrhea: specificity of abdominal CT for the diagnosis of Clostridium difficile disease. Radiology. 1994;191(1):103-6.

31. **Ans. C**

Mucormycosis

- Relatively uncommon opportunistic infection, primarily seen in immunocompromised patients.
- Rhinocerebral, pulmonary, cutaneous, gastrointestinal, and disseminated diseases.
- Stomach is the most common site, followed by colon and small bowel.
- Invasion of blood vessels, resulting in ischemia, hemorrhagic infarction and tissue necrosis.
- Diagnosis of angioinvasive fungus can be considered in immunocompromised patients with neutropenic fever and abdominal pain unresponsive to the antimicrobial treatment.

Ref:
1. Kim HJ, Rha SE. A patient with neutropenic fever and abdominal pain showing absent bowel wall on CT. Br J Radiol. 2011;84(1001):478-80.

32. **Ans. D**

- Histoplasmosis is an infective condition caused by a dimorphic, saprophytic fungus, *Histoplasma capsulatum*, and is acquired by inhalation of its spores. Soil rich in bird and bat dropping is its natural habitat, and it exists as a mycelium in the atmosphere.
- The disease is endemic in the United States, Africa, and Asia. Although most infections are asymptomatic, self-limiting acute pneumonitis and hilar lymphadenopathy may occur with inhalation of large aerosol.
- It may occur in disseminated form in some patients with impaired host defense mechanism and frequently involves liver, spleen, lymph node, bone marrow, and adrenal.
- Clinical manifestations in non-HIV positive resemble TB.
- Presents with fever, anorexia, night sweats, and features of adrenal insufficiency.
- In 99% cases, infection is subclinical.
- There are three major clinical presentations: pulmonary, progressive disseminated, and primary cutaneous histoplasmosis. Progressive disseminated form of the disease is rare and occurs in the immunocompromised patients in the endemic areas.
- Progressive disseminated disease may manifest as chronic disease in immunocompetent host or acute progressive disease in immunosuppressed hosts. In patients with disseminated histoplasmosis, abdominal imaging usually reveals mild to moderate hepatomegaly with or without splenomegaly. Abdominal lymphadenopathy and focal hypodense lesions in the spleen are also been described.

Adrenal involvement

- Adrenal infection is most frequently caused by hematologic dissemination.
- Most patients had symptoms, clinical signs, laboratory, and radiological features resembling adrenal neoplasms.
- On ultrasonography, they may show uniformly hypoechoic to heterogeneous echo pattern.
- Adrenal findings include mild enlargement with foci of calcification, moderate enlargement with focal low attenuation nodules, or massive enlargement with central necrosis or calcification which is bilaterally symmetrical, preserving the shape of adrenals.
- Differential diagnosis—TB, adenoma, metastasis, primary carcinoma, pheochromocytoma or post-inflammatory changes. Mycobacterium TB is the most common bacterial pathogen associated with adrenal destruction.

Ref:
1. Dwivedi MK, Piparsania B, Issar P. Disseminated histoplasmosis of adrenal gland. 2006;16(4):651-2.

2. Dylewski J. Acute pulmonary histoplasmosis. *CMAJ.* 2011;183(14):E1090.

33. Ans. A

Final diagnosis
- Microbiology report—*Staphylococcal* infection.

Pyogenic infections
- Two adjacent vertebrae with intervening disk
- Ill-defined marrow signal alternation, enhancement
- Loss of vertebral endplate cortex
- Obliteration of intranuclear cleft
- Disk space narrowing, disc enhancement
- Vertebral collapse
- Lumbar > thoracic > cervical spine
- Paraspinal ± epidural infiltrative soft tissues ± abscesses.

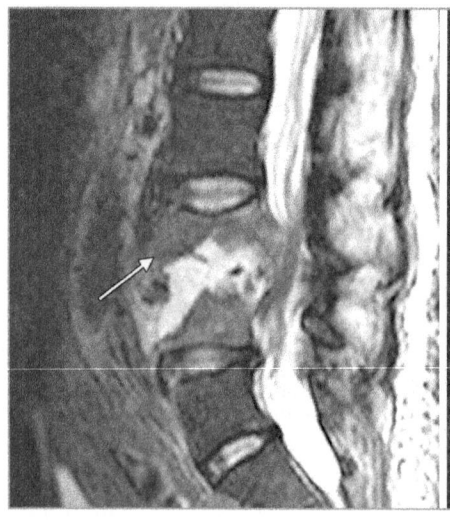
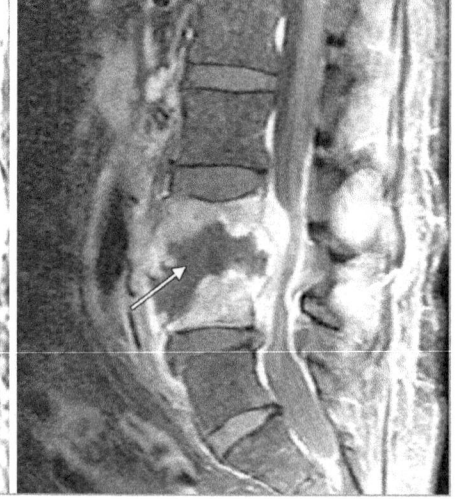

Advantages of MRI:
- Better definition of epidural extension of the inflammatory process and compression of the spinal cord and dural sac than other imaging modalities do.
- Paravertebral and epidural extension may appear in the form of either a phlegmon or an abscess with mixed signal intensity on both T1- and T2-weighted images.
- On contrast-enhanced images, either diffuse or rim-like enhancement is seen in paravertebral and epidural soft-tissue lesions.

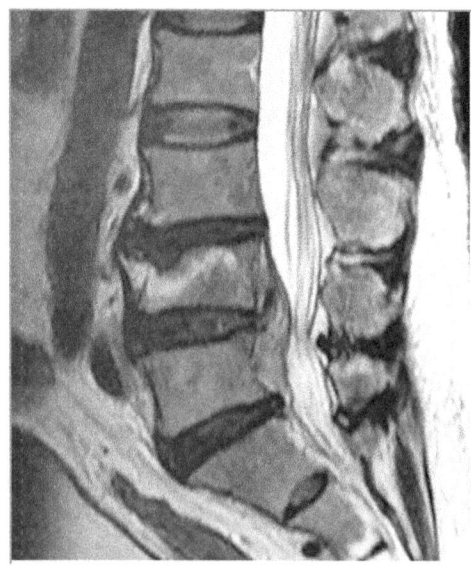
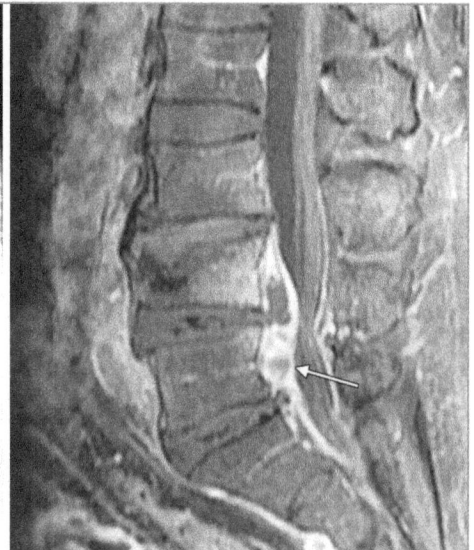

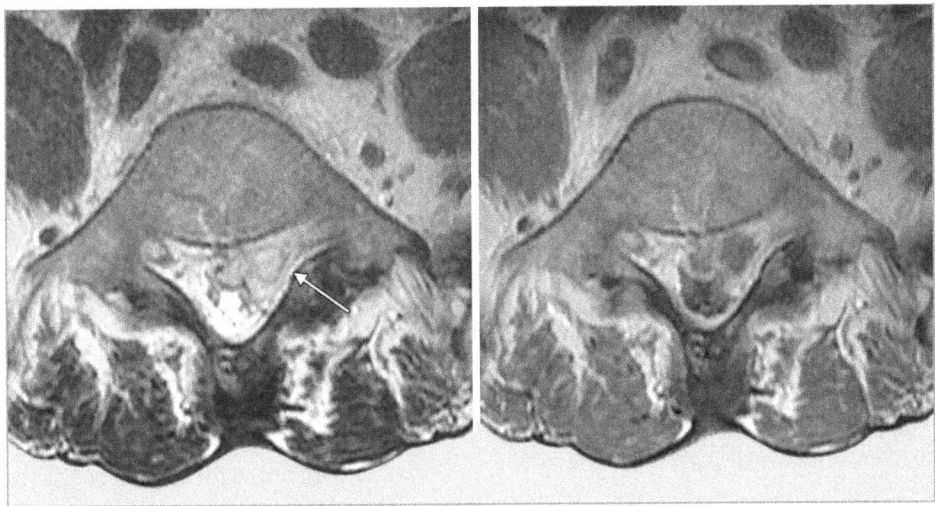

Ref:
1. Jung NY, Jee WH, Ha KY, Park CK, Byun JY. Discrimination of tuberculous spondylitis from pyogenic spondylitis on MRI. Am J Roentgenol. 2004; 182(6):1405-10.
2. Lee KY. Comparison of pyogenic spondylitis and tuberculous spondylitis. Asian Spine J. 2014;8(2):216-23.

34. Ans. B

Tuberculous spondylitis
- Tuberculous spondylitis, also known as Pott's disease, refers to vertebral body osteomyelitis and intervertebral discitis from TB.
- The spine is the most frequent location of musculoskeletal tuberculosis.
- Irregularity of both the endplate and anterior aspect of the vertebral bodies, with bone marrow edema and enhancement.
- Lack of proteolytic enzymes in Mycobacteria infections is cause of the relative preservation of the intervertebral disc and of the subligamentous spread of infection.
- The presence of skip lesions and of a large paraspinal cold abscess.
- Barely penetrate the anterior longitudinal ligament, neither an anterior paraspinal phlegmon nor an abscess encases the intercostal arteries in thoracic spinal tuberculosis.

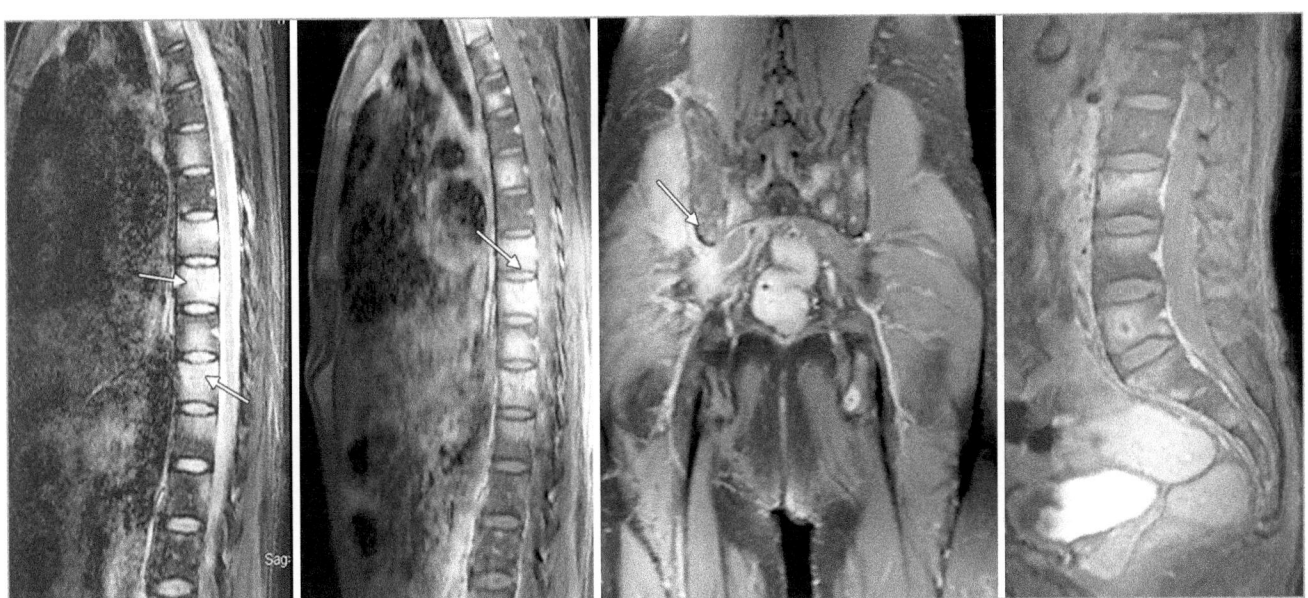

Multifocal tuberculosis.

Spinal infections

Pyogenic	Tuberculous
Abscess with thick irregular walls	Well-defined paraspinal region with abnormal signal intensity, a thin, smooth abscess wall
Small abscesses	Large cold abscesses
Involvement of one vertebral segment (two vertebral bodies and intervening disc)	Subligamentous spread to three or more vertebral levels
Early destruction of disc due to proteolytic enzymes	Multiple vertebral, skip lesions or entire-body involvement

Ref:
1. Burrill J, Williams CJ, Bain G, Conder G, Hine AL, Misra RR. Tuberculosis: a radiologic review. Radiographics. 2007;27(5):1255-73.
2. Harisinghani MG, Mcloud TC, Shepard JA, Ko JP, Shroff MM, Mueller PR. Tuberculosis from head to toe. Radiographics. 2000;20(2):449-70.
3. Jung NY, Jee WH, Ha KY, Park CK, Byun JY. Discrimination of tuberculous spondylitis from pyogenic spondylitis on MRI. Am J Roentgenol. 2004;182(6):1405-10.

35. **Ans. A**

Tuberculous arachnoiditis
- Thickening with enhancement of spinal meninges
- Multiple enhancing granulomas along surface of cord
- Thickening with clumping of thecal nerve roots
- Cord compression or edema may be present.

Ref:
1. Burrill J, Williams CJ, Bain G, Conder G, Hine AL, Misra RR. Tuberculosis: a radiologic review. Radiographics. 2007;27(5):1255-73.
2. Harisinghani MG, Mcloud TC, Shepard JA, Ko JP, Shroff MM, Mueller PR. Tuberculosis from head to toe. Radiographics. 2000;20(2):449-70.

36. **Ans. A**

Brodies abscess
- Subacute pyogenic osteomyelitis —smoldering indolent infection
- *Staphylococcus aureus*—most common
- *Histo*: Granulation tissue with eburnation of bone
- Males > females
- Predilection for ends of bones (proximal and distal tibial metaphyses)
- Metaphysis > epiphysis
- Central lucency surrounded dense rim of reactive sclerosis
- Lucent channel/tongue-like extension into growth plate
- May persist for many months to years
- MRI—Double line effect, high signal intensity T2 lesion with surrounding low signal.

Ref:
1. Brant WE, Helms CA. Fundamentals of Diagnostic Radiology. Philadelphia: Lippincott Williams & Wilkins; 2007.
2. Afshar A, Mohammadi A. The "Penumbra Sign" on Magnetic Resonance Images of Brodie's Abscess: A Case Report. Iran J Radiol. 2011;8(4):245-8.

CHAPTER 32

COVID-19

Rahul Bahot, Om Shrivastav

INTRODUCTION

The pandemic of an RNA virus named as coronavirus disease 2019 (COVID-19) or severe acute respiratory syndrome coronavirus 2 (SARS-CoV-2) brought the entire nations of the world to stand still. Economies collapsed and people were forced to stay indoors. This virus changed the way of living forever. The verses below summarize and pickup positive impact of this pandemic.

COVID WUHAN

A VIRUS WITH A CROWN
HAS FORCED THE WORLD TO PACE DOWN
CREATING GREAT FEAR
FILLING EYES WITH TEARS
WITH ITS FROWN
CAUSING NATIONS TO DROWN

THE RELIGION HAS LOST ITS IMPORTANCE
AS THE VIRUS KILLS HUMANS LIKE ACE
MUTATING FAST IT CHANGES ITS FACE
MAKING IT DIFFICULT TO IDENTIFY A CASE

THE GOVERNMENTS TAKE A STAND
AND EVERYONE JOIN THEIR HANDS
TO DO THEIR BIT
SO THAT THE TRANSMISSION OF VIRUS IS HIT

THE MEDICAL FATERNITY TAKES THE FRONT LINE
RISKING AND SACRIFICING THEIR LIVES
TO SAVE A LIFE
AND RESEARCHERS STAND ALONG IN SLEEPLESS NIGHT
TRYING FIND A WAY TO WIN THIS FIGHT

THE BOND OF LOVE GROWS STRONG
HANDS JOIN TO SAVE LIVES IN THIS STORM
WITH A STRONG ZEAL TO PERSIST
WE WILL WIN THIS FIGHT TO EXIST

—DR RAHUL BAHOT

THE VIRUS

The Structure of the Virus[1,2]

Coronaviruses are spherical single-stranded RNA viruses with club-like projections from the surface making them look like a crown. SARS-CoV-2 has five structural components:

1. *Spike (S)*: The S protein is the chief determinant for pathogenicity and host selection. It has further two subunits as S1 and S2. S1 is responsible for receptor recognition and S2 is responsible for anchoring and injection of the viral material into the host cell. The S protein's receptor-binding domain (RBD) is reported to have a crystal structure.
2. *Envelope (E)*: It has a role in assembly and release of the virus.
3. *Membrane protein (M)*: The curvature of the virus surface is maintained by membrane protein.
4. *Nucleocapsid (N)*:
   The N as two RNA substrates:
   - The transcriptional regulatory sequence (TRS)
   - The genomic packaging signal

   It helps in cell signaling and packaging of the viral genome.

   It is a structural protein, which helps the virus to enter the host and mucosal spread.
5. *The nuclear material hemagglutinin-esterase (HE)*: It is made of single-stranded, positive-sense RNA genome, which is devoid of any segments measuring 30 kb. COVID-19 has complex structure of B_0AT1, an amino acid transporter protein, with human host cell-binding receptor angiotensin-converting enzyme 2 (ACE2). The viral architecture of SARS-CoV-2 with post-fusion spike was observed by cryogenic electron microscopy (cryo-EM), which showed the image of disassociated spikes.

The Strains

The predominant strains of the virus have been classified into two varieties based on the mutations:
1. The "S"-strain
2. The "L"-strain

The L-strain is the predominant strain of virus contributing to approximately 70% of the total virus population and S-strain contributes to 30% of the total viral population. The L variant of the virus is contemplated more aggressive and more contagious and S variant of virus is assumed to be less aggressive and less contentious compared to its contemporary.[3]

Modes of Transmission

The transmission of virus happens via:
- Droplet nuclei
- Fecal oral
- Fomites

The SARS-CoV-2 is excreted in the body fluids of the patient such as respiratory droplets, saliva, feces, and urine.

The Basic Reproduction Number (R_0)

It is the average number of contacts[4] infected by a single case. R_0 value of more than 1 indicates that in the absence of external influences, the virus will continue to propagate among the susceptible host. Conversely, R_0 value of 0 means the virus will become extinct in the present environmental conditions. The influenza virus has R_0 value of approximately 1.3 and COVID-19 has R_0 value of approximately 2.3. This means that each patient suffering from COVID-19 can spread infection 1.8 times more than compared to the influenza patient.

The Viability of the Virus on Different Surfaces

The virus remains viable in aerosol for period of >3 hours at the relative humidity of 60% with the reduction in tissue-culture infectious dose ($TCID_{50}$) per milliliter from $10^{3.7}$ to $10^{2.7}$ with the half-life of 1.2 hours. The viable virus was detected up to 72 hours in the relative humidity of 40% on plastic (half-life of 6.8 hours) and 48 hours on stainless steel (half-life of 5.6 hours) battery for 29 over the world. The viable virus, however, was not found beyond 3 hours on copper surfaces.[5]

The virus gets inactivated rapidly in 30 seconds of exposure to World Health Organization (WHO) recommended handrub formulation I consisting of 80% (vol/vol) ethanol, 1.45% (vol/vol) glycerol, and 0.125% (vol/vol) hydrogen peroxide, and formulation II consists of 75% (vol/vol) 2-propanol, 1.45% (vol/vol) glycerol, and 0.125% (vol/vol) hydrogen peroxide along with the modified isopropyl-based WHO formulation II contains 75% (wt/wt) 2-propanol, 0.725% (vol/vol).[6]

HEALTHCARE FACILITY AS A RESERVOIR OF INFECTION IN THE SOCIETY

In a study from China, Wuhan between February 19th and March 2nd, 2020, sampling was done in hospitals[7] to check contamination of air and surface with COVID-19 virus. It was observed that the rate of positivity for floor swab samples was as high as 70% in intensive care unit (ICU), 15% in general ward while the pharmacy floor was 100% positive. This highlights the fact that the droplets settle on the floor. The results of the study are summarized in **Figure 1**.

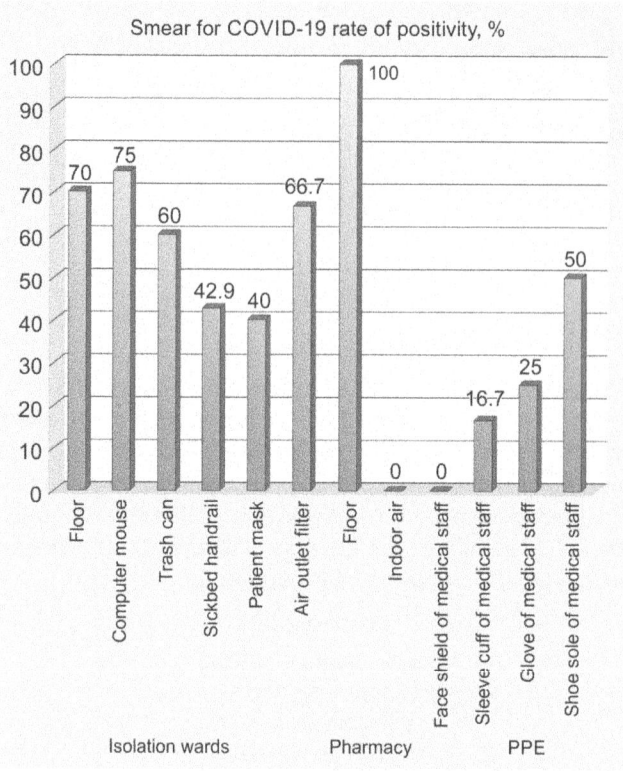

Fig. 1: The areas of the hospital showing contamination with coronavirus disease 2019 (COVID-19) virus.
(PPE: personal protective equipment)

INFECTION

The median age of individuals infected with COVID-19 was 43.5 years from a study in India. This was lesser than those compared from China (Wang et al., 56.0 years, Chen et al., 55.5 years, and Huang et al., 49.0 years).[1] About 80% of patients were <60 years of age. The disease had a male predominance (66.66%). 19.4% of the affected were healthcare workers.

As per the National COVID-19 tracker, the majority of the cases in India are seen in the age group of 31–40 years, which is followed by 21–30 years. This is in sharp contrast with the data is that the world where the elderly is more affected than the younger population.

In the state of Maharashtra, highest number of cases are seen in the age group of 21–30 years, which is followed by 31–40 years of age.

The incubation period for COVID-19 ranges from 2 to 14 days.[8]

SARS-CoV-2 binds to ACE2 receptor on the host cell membrane to gain entry into the host cell. The S protein of the virus has a high binding affinity to ACE2 receptor.

ACE2 receptor is present abundantly on the alveolar II cells and the goblet cells in the respiratory tract. These receptors are also expressed by the vascular endothelium and myocardium.

INTERACTION WITH THE HOST IMMUNE SYSTEM

COVID-19 invades the alveolar type II epithelial cells in the respiratory tract via ACE2 receptor. While in the epithelial cells, COVID-19 inhibits the tumor necrosis factor receptor-associated factors (TRAFs) 6 and 3.[9] As a result, activation of transcription factors NFκB and IRF-3 and -7 is limited. This suppresses the early proinflammatory responses through type I interferons (IFNs) and proinflammatory effector Interleukin-1 (IL-1), IL-6, and tumor necrosis factor-alpha (TNF-α). The infected epithelial cells with suppressed innate immunity promote the multiplication of the virus.

The virus multiplies in the cell and finally bursts open the cell thereby killing it and releasing young virions. Moreover, the virus-mediated death of epithelial cells causes endothelial damage, which affects the integrity of the epithelium of the lungs and the blood vessels. This further adds to inflammatory cytokine expression and immune cell recruitment with the activation.

These virus particles along with intracellular components of the dead cells trigger innate immunity. The viral particles and cell debris are ingested by the macrophages. Now in the macrophages, the virions inhibit interferon-1 signaling thereby resulting in excessive release of proinflammatory cytokines IL-1, IL-6, and TNF-α. IL-1, IL-6, and TNF-α undergo autoamplification through positive feedback loop.

The antibody-dependent enhancement happens is because of viral particles bound element complexes into the cells to the Fc-gamma receptor. In some immune cells (along with antigen presenting cells), there is persistent viral replication and immune-complex-mediated inflammatory response that further contributes to organ damage and tissue damage.

Hyperinflammatory response[10] undergoes loss of regulation giving rise to hypercytokinemia. The TNF and IL-1, IL-8 with MCP-1 levels rise, causing stained increasing IL-6. The pathophysiology of cytokine storm is summarized in **Figure 2**.

CLINICAL FEATURES

The median age of individuals infected with COVID-19 was 43.5 years from a study in India. This was lesser than those compared from China (Wang et al.: 56.0 years, Chen et al.: 55.5 years, and Huang et al.: 49.0 years).[1] 80% of patients were <60 years of age. The disease had a male predominance (66.66%). 19.4% of the affected were healthcare workers.

As per the National COVID-19 tracker, the majority of the cases in India are seen in the age group of 31–40 years, which is followed by 21–30 years. This is in sharp contrast with the data is that the world where the elderly is more affected than the younger population.

The incubation period for COVID-19 ranges from 2 days to 14 days. COVID-19 generally progresses as gradual course as compared to flu. Fever is the predominant complaint in COVID-19 as compared to common cold. Rhinorrhea and nasal congestion are rarely seen in COVID-19, which is a predominant complaint in common cold. **Figure 3** shows the progression of COVID-19.

The signs and symptoms as per the system are as follows.[11]

Table 1 gives organ-wise signs and symptoms of COVID-19.

Special Populations

Pregnancy

Fever is the most common symptom observed followed by cough, myalgia, breathlessness, and diarrhea in the order of decreasing frequency.

Diabetes and hypertension are significant comorbidities even in pregnant women.

Fetal distress was most commonly observed, which prompted the delivery by cesarean section in 89% of females. This was followed by the term labor (22%) and premature rupture of membranes (8%).

The neonatal complications include preterm birth (23%), lower respiratory tract infection (14% pneumonia), respiratory distress syndrome (14%), low-birth weight (11%), and small for gestational age (3%).

High Risk of Mortality

Comorbidities, which have been definitively shown to have a risk of mortality, are:
- Hypertension [odds ratio 2.36 (95% confidence interval 1.46–3.83)]
- Respiratory Disease [odds ratio 2.46 (1.76–3.44)]
- Clinical syndromes such as acute respiratory distress syndrome and sepsis were associated with high-mortality rates followed by cardiac injury, heart failure, acute kidney injury, and encephalopathy.[12]
- As per the government data, overall mortality in India is 3.34%; whereas in Maharashtra state, it is 6.41%.

INVESTIGATIONS

The investigations of COVID-19 are as follows.

Diagnostic Investigation

The diagnostic test with the number of days, which will come positive, is shown in **Figure 4**.

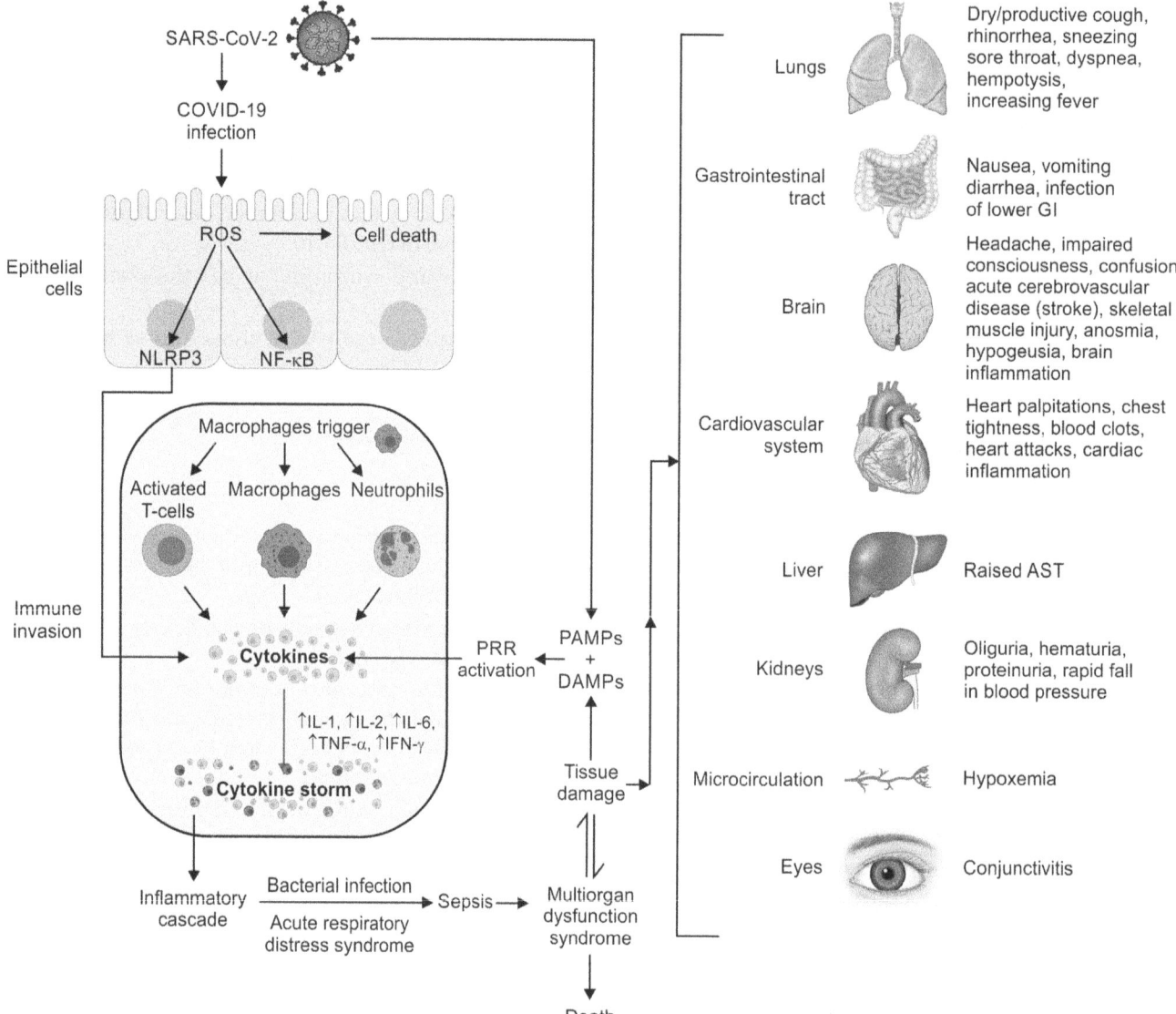

Fig. 2: Mechanisms of SARS-CoV-2-associated cytokine storm and associated damages. Infection with SARS-CoV-2 can stimulate a hyperinflammatory immune response wherein epithelial-cell-mediated production of reactive oxygen species (ROS) can cause cell death. ROS can also stimulate the synthesis of NLRP3 and NF-κB which contribute to increased cytokine levels, and thus, the cytokine storm. This essentially causes immune invasion which can lead to clinically relevant conditions such as ARDS, sepsis, MODS and potentially even death. The organs affected as a result of MODS, and their associated symptoms, have been shown. Lower gastrointestinal (GI) is rich in ACE2 receptors and hence at higher risk of infection due to COVID-19. 20% of COVID-19 patients have diarrhea as symptoms. [SARS-COV-2: severe acute respiratory syndrome coronavirus 2; COVID-19: coronavirus disease 2019; ROS: reactive oxygen species; NLRP3: (NOD)-like receptor protein 3 inflammasome; NF-κB: nuclear factor kappa-light-chain-enhancer of activated B-cells; IL: interleukin; TNF: tumor necrosis factor; IFN: interferon; PAMPs: pathogen-associated molecular patterns; DAMPs: damage-associated molecular patterns; PRR: pattern recognition receptors; AST: aspartate aminotransferase; MODS: multiple organ dysfunction syndrome]

Source: Bhaskar S, Sinha A, Banach M, Mittoo S, Weissert R, Kass JS, et al. Cytokine Storm in COVID-19—Immunopathological Mechanisms, Clinical Considerations, and Therapeutic Approaches: The REPROGRAM Consortium Position Paper. Front Immunol. 2020;11:1648.

RT-PCR of Body Secretions[13]

This is the primary mode of diagnosing COVID-19. Different varieties of reverse transcriptase polymerase chain reaction (RT-PCR) tips are available for diagnosis of COVID-19. As the name suggest, it is based on reverse transcription of COVID-19 RNA into complementary DNA strands. The specific regions of the DNA are amplified and detected. The regions on the viral genome utilized for identification are:

- The open reading frame (ORF1ab) region
- The *N* gene (nucleocapsid protein gene); it has poor analytical sensitivity
- The *E* gene (envelope protein gene)
- The RdRP gene (RNA-dependent RNA polymerase gene)

Has high analytical sensitivity

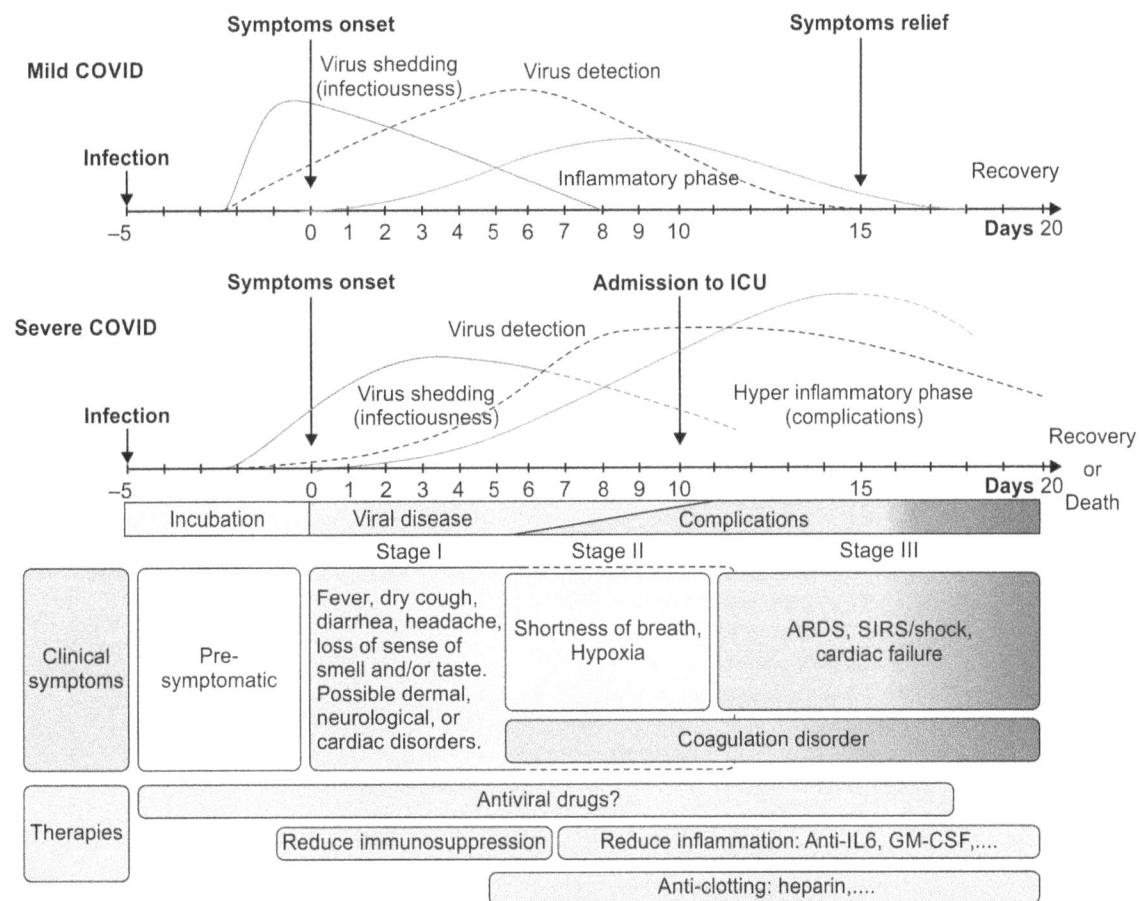

Fig. 3: Progresssion of coronavirus disease 2019 (COVID-19).

Table 1: Coronavirus disease 2019 (COVID-19) as per severity in various organ systems.

Organ system	Mild disease	Moderate disease	Severe disease	Diagnostic signs
Lung/Respiratory–Pulmonary	Cough, sore throat, rhinorrhea, sneezing, dry cough	Pneumonia, dyspnea, moderate hypoxemia	Severe hypoxemia, acute respiratory distress syndrome (ARDS), respiratory failure and death (if untreated)	Decreased PO_2, chest X-rays show ground-glass opacities
Heart/Cardiac	Chest pain, arrhythmia, sinus tachycardia	Cardiac inflammation, immunocytic infiltration	Cardiomayopathy, acute heart failure	Elevated cardiac enzymes, abnormal EKG (Prolonged QTc intervals, elevated ST), cardiac-specific troponin and brain natriuretic peptide
Blood vessels	Blood coagulation	Arterial or venous thromboembolism, cytokine storms	Pulmonary embolism, large vessel occlusions, disseminated intravascular coagulation	Elevated D-dimer, interleukin-6, other cytokines, ferritin, and lactate dehydrogenase, prolonged PT/PTT
Brain/Neurological	Hyposmia–Anosmia, hypogeusia–Ageusia, visual disturbance, fatigue, somnolence	Headaches, nausea and vomiting, dizziness, myalgia, ataxia, encephalopathy	Cerebrovascular disease (large vessel strokes), seizures, meningoencephalitis, neuropathy, Guillain–Barré syndrome, neurogenic ARDS, coma	Elevated creatine kinase with myalgia, brain MRI show hyperintensities in regions with infarction or encephalitis, SARS-CoV-2 detection in cerebrospinal fluid or brain tissues in some patients
Gastrointestinal	Nausea, vomiting, diarrhea, heartburn	Loss of appetite, abdominal pain and bloating	Gastrointestinal (GI) bleeding, GI viral dissemination	Elevated liver enzymes and bilirubins, SARS-CoV-2 detection in stool samples
Kidney/Renal	Proteinuria	Acute renal injury	Renal failure	Cardiac-specific troponin and brain natriuretic peptide, tubular necrosis and SARS-CoV-2 detection in kidney
Mental/Psychiatric	Depressed mood, anxiety, insomnia, anger, fear	Depression, post-traumatic stress disorder	Exacerbation of neurological or psychiatric disorders (e.g., Alzheimer's or addiction)	Elevated plasma, calcium and phosphorus (indicative of stress)

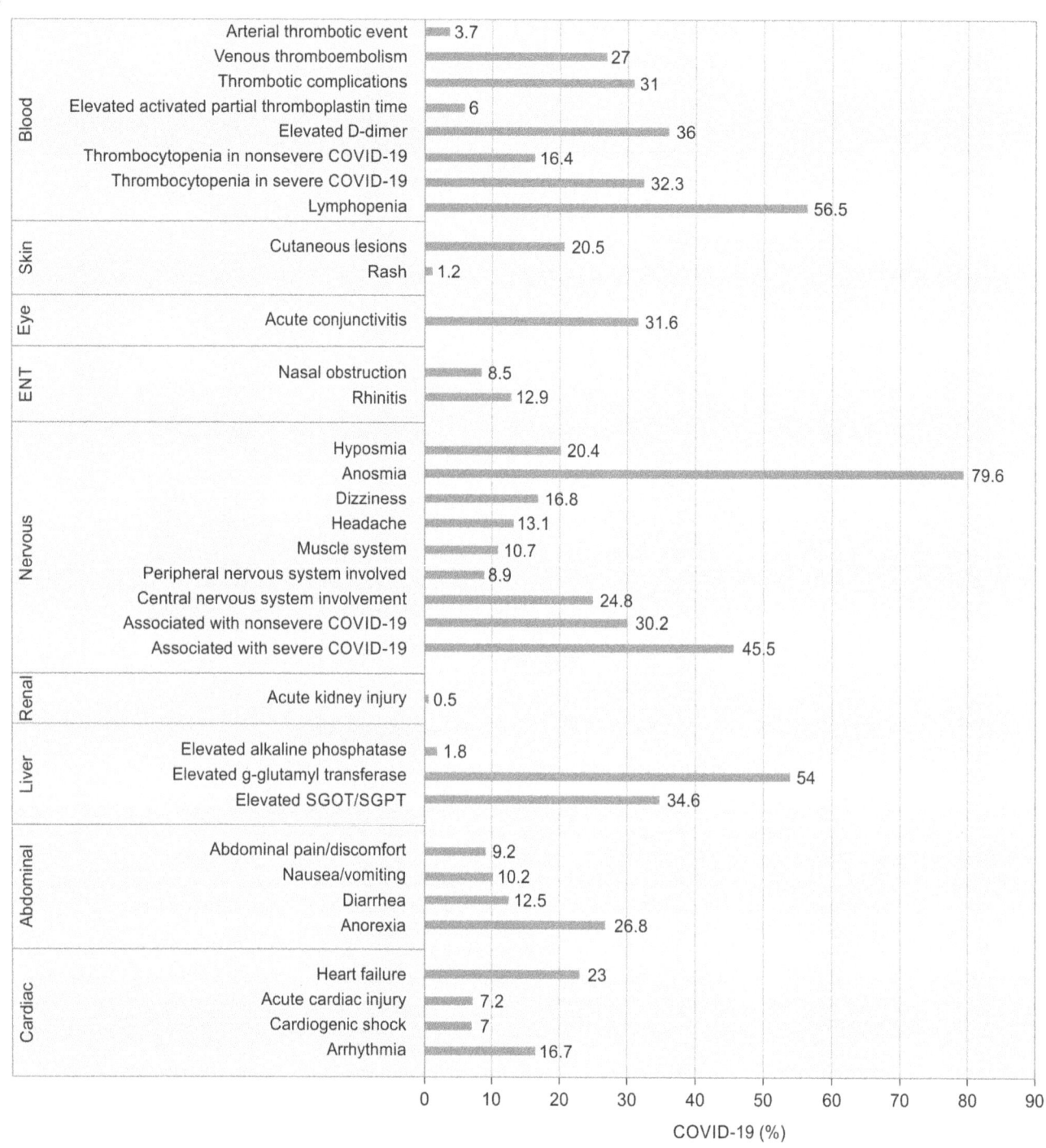

Fig. 4: Frequency of diseases organize involved in COVID-19.
Source: Adapted from Laia CC, Kob WC, Leec PI, Jeand SS, Hsuehf PR.

The common sites for sampling of specimen for RT-PCR are the oropharynx and the nasopharynx. **Figure 5** shows the workflow of the RT-PCR.

The sensitivity and specificity of RT-PCR for COVID-19 from various specimens are given in **Figure 6**.

At present, recommendation is to collect the specimen as soon as possible monthly decision irrespective of the symptom onset. The viral load is greatest at the time of viral onset and it decreases with time.

Loop-mediated Isothermal Amplification[14]

It amplifies the genomic material at a constant temperature of 60–65° in the presence of primer and the enzymes. Within less than an hour 10^9 copies of viral genomic material are made. It is user-friendly, more specific, and sensitive and faster with less power consumption than the conventional techniques.

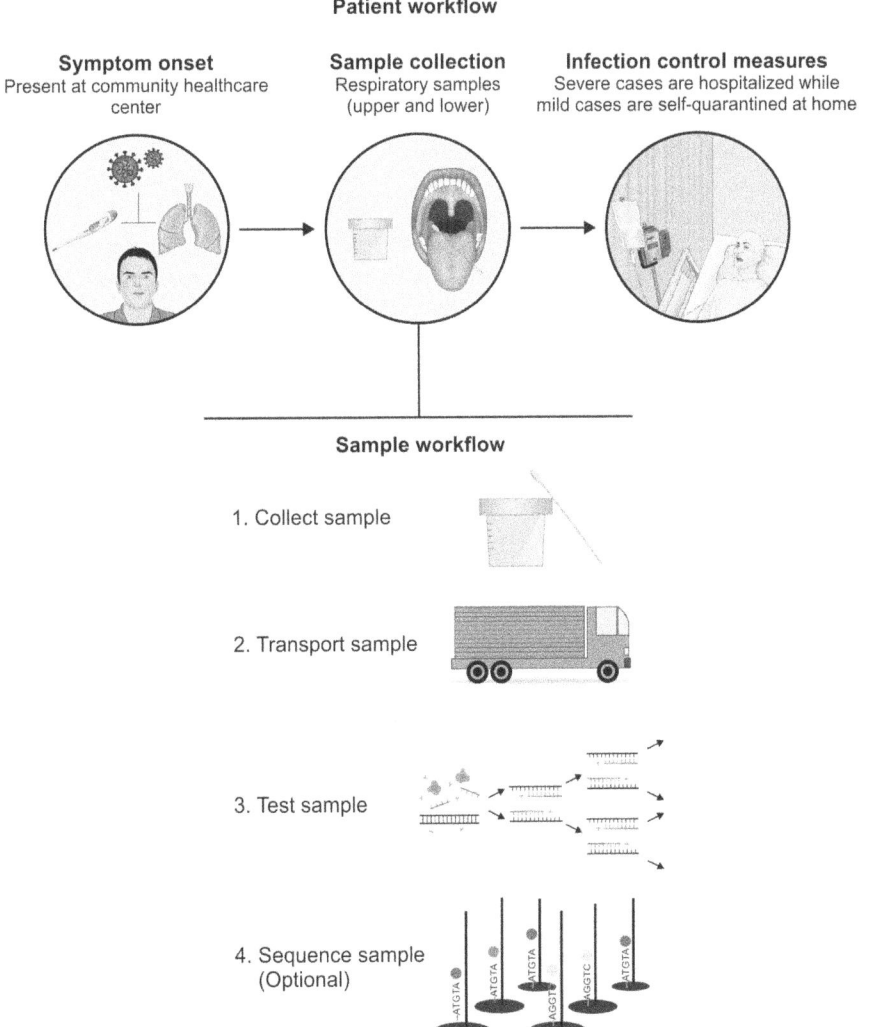

Fig. 5: Example of patient and sample workflow during the COVID-19 outbreak. Patients present at a healthcare facility for triage. The collected samples are tested on-site, if possible, or transported for molecular testing and sequencing. Patients are then managed appropriately.

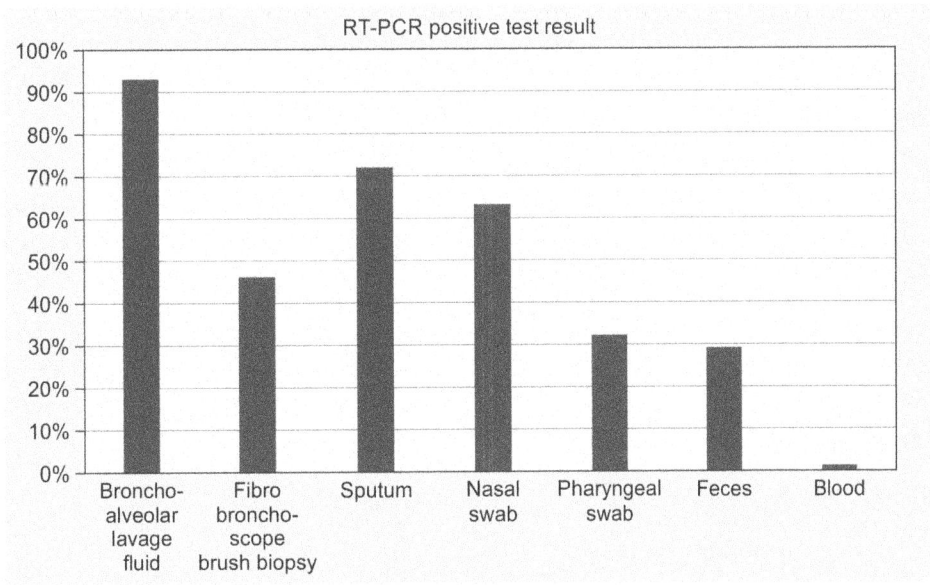

Fig. 6: Reverse transcription polymerase chain reaction (RT-PCR) positive result from various body samples.

Table 2: Interpretation of antibody tests.[17]

IgM	IgG	Interpretation
Negative	Negative	Antibodies are not produced, which indicate less probability of patients subject of having contracted COVID-19
Positive	Negative	COVID-19 infection has recently acquired and immune system is producing antibodies against it
Positive	Positive	COVID-19 infection has happened probably prior to 14 days below
Negative	Positive	Previous infection with COVID-19

Direct Antigen Test[15,16]

It is a fluorescent immunochromatographic assay for detecting and protein of SARS-CoV-2. The values are measured as per cycle threshold. Lower the cycle threshold higher is the viral load and higher the cycle threshold lower is the viral load. The cycle threshold (CT) <40 is considered to be positive. However, the sensitivity of the test declines by the 3rd week and becomes negative thereafter.

Antibody Test[17] (Table 2)

The antibodies appear in approximately <40% patients within the 1st week. By the end of 2 weeks, 94.3% patients demonstrate IgM and 79.8% patients have IgG antibody. The IgM antibodies rise in-between 5 and 7 days from the time of symptom onset. There is a fall in the level of IgM antibody at around 14 days. The IgG antibody appears around 14 days from the onset of symptoms and continues to rise for 28–35 days. IgG has a long half-life and can be detected even for years after resolution of infection.

The accuracy of various antibody tests is depicted in **Figure 7**.

The Radiological Investigations

CT Scan of the Chest

The high-resolution CT (HRCT) scan of the chest is the 1st investigation to pick up any abnormality in the COVID-19 infection. The HRCT chest shows ground-glass appearance as early as 2–4 days after acquisition of infection **(Figs. 8A and B)**.

Summary of all the test diagnosis of COVID-19 is given in **Table 3**.

Inflammatory Markers (Fig. 9)

The markers of inflammation rise up COVID-19

TREATMENT

The treatment is based on the severity of symptoms. As per Indian Council of Medical Research (ICMR), **Table 4** describes stages of infection as per severity.[20]

General Care

- Supportive care and symptomatic treatment, optimal nutritional support, maintain fluid and electrolytes balance, and close monitoring
- Monitor vital signs (BP/PR/RR/SpO_2) 12–8 hourly with increase in monitoring during intensive care.
- Blood investigations, e.g., full blood count (FBC), C-reactive protein (CRP), liver function test (LFT), RP, coagulation, blood culture, ferritin, D-dimer, fibrinogen, and procalcitonin according to clinical indications.
- Arterial blood gas (ABG) if needed according to severity of disease, inform laboratory staff before sending specimens
- Supplemental oxygen according to SpO_2
- Monitor sugar when needed
- For children who needs bronchodilator therapy, e.g., salbutamol; avoid using nebulizer. Instead use MDI with spacer
- Ensure good hydration in children by encouraging their usual milk/diets.

Supplemental Oxygen

The goal of oxygen therapy is to maintain an oxygen saturation of >90% and 92–95% in pregnant women.[21] The supplemental oxygen therapy is guided by the phenotype of pneumonia in the patient.[22] The phenotypes of pneumonia are mentioned in **Table 5**.

The L-pneumonia responds well to noninvasive modes of ventilation.[22] For SpO_2 < 90% with mild to moderately increased work breathing, non-rebreathing mask with goal of SpO_2 > 90%. For those increasing work of breathing, worsening hypoxia or failure to maintain O_2 > 90%, consider high-flow oxygen.[21]

High-flow nasal oxygen (HFNO) can achieve a flow rate of up to 60 L/min. HFNO reduces dead space, decreases the work of breathing and breathing frequency. It is associated with decreased mortality in hypoxemic respiratory failure. It is associated with decreased risk of progression to intubation and ICU admission.[21]

The success of HFNO is predicated by "ROX" index. ROX index is ratio of oxygen saturation as measured by pulse oximetry/FiO_2 to respiratory rate. It is calculated at 2, 6, and 12 hours. A ROX index > 4.88 is predictive of success, meaning the patient is unlikely to progress to needing mechanical ventilation.[23]

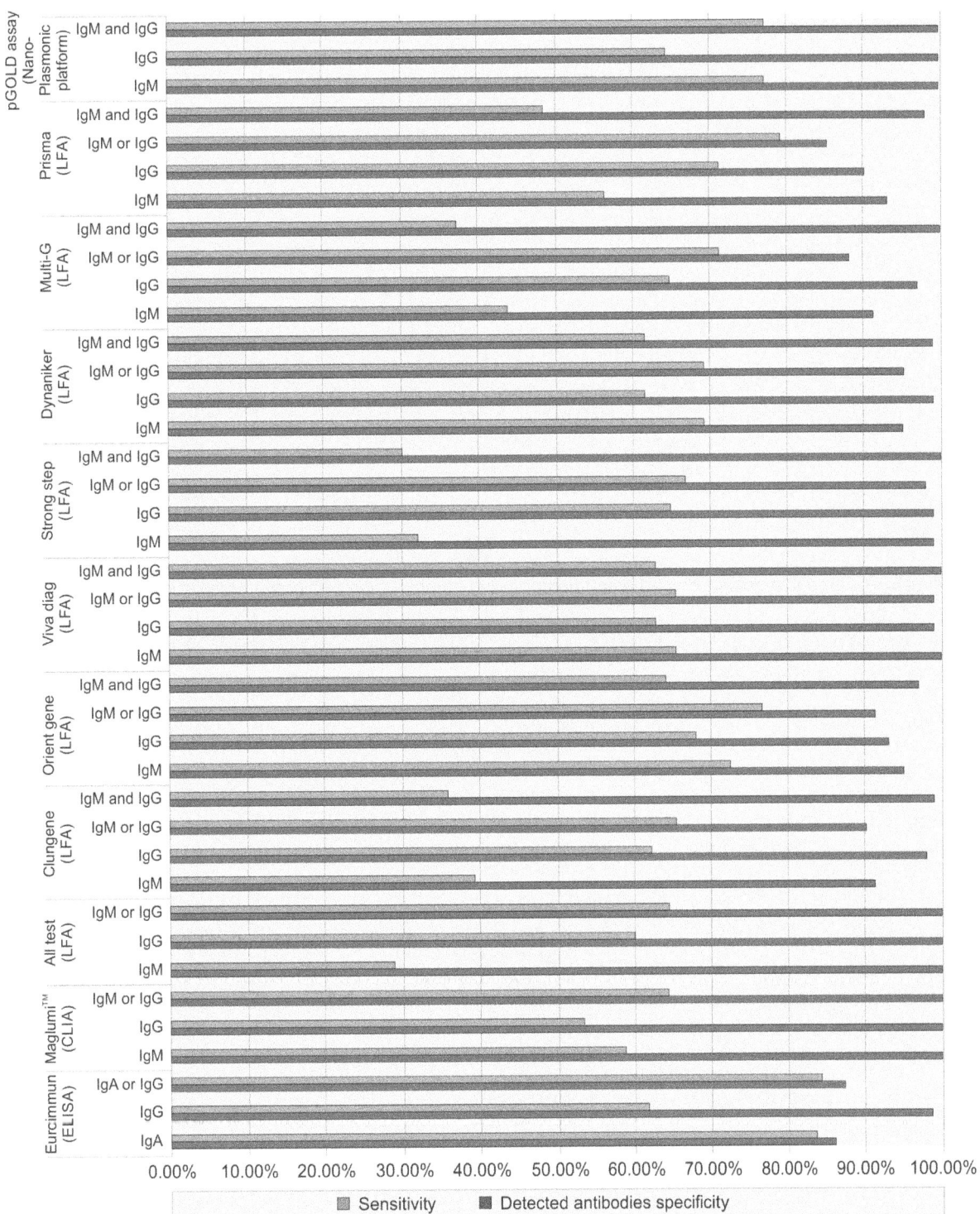

Fig. 7: Diagnostic accuracy of various commercially available antibody tests.[18]

Mechanical ventilation is indicated in patients with H-phenotype and those who do not respond to high-flow oxygen (HFNO/HVNI) in the first 2 hours and the following:
- Need of vasopressor support
- Persistently high respiratory rate
- Persistent thoracoabdominal asynchrony
- Low ROX index

Once intubated and deeply sedated, the type L patients, if hypercapnic, can be ventilated with volumes greater than 6 mL/kg (up to 8–9 mL/kg), as the high compliance results in tolerable strain without the risk of VILI. Prone positioning should be used only as a rescue maneuver, as the lung conditions are "too good" for the prone position effectiveness, which is based on improved stress and strain redistribution.[22]

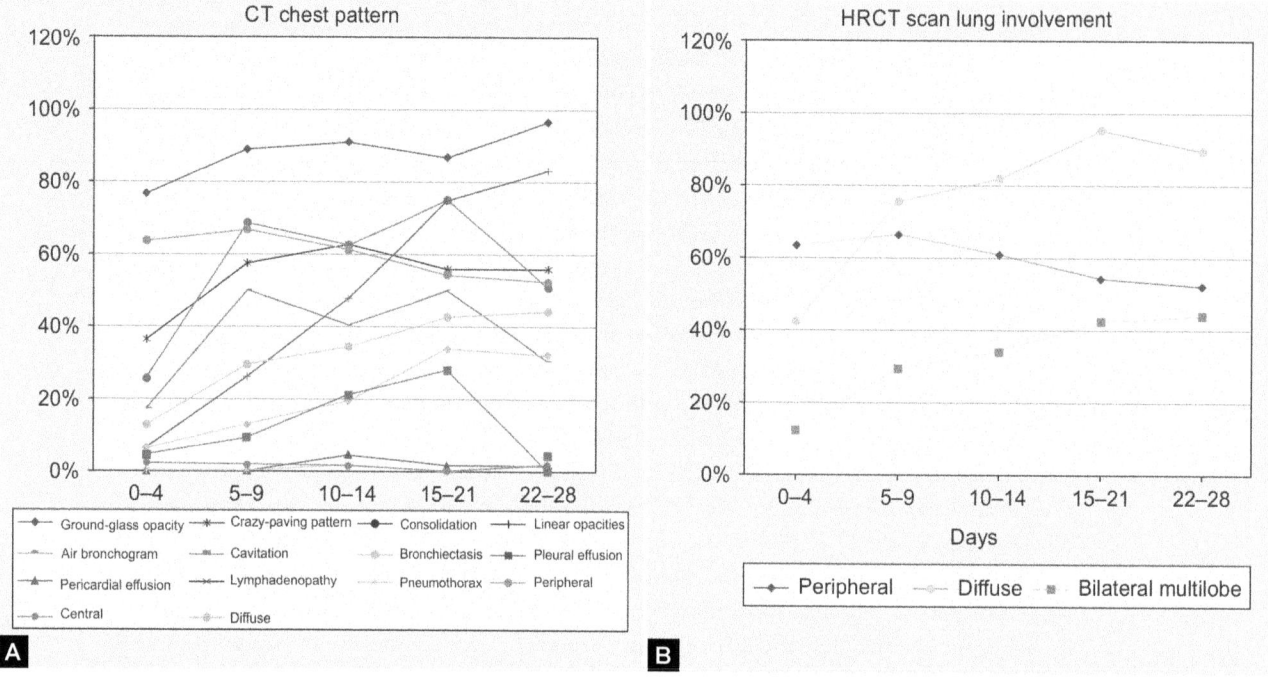

Figs. 8A and B: (A) Computed tomography (CT) chest pattern as per number of days; (B) Lung involvement as per number of days.

Table 3: Summary of various clinical tests available for diagnosis of COVID-19.

Method available	Working principle	Advantages	Time required	Disadvantages
Next-generation sequencing (NGS)	Whole genome sequencing	• Highly sensitive and specific • Provide all related information • Can identify novel strain	1–2 days	• High expertise • Equipment dependency and high cost • Highly sophisticated Lab required
RT-PCR	Specific primer- and probe-based detection	• Fast results • Higher sensitivity • Needs small amount of DNA • Can be performed in a single step • Well-established methodology in viral diagnostics	3–4 hours	• Higher costs due to the use of expensive consumables • Expensive lab equipment • Detection is also complex and time consuming
LAMP	More than two sets of specific primers pair-based detection	• Highly repeatable and accurate • Single working temperature	1 hour	• Too sensitive • Highly prone to false positives due to carryover or cross-contamination
Serological (traditional)	Antigen/Antibodies IgG/IgM	Sensitive and specific	4–6 hours	• Testing come after 3–4 days of infection • False positive
Rapid serological	Antigen/Antibodies IgG/IgM	POCT	15–30 min	• Testing come after 3–4 days of infection • False positive
CT scan	Chest images	Enhance sensitivity of detection if findings combined with RT-PCR results	1 hour	Indistinguishability from other viral pneumonia and the hysteresis of abnormal CT
Virus isolation	In vitro live virus isolation and propagation	• Highly (100%) specific • Gold standard	5–15 days	Low sensitivity

(CT: computed tomography; LAMP: loop-mediated isothermal amplification; RT-PCR: reverse transcription polymerase chain reaction)

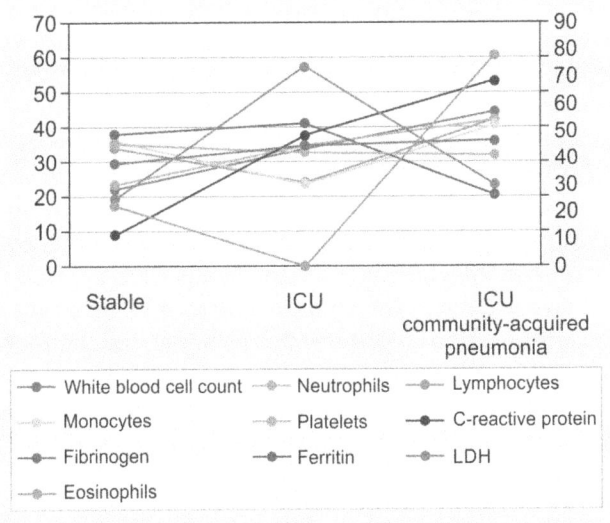

Fig. 9: The trends of inflammatory markers in accordance to severity of COVID-19.[19]

The positive end-expiratory pressure (PEEP) should be reduced to 8-10 cmH$_2$O, given that the recruitability is low and the risk of hemodynamic failure increases at higher levels. An early intubation may avert the transition to type H-phenotype.[22]

Type H patients should be treated as severe ARDS, including higher PEEP, if compatible with hemodynamics, prone positioning, and extracorporeal support.[22]

Anticoagulation

To reduce the risk of venous thromboembolism, use pharmacological prophylaxis (low molecular-weight heparin preferred, if available, or heparin 5,000 units subcutaneously twice daily) in adolescents and adults without contraindications. For those with contraindications, use mechanical prophylaxis (intermittent pneumatic compression devices).

Discharge Criteria[24]

- No fever spikes for 3 consecutive days
- Resolution of respiratory complaints

Table 4: Stages of infection as per severity in COVID-19.

Clinical		
1	Asymptomatic	No treatment required
2	Symptomatic, no pneumonia	Hydroxychloroquine 400 mg BD for 1 day and 200 mg BD for 4 days
		Alternative: Chloroquine 500 mg BD for 5 days
3	Symptomatic, pneumonia	Hydroxychloroquine 400 mg BD for 1 day and 200 mg BD
		In the presence of warning signs, add lopinavir/ritonavir 2 BD; duration: 7–14 days
4	Symptomatic, pneumonia, requiring supplemental oxygen	Hydroxychloroquine 400 mg BD for 1 day and 200 mg BD and lopinavir/ritonavir 2 BD; duration: 7–14 days
5	Critically ill with multiorgan	Hydroxychloroquine 400 mg BD for 1 day and 200 mg BD and lopinavir/ritonavir 2 BD
		Ribavirin 2.4 g stat and 1.2 g BD or SC; Interferon β-1b 250 mg/8 mIU EOD for seven doses
		Look for evidence of cytokine release syndrome

Stage 2 and 3 can be further classified based on the presence or absence of warning signs
Warning signs: Fever, dropping ALC, increasing CRP, and tachycardia

Table 5: The phenotypes of pneumonia.

	L-pneumonia	H-pneumonia
Elastance	Low	High
	The lung compliance is nearly normal	There is decrease in gas volume due to increased pulmonary edema
Ventilation–perfusion ratio	Low	High
	Loss of hypoxic vasoconstriction results in dysregulation of perfusion. The pulmonary artery pressures are normal	Perfusion of nonaerated (increasing edema) dependent region of the lungs
Lung weight	Moderate increase in lung weight. Subpleural and perifissural ground-glass opacities seen on CT scan of the chest	High
		Determined by quantitative analysis on CT scan
Recruitability	Low	High
	As the nonaerated lung tissue is low	Due to increased amount of nonaerated lung tissue

- Two serial, 24 hours apart, RT-PCR for COVID-19 negative from nasopharyngeal swab
- CT scan demonstrating resolution of lesions

Drugs for COVID-19

There is no sure treatment for COVID-19. Since there are a large number of people dying because of COVID-19, faster approvals have been given to these drugs showing one modest benefit.

Remdesivir

Remdesivir, a failed product of Gilead, gained attention in COVID-19 pandemic because of favorable effects documented in the most small sets of critical patients for compassionate use. The US FDA permitted emergencies of use of remdesivir on May 1st, 2020.

The Adaptive COVID-19 Treatment Trial (ACTT) having 1,063 patients showed rapid recovery 31% faster than the placebo. The median time to recovery and statistically insignificant benefit in mortality rate was 11 days and 7.1%, respectively in the remdesivir arm.[25]

In a phase 3 open-labeled randomized controlled trial (RCT), the number of subjects in the control arm was more than two times the subjects in the remdesivir treatment arm. With severe COVID-19 patients requiring mechanical ventilation, improvement in 5 days was observed in remdesivir arm. The data showed 62% reduction in mortality compared to standard care similarly 5 days clinical improvement for seen 65% patients.

The compassionate use of remdesivir without: control arm 80% children ventilator showed recovery while it is 87% on noninvasive oxygen for recovery.

This wonder drug miserably failed in a double-blind, placebo-controlled, multicenter trial at 10 hospitals in China.[26] This was only double-blind RCT done for remdesivir. It did not show any statistical significant benefit over the placebo in terms of clinical improvement. However, 66% of the patients had severe adverse drug reactions with remdesivir as compared to 64% with the placebo. The drug was discontinued in 12% of the patients in the treatment arm due to adverse drug reactions.

In the midst of conflicting evidence, more double-blind, prospective, RCTs are needed to definitively support the hype of usefulness as claimed. The seasonal flu since the seasonal flu seems to overtake sales to complicate the picture of COVID-19.

Favipiravir

Favipiravir is oral antiviral approved in Japan for treatment of influenza and in Russia for COVID-19. It is RNA polymerase selective inhibitor. By inhibiting RNA polymerase, it stops viral replication. On comparison with lopinavir/ritonavir, it did not show any advantage in improvement of any clinical symptoms as compared to latter regimen.[27] An, open-labeled, prospective randomized control of 236 patient with moderate-to-severe COVID-19 infection also showed no significant benefit of favipiravir as compared to arbidol at day 7 in terms of clinical recovery.[28]

In an open-label control study[29] with 80 patients having mild-to-moderate severity of COVID-19 infection, favipiravir showed some better results as compared to lopinavir/ritonavir. The viral clearance and improvement on chest imaging was better with favipiravir as compared to lopinavir/ritonavir combination.

However, conflicting results of the clinical trials mandate information of results in a proper prospective, randomized, double-blind controlled trial.

Lopinavir/Ritonavir

They are antiretroviral drugs, which have shown efficacy against flu and HIV in February 2020. The combination reduced viral load and improved clinical outcomes in SARS infection. Hence, this combination was tried in COVID-19.

Cao et al.[30] compared the combination in 99 patients with respect to standard care in 100 patients with COVID-19 pneumonia having oxygen saturation <94% with ratio of partial pressure of oxygen to fractional inspired oxygen <300 mm Hg. The primary endpoint of median time to clinical improvement (16 days) was achieved in both the treatment and the control arms. No difference was observed in mortality at 28 days. However, the combination reduced the length of ICU stay 6 days against the standard care of 11 days. The adverse events were more in the combination group as compared with the standard care.

Li et al.[31] compared lopinavir (200 mg)/ritonavir (50 mg) twice daily with arbidol (200 mg) thrice daily and standard treatment in a RCT. It was observed that lopinavir–ritonavir combination was nonsuperior to the other arms. There was no benefit of the combination with respect to reduction in clinical worsening, symptoms, or radiological improvement.

Chloroquine and Hydroxychloroquine

Remdesivir exhibits its effect at the entry of virus into the cell whereas chloroquine shown to exhibit antiviral action at the entry and postentry level.

Hydroxychloroquine is known to have anti-inflammatory properties. The mechanism of action of hydroxychloroquine is as follows:[32]

It is known to reduce:

- *Inflammatory cytokines*: Interleukin (IL)-6, IL-17, IFN-α, IFN-l, TNF-α
- *Toll-like receptors (TLRs)*: TLR-3, TLR-7, and TLR-9
- Prostaglandin and phospholipid

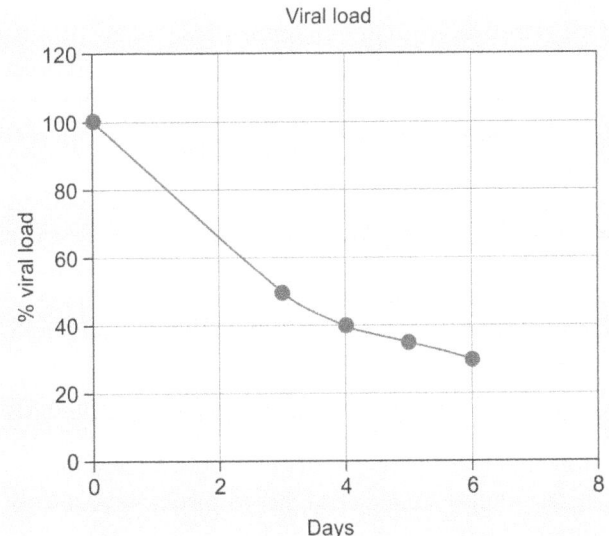

Fig. 10: Reduction in viral load following hydroxychloroquine.[33]

It is known to increase the endosomal and lysosomal pH, stabilize the lysosomal enzymes, and inhibit the extracellular matrix metalloproteinases.

It is also known to reduce oxidative stress.

It is one of the most widely studied molecules to treat COVID-19. A nonrandomized open-label trial showed 70% reduction of viral load by day 7 as shown in **Figure 10**.

Chloroquine causes QT prolongation in susceptible individuals. Risk of retinal damage, especially with long-term use. It can cause hemolysis in patients with G6PD deficiency. Caution is to be exercised in diabetics.[34]

It is interesting that azithromycin is prescribed for "bacterial superinfection prevention" in six patients. Researchers found that viral eradication was statistically better in this subgroup (6/6, 100%) than in those receiving hydroxychloroquine alone (8/14, 57%). The authors conclude that the SARS-CoV-2 emitted by azithromycin hydroxychloroquine "reinforces the viral load." Although this data is convenient, some limitations of this dataset must be accepted.

First, although viral eradication is an important endpoint, the authors did not report clinical outcomes in these patients. Second, the cohort initially included 26 hydroxychloroquine patients, but six of them were excluded from the analysis due to early discontinuation of hydroxychloroquine therapy, in which three PCR-positive patients were transferred to the ICU, with 1% RCR negative. Those who passed and one PCR-positive patient discontinued hydroxychloroquine due to nausea. Finally, there are fewer patients with hydroxychloroquine monotherapy who have lower bicycle threshold (CT) values than those who receive combination therapy. Hydroxychloroquine monotherapy patients with CT values <23 had significantly higher (1/5, 20% vs. 7/9, 78%) differences in viral elimination rate compared with CT values. The treatment was performed when a combination of hydroxychloroquine and azithromycin was reached, where the CT value was 6% in all patients.

In this finding, we caution clinicians because of the small number of studies, the lack of presented clinical results, the toxicity of additives with hydroxychloroquine and azithromycin, and the need to follow good antimicrobial standards during the COVID-19 pandemic. These data support combination therapy.

In addition, the hydroxychloroquine effect is even more potent when patients are combined with azithromycin to suit their clinical need. However, the incidence of clinical follow-up and adverse effects has not been discussed; further efforts should be made to reduce the morbidity and mortality of COVID-19. Although these two drugs have shown good efficacy against SARS-CoV-2, there is a risk of arrhythmia with their administration.

Corticosteroids

Corticosteroids are endogenously produced hormones by the adrenal cortex. They are powerful anti-inflammatory hormones. They act by entering the cells and causing DNA transcription to produce new proteins on the cytoplasmic ribosomes. These proteins produced by the glucocorticoids exert the biological effects.

They exert immunosuppressive effect by inhibition of cytokine production by inhibiting kinases and partly from inhibition of nuclear transcription factor (NF-kB). NF-kB stimulates the transcription of cytokines, chemokines, and also activates histone deacetylase (causing increased genetic transcription). They are also responsible for increasing apoptosis in the inflammatory cells like eosinophils, T-lymphocytes, mast cells, and macrophages resulting in blunting in cell-mediated immune response and production of cytokines.

The biological half-life of dexamethasone is 36–54 hours, which is nearly twice the half-life of prednisolone.

Zhikang Ye et al.[35] in the month of May, 2020 published a review article on safety and efficacy of corticosteroid in COVID-19. As per them, corticosteroids reduce mortality for patient with COVID-19 and ARDS. However, this beneficial effect was inconsistent when patients suffered from severe COVID-19 with the absence of ARDS.

After this initial review and recovery trial showing positive benefits of use of corticosteroids in COVID-19, two systemic reviews published recently have different viewpoint of examining the data more comprehensively.

Recently published review in June, 2020[36] analyzed four retrospective studies and one quasi prospective study. The investigators concluded that out of the five studies, three showed some benefit whereas the other two studies did not show any benefit but instead a significant clinical harm.

Tlayjeh H et al.[37] published a review and meta-analysis in August 2, 2020. They found the following:
- Corticosteroids lack efficacy in reducing short-term mortality
- There is delay in viral clearance in the following corticosteroid group
- There is discordance of results observed in the clinical trials with corticosteroids; hence, a large RCT is required for asserting the benefit of corticosteroids in COVID-19.

Ivermectin

Ivermectin has been shown to have antibacterial, antiparasitic, and antiviral (including coronavirus family) properties. It is a lipid-soluble molecule with immunomodulatory effect in the host. A recent in vitro study tested the efficacy of ivermectin on SARS-CoV-2-infected Vero/hSLAM cells. At concentration as low as 5 mm (millimoles) in 48 hours, ivermectin resulted in 5,000-fold reduction in the viral load as compared with control.[38] Thus, ivermectin nearly effectively killed the entire viral particles in 48 hours.

Ivermectin crosses the intestinal epithelium to get concentrated in the blood without any toxicity. It has been shown that a drug cannot close a pleasant barrier; hence, it is safe to be used in pregnant females.

A retrospective cohort study of 280 hospitalized patient at four centers in Florida confirmed lower mortality rate of 15% in people receiving ivermectin compared to the usual care (25% mortality rate). And in severe pulmonary disease, the mortality rate was 38.8% against 80.7% in those who received standard care.[39]

In a study from Bangladesh,[40] ivermectin in combination with doxycycline had 66% virus clearance on day 5, and 83.5% on day 6 of treatment. In comparison to this, hydroxychloroquine and azithromycin had viral clearance of 77% at day 11 and 81.5% at day 12. In the doxycycline group, 16.5% individuals remain PCR positive after 6 days of ingestion as compared to 18.5% at day 12 of the hydroxychloroquine/azithromycin.

Study reveals that doxycycline and ivermectin are a better combination as compared to hydroxychloroquine and azithromycin.

Based on the evidence in treatment of COVID-19, Patri and his associates hypothesized that combination of hydroxychloroquine and ivermectin would exhibit of consequential synergistic action. As per them, hydroxychloroquine would first ban the entry of virus into the host cell, while ivermectin would reduce viral replication of the viruses escaping the effect of hydroxychloroquine and entering the cell. Ivermectin has been found safe with negligible adverse drug reactions, which were well tolerated.[41]

Tocilizumab

Interleukin-6 (IL-6) is proinflammatory cytokine. It is the major cytokine responsible for cytokine storm. IL-6 affects the functioning of the cell-mediated immunity. It causes increasing CRP.[42]

Observational study of 239 patients with severe COVID-19 disease showed the survival rate of patients treated with tocilizumab was the same as the control group. However, in the tocilizumab group, 75% patients on mechanical ventilation survived. In New Jersey, tocilizumab improved the survival rate by 56% as compared with the standard line of care.

However, an Italian study with tocilizumab was terminated, as the molecule failed to show appreciable improvement on all the parameters in consideration.

Large phase-3 legal trial was conducted under the funding of Roche. Tocilizumab failed miserably to meet the primary and secondary endpoints. Similarly, another IL-6 inhibitor sarilumab failed to meet the primary endpoint in the phase-III clinical trials conducted by Sanofi and Regeneron.

In view of conflicting evidence, it is necessary to have double-blind RCT on a larger scale to validate the claims.

Convalescent Plasma Treatment for COVID-19

The mortality in COVID-19 ranges from 10 to 80% despite of all the available treatment options.[43,44] Convalescent plasma is obtained from the person who has recovered from COVID-19 sickness and has developed humoral immunity. This plasma has high titers of neutralizing antibodies against the COVID-19 virus. This is to treat a person having COVID-19 infections by passive transfer of immunity.[45] The antibodies from the convalescent blood product neutralize the virus in the patient's blood by binding to it and opsonization.

Mechanism of Action[46]

The direct antiviral action of convalescent plasma by the neutralizing antibodies found COVID-19 virus in the recovered patient who acted as a donor. The antiviral action is also reputed by modulation by complement pathway, cytokines, and autoantibodies. The composition of convalescent plasma and mechanism of action are illustrated in **Figures 11A to C**.

Figure 12 briefly outlines the process of convalescent plasma collection to its administration.

A prospective study from Houston Methodist Hospital[47] studied the effects of convalescent plasma in 316 patients. **Figures 13A to D** shows the results of the trial.

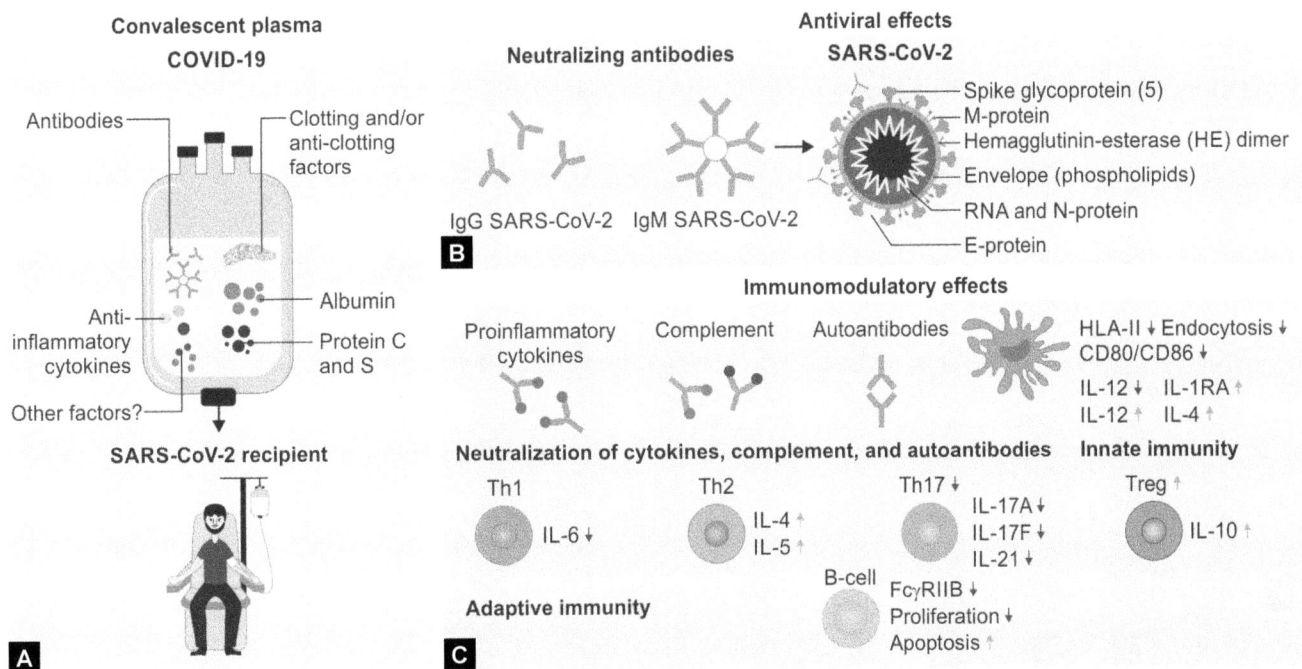

Figs. 11A to C: Schematic representation of convalescent plasma components and its mechanisms of action. (A) Main convalescent plasma components; (B) Antiviral effects of neutralizing antibodies (NAbs). IgG and IgM are the main isotypes, although IgA may be also important, particularly in mucosal viral infections. Other non-NAbs may exert a protective effect. The humoral immune response is mainly directed toward spike (S) protein; (C) Anti-inflammatory effects of CP include network of autoantibodies and control of an overactive immune system (*i.e.*, cytokine storm, Th1/Th17 ratio, complement activation, and regulation of a hypercoagulable state). (N: nucleoprotein; M: membrane; E: envelop).

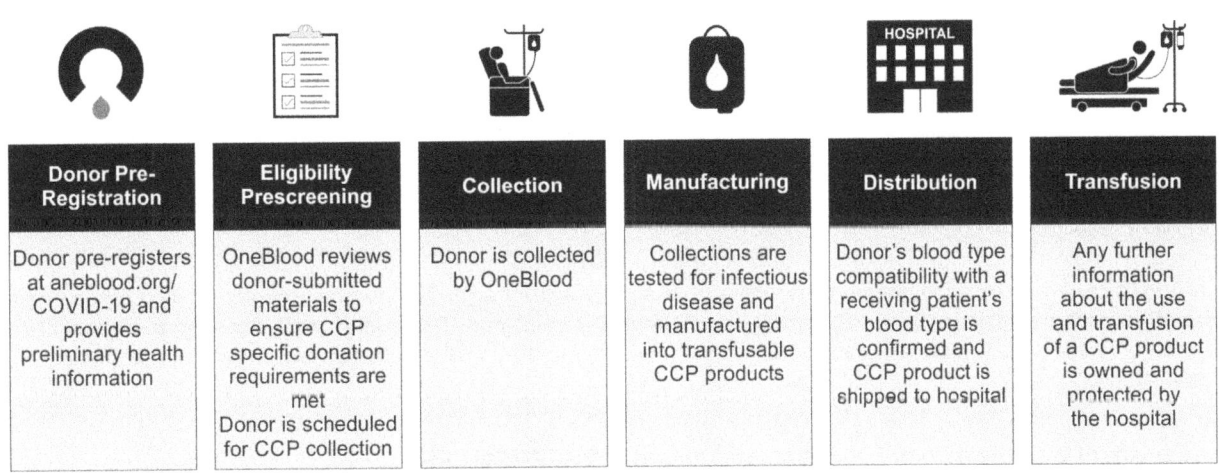

Fig. 12: Convalescent plasma process.

This study clearly shows mortality benefit with use of convalescent plasma as treatment for severe cases of COVID-19.

The updated Cochrane review[48] analyzed 19 studies of convalescent plasma with total of 38,160 participants. The investigators concluded convalescent plasma therapy caused no significant improvement in symptoms at 7 days, but some improvements may be seen from 15 days up to 30 days. The therapy did not show any mortality benefit.

Cochrane review observed a bias in the reporting of adverse events. Most of the studilaes did not report the grade of adverse events. 14 studies (566 participants) documented

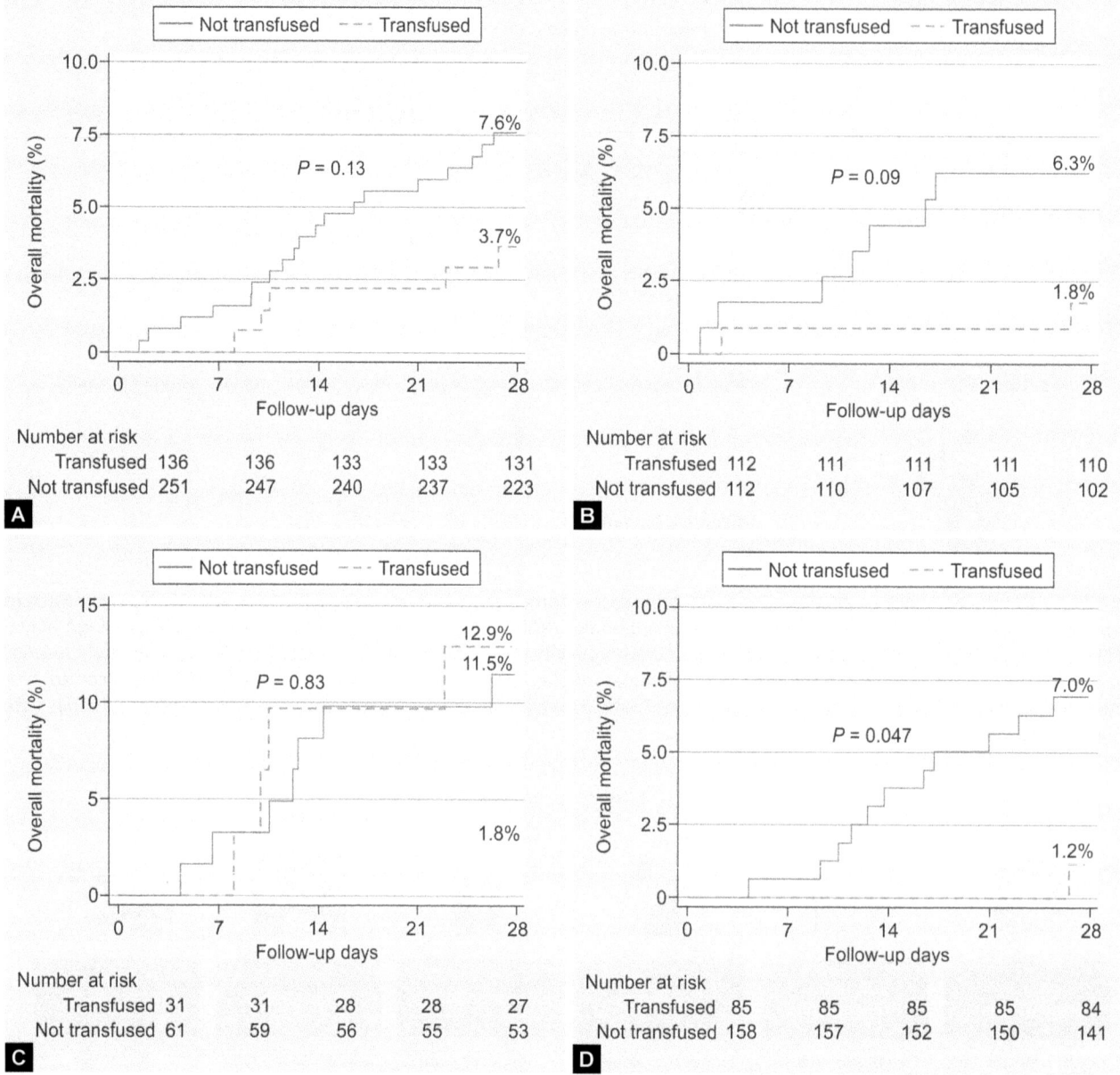

Figs. 13A to D: Kaplan–Meier curves for mortality within 28 days post-day 0 for secondary matched cohorts. (A) All secondary matched patients; (B) Secondary matched patients transfused within 72 hours of admission; (C) Secondary matched patients transfused >72 hours after admission; (D) Secondary matched patients transfused within 72 hours of admission with plasma with antireceptor-binding domain IgG titer ≥ 1:1,350.

adverse events of grade 3–4 severity. Nine nonrandomized controlled trials amounting to 20,662 participants reported the adverse events, which included 63 deaths.

The investigators also documented 146 serious adverse drug events in the first 4 hours and 1,136 serious adverse drug events in the span of 7 days following convalescent plasma transfusion.

However, 73 RCTs studying the effect of convalescent plasma in COVID-19 are already underway. Therefore, the interpretation of data must be done with caution.

REFERENCES

1. Felsensteina S, Herbertb JA, McNamarab PS, Hedrich CM. Review article: COVID-19: immunology and treatment options. Clin Immunol. 2020;215:108448.
2. Liang Y, Wang ML, Chien CS, Yarmishyn AA, Yang YP, Lai WY, et al. Highlight of immune pathogenic response and hematopathologic effect in SARS-CoV, MERS-CoV, and SARS-Cov-2 infection. Front Immunol. 2020;11:1022.
3. Jin Y, Yang H, Ji W, Wu W, Chen S, Zhang W, et al. Virology, epidemiology, pathogenesis, and control of COVID-19. Viruses. 2020;12(4):372.

4. Domingo E. Long-term virus evolution in nature. Virus as Populations. 2020:225-61.
5. van Doremalen N, Bushmaker T, Morris DH, Holbrook MG, Gamble A, Williamson BN, et al. Aerosol and surface stability of SARS-CoV-2 as compared with SARS-CoV-1. N Engl J Med. 2020;382:1564-7.
6. Kratzel A, Todt D, V'kovski P, Steiner S, Gultrom M, Thao TTN, et al. Inactivation of severe acute respiratory syndrome coronavirus 2 by WHO-recommended hand rub formulations and alcohols. Emerg Infect Dis. 2020;26(7):1592-5.
7. Guo ZD, Wang ZY, Zhang SF, Li X, Li L, Li C, et al. Aerosol and surface distribution of severe acute respiratory syndrome coronavirus 2 in hospital wards, Wuhan, China, 2020. Emerg Infect Dis. 2020;26(7):1583-91.
8. Kakodkar P, Kaka N, Baig M. A Comprehensive literature review on the clinical presentation, and management of the pandemic coronavirus disease 2019 (COVID-19). Cureus. 2020;12(4):e7560.
9. Kindler E, Thiel V, Weber F. Interaction of SARS and MERS coronaviruses with the antiviral interferon response. Adv Virus Res. 2016;96:219-43.
10. Bhaskar S, Sinha A, Banach M, Mittoo S, Weissert R, Kass JS, et al. Cytokine storm in COVID-19—Immunopathological mechanisms, clinical considerations, and therapeutic approaches: The REPROGRAM Consortium Position Paper. Front Immunol. 2020;11:1648.
11. Machhi J, Herskovitz J, Senan AM, Dutta D, Nath B, Oleynikov MD, et al. The natural history, pathobiology, and clinical manifestations of SARS-CoV-2 infections. J Neuroimmune Pharmacol. 2020;15(3):1-28.
12. Chen T, Wu D, Chen H, Yan W, Yang D, Chen G, et al. Clinical characteristics of 113 deceased patients with coronavirus disease 2019: Retrospective study. BMJ. 2020;368:m1091.
13. Udugama B, Kadhiresan P, Kozlowski HN, Malekjahani A, Osborne M, Li VYC, et al. Diagnosing COVID-19: the disease and tools for detection. ACS Nano. 2020;14(4):3822-35.
14. Kumar R, Nagpal S, Kaushik S, Mendiratta S. COVID-19 diagnostic approaches: different roads to the same destination. Virusdisease. 2020;31(2):97-105.
15. La Marca A, Capuzzo M, Paglia T, Roli L, Trenti T, Nelson SM. Testing for SARS-CoV-2 (COVID-19): a systematic review and clinical guide to molecular and serological in-vitro diagnostic assays. Reprod Biomed Online. 2020;41(3):483-99.
16. Sethuraman N, Jeremiah SS, Ryo A. Interpreting diagnostic tests for SARS-CoV-2. JAMA. 2020;323(22):2249-51.
17. Jacofsky D, Jacofsky EM, Jacofsky M. Understanding antibody testing for COVID-19. J Arthroplasty. 2020;35(7S):S74-S81.
18. Li C, Zhao C, Bao J, Tang B, Wang Y, Gu B. Laboratory diagnosis of coronavirus disease-2019 (COVID-19). Clin Chim Acta. 2020;510:35-46.
19. Elvaney OJ, McEvoy NL, McElvaney OF, Carroll TP, Murphy MP, Dunlea DM, et al. Characterisation of inflammatory response to severe COVID-19 illness. AJRCCM. 2020;202(6):812-21.
20. Ministry of Health, Malaysia (MOH) (2020). Clinical Management of Conrmed Case. Annex 2e. [online] Available from: https://www.moh.gov.my/moh/resources/Penerbitan/Garis%20Panduan/COVID19/Annex_2e_Clinical_Management_22032020.pdf [Last accessed December, 2020].
21. Whittle JS, Pavlov I, Sacchetti AD, Atwood C, Rosenberg MS. Respiratory support for adult patients with COVID-19. JACEP Open. 2020;1(2):95-101.
22. Gattinoni L, Chiumello D, Caironi P, Busana M, Romitti F, Brazzi L, et al. COVID-19 pneumonia: different respiratory treatment for different phenotypes? Intensive Care Med. 2020;46(6):1099-102.
23. Roca O, Caralt B, Messika J, Samper M, Sztrymf B, Hernández G, et al. An index combining respiratory rate and oxygenation to predict outcome of nasal high-flow therapy. Am J Respir Crit Care Med. 2019;199(11):1368-76.
24. European Center for Disease Prevention and Control (2020). Discharge criteria for confirmed COVID-19 cases—When is it safe to discharge COVID-19 cases from the hospital or end home isolation? [online] Available from: https://www.ecdc.europa.eu/sites/default/files/documents/COVID-19-Discharge-criteria.pdf [Last accessed December, 2020].
25. Beigel JH, Tomashek KM, Dodd LE, Mehta AK, Zingman BS, Kalil AC, et al. Remdesivir for the Treatment of COVID-19—Preliminary Report (ACTT-1 Study). N Engl J Med. 2020;383(19):1813-26.
26. Yeming W, Zhang D, Du G, Du R, Zhao J, Jin Y, et al. Remdesivir in adults with severe COVID-19: a randomised, double-blind, placebo-controlled, multicentre trial. Lancet. 2020;395(10236):1569-78.
27. Lou Y, Liu L, Qiu Y. Clinical outcomes and plasma concentrations of Baloxavir Marboxil and Favipiravir in COVID-19 patients: an exploratory randomized, controlled trial. Eur J Pharm Sci. 2021;157:105631.
28. Chen C, Zhang Y, Huang J, Yin P, Cheng Z, Wu J, et al. Favipiravir versus arbidol for COVID-19: a randomized clinical trial. medRxiv; 2020. [online] Available from: https://doi.org/10.1101/2020.03.17.20037432.
29. Cai Q, Yang M, Liu D, Chen J, Shu D, Xia J, et al. Experimental treatment with Favipiravir for COVID-19: an open-label control study. Engineering (Beijing). 2020;6(10):1192-8.
30. Cao B, Wang Y, Wen D, Liu W, Wang J, Fan G, et al. A trial of lopinavir-ritonavir in adults hospitalized with severe Covid-19. N Engl J Med. 2020;382:1787-99.
31. Li Y, Xie Z. Efficacy and safety of lopinavir/ritonavir or arbidol in adult patients with mild/moderate COVID-19: An exploratory randomized controlled trial. Med (NY). 2020;1(1):105-13.e4.
32. Drożdżal S, Rosik J, Lechowicz K, Machaj F, Kotfis K, Ghavami S, et al. FDA approved drugs with pharmacotherapeutic potential for SARS-CoV-2 (COVID-19) therapy. Drug Resist Updat. 2020;53:100719.
33. Gautret P, Lagier J-C, Parola P, Hoang VT, Meddeb L, Mailhe M, et al. Hydroxychloroquine and azithromycin as a treatment of COVID-19: results of an open-label non-randomized clinical trial. Int J Antimicrob Agents. 2020;56(1):105949.
34. Smith T, Bushek J, Prosser T. (2020). COVID-19 Drug Therapy—Potential Options. [online] Available from: elsevier.com/__data/assets/pdf_file/0007/988648/COVID-19-Drug-Therapy_2020-8-28.pdf [Last accessed December, 2020].

35. Ye Z, Wang Y, Colunga-Lozano LE, Prasad M, Tangamornsuksan W, Rochwerg B. Efficacy and safety of corticosteroids in COVID-19 based on evidence for COVID-19, other coronavirus infections, influenza, community-acquired pneumonia and acute respiratory distress syndrome: a systematic review and meta-analysis. CMAJ. 2020;192(27):E756-E767.

36. Singh AK, Majumdar S, Singh R, Misra A. Role of corticosteroid in the management of COVID-19: A systemic review and a Clinician's perspective. Diabetes Metab Syndr. 2020;14(5):971-8.

37. Tlayjeh H, Mhish O, Enani M, Alruwaili A, Tleyjeh R, Thalib L, et al. Efficacy of Corticosteroids in COVID-19 Patients: A Systematic Review and Meta-Analysis. medRxiv. 2020.08.13.20174201; doi: https://doi.org/10.1101/2020.08.13.20174201.

38. Caly L, Druce JD, Catton MG, Jans DA, Wagstaff KM. The FDA-approved drug ivermectin inhibits the replication of SARS-CoV-2 in vitro. Antiviral Res. 2020;178:104787.

39. Rajter JC, Sherman M, Fatteh N, Vogel F, Sacks J, Rajter JJ. ICON (Ivermectin in COvid Nineteen) study: Use of ivermectin is associated with lower mortality in hospitalized patients with COVID-19. medRxiv; 2020. [online] Available from: https://doi.org/10.1101/2020.06.06.20124461.

40. Rahman MA, Iqbal S, Islam MA, Niaz MK, Hussain T, Siddiquee T. Comparison of Viral Clearance between Ivermectin with Doxycycline and Hydroxychloroquine with Azithromycin in COVID-19 Patients. J Bangladesh Coll Phys Surg. 2020;38:5-9.

41. Patrì A, Fabbrocini G. Hydroxychloroquine and ivermectin: a synergistic combination for COVID-19 chemoprophylaxis and treatment? J Am Acad Dermatol. 2020;82(6):e221.

42. Higgins PJ, Rider P, Carmi Y, Cohen I. Biologics for targeting inflammatory cytokines, clinical uses, and limitations. Int J Cell Biol. 2016;2016:9259646.

43. Zeng QL, Yu ZJ, Gou JJ, Li GM, Ma SH, Zhang GF, et al. Effect of convalescent plasma therapy on viral shedding and survival in patients with coronavirus disease 2019. J Infect Dis. 2020;222(1):38-43.

44. Guan WJ, Ni ZY, Hu Y, Liang WH, Ou CQ, He JX, et al. Clinical characteristics of coronavirus disease 2019 in China. N Engl J Med. 2020;382:1708-20.

45. Long K CV, Sayed A, Karki P, Acharya Y. Convalescent blood products in COVID-19: a narrative review. Ther Adv Infect Dis. 2020;7:2049936120960646.

46. Manuel R, Yhojan R, Diana M, Yeny AA, Bernardo C, Esteban GJ, et al. Convalescent plasma in COVID-19: Possible mechanisms of action. Autoimmun Rev. 2020;19(7):102554.

47. Salazar E, Christensen PA, Graviss EA, Nguyen DT, Castillo B, Chen J, et al. Treatment of COVID-19 patients with convalescent plasma reveals a signal of significantly decreased mortality. Am J Pathol. 2020;190(11):2290-303.

48. Chai KL, Valk SJ, Piechotta V, Kimber C, Monsef I, Doree C, et al. Convalescent plasma or hyperimmune immunoglobulin for people with COVID-19: a living systematic review. Cochrane Database Syst Rev. 2020(10):CD013600.

Index

A

Abacavir 73, 78, 170
    case of hypersensitivity reaction 173
Abdominal bloating 2
Abdominal examination 215
Abdominal hysterectomy 148
Abdominal infections 398
    case study 377-382
Abdominal lymphadenopathy 63
Abdominal pain 56, 216, 218, 230, 380
    diffuse 279
    upper 212
Abdominal sonography 341
Abscess 2
    rupture of 179
Acanthamoeba 326, 333
Acetabulum 162, 391
Acid-fast bacilli 95, 86, 125, 266
    detection of 289
Acid-fast structures 204
Acidosis disrupts 191
Acinetobacter 27, 152, 153, 257, 271
Acinetobacter baumannii 17, 257
Acinetobacter junii 257
Acquired cytomegalovirus 120
Acquired immunodeficiency syndrome 25, 91, 123, 209, 272, 336, 358, 397
Actinomycosis, osseous lesions in 122
Activated partial thromboplastin 342
Acute respiratory distress syndrome 3, 129, 230, 271, 300
    develop 19
Acute retroviral syndrome 219
Acyclovir 120, 253, 297
Adenosine monophosphate 188
Adrenal infection 401
Adrenal insufficiency in infection 183
Adrenal masses, bilateral 383
Aedes aegypti 231, 353, 357
Aedes albopictus 346
Aeromonas species 21
Afebrile 305
African eye worm 221
African tumbu fly 223
Agranulocytic angina 19
AIDS dementia complex 119
Airway invasive aspergillosis 396
Albendazole 198, 222, 307, 351
Alcohol induced 213
Alcoholic liver cirrhosis 12, 110
Allergic bronchopulmonary aspergillosis 229, 352, 396
Allergic conjunctivitis 332
Allergic granulomatosis 229
Allogeneic bone marrow transplant 373
Allogeneic stem cell transplant 314
Allograft biopsy 281

Allopurinol 56
Alpha-1 antitrypsin deficiency 181
Alpha-blockers and catheterization 152
Alphavirus 348
Alveolar-arterial oxygen tension 129
Alveolar haemorrhage, diffuse 320
Amblyomma aureolatum 222
Amblyomma cajennense 222
Amebic hepatic abscesses 398
Amebic liver abscess 176, 398
Amebic meningoencephalitis, primary 205, 211
American College of Obstetricians and Gynecologists 359
American College of Rheumatology 60
American Society of Transplantation 312
American Thoracic Society 16
Amikacin 18, 312
Aminoglycoside 18, 228, 264, 289, 305
    synergy 304
Ammonium compounds, quaternary 23
Amoxicillin 261, 270
Amphotericin B 31, 305
    lipid formulation of 299
Amphotericin B deoxycholate 30, 311
Ampicillin 270, 363
    plus azithromycin 367
Amyloidosis 181
    primary 317
Ancylostoma braziliense 222
Ancylostoma duodenale 209, 210
Anemia
    cause of 208
    etiology of 297
Angioedema 210, 221
Angioimmunoblastic lymphoma 274, 277
Angiotensin converting enzyme inhibitors 297
Angiotensin receptor blockers 297
Anidulafungin 299, 306
Antibiotic 304
    broad spectrum 26, 28, 29
    coverage 19
    lock therapy 248
    treatment risks 18
Antibodies, titration of 136
Antibody test 36, 412
Anti-cyclic citrullinated peptide 213
Antifungal agents
    selection of 268
    titration of 78
Antifungal prophylaxis 46, 49, 267, 273
Antifungal susceptibility 305
Antigen detection 36
Antigen test, direct 412
Anti-histone antibodies 59
Antimicrobial prophylaxis 320
Antinuclear antibody 63, 90, 161
Antioxidant enzymes 186

Antiretroviral therapy 86, 167, 416
Antithymocyte globulin 279
Antitubercular
    chemotherapy 158
    treatment 168, 225, 289
Aphasia 296
Arginine deiminase 173
Arlt's line 332, 333
Artemether-lumefantrine, combination therapy 229
Arterial blood gas 283, 338
Artesunate 218, 340
    amodiaquine, combination therapy 229
    mefloquine, combination therapy 229
Arthralgia 170, 190, 212, 217, 339
Arthritis, pyogenic 156
Arthrocentesis 56
Arthroplasty, permanent resection 263
Ascaris lumbricoides 209
Aspartate aminotransferase 215, 303, 408
Aspartate transaminase 15
Aspergilloma 396
Aspergillosis 1, 29, 191, 310
    invasive 25
    mild form of 396
    treatment 316
Aspergillus bronchiolitis 396
Aspergillus fumigatus 25, 64, 301, 305
Aspergillus galactomannan 43, 51
Aspergillus infection 26, 310
Aspergillus pneumonia 17
Aspergillus species 94, 292, 304
Asthma-like attacks 229
Atenolol 56
Atorvastatin 187
Autoimmune diseases 350
Autoimmune exocrine disorder 189
Autoimmune mesenteric vasculature 203
Autologous stem cell transplant 314
Autosomal dominant polycystic disease 287
Azathioprine 60, 68, 124, 137, 293
Azithromycin 20, 48, 417
Azole 191, 312, 321
    causes resistance to 185
    developing breakthrough candidemia 47
    resistant *Candida* species 267

B

Bacille Calmette-Guérin vaccination 143
Bacillus anthracis 224
Bacteria
    intracellular killing of 135
    conjunctivitis 332
Bacterial infection 24, 278
Bacterial pneumonia 225
Bacterial ulcers 334

Index

Bacterial vaginosis 90
  risk factor for 356
Bactericidal agent, backbone of 196
Bacteriuria 364
  absence of 147
  asymptomatic 149, 354
Bacteroides 22
Bacteroides fragilis 80
Bacteroides species 398
Bartonella henselae 7
Basal ganglia 106, 108
Basophilic nuclear 145
Bedaquiline 289
Behçet's disease 189
Benign quartan 209
Beta-lactam 151
Bevacizumab 187
Bevacizumab blocks vascular endothelial growth factor 142
Bladder cancer 152
Blastomyces dermatitidis 387
Bleeding problems 195
Bleeding upper gastrointestinal ulceration 203
Blood cerebrospinal fluid 311
Blood test reveals, routine 369
Blood urea nitrogen 15
Bodyache, severe 340
Bone and joint infections 155
Bone marrow 196, 272
  biopsy 303
  transplant 4, 240
    infections in 314
Bony ankylosis 390
Bordetella pertussis 20, 186
Borrelia burgdorferi, serology test 73
Bovine tuberculosis 196
Bowel-associated dermatosis-arthritis syndrome 55
Bowel predominantly transverse colon 381
Brain biopsy 91
Brain stem cerebrum 118
Brainerd diarrhea 218
Braziliensis 209
Breast cancer
  adjuvant high risk 318
Breathlessness 40, 369, 371
Brincidofovir 296
British Society for Medical Mycology 31
British Thoracic Society, guideline 138
Brodie abscess 161, 404
Bronchial asthma 256
Bronchial breath sounds 125
Bronchiectasis
  chronic 125
  develops headache 29
  therapy for 135
Bronchoalveolar lavage 25, 48, 64, 123, 255, 266, 279, 303
Bronchodilators 124
Bronchopneumonia 396
Brown and Hopps stain 328
Brucella 192, 230
  from tuberculosis 165
  melitensis relapse 192
  positive for 216
  spondylitis 165

Brucellar spondylodiskitis 157
Brucellosis melitensis 196
Brugia malayi 351
Budd-Chiari syndrome 181
Burkholderia pseudomallei 224
Burkitt lymphoma 318
Buruli ulcer 226
Byler's disease 181

C

Calabar swellings 210, 221
Calcineurin inhibitors 31, 267, 312
Calcium pyrophosphate dihydrate 59
Calymmatobacterium granulomatis 87
Campylobacter gastroenteritis 243
Campylobacter jejuni 243, 246
Campylobacter, livestock transmission of 197
Candida 91, 292, 298
Candida albicans 1, 26, 85, 147
Candida auris 37, 38, 154, 257, 258, 270, 305
Candida chorioretinitis 268
Candida glabrata 85, 90, 154, 283
Candida infection 28, 47, 298
Candida krusei 39, 43, 299
Candida nonalbicans 84
Candida species 27, 30, 39, 247, 254, 267, 299, 307
  clearance of 268
Candida strain 283
Candida superbug 258
Candida urosepsis, treatment of 283
Carbamate kinase 173
Carbapenem therapy 146
Carbapenem-resistant *Klebsiella pneumoniae* 286
Carbapenems 18
Carbuncles 81
Carcinoma lung 249
Card agglutination test for trypanosomes 220
Cardiac implantable electronic device 263
Cardiovascular system 215
Caroli's disease 181
Carpal tunnel syndrome, diagnosis of 341
Cartridge-based nucleic acid amplification test 97
Casoni's test 20, 205
Caspofungin 25, 31, 35, 41, 44, 154, 299, 301, 306, 312, 313
Cataract, congenital 363
Cataract surgery 331
Catheter-associated asymptomatic bacteriuria 258
Catheter-associated urinary tract infection 257
Catheter-related blood stream infection 20
  suspected 259
Cat-scratch disease 7
Causative agents 242, 323, 324
Cefazolin 260, 262
Cefepime 18
Cefoperazone-sulbactam 249, 261
Cefotaxime 20, 367
Ceftaroline 309
Ceftazidime 18
Ceftriaxone 12, 15, 132, 340, 363, 367
Cell death 188, 408

Cell debris 407
Cellular dysfunction 186
Cellular immunosuppression 266
Centers for Disease Control and Prevention 138, 229, 289, 312, 350, 354
Central nervous system 211, 215, 220, 292, 308, 345
  examination 216
  infection 33, 100
Central perihilar regions 376
Central venous catheter 31
  infection 47
Cephalosporin
  first-generation 262
  third-generation 20
Cephalosporins 18, 305
Cerebellum 118
Cerebral atrophy 358
Cerebral malaria 346
Cerebrospinal fluid 4, 13, 65, 100, 339
Cervical lymphadenopathy 52, 58, 65
Cervicofacial actinomycosis 121
Chancroid 87, 89, 91
Charcot's triad 23
Charcot-Leyden crystals 211
Chemiluminescence immunoassay 306
Chemoprophylaxis 365
  in malaria 347
Chest 393
  pain 128, 369
    severe 127
  radiography 5
Chikungunya 346
  active 69
  cocirculation of 348
  virus infection 349
Childhood asthma 1
Childhood pneumonia, multiple episodes of 125
Chills 12, 13, 29, 37, 55, 125, 129, 146, 217
Chlamydia 22, 226
Chlamydia infection 90, 137
Chlamydia trachomatis 90
  infection 89
Chlamydophila pneumoniae 127
Chlorhexidine 155, 306
Chloroquine 228, 347, 416
Cholangiocarcinoma 181
Cholangitis, acute 16, 23
Choledochojejunostomy 307
Cholestatic liver diseases 181
Chorioamnionitis 363, 364
Chorioretinitis 291, 358
Choroidal exudates 337
Churg-Strauss syndrome 52, 190, 352
Cidofovir 308
Ciprofloxacin 12, 18, 162, 230
Cirrhosis 181
Clarithromycin 126
Clavulanate 18
Clinical and Laboratory Standards Institute 37, 305
Clinical Microbiology and Infectious Diseases, guidelines 310
Clostridioides difficile 18, 290, 303, 308, 312
  colitis 401
  infection 265
  toxin A and B, stool for 279

Clostridium perfringens 223
Clostridium species 398
Coagulase-negative *Staphylococci* 256, 259
Coarse crepitations 184
Coccidioides immitis 34, 387
Coccidioidomycosis 225
Coccobacillus 22
Cognitive impairment 296
Cold antibody hemolytic anemia 9
Collapse, vertebral 390
Colloidal vesicular 116
Colon, inflammation in 381
Colorectal metastasis 178
Community-acquired pneumonia 133
Conductive deafness, bilateral 52
Condyloma acuminata 88, 361
   infection 354
Congenital rubella syndrome 363
Congenital varicella syndrome 358
Conjunctiva 324, 332
Conjunctival flora 337
Contact precautions continue 38
Coombs' test 4, 10, 137
Cordylobia anthropophaga 223
Cornea 325, 333
Corneal Herbert's Rosettes 325
Coronary artery bypass grafting 25
Coronary artery disease 341
Corticosteroids 417
Cotrimoxazole 139, 293
Cough 12, 370
   episode of 285
COVID-19 405
   basic reproduction number 406
   clinical features 407
   clinical tests 414
   computed tomography chest pattern 414
   convalescent plasma
      components 419
      treatment for 418
   diagnostic accuracy of 413
   different surfaces 406
   discharge criteria 415
   drugs for 416
   frequency of diseases organize 410
   healthcare facility 406
   infection 406
   interaction with host immune system 407
   investigations 407
   modes of transmission 406
   outbreak 411
   progresssion of 409
   radiological investigations 412
   reservoir of infection in society 406
   reverse transcriptase polymerase chain reaction 408, 411
   severity in various organ systems 409
   special populations 407
   stages of infection 415
   strains 405
   structure of 405
   supplemental oxygen 412
   treatment 412
Coxiella burnetii 197
Coxiella, transmission of 198
Cranial nerve deficits 296

Crescent sign 51
Creutzfeldt-Jakob disease 120
   familial 120
   iatrogenic 120
   sporadic 120
   variant 120
Crigler-Najjar syndrome 181
Crohn's disease 189, 318
   case of 39
Cryogenic electron microscopy 405
Cryptococcal meningitis 39, 91
Cryptococcosis 118, 300, 313
Cryptococcus neoformans 118
Cryptococcus spp. 300
Cryptosporidium 209, 231
Culex mosquito 198
Cumbo sign 397
Cunninghamella bertholletiae 305, 311
Cunninghamella spp. 311
Cushing's disease 298
Cyclophosphamide 79
Cyclospora 209, 218, 231
Cyst 198, 386
   rupture and fatal complications 390
Cystic fibrosis 124, 133, 181
Cystic lesions, multiple 379
Cysticerci 116, 198, 392
Cystitis 225
   organism causing 287
   treatment of 147
   uncomplicated, risk factor for 151
Cytokine storm 408
Cytomegalovirus 276, 285, 286, 291, 308, 309, 319, 364
   disease 292, 293
   immune globulin 294
   infection 8, 292, 400
      maternal 355
   prevention 292
   reactivation disease 364
   retinitis of 336
   viral 303
Cytotoxic T lymphocyte associated antigen 4 188

D

Dacryocystitis 331
Damage-associated molecular patterns 408
Daptomycin 270, 304
Debridement and implant retention 263
Deep vein thrombosis 21
Dematiaceous fungi 301
Dengue 350
   antibodies 349
   fever 230, 231
   serology 226
   virus 345
Dentate nuclei 105
Deoxyribonucleic acid 36, 77
Dermacentor andersoni 222
Dermacentor variabilis 222
Descemet's folds 327
Diabetes, case of 75
Diabetes develops erysipelas, case of 75
Diabetes mellitus 368
   controlled 111, 146
   type 2 27, 144, 188, 341

Diabetic nephropathy 279
Diarrhea
   multiple episodes of 279
   nonsevere 290
   respiratory complications 270
   specific cause of 218
   worsening 194
Dientamoeba fragilis 218
Diethylcarbamazine 207, 221, 343
   sign of 3
Diffuse wheeze, bilateral 184
Dihydroartemisinin-piperaquine 229
Dimorphic fungi 39, 43
Diphyllobothrium latum 218
Diplococci 13, 257, 325
   gram-negative 26
   gram-positive 132
Direct immunofluorescent antibody testing 231
Dirofilaria 210
Disease modifying antirheumatic drug 54, 55, 61
Disease, severe 291
Diseases Society of America 30
Disseminated candidiasis, cases of 299
Disseminated gonococcal infection 89
Disseminated intravascular coagulation 19, 272
Disseminated varicella zoster virus 49
Distal interphalangeal joints 75
DNA antibodies, anti-single-stranded 59
Donor platelets, random 3
Donovanosis 87
Doripenem 18
Doxorubicin 79
Doxycycline 117, 132, 196, 222, 230, 347
Drug-induced lupus erythematosus 59
Drug-susceptibility testing 261
Dyskaryotic cell lines 3
Dyspareunia 84
Dysphagia, severe 65
Dyspnea
   acute 4
   sudden onset 194
Dysuria 12
   and urinary frequency 146

E

Eastern Cooperative Oncology Group 142
Ebola virus disease 196
Echinocandin 31, 40, 259
Echinococcus granulosus 175, 209, 397, 400
Ecthyma gangrenosum 81, 269
Edema 115
   in adjacent liver parenchyma 377
Efavirenz 85
Emphysematous pyelonephritis 152
   cause of 146
   treatment of 152
Enalapril 56
Encapsulated bacteria, risk of 68
Encephalitis syndromes 270
Endocarditis 260
Endogenous candidemia, cause of 1
Endophthalmitis 330, 331, 337

Endoscopic gastrostomy, percutaneous 192
Endoscopic retrograde cholangiopancreatography 219, 264
Endosymbiont rickettsiae 351
Endothelial damage syndromes 320
Endovascular infection 197
Engraftment syndrome 320
Entamoeba histolytica 208
Enterobacter 264
Enterobacter cloacae 286
Enterobacter species 17
Enterobacteriaceae species 17
Enterobius vermicularis 210
Enterococcal infection, treatment of 257
Enterococcus 309
Enterococcus faecalis 151, 287
Enterococcus faecium 287
Enterococcus species 261, 249
Environmental health assessment 242
Environmental hygienic measures 94
Enzyme-linked immunosorbent assay 2, 290
Eosinophilic pneumonia
    acute 136, 352
    chronic 352
Epidural extension 402
Epidural soft-tissue lesions 402
Epiglottitis 17, 155
Episcleritis 349
Epithelial cells 145, 407
Epithelioid hemangioendothelioma 181
Epstein-Barr virus 272, 274, 285, 286
    associated lymphomas 277
    infection 8
Ergosterol 33
Ertapenem 367
Erysipelas bacterial skin infection 80
Erythema infectiosum 6, 70, 364
Erythema, mucosal 84
Erythema multiforme 27, 214, 219
Erythema nodosum 189
Erythematous oral mucosa 52
Erythrocyte sedimentation rate 103
Erythrocytic schizogony 206
Erythromycin 132, 137
Escherichia coli 23, 81, 84, 145, 151, 246, 247, 264, 287, 362, 366, 391, 398
Esophagoduodenoscopy 342
Ethambutol 126, 128, 132, 135, 139, 148, 166, 261, 289
European Association for Study of Liver 50
European Committee on Antimicrobial Susceptibility Testing 37
Ewing's sarcoma, high risk 318
Exoerythrocytic schizogony 206
Exserohilum 36
Extracorporeal membrane oxygenation 125
Extrahepatic prodromal 176
Extrapulmonary manifestations 130

F

Falciparum, antigen for 346
Falciparum malaria 365
Famciclovir 298
Fanconi's anemia 318
Fasciola hepatica 218
Fascioliasis, diagnosis of 218
Fatty acid oxidation 188
Fatty acid, short-chain 290
Favipiravir 416
Febrile 370
    agglutinins 234
    illness associated 272
    neutropenia 47
    neutropenia, risk of 46
Feline immunodeficiency virus infection 197
Felty's syndrome 58
Fetal distress, features of 66
Fetal infection 364
    diagnosis of 364
    route of 355
Fever 184, 305, 370
    cause of 275
    factitious 234, 239
    familial Mediterranean, 238
        features of 234
    high-grade 65, 212, 217, 339, 340
    history of 3
    in non-infection settings 52
    in returning traveler 212
    low-grade 306
    spikes started reducing 255
    symptoms of 285
    tick-borne relapsing 228
Fibrinogen levels 274
Fibrosis scar, sign of 333
Fidaxomicin 265, 291
Filarial tropical pulmonary eosinophilia 343
Fine-needle aspiration cytology 85
Finger necrosis 54
Fingernails 203
Flagellated protozoan parasites 219
Flaviviruses 348
Flavobacterium meningosepticum 264
Fluconazole 28, 32, 33, 40, 51, 78, 298, 301
Fluid-attenuated inversion recovery 113
Flu-like symptoms 2
Fluorescent in situ hybridization 301
Fluorescent treponemal antibody absorption 306
Fluoroquinolone prophylaxis 315
Fog, headlight in 337
Follicular lymphoma 317
Follicular trachoma 332, 333
Food and Drug Administration 362
Foodborne disease 241
    outbreak 242
Foodborne illness 245
Foodborne outbreak investigation 241, 243
Fosfomycin 153, 270
    use of 146
Fulminant colitis, severe 290
Fulminant disease 291
Fungal
    abscess 400
    diseases, invasive 322
    etiology and miliary metastasis 389
    infection 282
        causes of breakthrough 316
        endemic 39
        invasive 26, 315
        risk factor for 34
    septicemia 64
Fusarium infection 313
Fusarium species 64, 191, 313
    testing of 306

G

Galactomannan 268
    positive for 25
Galactosemia 181
Gallbladder sludge 339
Gambiense 219, 220
Gametocytes 205
Ganciclovir ocusert 336
Ganciclovir, short-chain 293
Gardasil 9 361
Gardnerella vaginalis 90, 365
Gastroenteritis, cases of 243
Gastrointestinal tract disease 292
GeneXpert 249, 305
    for TB 94, 97
    blood sample 192
Genital herpes 225
Genital ulcers 72
Genital wart 88, 361
Genitourinary tract infections 144
Genitourinary tracts 355
Genotypic testing 294
Gentamicin 18, 160
Germ cell tumor
    refractory 318
    relapse 318
German measles infection 355
Giant pronormoblasts 272
Giardia 218
    intestinal 267
Giardia lamblia 253
Giemsa stain 228
Glasgow Coma Scale 3, 240, 367
Glomerulonephritis 58
    chronic 284
Glucocorticoids, high level of 292
Glucose-6-phosphate dehydrogenase 338
Glutamate dehydrogenase antigen 303
Glycogen storage disease 181
Glycopeptides 260, 262
Glycosylated ferritin, percentage of 59
Gnathostoma spinigerum 221
Gnathostomiasis 220, 221
Goblet cells 406
Gonococcal urethritis, typical of 90
Gonococcus species 391
Gonorrhea 89, 225, 356
    in pregnancy, developing 366
Goodpasture's disease 137
Graft transmission 308
Gram-negative bacilli 13, 224, 286, 264
Gram-negative bacteria 16
Gram-negative bipolar staining bacilli 224
Gram-negative crisis 12
Gram-negative infections 309
Gram-positive bacilli 224
Granular nodular 116
Granulomas 148
    multiple 384
Granulomatous
    anterior uveitis 349
    disease 239

fungal disease, chronic 161
 inflammation 266
 uveitis 334
Grocott-Gomori's Methenamine Silver nitrate 123
Guillain-Barré syndrome 193

H

H1N1 infection 1
H1N1 influenza, epidemic 355
Haemophilus ducreyi 87, 362
Haemophilus influenzae 19, 135, 337
Hairless spot 195
Halo sign 51
Hand hygiene 365
Haufen 295
HBV infections 175
Head of femur, osteonecrosis of 371
Headache 71, 105, 194, 212, 217, 305
Healthcare-associated pneumonia 12
Healthcare-associated urinary tract infection 18
HELLP syndrome 274
Hematemesis 217
Hematogenous dissemination 389
Hematogenous osteomyelitis 155, 156, 160
Hematological malignancy 238
Hematopoietic cell transplantation 309
 indication for 316
Hematopoietic stem cell transplant 51, 241, 316
Hematuria 12
Hemiparesis 296
Hemodialysis, maintenance 248
Hemolytic uremic syndrome 291
Hemophagocytic lymphohistiocytosis 8, 350
Hemorrhagic cystitis 320
Henderson-Patterson bodies 354, 362
Henoch-Schönlein purpura 58
Hepatic artery thrombosis 177, 180
Hepatic dysfunction 289
Hepatic trauma 181
Hepatitis B vaccine 176, 179, 285, 286, 310, 358, 359
Hepatitis, type of 179
 B virus
  features of 176
  infection 353, 358
 C virus 175, 177, 180, 285, 286
  chronic 4
  history of 15
 D virus 179
 E infection with genotype 1 10
 E virus, compartment of 4
Hepatocellular carcinoma, diagnosis of 180
Hepatomegaly 342
Hepatosplenic candidiasis 254, 267
Hepatosplenomegaly 217, 383
Herbert pits 333
Hereditary hemochromatosis 181
Herniated disk 262
Herpes progenitalis 87
Herpes simplex 2 genital lesions 361
Herpes simplex encephalitis 119
Herpes simplex virus 100, 303, 334
Herpes zoster 226, 297
 ophthalmicus, opportunistic infection of 330

Herpetic genital infections 82
Herpetic uveitis 334
Hexachlorophene 23
Hickman catheter, presence of 64
Highly active antiretroviral therapy 4, 274
Hilar adenopathy 375
Hilar nodal enlargement 397
Hip joint, left 391
Histoplasma 36, 37
Histoplasma capsulatum 387, 401
Histoplasma specific antibodies 37
Histoplasmosis 225, 401
 disease 37
HIV transmission, risk of 359
Hodgkin lymphoma 317
Hot tub lung 94, 96
Human African trypanosomiasis 219
Human immunodeficiency virus 27, 68, 132, 144, 167, 204, 233, 272, 275, 285, 286, 314, 340, 353, 358
Human leukocyte antigen 78
 increased 295
Human papillomavirus 361
 infection 354
Humoral immune response 419
Humoral immunodeficiency 273
Hutchinson's teeth 362
Hyaline cartilage 392
Hyaline membrane 393
Hydatid disease 386
Hydralazine 190
Hydrogen peroxide 406
Hydronephrosis 358
Hydrops fetalis 70
Hydroxychloroquine 4, 53, 54, 59, 416, 417
Hydroxyurea 79
Hymenolepis nana 210
Hyperbilirubinemia 340
Hypereosinophilic syndrome 221
Hyperglycemia 298
Hyperinflammatory response 407
Hypertension 407
Hypodense conglomerate lesions, multiple 378
Hypogammaglobulinemia 286
Hypopyon corneal ulcer, cause of 326
Hypothesis, development of 245
Hypothyroidism 341
Hypoxic hepatitis 188

I

Icosahedral aggregates 295
Idiopathic hypereosinophilic syndrome 352
Idiopathic pneumonia syndrome 320
Idiopathic thrombocytopenic purpura 274
Ileosacral osteomyelitis 253
Illness
 severity of 322
 timing of 217
 travel-related 212
Imipenem 18, 28
Immune dysfunction and infections 63
Immune reconstitution inflammatory syndrome 168, 172
Immune system suppression 5

Immune-complex-mediated inflammatory 407
Immune-mediated reactions 180
Immunity, immunological evidence of 177
Immunocompetent male 123
Immunodeficiency, severe combined 314, 316
Immunoglobulin 61
 G 65, 286, 302, 339
 M 357
Immunomodulating drugs 271
Immunoproliferative small intestinal disease 47, 50
Immunosuppression 298, 350
 agents, reduction of 294
 chronic 294
 high-dose 295
 receives interferon 71
Immunosuppressive therapy 285
 triple 279, 281
In vitro fertilization 359
Inactivated influenza vaccine 46
Indian Council of Medical Research 412
Indirect fluorescent antibody test 271
Indirect ophthalmoscopy 328
Infantile osteomyelitis 160
Infection
 atypical 137
 in eye 323
 in transplant, risk of 314
 metastatic spread of 248, 260
 multiple, risk for 12
 related malignancies 46
 risk factor for 231
 risk of 278, 286
 severe 96
 source of 337
 typical 315
Infectious complications 319
Infectious Disease Society of America 307
Infectious diseases
 imaging cases 368-403
  abdominal infections 277-283
  X-ray 368-371
 outpatient department 302
Infectious mononucleosis 2, 219
 worsening of 65
Infective endocarditis 190
Inflammatory bowel disease 291
 diagnosis of 242
Inflammatory cytokines 416
Inflammatory disorders 238
Inflammatory exudates 328
Inflammatory lesion, self-limited 220
Inflammatory markers 412
Inflammatory pathways 275
Inflammatory tissue 161
Influenza 134
 vaccination 46, 142
 virus 319
  vaccine 363
Inhibitory quotient 264
Injection benzathine penicillin 222
Injection ceftriaxone 222
Inspiratory oxygen fraction 129
Inteneron genes, stimulator of 188
Intensive care unit 12, 30, 64, 145, 194, 248, 406
Interferon 408

Intermittent pneumatic compression devices 415
Interstitial keratitis 335
Interstitial lung disease 137
Intestinal epithelium 418
Intestinal giardiasis 267
Intestinal hookworms 200
Intra-abdominal
   fungal infections 28
   infection, etiology of 34
Intracameral moxifloxacin 337
Intracranial calcification 364
Intradermal leishmanin test 274
Intradermal skin test 210
Intrahepatic bile duct 264
Intraventricular antibiotic, administration 252
Invasive candidiasis, treatment of 48
Ipillmumab 187
Irritable bowel syndrome 218
Isavuconazole 300
Ischemic bowel segment 28
Ischemic cardiomyopathy 341
Isolated hepatic tuberculosis 398, 400
Isoniazid 4, 126, 128, 135, 139, 148, 166, 192, 261, 289
Isospora 209
Itraconazole 154, 298, 305
Ivermectin 307, 418
Ixodes tick 230

J

Japanese encephalitis virus 198, 345
Jarisch-Herxheimer reaction 228
Jaundice 195, 230
Jejunum resection 39
Joint
   infections 17
   pain 63
   replacement surgery 157
Juvenile idiopathic arthritis 59

K

Kala azar 350
Kaplan-Meier curves for mortality 420
Kaposi's sarcoma 91
Katayama fever 148
Kawasaki disease 58
Keratitis 334, 362
Ketoconazole shampoo 298
Kidney bilateral bulky 247
Kidney function test 327
Kingella kingae 24
Klebsiella 17, 264, 309
Klebsiella oxytoca 240, 287
Klebsiella pneumoniae 151, 251, 286, 287, 304
Knee replacements, bilateral 53
Kyasanur forest disease transmission 199

L

Lactic acidosis 73, 279
Lactobacilli 365
Lamivudine 85
Larva migrans, cutaneous 201, 222

Laryngeal edema 67
Legionella 141, 227
   infection 46, 138
   pneumonia 131
      suspicion of 141
   pneumophila 24
      diagnostic test for 125
Legionnaires' disease 227
   presence of 137
Leishmania 208, 226
Leishmania donovani 206
Leishmaniasis 208, 226
Lepromin test 336
Leptomeningitis 113
Leptospira 229, 342
Leptospirosis 201, 229, 344
Lesions, worsening of 213
Leukocyte adhesion deficiency 135
Leukocytosis 275
Leukopenia 227, 230, 275, 293, 298, 347
Levofloxacin 18, 132, 141
Libman-Sacks vegetations 190
Lichen planus 88
Limb hypoplasia 358
Limulus amebocyte lysate 17, 23
Linezolid 261, 270, 304
Lipid amphotericin B formulation 26
Lipoprote, low-density 188
Liposomal amphotericin 301
Listeria 285, 307
Listeria meningitis 21
Listeriosis 198
Liver 342
   abscess 180
      pyogenic 177
   benign lesions of 175
   biopsy 180
   cysts, multilocular 400
   damage, severe 176
   diseases, chronic 181
   dysfunction in sepsis 183
   infections of 175
   lesions in both lobes of 377
   malignant diseases of 181
   metastases 131
   pyogenic abscess of 175
   transplant 177, 309
      deceased-donor 302
      indication for 177, 181
      infections in 302
      living donor 304
Liver function test 86, 234, 412
Loa loa 210, 221
Lobular consolidation 396
Löffler syndrome 229
Loiasis 221
   treatment of 7
Loop-mediated isothermal amplification 410, 414
Lopinavir 416
Louse-borne relapsing fever 228
Lovastatin 187
Low intraocular pressure 333
Lower lobe tubular bronchiectasis 125
Lumbar pain, lower 368

Lung
   air sounds 368
   cavitation, radiological evidence of 96
   diffuse ground-glass attenuation 376
   injury, acute 393
   masses, solitary 393
Lupu-like syndrome 190
Lutzomyia verruca rum 23
Lyme disease 55
Lymph nodes, multiple 192
Lymphadenopathy 98, 170, 230, 270, 341, 354
Lymphatic filariasis, elimination of 343
Lymphatic filariasis, treatment of 343
Lymphedema 343, 351
Lymphoblastic leukemia, acute 317
Lymphocyte transforming virus 277
Lymphogranuloma venereum 351
Lymphoma 47, 117
Lymphoplasmacytic lymphoma 318

M

Macrophage dysfunction 68
Madura foot 156
Magnetic resonance spectroscopy 113
Malaise 184
Malaria 365
   acute 229
   case of 202
   control and prevention 365
   parasite life cycle 206
   serology 226
   severe 229
Malassezia furfur 298
Malassezia species 78
Malassezia, presence of 298
Malignancies 350
Malignant otitis externa 121
Mandibular mass, presence of 275
Mantle cell lymphoma 317
Marginal keratitis 334
Mastitis 364
Mastoid, massive bone destruction of 111
Maternal sepsis, risk factor for 356
Mazzotti reaction 207, 351
Mefloquine 347, 365
Melena 217
Membrane protein 405
Membranoproliferative glomerulonephritis 123
Meningeal enhancement 104
Meningococcal disease 21
Meningococcemia 22
Meningoencephalitis 291
   cause of 341
Meropenem 12, 18, 222, 261
   minimum inhibitory concentration 305
Metabolic liver disease 181
Metabolic perturbations 189
Metacarpophalangeal joints 52, 54, 56
Meta-diaphyseal region of left femur 385
Metformin 187
Methicillin-resistant *Staphylococcus aureus* 17, 80, 156, 240, 244, 262, 302, 356
Methicillin-sensitive *Staphylococcus aureus* 244

Methotrexate 53
Methylprednisolone therapy 279, 285
Metronidazole 90, 265, 280, 291
Micafungin 31, 299, 306
Microbial resistance 191
Microcephaly 364
Microfilariae 221, 222
    number of 351
Microgametocytes 207
Microhemagglutination test for antibodies 306
Microphthalmia 358
Microsporidia 209
Microsporidial keratitis 335
Micturition, urgency of 12
Miliary mottling 389
Miliary tuberculosis 171, 397
Minocycline 79
Mobiluncus species 365
Molds, prevention of 38
Molecular patterns, pathogen-associated 408
Molecular typing 240
Moll's sweat gland 332
Molluscum 332, 362
Molluscum contagiosum 77, 88, 362
    features of 83
Molluscum lesions 362
Monoarticular arthritis 189
Monocytosis 275
Mononucleosis syndromes, prolonged 233
Moraxella 333, 334
Moraxella axenfeld 332
Moraxella catarrhalis 135
Morganella morganii 153, 286, 287
Mosquito bites 342, 350
Mosquito-borne infection 231
Moxifloxacin 141, 289
Mucor spp. 300
Mucorales 191, 299
Mucormycosis 39, 185, 401
    diagnosis of 300
    infections 299
    management of 39
    treatment of 38, 300
Mucositis 170
    severe 47
Multidrug-resistant *Enterobacteriaceae* infection 16
Multidrug-resistant organisms 252
Multiorgan failure 271
Multiple organ dysfunction syndrome 408
Multiple scoring systems 267
Mupirocin, intranasal application of 306
Muscle tenderness 230
Musculoskeletal
    cases and imaging 383
    tuberculosis 388
        location of 403
Mutations, testing of 128
Myalgia 184, 190, 230
    severe 212, 216, 217
Mycobacteria, cultural growth of 136
Mycobacterium abscessus 94, 261
Mycobacterium avium complex 5, 11, 93, 96, 98, 172
Mycobacterium chelonae 4, 266
Mycobacterium fortuitum 96, 261
Mycobacterium kansasii 92, 98

Mycobacterium leprae 336
Mycobacterium smegmatis 148
Mycobacterium tuberculosis 114, 123, 144, 158, 249
    complex 98, 388
Mycobateriae 139
Mycophenolate mofetil 253, 273, 276, 281, 283, 293
Mycophenolate, use of 292
Mycoplasma hominis 90, 365
Mycoplasma infection 136
Mycoplasma pneumoniae, diagnosis of 126, 140
Mycotic organisms, secondary 387
Mycotoxins 69
Myelodysplastic syndromes 317
Myelofibrosis and myeloproliferative diseases 317
Myeloid leukemia
    acute 38, 240, 316
    chronic 317
Myeloma 267
    initial response 317
    multiple 253
    refractory 317
    sensitive relapse 317
Myeloperoxidase stains primary 276
Myiasis 226
Myocarditis 230

N

Naegleria fowleri 211
Nasal
    endoscopy 284
    oxygen, high-flow 412
    polyposis 133
National AIDS Control Organization 359
National Comprehensive Cancer Network 142, 276
National Healthcare Safety Network, operation procedure 256
Nausea 270
Necator americanus 210
Neck pain 370
Neck rigidity 100, 341
Necrotic lymphadenopathy 380
Necrotic mediastinal 375
Necrotic pancreas 16
Necrotic ulcers, developed 76
Necrotizing granuloma 94, 97
Neisseria gonorrhoeae 225
Neisseria meningitidis 20
Neoplasms, malignant 175
Nephrectomy 152
Neurocysticercosis 116
Neurological deficits 296
Neuromyelitis optica 342
Neuropathy, peripheral 230, 289
Neuroretinal involvement 329
Neutropenia 31
    antimicrobial treatment for 315
    combination of 48
Neutropenic enterocolitis 46
Neutropenic fever
    risk stratification in 47
    treatment of 19, 47

Neutrophil leukocytosis 127
Nitazoxanide 218, 310
Nitrofurantoin 270
Nivolumab 187
Nocardia 285, 311
Nocardia nova complex 305
Nocardia species of 311
Nocardiosis, diagnosis of 279
Nodular calcified 116
Nodular regenerative hyperplasia 181
Nonbile stained eggs 210
Nongranulomatous anterior uveitis 349
Non-Hodgkin's lymphoma 168, 274
Noninfectious inflammatory disease 238
Non-*Salmonella typhi*, suspicion of 241
Nonsteroidal anti-inflammatory drugs 63, 187, 188, 346
Nontuberculous mycobacteria 93, 261
Norovirus 304, 310
Nosocomial infections 247
Nosocomial pneumonia, treatment of 16
Nuclear material hemagglutinin-esterase 405
Nucleic acid amplification test 289, 358
Nucleic acid assays 196
Nucleic acid screening test 350
Nucleocapsid 405, 408
Nucleoside reverse transcriptase inhibitors 149

O

Obstructive airway disease 229
Obstructive lung disease
    chronic 130
Obstructive pulmonary disease
    advanced chronic 248
    chronic 25, 134
Ocular toxicity 289
Ofloxacin 289
Ommaya reservoir, insertion of 252
Onion peel sign 397
Opacity, corneal 332
Ophthalmia neonatorum 333
Opravil scoring in H1N1 394
Optical coherence tomography 330
Oral *viridans streptococci*, predictor of 50
Orbit and lid 331
Organ transplantation, multiple 292
Ornithine transcarbamoylase 173
Osteoarthritis 58
    case of 251
Osteomyelitis 156, 197, 364
    acute 155, 160
    changes of 155
    chronic 156
    subacute 161
    vertebral 260
Otitis media 58
Outer retinal necrosis, progressive 330
Oxygen administration 139

P

Pacemaker insertion, permanent 250
Pain, development of 52
Painless papule, pccurrence of 72
Palpable purpura 57

Pancreatitis 291
Pancytopenia 202
Pannus, superior 324, 332
Panuveitis 349
Paracoccidioides brasiliensis 387
Paragonimus ova 211
Parainfluenza virus 319
Parasite, intracellular 360
Parasitemia, high level of 229
Parasitic infection 178, 202
Paravertebral abscesses, large bilateral 384
Paravertebral shadows 391
Parenteral gold 53
Parkinson's disease 220
Parogonimus spp. 218
Parvovirus B19 364
    infection 273
Pattern recognition receptors 408
Peculiar infection 324
Pedal edema 208
Pelvic examination, bimanual 16
Pelvic infections 261
Pembrolizumab 187
Penicillamine 53
Penicillin 364
Penicillin-allergy 76, 356
    for syphilis 78
Perianal itching 203
Perinephric region, left 305
Periodontitis 356
Peripheral anterior synechiae 289
Peripheral vascular 47
Periprosthetic joint infection 155
Peritoneal, abnormal 400
Personal protecting equipment 291, 406
Pharyngitis 230
Phlebotomus argentipes 209
Phlyctenular conjunctivitis 327
Phlyctenular keratoconjunctivitis 334
Phlyctenular reaction 332
Phosphatidylinositol-3-kinase 188
Photophobia 184
Phthiriasis 332
Phthiriasis palpebrarum 332
Piperacillin 12, 18
Pityriasis rosea, case of 74
Plasma blood glucose 145
Plasma viral load 359
Plasmablastic lymphoma 318
Plasmodium falciparum 186, 215, 338-340, 356
    gametocyte 365
    infections 393
    malaria 228
Plasmodium ovale 347
Plasmodium vivax 276, 347
    infects 273
    malaria 273
    trophozoites of 340
Platelet 69
    components, single-donor 65
    effusion 387
        bilateral 128
        right-sided 130
    transfusion 232
Pleural fluid analysis 136
Pneumococcal polysaccharide vaccine 141
Pneumococcus 334

Pneumocystis carinii 49
    pneumonia 46
Pneumocystis infection 143
Pneumocystis jirovecii 1, 40, 97, 167, 285, 319, 387
    infection 316, 299
    pneumonia 387, 397
    treatment of 4
Pneumocystis pneumonia 123, 307, 397
Pneumomediastinum 397
Pneumonia 273
    aspiration 19
    causing agents 17
    phenotypes of 415
    round 388
Pneumonitis, bilateral 185
Polyarteritis nodosa 58
Polydrug-resistant TB 98
Polymerase chain reaction 2, 30, 36, 63, 229, 289
    quantitative 149
    testing 130
Polymethyl methacrylate 156
Polymyositis-dermatomyositis 318
Polyomaviridae family 296
Polyomavirus particles 295
Polyurethane catheters 153
Polyvinylchloride 153
Posaconazole 300
    antifungal prophylaxis 254
    prophylaxis 253
Positive end-expiratory pressure 415
Positron emission tomography scan 167, 287
Posterior reversible encephalopathy syndrome 296
Postrenal transplant 76, 285
Postsplenectomy infection 274
Poststreptococcal reactive arthritis 55, 61
Posttransplant lymphomas, cause of 273
Posttransplant lymphoproliferative disorder, risk of developing 304
Potassium hydroxide 306
Potential soil 262
Pravastatin 187
Praziquantel 218
Prednisolone 281, 283
Pretransplant decolonization 306
Prevotella species 22
Primaquine 347
Procainamide 190
Progressive multifocal leukoencephalopathy 296
    diagnosis of 281
Promyelocyte leukemia, acute 317
Propionibacterium 337
Prostatitis, acute 151
    treatment of 146
Protease inhibitor 360
Protein derivative test 289
Protein kinase, activated 188
Proteolytic enzymes, lack of 403
Proteus 81,152
Proteus mirabilis 287
Protozoa transmitted sexually 205
Protozoan, intracellular 328
Proximal interphalangeal joints 54
Pruritus, mild 298

Pseudomembranous colitis 401
Pseudomonas 21, 22, 152, 264, 310
Pseudomonas aeruginosa 17, 260, 286, 287, 305
    bacteremia 81
Pseudomonas infection 133, 139
Pseudo-outbreaks 240, 243
Psoas abscess 260
Psoriatic arthritis 55
Pulmonary angiography 255
Pulmonary aspergillosis 241, 256
Pulmonary cryptococcosis 300
Pulmonary disease 93
Pulmonary eosinophilia, tropical 229, 351
Pulmonary exacerbation 133
Pulmonary function test 4, 229
Pulmonary hemorrhage 230
Pulmonary hydatid disease 397
Pulmonary infections 182
Pulmonary manifestations
    acute 29
    severe 29
Pulmonary microcirculation 352
Pulmonary nocardiosis 393
Pulmonary *Pneumocystis jirovecii* infection 387, 397
Pulmonary tuberculosis 144, 396
Pulse methylprednisolone therapy, dose of 284
Pulse steroid therapy 295
Punctate calcifications 357
Pure red cell aplasia 274
Purified protein derivative tests 234
Pus cells 278
Pus-containing blisters 223
Pyelonephritis 151, 363, 364
    in pregnancy 146, 153
    organism, causing 287
Pyoderma gangrenosum 189, 223
Pyogenic abscess 178, 398
Pyogenic hepatic abscess, therapy for 175
Pyrazinamide 4, 128, 132, 135, 139, 148, 166, 289
Pyrexia of unknown origin 103, 233
    causes of 233
    drug-induced fever 234
    granulomatous causes of 235
    malignancies associated with 233
    malignancy in 233
    noninfectious causes of 234
Pyrimethamine 171

Q

Q fever 197, 198, 235
Quinacrine 60
Quinine plus clindamycin 229
Quinolone 367
    long-term 137
    prophylaxis 46, 49
Quinupristin-dalfopristin, combination of 270

R

Rabies vaccine, period of 70
Radius-ulna, pathological fracture of 2
Rapamycin 312
    mammalian target of 188
    mechanistic target of 296

Rapid fever clearance time 346
Rapid malaria antigen test 339, 346
Rapid plasma reagin 302, 323
Rapidly progressive dementia 109
Raynaud's phenomenon 54
Raynaud's syndrome 137
Reactive arthritis 62
Receptor-binding domain 405
Recombinant human DNAs, inhalation therapy 124
Refractory disease 93, 96
Reiter's disease 89
Remdesivir 416
Renal biopsy 281, 296
Renal cancer, metastatic 318
Renal failure 230
    acute 72
Renal infarction 260
Renal parenchymal infections 299
Renal replacement therapy 145
    continuous 28
Renal stones 152
Renal transplant 278, 279, 287, 288
Renin-angiotensin system blockers 149
Resistance temperature detectors 349
Respiratory disease 407
    lower 58
Respiratory distress syndrome 344
Respiratory failure 28
Respiratory flora, upper 129
Respiratory fluoroquinolone 141
Respiratory infection 123
    upper 15
Respiratory secretions 292
Respiratory syncytial virus 319
Respiratory tract infection, lower 281
Resveratrol 187
Reticulocytopenia 272
Retinal damage, risk of 417
Retinoic acids 296
Retro-orbital headache, severe 216
Retro-orbital pain 339, 340
Retroviral disease 168, 368
Retroviral infection 1, 169
Reveal tenderness 217
Reverse transcriptase-polymerase chain reaction 230, 363, 344, 414
Reye syndrome 181
Reynolds' pentad 23
Rhabdomyolysis 230
Rheumatoid arthritis 58, 213, 318, 327
    treatment of 296
Rheumatoid factor 61
Rheumatoid vasculitis, marker of 55
Rhinitis 58
Rhinocerebral, pulmonary 300
Rhizopus spp. 311
Rickettsia infection, treatment of 351
Rickettsia rickettsii antigen 237
Rifampicin 4, 126, 128, 132, 135, 139, 166, 192, 196, 228, 261, 289, 312
Right orbit, compartment of 110
Ringworm 201
Ritonavir 416
Rituximab 47, 49
RNA viruses, spherical single-stranded 405

Rocky mountain spotted fever 222, 234
Roundworm 209
Rubella in pregnancy 355

S

Sabin-Feldman dye test 328
Sacroiliac joint, left 392
Salmonella bacteria 7
Salmonella invasion 161
Salmonella nontyphoidal, outbreak of 241
Salmonella septicemia 7
Salmonella typhi 192, 226
Salmonellosis, episode of 169
Salt and pepper retinopathy 329
Sarcoidosis 181, 190, 334
Schistosoma haematobium, eggs of 144
Schistosoma mansoni 148
Schistosomiasis, acute 148
Schizogony 209
Schizonts 202, 205
Sclerosis, multiple 318
Seasonal influenza, treatment of 257
Selenium 183, 188
Selenium sulfide 78
Sensitive test 157
Sensorium 109
Sepsis 182, 183, 366, 408
    biliary source of 180
    cause of 356
    maternal 366
    pathogenesis of 182
    puerperal 364
Septate hyphae 306
Septic arthritis 64, 162
    pyogenic 391
Septic emboli 260
Septic shock 3, 182, 188, 273
Septicemia 225
Septicemic shock, maternal 356
Sequential organ failure assessment score 366
Serology 292
Serum glutamic oxaloacetic transaminase 338
Serum glutamic pyruvic transaminase 86, 204
Severe acute respiratory syndrome coronavirus 2 405, 408
Severe pulmonary hemorrhage syndrome 344
Sexual intercourse 151
Sexual intercourse, unprotected 85
Sexual transmission, risk of 359
Sexually transmitted disease 82, 327
Shake and bake 29
Shigella species 246
Sicca syndrome 190
Sigmoidoscopy reveals 290
Simian virus 40 149
Simulium damnosum 209
Simvastatin 187
Sinusoidal obstruction syndrome 320
Sirolimus 312
Sjögren's syndrome 62, 189
Skin infection 72
Skin lesions 83
Soft tissue
    adjacent 111
    diffuse 112
    infections, approach to 71

Solid organ transplant 278
Spectrum beta-lactamase, extended 310, 315, 319
Spinal infections 404
Spinal tuberculosis, diagnosis of 165
Spindle cells, large 168
Spirochetes 228
Spirometry, normal 125
Spleen 379
Splenomegaly 203, 230
Spondylodiscitis 390
Spontaneous bacterial peritonitis 17
Sputum cytology 284
Squamous cell carcinoma 131
Squamous temporal bone 111
Staining pattern 326
Staphylococcal pneumonia, risk factor for 224
Staphylococcus aureus 80, 155, 180, 244, 248, 260, 262, 391
Staphylococcus epidermidis 159, 256, 268
Staphylococcus lugdunensis 268
Staphylococcus saprophyticus 151, 268
Staphylococcus schleiferi 268
Staphylococcus species 23
Statins 187
Stem cell transplant 315
    principle of 314
    source of stem cells 314
Stenotrophomonas 153
Steroids increases 47
Stevens-Johnson syndrome 174
Still's disease 59, 189, 234, 237
Strawberry tongue 58
Streptococcus 152, 155
Streptococcus agalactiae 364, 365
Streptococcus milleri group 180
Streptococcus pneumoniae 3
Streptomycin 4, 132
Strongyloides 302, 307
Subclavian Permcath catheter, right 26
Sulfa allergy 299
Sulfamethoxazole 12
Sulfonamides 228
Swelling 52, 342
    of eyes, bilateral 325
Swine flu virus 363
Synovial fluid analysis 53
Synovial fluid examination 263
Syphilis 219, 334
    in pregnant woman 354
    late latent 84
    secondary 88
    treatment of 73
Syphilitic neuroretinitis 336
Systemic lupus erythematosus 57, 61, 184, 318, 368
Systemic sclerosis 318
Systemic vasculitides 229

T

Tachypneic 215
Tacrolimus 253, 281, 283
Taenia solium 209
Tamm-Horsfall protein 295
Tazobactam 12, 18
T-cell dysfunction, diagnosis of 65

T-cell lymphoma 317
Teicoplanin 28, 222, 304
Temoniera 319
Temporal neocortex, left 108
Tender lymphadenopathy 275
Tenofovir disoproxil fumarate 85
Tetracyclines 143
Thalami 106
    hyperintensities, bilateral 118
Thioacetazone 289
Thoracic segments 391
Thrombocytopenia 6, 293, 347
    severe 230
Thrombotic thrombocytopenic purpura 19
Thyroid-stimulating hormone 341, 237
Ticarcillin 18
Tigecycline 304
Tissue
    culture infectious dose 406
    transplantation of 314
Tobramycin 18
Tocilizumab 418
Toll-like receptors 416
Toothbrushes, sharing of 180
Toxoplasma 307, 308
Toxoplasma gondii 7, 360
    in serum 91
Toxoplasma immunoglobulin g 86
Toxoplasma infection 167, 173
Toxoplasmosis 2, 117
Toxoplasmosis, congenital 7
Trachomatous inflammation 332
Trachomatous scarring 332
Transbronchial biopsy 225
Transcriptional regulatory sequence 405
Transplant-associated microangiopathy 320
Transplant community 320
Transplant infectious diseases 302
Travelers' diarrhea, cases of 217
Treponema pallidum 87, 306, 336, 361
Trichinosis 209
Trichomonas vaginalis 89, 90
Triclabendazole 218
Tricuspid regurgitation, quantification of 263
Triiodothyronine, serum levels of 186
Trimethoprim 12
Trimethoprim-sulfamethoxazole 40, 46, 143, 288, 302
Trophozoites 205
Truncal rash 339
Trypanosomal chancre 220
Trypanosomes 220
Tsetse fly 209
Tubercular osteomyelitis 156, 162
Tubercular spondylodiskitis, diagnosis of 157
Tuberculin skin test 124, 165
Tuberculomas 116
Tuberculosis 91, 93, 334, 388, 400
    and syphilis of orbit 331
    arthritis, chronic 162
    causing 94
    incidence of multidrug-resistant 158
    infection, latent 188
    lymphadenopathy, diagnosis of 95
    multifocal 403
    osteomyelitis 156
    postprimary 396
    prevention of spread of 95
    treatment of 95
Tuberculous 404
    abscess 399
    arthritis
        changes of 156
        presentation of 157
        rarefaction of 157
    peritonitis 400
    spondylitis 165, 387, 403
    spondylodiskitis, case of 157
Tubo-ovarian abscess 226
Tumor necrosis factor 59, 311, 407, 408
Tumors, solid 238, 318

U

Ulceration, mucosal 148
Ulcers, corneal 337
Ureaplasma urealyticum 89
Urethral stricture 152
Uric acid, levels 61
Urinalysis, normal 183
Urinary incontinence, worsening 3
Urinary schistosomiasis 144
Urinary tract infection 147, 286, 354, 362
    epithelium of 149
Urine cultures 128
Urticaria 221
Uvea 328, 335
Uveitis 230

V

Vaccines 217
Vaccines-like influenza 307
Vaginal ulcers 84
Vaginal whitish discharge 84
Valacyclovir 298
    prophylaxis 280
Vancomycin 160, 265, 280, 291, 304, 365
    resistant *Enterococci* 309
Varicella antigen, detection of 297
Varicella zoster virus 285, 303, 319, 358
    infection 88, 353
Vascular catheters 39, 181
Vascular endolhelial growth factor 188
Vasculitis, occlusive 323
Vector-borne diseases 338
Venereal disease 325
Venereal Disease Research Laboratory 84, 324
Venoocclusive disease 181, 320
Venous thromboembolism, risk of 415
Venovenous hemodialysis, continuous 3
Ventilation ducts 244
Ventricular drain, external 252
Ventriculomegaly 357
Ventriculoperitoneal shunt 240
Vibrio species 21
Vibrio vulnificus 223, 224
Vietnam 2
Viral
    conjunctivitis 332
    hepatitis 176, 345
    infections 65
Virchow-Robin spaces 105
Virus, predominant strain of 405
Visceral, complications 59
Visceral leishmaniasis 209, 272, 350
Vision
    blurring of 284
    loss of 329
    mild blurring of 330
Visual
    acuity, decreased 184
    disturbance, worsening of 343
    field deficits 296
Vitrectomy 268
Vivax malaria, severe 275
Vomiting 15, 194, 217, 270
Voriconazole 32, 36, 40, 154, 259, 301, 305, 310
    efficacy of 26
    refractory IA 316
    toxicity, sign of 26
Vulvovaginal candidiasis 90

W

Warburg effect in sepsis 182
Waterhouse-Friderichsen syndrome 22
Wegener granulomatosis 57, 58, 190
West Nile virus 345
Western blot 219
Wheezing 229
Whipple disease 55
White blood cell 303
Wilson's disease 181
Wood's lamp examination 282
World Health Organization 138, 172, 332, 359
Wound 268
    lavage 155
Wright stain 228
Wuchereria bancrofti 229, 351

X

X-linked agammaglobulinemia 135

Y

Yellow fever virus 345
Yersinia pestis 22
Yttrium-aluminum-garnet laser capsulotomy 330

Z

Zidovudine 79, 145, 359
    short course of 358
Ziehl-Neelsen stain 231, 328, 334
Zika infection 357
Zika virus 230, 349, 353
    risks of 357
    transmission 357
Zinc pyrithione 78
Zoonosis 192, 229, 246, 386
Zoonotic diseases 193
Zoonotic hookworm infections 201
Zoonotic transmitted tuberculosis 196
Zygomycetes 191, 301
Zygomycosis 33
Zygotes 207

EU GSPR Authorised Reprsentative
Logos Europe, 9 rue Nicolas Poussin
1700, La Rochelle, France
Phone: +33 (0) 6 67 93 73 78
E-mail: contact@logoseurope.eu

www.ingramcontent.com/pod-product-compliance
Ingram Content Group UK Ltd.
Pitfield, Milton Keynes, MK11 3LW, UK
UKHW050458150426
5217IPUK00025B/1745